Anticancer Drug Development and Clinical Response

Anticancer Drug Development and Clinical Response

Editor: Octavia Settle

AMERICAN
MEDICAL PUBLISHERS
www.americanmedicalpublishers.com

AMERICAN
MEDICAL PUBLISHERS
www.americanmedicalpublishers.com

Cataloging-in-Publication Data

Anticancer drug development and clinical response / edited by Octavia Settle.
p. cm.
Includes bibliographical references and index.
ISBN 978-1-63927-879-4
1. Drugs--Design. 2. Cancer--Chemotherapy. 3. Drug development.
4. Clinical pharmacology. 5. Antineoplastic agents--Development.
I. Settle, Octavia.
RS420 .A583 2023
615.19--dc23

American Medical Publishers,
41 Flatbush Avenue,
1st Floor, New York,
NY 11217, USA

ISBN 978-1-63927-879-4 (Hardback)

Contents

Preface

I am honored to present to you this unique book which encompasses the most up-to-date data in the field. I was extremely pleased to get this opportunity of editing the work of experts from across the globe. I have also written papers in this field and researched the various aspects revolving around the progress of the discipline. I have tried to unify my knowledge along with that of stalwarts from every corner of the world, to produce a text which not only benefits the readers but also facilitates the growth of the field.

Anticancer drugs are utilized in the treatment of cancerous growth or malignancies. These drugs can be administered in isolation, or they can be given along with other treatments, like radiation therapy or surgery. The development of novel anticancer drugs is a lengthy process that includes acquiring new compounds, testing for antitumor activity, formulation and manufacturing, animal toxicology, and lastly assessing the compound's toxicity as well as antitumor activity in humans. There are various medications that are utilized as anticancer drugs, such as L-asparaginase, amsacrine, platinum-based drugs and hydroxyurea. Preclinical models such as cell line model systems may be especially useful in predicting anticancer drug response. It also helps to understand the mechanisms of drug action in situations when clinical samples are unavailable, or the cost of obtaining clinical samples for studying drug response is expensive. The aim of this book is to present researches that have transformed anticancer drug development. Those in search of information to further their knowledge will be greatly assisted by this book.

Finally, I would like to thank all the contributing authors for their valuable time and contributions. This book would not have been possible without their efforts. I would also like to thank my friends and family for their constant support.

Editor

1

Potent Anti-Ovarian Cancer with Inhibitor Activities on Both Topoisomerase II and ^{V600E}BRAF of Synthesized Substituted Estrone Candidates

Mohamed El-Naggar [1], Abd El-Galil E. Amr [2,3,*], Ahmed A. Fayed [3,4], Elsayed A. Elsayed [5,6], Mohamed A. Al-Omar [2] and Mohamed M. Abdalla [7]

1 Chemistry Department, Faculty of Sciences, University of Sharjah, Sharjah 27272, UAE; m5elnaggar@yahoo.com
2 Drug Exploration & Development Chair (DEDC), Pharmaceutical Chemistry Department, College of Pharmacy, King Saud University, Riyadh 11451, Saudi Arabia; malomar1@ksu.edu.sa
3 Applied Organic Chemistry Department, National Research Center, Cairo 12622, Egypt; dr_ahmedfayed14@yahoo.com
4 Respiratory Therapy Department, College of Medical Rehabilitation Sciences, Taibah University, Madinah Munawara 22624, Saudi Arabia
5 Zoology Department, Bioproducts Research Chair, College of Science, King Saud University, Riyadh 11451, Saudi Arabia; eaelsayed@ksu.edu.sa
6 Chemistry of Natural and Microbial Products Department, National Research Centre, Cairo 12622, Egypt
7 Atos Pharma, Elkatyba Land, Belbis 44621, El Sharkya, Egypt; mmostafa201120@yahoo.com
* Correspondence: aamr@ksu.edu.sa;

Abstract: A series of 16-(α-alkoxyalkane)-17-hydrazino-estra-1(10),2,4-trien[17,16-c]-3-ol (**3a–l**) and estra-1(10),2,4-trien-[17,16-c]pyrazoline-3-ol derivatives (**4a–d**) were synthesized from corresponding arylidines **2a,b** which was prepared from estrone **1** as starting material. Condensation of 1 with aldehydes gave the corresponding arylidine derivatives **2a,b** which were treated with hydrazine derivatives in alcohols to give the corresponding derivatives **3a–l**, respectively. Additionally, treatment of **2a,b** with methyl- or phenylhydrazine in ethanolic potassium hydroxide afforded the corresponding N-substituted pyrazoline derivatives **4a–d**, respectively. All these derivatives showed potent anti-ovarian cancer both in vitro and in vivo. The mechanism of anti-ovarian cancer was suggested to process via topoisomerase II and ^{V600E}BRAF inhibition.

Keywords: estrone derivatives; hydrazine; N-substituted pyrazoline; anti-ovarian cancer; topoisomerase II inhibitor; kinase inhibitor

1. Introduction

Synthetic alterations of estrone lead to discovering of compounds with diverse biological activities, for example with antitumor effect [1], as anti-breast cancer agent [2] and with antioxidant activity [3]. Estrone derivatives with antitumor activities must be devoid completely of the estrogenic activities [4–6]. The inversion of the configuration at C-13 lead to estrone derivatives with antitumor activities devoid from hormonal actions due to conformational change for the overall molecule resulting from the cis junction of rings C and D [4,7]. Some recent publications report on the syntheses and in vitro biological evaluation of several 13α-estrone derivatives [8–11]. These derivatives exhibited biological activities with substantial anti-proliferative or enzyme inhibitory potentials. Most literature data are mainly focusing on 13α-estrone substitution in ring D, while modified derivatives with ring A substitutions are rarely reported [12].

Cancer is considered one of the most significant causes of death worldwide. Ovarian cancer is one of the major causes for death among adult females [13]. Cancer is characterized by abnormal cell proliferation bypassing normal cell growth and death mechanisms. Recently, DNA topoisomerase II inhibitors have been researched as a potential target, which interferes with cancer growth and development [14]. Topoisomerase II inhibition leads finally to cell cycle inhibition and apoptosis in abnormal cancer cells [15]. BRAF kinase inhibition is another possible control mechanism, which was also developed to interfere with cancer cell growth [16]. BRAF kinase constitutes a major signaling process integrated in the RAS-MEK proliferation process. The activation of MEK by BRAF signals finally induces cell proliferation and survival [17]. Inhibiting BRAF activity results in inhibition of the proliferation signals, and thus inhibiting cancer cell development and growth [18].

In view of these observations and in continuation of our previous work in heterocyclic chemistry [19–22], the current work aimed at evaluating the effect or remote long cage distortion caused by introducing some moieties in both 16 and 17 locations of ring D. We screened some of synthesized estrone candidates for their anti-ovarian cancer potential both in vitro and in vivo. Furthermore, the inhibitory effects of the synthesized compounds were investigated against topoisomerase II and ^{V600E}BRAF kinase inhibitors.

2. Results and Discussion

2.1. Results

2.1.1. Chenical Synthesis

A series of 17-hydrazino-estratrienol (**3a–l**) and pyrazolinestratrienol (**4a–d**) were synthesized from corresponding arylidines **2a,b** which was prepared from estrone **1** as starting material.

Treatment of aryledine derivatives **2a,b** with hydrazine hydrate, in refluxing methanol or ethanol afforded the corresponding 17-hydrazino-16-α-methoxymethane estrone derivatives **3a,b** and 17-hydrazino-16-α-ethoxyethane estrone derivatives **3c,d**, respectively.

Also, reaction of compounds **2a,b** with N-methyl hydrazine, in refluxing methanol or ethanol afford 17-N-methyl hydrazino-16-α-methoxymethane estrone derivatives **3e,f** and 17-*N*-methyl hydrazino-16-α-ethoxyethane estrone derivatives **3g,h** respectively.

Additionally, when compounds **2a,b** reacted with *N*-phenyl hydrazine, under the same conditions afford the corresponding 17-*N*-phenylhydrazino- 16-α-methoxymethane estrone derivatives **3i,j** and 17-*N*-phenylhydrazino- 16-α-ethoxyethane estrone derivatives **3k,l**, respectively. Finally, condensation of **2a,b** with CH_3NHNH_2 or $PhNHNH_2$ in refluxing dioxane afforded the corresponding N-substituted pyrazoline derivatives **4a–d**, respectively (Scheme 1).

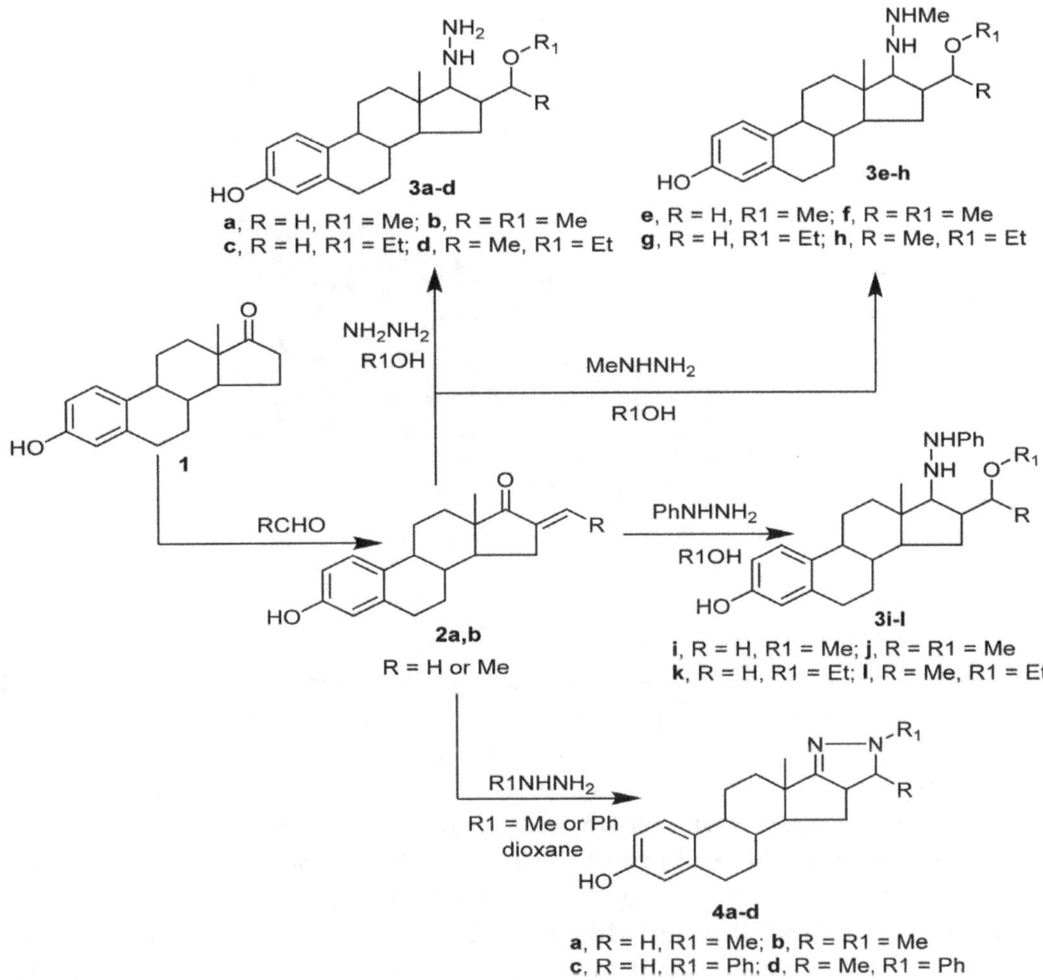

Scheme 1. Synthetic route for compounds **2–4**.

2.1.2. Biological Screening

In Vitro Cytotoxic Activities

The cytotoxicity of some synthesized derivatives against SKOV-3 cancer cell line in vitro was performed with the MTT assay. The obtained results showed that all synthesized compounds showed potent in vitro cytotoxic activities against SKOV-3 cells at the nanomolar level. Moreover, the effect of the synthesized compounds was dose-dependent. From the obtained IC_{50} values (Figure 1), prepared compounds can be arranged discerningly in the following order: **3a, 3b, 3c, 3d, 3e, 3f, 3g, 3h, 3i, 3j, 3k, 3l, 4a, 4b, 4c, 4d** (Figure 1). Compounds **3a–l** are characterized with the presence of hydrazine group rather than the pyrazoline group present in compounds **4a–d**. Furthermore, the alkyl group is found to be more active than the aromatic group. Generally Cpd. **3a** showed highest cytotoxic activity with IC_{50} value of 4.23 ± 0.12 nM, while Cpd. **4d** was the least active, where its IC_{50} value was about 9.5% of that obtained for Cpd. **3a**.

The effect of resveratrol (RES) and doxorubicin (DOX) on SKOV-3 showed IC_{50} of 55 and 250 nM, respectively.

The cytotoxicity of the newly synthesized compounds against fibroblast were as follow **IC_{50}** **3a** (1.2 μM), **3b** (2.45 μM), **3c** (5.67 μM), **3d** (7.44 μM), **3e** (8.11 μM), **3f** (9.20 μM), **3g** (11.18 μM), **3h**(16.22 μM), **3i** (15.13 μM), **3j** (16.20 μM), **3k** (17.78 μM), **3l** (20.21 μM), **4a** (23.34 μM), **4b** (24.55 μM), **4c** (25.55 μM), **4d** (30.34 μM).

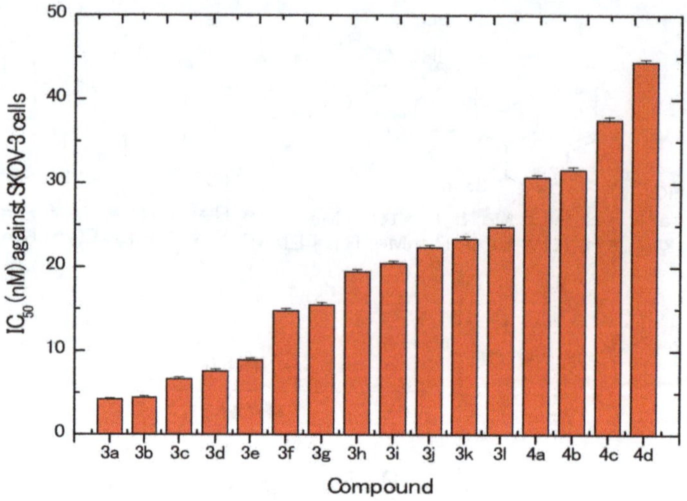

Figure 1. In vitro Cytotoxicity activities of the tested compounds against SKOV-3 cells.

In Vivo Anti-Ovarian Cancer

The in vivo anti-ovarian cancer activities of the tested compounds were evaluated using mouse xenograft model. Figure 2 represents the percentages of decrease in tumor growth upon treatment with different synthesized compounds. The obtained results showed that all compounds potentially reduced tumor growth over a period of 40 days of treatment, in comparison to control treatments, which showed normal tumor growth development. Moreover, it can be seen that the reduction in tumor size started directly from the 5th day of treatment, where the reduction percentage ranged from 45.7 ± 0.05% to 54.71 ± 0.01%. The reduction in tumor growth increased significantly reaching its maximal by the end of treatment period (40 days). The highest reduction in tumor growth was recorded for occurred Cpd. **3a**, which significantly decreased tumor growth by about 93.61 ± 0.7%. It can also be seen that Cpd. **3a**, was the most potent for in vivo treatment, where its effect was more obvious starting from day15 of treatment, where the reduction percentage in tumor size due to other compounds was more or less within the same range. We also can see that the in vivo results are coincided with those obtained for *in vitro* results, where the reduction in tumor size followed the same descending order: **3a**, **3b**, **3c**, **3d**, **3e**, **3f**, **3g**, **3h**, **3i**, **3j**, **3k**, **3l**, **4a**, **4b**, **4c**, and **4d**.

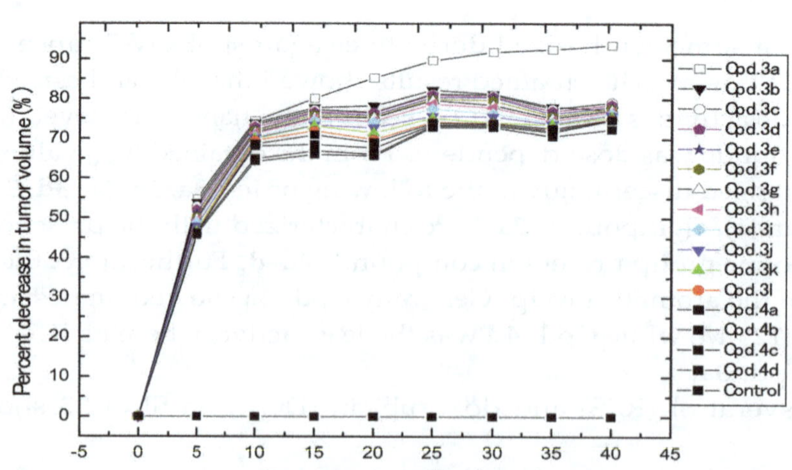

Figure 2. Percentages of decrease in tumor volume in nude mice in response to different synthesized derivatives.

2.1.3. Inhibition of Topoisomerase II Activities

In order to further investigate the possible mechanism of action of the newly synthesized derivatives, we investigated their inhibitory effects on topoisomerase II. Results obtained (Figure 3) showed that all synthesized compounds showed potential inhibitory effects against topoisomerase II. Furthermore, the inhibitory effect was also found to follow the same descending order obtained before during in vitro and in vivo investigation: **3a, 3b, 3c, 3d, 3e, 3f, 3g, 3h, 3i, 3j, 3k, 3l, 4a, 4b, 4c,** and **4d**. Cpd. **3a** showed the most inhibitory action for topoisomerase II with IC_{50} value of 3.45 ± 0.13 nM, which was about 7,9% of that obtained for the lest potent compound (IC_{50} for Cpd. **4d**: 43.56 ± 0.98 nM).

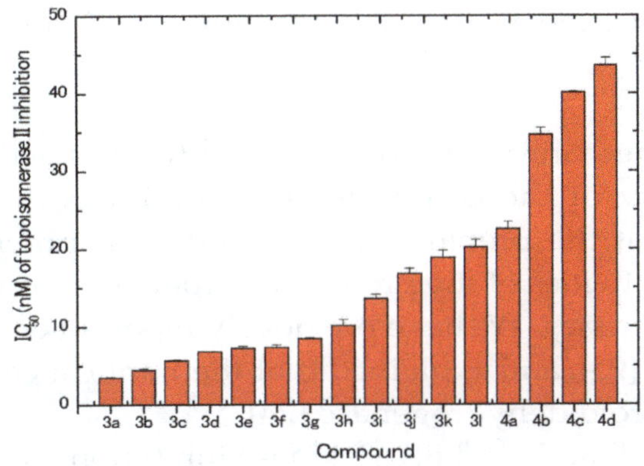

Figure 3. IC_{50} of Topoisomerase II Inhibitor activities of the tested compounds.

2.1.4. In Vitro Kinase Assay

The in vitro kinase assay of synthesized derivatives was investigated against both ^{WT}BRAF (BRAF kinase wild type) and ^{V600E}BRAF (mutant BRAF kinase). Results obtained in Figure 4 showed that all synthesized compounds were highly active inhibitors for ^{V600E}BRAF compared with moderate activities against ^{WT}BRAF. Again, the descending order of activities was as follow **3a, 3b, 3c, 3d, 3e, 3f, 3g, 3h, 3i, 3j, 3k, 3l, 4a, 4b, 4c,** and **4d**. Compound **3a** recorded the most active inhibition (IC_{50}: 0.041 ± 0.0016 and 4.23 ± 0.12 μM for mutant and wild type BRAF kinase, respectively. Furthermore, it can be seen that the inhibitory effect of Cpd. **3a** was much more superior to that obtained for different positive control drugs (0.48, 3.87 and 0.97 μM for Sorafenib, Dabrafenib and Vemurafenib, respectively.

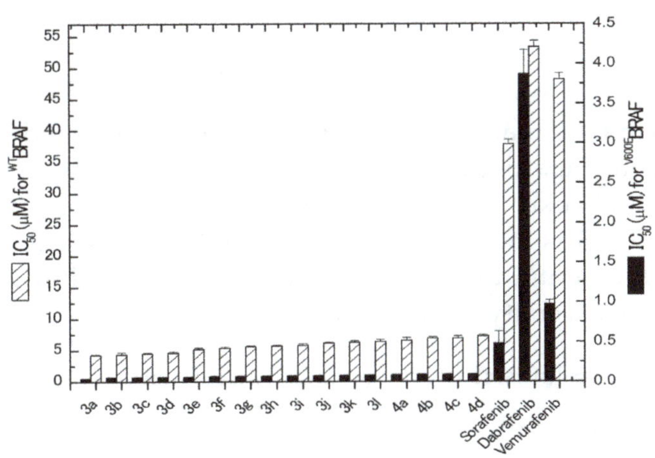

Figure 4. IC_{50} values of synthesized for both ^{WT}BRAF and ^{V600E}BRAF.

2.2. Discussion

Within the framework of the current work we synthesized new estrone derivatives from their corresponding arylidines. The newly synthesized derivatives showed potential cytotoxic activities against SKOV-3 cells. Moreover, in vivo investigations revealed that the synthesized compounds were able to potentially reduce tumor volume growth over a treatment period of 45 days.

The newly introduced 1-alkoxy benzyl moiety alone or combined with the 17- hydrazino- moities make remote destortion of the structure cage that completely elminate any hormonal activities of te estrone molceules and deviate the biological activities towards the aniticancer ones, so we investigated this property and tried to find the mechnisms of anticancer actions of these newly synthesized compounds.

In search for the possible mechanism of action of the anticancer activities of the tested compounds, we investigated the possibility of the compounds to inhibit both topoisomerase II and kinase enzymes. Results showed that the prepared compounds can potentially serve as inhibitors for these enzymes. The cytotoxic activities of the prepared estrone derivatives can be due to the inhibition of 17-hydroxysteroid dehydrogenases. We have previously reported on the anti-breast cancer activities of different estrone derivatives [23], and explained that their anticancer activities can be attributed to the inhibition of 17-hydroxysteroid dehydrogenase [24].

Concerning topoisomerase II and ^{V600E}BRAF kinase inhibition, our results suggest that the newly synthesized compounds exert their cytotoxic action against SKOV-3 cancer cells by interfering with the metabolic activity of these enzymes, thus preventing cancer cells from obtaining proliferation signaling molecules essential for their growth and survival [16,17]. Different activities of the prepared compounds may be attributed to the structure activity relationship of these compounds.

Hydrazine derivatives are generally potent than pyrazoline ones, due to their open chain structure as well as their higher electron density. Furthermore, it can be suggested that *N*-methyl derivatives are more active than *N*-phenyl ones. On the other hand, hydrazine derivatives can be divided into more active α-methoxyl derivatives and the less active α-ethoxyl, and then the least active *N*-phenyl derivatives. This can be explained due to the fact that phenyl group act as a withdrawing group. On the other hand, the weaker effect of α-ethoxyl derivatives than the α-methoxyl ones can be attributed to their bulky nature. This effect can be observed among different series of compound **3**. As the bulky nature of the substituted groups increase, accordingly more steric hindrance can be observed, leading to decreased cytotoxic activities.

3. Materials and Methods

3.1. Chemical Synthesis

"Melting points reported are inaccurate. IR spectra were registered on Shimadzu FT-IR 8300 E (Shimadzu Corporation, Kyoto, Japan) spectrophotometer using the (KBr) disk technique. The ^{1}H-NMR spectra were determined with bruker 600 MHz NMR spectrometer. The chemical shifts are expressed on the δ (ppm) scale using TMS as the standard reference. Mass spectra were recorded on Finnigan SSQ operating at 70 ev. Elemental analysis determined on a Perkin Elmer 240 (Microanalysis), Microanalysis Center, Cairo University, Cairo, Egypt".

3.1.1. Synthesis of 3-Hydroxy-16-[substituted]-estra-1(10),2,4-trien-17-ones (**2a**,**b**)

"A mixture of (**1**) (0.54 g, 20 mmol) and formaldehyde or acetaldehyde (20 mmol) in EtOH (50 mL) and aqueous KOH (10 mL, 30%) was stirred for 24 h at room temperature. The formed solid was collected by filtration, crystallized from ethanol to give compounds **2a** [25] and **2b**, respectively".

3-Hydroxy-16-[ethylene]-estra-1(10),2,4-trien-17-one (**2b**)

Yield 97%, mp 198–200 °C, $[\alpha]_D^{25}$ = + 71 (c 1, MeOH). IR (KBr, cm^{-1}): 3340 (OH), 2944 (CH, aliphatic), 1743 (C=O), 1642 (C=C). ^{1}H NMR: (600 MHz, $CDCl_3$): δ ppm 0.61 (1H, m, H-8β), 0.90 (3H, s, CH_3-18), 1.01 (1H, m, H-11β), 1.12 (1H, m, H-7α), 1.15 (1H, m, H-12α), 1.25 (1H, m, H-14α), 1.44 (1H, m, H-15β), 1.63 (1H, m, H-15α), 1.72 (1H, m, H-7β), 2.01 (1H, m, H-9α), 2.13 (1H, m, H-11α), 2.50 (1H, m, H-12β), 2.56 (1H, m, H-6α), 2.66 (1H, m, H-6β), 4.90 (1H, s, OH, disappeared with D_2O), 5.75 (1H, dd, H-2), 6.67 (1H, d, H-4), 2.08 (3H, d, CH_3, enone), 6.41 (1H, s, enone proton), 7.12 (1H, d, H-1). ^{13}C NMR: (150 MHz, $CDCl_3$): δ 13.52, 21.73, 25.51, 26.64, 27.48, 29.75, 36.35, 38.61, 43.81, 48.92, 50.43, 112.79, 115.53, 126.56, 128.48, 132.50, 137.02, 138.44, 153.82, 210.02 (20 C). MS (EI): *m/z* 296 (100%) [M^+]. Anal. Calcd for $C_{20}H_{24}O_2$ (296.40): Calcd C, 81.04; H, 8.16. Found C, 81.00; H, 8.10.

3.1.2. Synthesis of 16-(α-alkoxy-alkane)-17-hydrazino-estra-1(10),2,4-trien[17,16-c]-3-ol and their *N*-substituted derivatives (**3a–l**)

"A mixture of **2a,b** (14 mmol) and hydrazine derivatives, namely, hydrazine hydrate, methyl hydrazine or phenyl hydrazine (8 mmol) in absolute methanol or ethanol (30 mL) was refluxed for 5–10 h. The solvent was concentrated under reduced pressure, the formed precipitate was filtered off, washed with water, dried and crystallized from ethanol to give the corresponding derivatives **3a–l**, respectively".

16-(α-Methoxy-methane)-17-hydrazino-estra-1(10),2,4-trien-[17,16-c]-3-ol (**3a**)

Yield 80%, mp 199–201 °C, $[\alpha]_D^{25}$ = + 81 (c 1, MeOH). IR (KBr, cm^{-1}): 3444–3377 (NH, NH_2), 3345 (OH), 2951 (CH, aliphatic), 1638 (C=C). ^{1}H NMR: (600 MHz, $CDCl_3$): δ ppm 0.61 (1H, m, H-8β), 0.90 (3H, s, CH_3-18), 1.00 (1H, m, H-11β), 1.11 (1H, m, H-7α), 1.14 (1H, m, H-12α), 1.26 (1H, m, H-14 α), 1.39 (1H, m, H-15β), 1.58 (1H, m, H-15α), 1.68 (1H, m, H-7β), 2.01(1H, m, H-9α), 1.84 (1H, m, CH, 16-Hα), 2.11 (1H, m, H-11α), 2.49 (1H, m, H-12β), 2.61 (1H, m, H-6α), 2.66 (1H, m, H-6β), 2.83 (1H, d, H-17), 3.48 (3H, s, OCH_3), 4.65 (2H, m, NH_2, disappeared with D_2O), 4.80 (2H, d, CH_2-O), 4.87 (1H, s, OH, disappeared with D_2O), 5.70 (1H, dd, H-2), 6.61 (1H, d, H-4), 7.10 (1H, d, H-1), 7.70 (1H, br.s, NH, disappeared with D_2O). ^{13}C NMR: (150 MHz, $CDCl_3$): δ 13.58, 21.76, 25.57, 26.76, 28.00, 29.78, 36.38, 38.65, 43.89, 48.40, 50.45, 59.45, 69.11, 112.37, 115.56, 126.53, 132.81, 138.46, 153.84, 167.02 (20 C). MS (EI): *m/z* 330 (90%) [M^+]. Anal. Calcd for $C_{20}H_{30}N_2O_2$ (330.46): Calcd C, 72.69; H, 9.15; N, 8.48. Found C, 72.60; H, 9.10; N, 8.40.

16-(α-Methoxy-ethane)-17-hydrazino-estra-1(10),2,4-trien[17,16-c]-3-ol (**3b**)

Yield 57%, mp. 308–310 °C, $[\alpha]_D^{25}$ = + 112 (c 1, MeOH). IR (KBr, cm^{-1}): 3448-3377 (NH, NH_2), 3348 (OH), 2959 (CH, aliphatic), 1634 (C=C). ^{1}H NMR: (600 MHz, $CDCl_3$): δ ppm 0.59 (1H, m, H-8β), 0.91 (3H, s, CH_3-18), 1.01 (1H, m, H-11β), 1.12 (1H, m, H-7α), 1.14 (1H, m, H-12 α), 1.26 (1H, m, H-14 α), 1.39 (1H, m, H -15 β), 1.58 (1H, m, H-15α), 1.42 (3H, m, CH_3,C-16 ethane), 1.69 (1H, m, H-7β), 2.02(1H, m, H-9α), 1.83 (1H, m, CH, H-16α), 2.11 (1H, m, H-11α), 2.49 (1H, m, H-12β), 2.61 (1H, m, H-6α), 2.66 (1H, m, H-6β), 2.83 (1H, d, H-17), 3.48 (3H, s, OCH_3), 4.65 (2H, s, NH_2, disappeared with D_2O), 4.84 (1H, d, CH-O), 4.99 (1H, s, OH, disappeared with D_2O), 5.72 (1H, dd, H-2), 6.61 (1H, d, H-4), 7.11 (1H, d, H-1), 7.78 (1H, bs, NH, disappeared with D_2O). ^{13}C NMR: (150 MHz, $CDCl_3$): δ 13.58, 21.77, 22.22, 25.57, 26.47, 28.00, 29.78, 36.68, 38.47, 43.89, 48.69, 50.45, 59.45, 69.11, 112.37, 115.56, 126.55, 132.48, 138.46, 153.54, 167.76 (21 C). MS (EI): *m/z* 344 (11%) [M^+]. Anal. Calcd for $C_{21}H_{32}N_2O_2$ (344.49): Calcd C, 73.22; H, 9.36; N, 8.13. Found C, 73.18; H, 9.30; N, 8.10.

16-(α-Ethoxy-methane)-17-hydrazino-estra-1(10),2,4-trien-[17,16-c]-3-ol (**3c**)

Yield 56%, mp 219–221 °C, $[\alpha]_D^{25}$ = + 77 (c 1, MeOH). IR (KBr, cm^{-1}): 3445–3376 (NH, NH_2), 3346 (OH), 2951 (CH, aliphatic), 1638 (C=C). ^{1}H NMR: (600 MHz, $CDCl_3$): δ ppm 0.61 (1H, m, H-8β), 0.90 (3H, s, CH_3-18), 1.00 (1H, m, H-11β), 1.11 (1H, m, H-7α), 1.15 (1H, m, H-12α), 1.21 (3H, m, CH_3, ethoxyl), 1.25 (1H, m, H-14α), 1.36 (1H, m, H-15β), 1.57 (1H, m, H-15α), 1.68 (1H, m, H-7β), 2.01 (1H, m, H-9α), 1.84 (1H, m, CH, H-16α), 2.10 (1H, m, H-11α), 2.50 (1H, m, H-12β), 2.60 (1H, m, H-6α), 2.70 (1H, m, H-6β), 6.61 (1H, d, H-4), 2.80 (1H, d, H-17), 3.50 (2H, m, OCH_2), 4.70 (2H, m, NH_2, disappeared with D_2O), 4.80 (2H, d, CH-O), 4.87 (1H, s, OH, disappeared with D_2O), 5.70 (1H, dd, H-2), 7.10 (1H, d, H-1), 7.70 (1H, br.s, NH, disappeared with D_2O). ^{13}C NMR: (150 MHz, $CDCl_3$): δ 13.65, 18.74, 21.57, 25.17, 26.38, 28.04, 29.64, 36.54, 38.15, 44.11, 48.44, 50.54, 68.45, 69.11, 112.44, 115.67, 126.34, 131.11, 138.46, 153.84, 161.47 (21 C). MS (EI): *m/z* 344 (35%) [M^+]. Anal. Calcd for $C_{21}H_{32}N_2O_2$ (344.49): Calcd C, 73.22; H, 9.36; N, 8.13. Found C, 73.16; H, 9.30; N, 8.10.

16-(α-Ethoxy-ethane)-17-hydrazino-estra-1(10),2,4-trien-[17,16-c]-3-ol (**3d**)

Yield 90%, mp 223–225 °C, $[\alpha]_D^{25}$ = + 95 (c 1, MeOH). IR (KBr, cm^{-1}): 3440-3370 (NH, NH_2), 3350 (OH), 2951 (CH, aliphatic), 1631 (C=C). ^{1}H NMR: (600 MHz, $CDCl_3$): δ ppm 0.57 (1H, m, H-8β), 0.90 (3H, s, CH_3-18), 1.00 (1H, m, H-11β), 1.10 (1H, m, H-7α), 1.15 (1H, m, H-12α), 1.20 (3H, m, CH_3, ethoxyl), 1.24 (1H, m, H-14α), 1.36 (1H, m, H-15β), 1.45 (3H, m, CH_3,C-16 ethane), 1.59 (1H, m, H-15α), 1.71 (1H, m, H-7β), 1.96 (1H, m, H-9α), 1.82 (1H, m, CH, H-16α), 2.10 (1H, m, H-11α), 2.50 (1H, m, H-12β), 2.62 (1H, m, H-6α), 2.67 (1H, m, H-6β), 2.86 (1H, d, H-17), 3.48 (2H, m, OCH_2), 4.64 (2H, s, NH_2, disappeared with D_2O), 4.83 (1H, d, CH-O), 4.88 (1H, s, OH, disappeared with D_2O), 5.74 (1H, dd, H-2), 6.65 (1H, d, H-4), 7.12 (1H, d, H-1), 7.78 (1H, br.s, NH, disappeared with D_2O). ^{13}C NMR: (150 MHz, $CDCl_3$): δ 13.55, 18.79, 22.07, 22.28, 25.47, 26.52, 27.77, 28.09, 36.68, 37.97, 44.09, 48.11, 51.41, 68.43, 69.13, 112.56, 115.57, 126.37, 133.18, 137.87, 155.56, 162.74 (22 C). MS (EI): *m/z* 358 (45%) [M^+]. Anal. Calcd for $C_{22}H_{34}N_2O_2$ (358.51): Calcd C, 73.70; H, 9.56; N, 7.81. Found C, 73.64; H, 9.52; N, 7.75.

16-(α-Methoxy-methane)-17-[N-methyl-hydrazino]estra-1(10),2,4-trien[17,16-c]-3-ol (**3e**)

Yield 76%, mp 222–224 °C, $[\alpha]_D^{25}$ = + 66 (c 1, MeOH). IR (KBr, cm^{-1}): 3443–3371 (NH), 3344 (OH), 2953 (CH, aliphatic), 1634 (C=C). ^{1}H NMR: (600 MHz, $CDCl_3$): δ ppm 0.61 (1H, m, H-8β), 0.92 (3H, s, CH_3-18), 1.03 (1H, m, H-11β), 1.10 (1H, m, H-7α), 1.14 (1H, m, H-12α), 1.25 (1H, m, H-14α), 1.37 (1H, m, H-15β), 1.57 (1H, m, H-15α), 1.66 (1H, m, H-7β), 2.00 (1H, m, H-9α), 1.84 (1H, m, CH, H-16α), 2.13 (1H, m, H-11α), 2.32 (3H, s, NCH_3), 2.48 (1H, m, H-12β), 2.63 (1H, m, H-6α), 2.68 (1H, m, H-6β), 2.84 (1H, d, H-17), 3.49 (3H, s, OCH_3), 4.86 (2H, d, CH-O), 4.87 (1H, s, OH, disappeared with D_2O), 5.72 (1H, dd, H-2), 6.63 (1H, d, H-4), 7.11 (1H, d, H-1), 7.76 (1H, brs, NH, disappeared with D_2O), 7.99 (1H, bs, NH, disappeared with D_2O). ^{13}C NMR: (150 MHz, $CDCl_3$): δ 13.53, 21.44, 25.67, 26.36, 28.03, 29.23, 36.33, 38.43, 43.83, 47.47, 48.43, 50.34, 59.35, 69.31, 112.36, 115.67, 126.52, 132.32, 138.21, 153.45, 162.32 (21 C). MS (EI): *m/z* 344 (45%) [M^+]. Anal. Calcd for $C_{21}H_{32}N_2O_2$ (344.50): Calcd C, 73.22; H, 9.36; N, 8.13. Found C, 73.15; H, 9.31; N, 8.09.

16-(α-Methoxy-ethane)-17-[N-methyl-hydrazino]-estra-1(10),2,4-trien-[17,16-c]-3-ol (**3f**)

Yield 57%, mp 310–312 °C, $[\alpha]_D^{25}$ = + 112 (c 1, MeOH). IR (KBr, cm^{-1}): 3443–3374 (NH), 3344 (OH), 2955 (CH, aliphatic), 1628 (C=C). ^{1}H NMR: (600 MHz, $CDCl_3$): δ ppm 0.58 (1H, m, H-8β), 0.90 (3H, s, CH_3-18), 1.00 (1H, m, H-11β), 1.10 (1H, m, H-7α), 1.14 (1H, m, H-12α), 1.26 (1H, m, H-14 α), 1.39 (1H, m, H-15 β), 1.60 (1H, m, H-15α), 1.44 (3H, m, CH_3, C-16 ethane), 1.70 (1H, m, H-7β), 2.00 (1H, m, H-9α), 1.82 (1H, m, CH, H-16α), 2.11 (1H, m, H-11α), 2.36 (3H, s, NCH_3), 2.51 (1H, m, H-12β), 2.62 (1H, m, H-6α), 2.65 (1H, m, H-6β), 2.85 (1H, d, H-17), 3.44 (3H, s, OCH_3), 4.83 (1H, d, CH-O), 4.99 (1H, s, OH, disappeared with D_2O), 5.74 (1H, dd, H-2), 6.65 (1H, d, H-4), 7.13 (1H, d, H-1), 7.73 (1H, br.s, NH, disappeared with D_2O), 7.99 (1H, m, NH, disappeared with D_2O). ^{13}C NMR: (150 MHz, $CDCl_3$): δ 13.78, 21.54, 22.27, 25.97, 26.69, 28.03, 29.43, 36.45, 38.54, 43.68, 47.88, 48.57, 50.86, 59.46, 69.15, 112.54, 115.69, 126.46, 132.90, 138.75, 153.45, 163.60 (22 C). MS (EI): *m/z* 358 (100%) [M^+]. Anal. Calcd for $C_{22}H_{34}N_2O_2$ (358.50): Calcd C, 73.70; H, 9.56; N, 7.81. Found C, 73.60; H, 9.49; N, 7.75.

16-(α-Ethoxy-methane)-17-[N-methyl-hydrazino]-estra-1(10),2,4-trien-[17,16-c]-3-ol (**3g**)

Yield 90%, mp 286–288 °C, $[\alpha]_D^{25}$ = + 121 (c 1, MeOH). IR (KBr, cm^{-1}): 3441–3379 (NH), 3348 (OH), 2957 (CH, aliphatic), 1636 (C=C). ^1H NMR: (600 MHz, $CDCl_3$): δ ppm 0.61 (1H, m, H-8β), 0.91 (3H, s, CH_3-18), 1.01 (1H, m, H-11β), 1.13 (1H, m, H-7α), 1.15 (1H, m, H-12α), 1.22 (3H, m, CH_3, ethoxyl), 1.25 (1H, m, H-14α), 1.37 (1H, m, H-15β), 1.58 (1H, m, H-15α), 1.69 (1H, m, H-7β), 2.00 (1H, m, H-9 α), 1.81 (1H, m, CH, H-16α), 2.12 (1H, m, H-11α), 2.33 (3H, s, NCH_3), 2.54 (1H, m, H-12β), 2.65 (1H, m, H-6α), 2.76 (1H, m, H-6β), 2.87 (1H, d, H-17), 3.50 (2H, m, OCH_2), 4.85 (2H, d, CH_2-O), 4.98 (1H, s, OH, disappeared with D_2O), 5.74 (1H, dd, H-2), 6.65 (1H, d, H-4), 7.10 (1H, d, H-1), 7.76 (1H, br.s, NH, disappeared with D_2O), 7.95 (1H, m, NH, disappeared with D_2O). ^{13}C NMR: (150 MHz, $CDCl_3$): δ 13.35, 18.45, 21.43, 25.78, 26.80, 28.14, 29.88, 36.47, 38.90, 44.41, 47.37, 48.34, 50.54, 68.66, 69.67, 113.34, 115.55, 125.54, 131.53, 137.99, 154.44, 162.27 (22 C). MS (EI): *m/z* 358 (100%) [M^+]. Anal. Calcd for $C_{22}H_{34}N_2O_2$ (358.50): Calcd C, 73.70; H, 9.56; N, 7.81. Found C, 73.62; H, 9.50; N, 7.74.

16-(α-Ethoxy-ethane)-17-[N-methyl-hydrazino]-estra-1(10),2,4-trien-[17,16-c]-3-ol (**3h**)

Yield 78%, mp 280–282 °C, $[\alpha]_D^{25}$ = + 135 (c 1, MeOH). IR (KBr, cm^{-1}): 3441–3371 (NH), 3351 (OH), 2951 (CH, aliphatic), 1631 (C=C). ^1H NMR: (600 MHz, $CDCl_3$): δ ppm 0.60 (1H, m, H-8β), 0.93 (3H, s, CH_3-18), 1.04 (1H, m, H-11β), 1.11 (1H, m, H-7α), 1.16 (1H, m, H-12α), 1.19 (3H, m, CH_3,ethoxyl), 1.23 (1H, m, H-14α), 1.37 (1H, m, H-15β), 1.46 (3H, m, CH_3,C-16 ethane), 1.61 (1H, m, H-15α), 1.72 (1H, m, H-7β), 1.82 (1H, m, CH, H-16α), 1.93 (1H, m, H-9α), 2.10 (1H, m, H-11α), 2.50 (1H, m, H-12β), 2.34 (3H, s, NCH_3), 2.63 (1H, m, H-6α), 2.62 (1H, m, H-6β), 2.85 (1H, d, H-17), 3.43 (2H, m, OCH_2), 4.64 (1H, s, OH, disappeared with D_2O), 4.83 (1H, d, CH-O), 5.72 (1H, dd, H-2), 6.64 (1H, d, H-4), 7.10 (1H, d, H-1), 7.75 (1H, br.s, NH, disappeared with D_2O), 7.88 (1H, s, NH, disappeared with D_2O). ^{13}C NMR: (150 MHz, $CDCl_3$): δ 13.53, 18.67, 22.43, 22.90, 25.67, 26.78, 27.45, 28.29, 36.89, 37.65, 44.65, 47.35, 48.68, 51.90, 68.78, 69.13, 112.56, 115.56, 126.34, 133.55, 137.43, 155.34, 163.34 (23 C). MS (EI): *m/z* 372 (100%) [M^+]. Anal. Calcd for $C_{23}H_{36}N_2O_2$ (372.54): Calcd C, 74.15; H, 9.74; N, 7.52. Found C, 74.05; H, 9.68; N, 7.48.

16-(α-Methoxy-methane)-17-[N-phenyl-hydrazino]-estra-1(10),2,4-trien-[17,16-c]-3-ol (**3i**)

Yield 67%, mp 312–314 °C, $[\alpha]_D^{25}$ = + 95 (c 1, MeOH). IR (KBr, cm^{-1}): 3430–3367 (NH), 3345 (OH), 3068 (CH, aromatic), 2951 (CH, aliphatic), 1638 (C=C). ^1H NMR: (600 MHz, $CDCl_3$): δ ppm 0.61(1H, m, H-8β), 0.91 (3H, s, CH_3-18), 1.00 (1H, m, H-11β), 1.12 (1H, m, H-7α), 1.15 (1H, m, H-12α), 1.28 (1H, m, H-14α), 1.40 (1H, m, H-15β), 1.60 (1H, m, H-15α), 1.68 (1H, m, H-7β), 2.02 (1H, m, H-9α), 1.86 (1H, m, CH, H-16α), 2.12 (1H, m, H-11α), 2.49 (1H, m, H-12 β), 2.59 (1H, m, H-6α), 2.65 (1H, m, H-6β), 2.84 (1H, d, H-17), 3.47 (3H, s, OCH_3), 4.80 (2H, d, CH-O), 4.87 (1H, s, OH, disappeared with D_2O), 5.70 (1H, dd, H-2), 6.61 (1H, d, H-4), 7.10 (1H, d, H-1), 7.28-7.48 (5H, m, Ar-H), 7.76 (1H, br.s, NH, disappeared with D_2O), 7.99 (1H, s, NH, disappeared with D_2O). ^{13}C NMR: (150 MHz, $CDCl_3$): δ 13.45, 21.76, 25.76, 26.67, 28.45, 29.66, 36.43, 38.65, 43.45, 48.40, 50.87, 59.45, 69.67, 112.43, 112.76, 115.66, 119.11, 126.68, 129.45, 132.67, 138.53, 152.55, 153.79, 161.02 (26 C). MS (EI): *m/z* 406 (77%) [M^+]. Anal. Calcd for $C_{26}H_{34}N_2O_2$ (406.56): Calcd C, 76.81; H, 8.43; N, 6.89. Found C, 76.75; H, 8.40; N, 6.80.

16-(α-Methoxy-ethane)-17-[N-phenyl-hydrazino]-estra-1(10),2,4-trien-[17,16-c]-3-ol (**3j**)

Yield 66%, mp 229–231 °C, $[\alpha]_D^{25}$ = + 147 (c 1, MeOH). IR (KBr, cm^{-1}): 3433–3363 (NH), 3346 (OH), 3066 (CH, aromatic), 2955 (CH, aliphatic), 1635 (C=C). ^1H NMR: (600 MHz, $CDCl_3$): δ ppm 0.62 (1H, m, H-8β), 0.92 (3H, s, CH_3-18), 1.02 (1H, m, H-11β), 1.13 (1H, m, H-7α), 1.18 (1H, m, H-12α), 1.26 (1H, m, H-14α), 1.39 (1H, m, H-15β), 1.42 (3H, m, CH_3, C-16 ethane), 1.58 (1H, m, H-15α), 1.69 (1H, m, H-7β), 1.83 (1H, m, CH, H-16α), 2.03 (1H, m, H-9α), 2.10 (1H, m, H-11α), 2.52 (1H, m, H-12β), 2.62 (1H, m, H-6α), 2.65 (1H, m, H-6β), 2.85 (1H, d, H-17), 3.49 (3H, s, OCH_3), 4.86 (1H, d, CH-O), 4.89 (1H, s, OH, disappeared with D_2O), 5.71 (1H, dd, H-2), 6.61 (1H, d, H-4), 7.12 (1H, d, H-1), 7.27-7.49 (5H, m, Ar-H), 7.77 (1H, br.s, NH, disappeared with D_2O), 7.97 (2H, s, NH, disappeared with D_2O). ^{13}C NMR:

(150 MHz, $CDCl_3$): δ 13.52, 21.78, 22.92, 25.67, 26.45, 28.10, 29.90, 36.17, 38.47, 43.80, 48.69, 50.55, 59.25, 69.11, 112.12, 112.78, 115.54, 119.17, 126.46, 129.53, 132.79, 138.78, 152.42, 153.76, 163.11 (27 C). MS (EI): *m/z* 420 (81%) [M^+]. Anal. Calcd for $C_{27}H_{36}N_2O_2$ (420.58): Calcd C, 77.10; H, 8.63; N, 6.66. Found C, 77.00; H, 8.58; N, 6.60.

16-(α-Ethoxy-methane)-17-[N-phenyl-hydrazino]-estra-1(10),2,4-trien-[17,16-c]-3-ol (**3k**)

Yield 60%, mp 338–340 °C, $[\alpha]_D^{25}$ = + 155 (c 1, MeOH). IR (KBr, cm^{-1}): 3431–3362 (NH), 3343 (OH), 3064 (CH, aromatic), 2956 (CH, aliphatic), 1637 (C=C). ^{1}H NMR: (600 MHz, $CDCl_3$): δ ppm 0.63 (1H, m, H-8β), 0.90 (3H, s, CH_3-18), 1.01 (1H, m, H-11β), 1.11 (1H, m, H-7α), 1.16 (1H, m, H-12α), 1.21 (3H, m, CH_3, ethoxyl), 1.24 (1H, m, H-14α), 1.36 (1H, m, H-15β), 1.59 (1H, m, H-15α), 1.68 (1H, m, H-7β), 2.00 (1H, m, H-9α), 1.84 (1H, m, CH, H-16α), 2.11 (1H, m, H-11α), 2.50 (1H, m, H-12β), 2.61 (1H, m, H-6α), 2.70 (1H, m, H-6β), 6. disappeared (1H, d, H-4), 2.80 (1H, d, H-17), 3.53 (2H, m, OCH_2), 4.80 (2H, d, CH-O), 4.84 (1H, s, OH, exchangeable with D_2O), 5.70 (1H, dd, H-2), 7.15 (1H, d, H-1), 7.26-7.47 (5H, m, Ar-H), 7.76 (1H, br.s, NH, disappeared with D_2O), 7.98 (1H, m, NH, disappeared with D_2O). ^{13}C NMR: (150 MHz, $CDCl_3$): δ 13.64, 18.74, 21.57, 25.17, 26.30, 28.05, 29.64, 36.54, 38.15, 44.18, 48.46, 50.55, 68.43, 69.13, 112.49, 112.72, 115.60, 119.11, 126.34, 129.50, 131.11, 138.49, 152.40, 153.84, 162.47 (27 C). MS (EI): *m/z* 420 (88%) [M^+]. Anal. Calcd for $C_{27}H_{36}N_2O_2$ (420.58): Calcd C, 77.10; H, 8.63; N, 6.66. Found C, 77.02; H, 8.57; N, 6.61.

16-(α-Ethoxy-ethane)-17-[N-phenyl-hydrazino]-estra-1(10),2,4-trien-[17,16-c]-3-ol (**3l**)

Yield 96%, mp 288–300 °C, $[\alpha]_D^{25}$ = + 95 (c 1, MeOH). IR (KBr, cm^{-1}): 3431–3367 (NH), 3343 (OH), 3068 (CH, aromatic), 2951 (CH, aliphatic), 1631 (C=C). ^{1}H NMR: (600 MHz, $CDCl_3$): δ ppm 0.58 (1H, m, H-8β), 0.91 (3H, s, CH_3-18), 1.00 (1H, m, H-11β), 1.10 (1H, m, H-7α), 1.14 (1H, m, H-12α), 1.21 (3H, m, CH_3, ethoxyl), 1.24 (1H, m, H-14α), 1.36 (1H, m, H-15β), 1.44 (3H, m, CH_3, C-16 ethane), 1.60 (1H, m, H-15α), 1.71 (1H, m, H-7β), 1.97 (1H, m, H-9 α), 1.83 (1H, m, CH, H-16α), 2.11 (1H, m, H-11α), 2.51 (1H, m, H-12β), 2.62 (1H, m, H-6α), 2.67 (1H, m, H-6 β), 2.88 (1H, d, H-17), 3.49 (2H, m, OCH_2), 4.84 (1H, d, CH-O), 4.87 (1H, s, OH, disappeared with D_2O), 5.73 (1H, dd, H-2), 6.62 (1H, d, H-4), 7.13 (1H, d, H-1), 7.23-7.47 (5H, m, Ar-H), 7.77 (1H, br.s, NH, disappeared with D_2O), 7.87 (1H, m, NH, disappeared with D_2O). ^{13}C NMR: (150 MHz, $CDCl_3$): δ 13.56, 18.77, 22.27, 22.32, 25.76, 26.78, 27.34, 28.29, 36.54, 37.90, 44.21, 48.23, 51.32, 68.34, 69.56, 112.67, 112.77, 115.56, 119.10, 126.45, 129.50, 133.47, 137.23, 152.55, 155.51, 163.73 (28 C). MS (EI): *m/z* 434 (93%) [M^+]. Anal. Calcd for $C_{28}H_{38}N_2O_2$ (434.61): Calcd C, 77.38; H, 8.81; N, 6.45. Found C, 77.30; H, 8.75; N, 6.40.

3.1.3. Synthesis of pyrazoline-3-ol derivatives (**4a–d**)

A mixture of **2a,b** (4 mmol) and hydrazine derivatives, namely, methy hydrazine or phenyl hydrazine (16 mmol) in dioxane (25 mL) was refluxed for 5 h. The mixture was evaporated under vacuum, the residue formed was triturated with water, filtered off, washed with water, dried and crystallized from MeOH to give derivatives **4a–d**, respectively.

1′-Methyl-1′H-estra-1(10),2,4-trien-[17,16-c]pyrazoline-3-ol (**4a**)

Yield 96%, mp 117–119 °C, $[\alpha]_D^{25}$ = + 109 (c 1, MeOH). IR (KBr, cm^{-1}): 3351 (OH), 2946 (CH, aliphatic), 1627 (C=C), 1610 (C=N). ^{1}H NMR: (600 MHz, $CDCl_3$): δ ppm 0.61 (1H, m, H-8β), 0.94 (3H, s, CH_3-18), 1.08 (1H, m, H-11β), 1.13 (1H, m, H-7α), 1.18 (1H, m, H-12α), 1.27 (1H, m, H-14α), 1.41 (1H, m, H-15β), 1.66 (1H, m, H-15α), 1.74 (1H, m, H-7β), 1.84 (1H, m, CH, H-16α), 2.01 (1H, m, H-9α), 2.10 (3H, s, NCH_3), 2.22 (1H, m, H-11α), 2.42 (1H, m, H-12β), 2.52 (1H, m, H-6α), 2.66 (1H, m, H-6β), 2.84 (2H, d, pyrazoline-5′), 4.95 (1H, s, OH, disappeared with D_2O), 5.75 (1H, dd, H-2), 6.65 (1H, d, H-4), 7.15 (1H, d, H-1). ^{13}C NMR: (150 MHz, $CDCl_3$): δ 14.60, 22.56, 25.35, 26.46, 28.77, 29.56, 36.68, 38.68, 43.34, 45.36, 48.21, 50.24, 64.45, 112.46, 115.57, 126.44, 132.56, 138.45, 152.67, 156.46 (20 C). MS (EI): *m/z* 310 (100%)

[M+]. Anal. Calcd for $C_{20}H_{26}N_2O$ (310.43): Calcd C, 77.38; H, 8.44; N, 9.02. Found C, 77.29; H, 8.36; N, 8.98.

1′-Methyl -1′H-5′-methyl-estra-1(10),2,4-trien-[17,16-c]pyrazoline-3-ol (**4b**)

Yield 88%, mp 216–218 °C, $[\alpha]_D^{25}$ = + 111 (c 1, MeOH). IR (KBr, cm^{-1}): 3351 (OH), 2946 (CH, aliphatic), 1627 (C=C), 1617 (C=N). ^{1}H NMR: (600 MHz, $CDCl_3$): δ ppm 0.62 (1H, m, H-8β), 0.92 (3H, s, CH_3-18), 1.02 (1H, m, H-11β), 1.05 (3H, s, CH_3-5′-methyl), 1.10 (1H, m, H-7α), 1.14 (1H, m, H-12α), 1.25 (1H, m, H-14α), 1.40 (1H, m, H-15β), 1.66 (1H, m, H -15α), 1.77 (1H, m, H-7β), 1.88 (1H, m, CH, H-16α), 2.00 (1H, m, H-9α), 2.17 (3H, s, N-CH_3), 2.20 (1H, m, H-11α), 2.47 (1H, m, H-12β), 2.57 (1H, m, H-6α), 2.66 (1H, m, H-6β), 2.84 (1H, m, pyrazoline-5′), 4.88 (1H, s, OH, disappeared with D_2O), 5.79 (1H, dd, H-2), 6.68 (1H, d, H-4), 7.19 (1H, d, H-1). ^{13}C NMR: (150 MHz, $CDCl_3$): δ 13.35, 21.80, 24.27, 25.30, 26.07, 28.20, 29.77, 36.76, 38.70, 43.67, 45.67, 48.50, 50.70, 64.45, 112.37, 115.54, 126.46, 132.40, 138.77, 153.44, 155.42 (21 C). MS (EI): *m/z* 324 (100%) [M+]. Anal. Calcd for $C_{21}H_{28}N_2O$ (324.45): Calcd C, 77.74; H, 8.70; N, 8.63. Found C, 77.66; H, 8.64; N, 8.58.

1′-Phenyl-1′H-estra-1(10),2,4-trien-[17,16-c]pyrazoline-3-ol (**4c**)

Yield 70%, mp 255–257 °C, $[\alpha]_D^{25}$ = + 128 (c 1, MeOH). IR (KBr, cm^{-1}): 3347 (OH), 3071 and 3061 (CH, aromatic), 2931 (CH, aliphatic), 1633 (C=C), 1614 (C=N). ^{1}H NMR: (600 MHz, $CDCl_3$): δ ppm 0.60 (1H, m, H-8β), 0.90 (3H, s, CH_3-18), 1.00 (1H, m, H-11β), 1.10 (1H, m, H-7α), 1.20 (1H, m, H-12α), 1.28 (1H, m, H-14α), 1.49 (1H, m, H-15β), 1.68 (1H, m, H-15α), 1.77 (1H, m, H-7β), 1.86 (1H, m, CH, H-16α), 2.04 (1H, m, H-9α), 2.26 (1H, m, H-11α), 2.48 (1H, m, H -12β), 2.54 (1H, m, H-6α), 2.64 (1H, m, H-6β), 2.84 (2H, d, pyrazoline-5′), 5.00 (1H, s, OH, disappeared with D_2O), 5.71 (1H, dd, H-2), 6.70 (1H, d, H-4), 7.10 (1H, d, H-1), 7.28-7.40 (5H, m, Ar-H). ^{13}C NMR: (150 MHz, $CDCl_3$): δ 13.49, 21.24, 25.55, 26.46, 28.51, 29.67, 36.64, 38.45, 43.35, 50.73, 58.26, 64.45, 112.10, 112.48, 115.46, 119.31, 126.10, 129.20, 132.52, 138.79, 152.20, 153.13, 163.48 (25 C). MS (EI): *m/z* 372 (81%) [M+]. Anal. Calcd for $C_{25}H_{28}N_2O$ (372.50): Calcd C, 80.61; H, 7.58; N, 7.52. Found C, 80.52; H, 7.50; N, 7.48.

1′-Phenyl-1′H-5′-methyl-estra-1(10),2,4-trien-[17,16-c]pyrazoline-3-ol (**4d**)

Yield 75%, mp 214–216 °C, $[\alpha]_D^{25}$ = + 127 (c 1, MeOH). IR (KBr, cm^{-1}): 3345 (OH), 3068 (CH, aromatic), 2949 (CH, aliphatic), 1625 (C=C), 1614 (C=N). ^{1}H NMR: (600 MHz, $CDCl_3$): δ ppm 0.62 (1H, m, H-8β), 0.93 (3H, s, CH_3-18), 1.02 (1H, m, H-11β), 1.05 (3H, s, CH_3-5′-methyl), 1.12 (1H, m, H-7α), 1.17 (1H, m, H-12α), 1.27 (1H, m, H-14α), 1.41 (1H, m, H-15β), 1.71 (1H, m, H -15α), 1.77 (1H, m, H-7β), 1.87 (1H, m, CH, H-16α), 2.02 (1H, m, H-9α), 2.22 (1H, m, H-11α), 2.46 (1H, m, H -12β), 2.54 (1H, m, H-6α), 2.65 (1H, m, H-6β), 3.83 (1H, s, pyrazoline-5′), 4.91 (1H, s, OH, disappeared with D_2O), 5.81 (1H, dd, H-2), 6.73 (1H, d, H-4), 7.21 (1H, d, H-1), 7.28-7.48 (5H, m, Ar-H). ^{13}C NMR: (150 MHz, $CDCl_3$): δ 13.81, 21.89, 24.25, 25.80, 26.35, 28.34, 29.23, 36.56, 38.67, 43.34, 48.55, 50.67, 64.44, 112.70, 115.34, 119.10, 126.76, 129.50, 132.45, 138.56, 152.40, 154.36, 163.56, 164.55 (26 C). MS (EI): *m/z* 386 (23%) [M+]. Anal. Calcd for $C_{26}H_{30}N_2O$ (386.52): Calcd C, 80.79; H, 7.82; N, 7.25. Found C, 80.70; H, 7.76; N, 7.20.

3.2. Biological Screening

3.2.1. In Vitro Cytotoxic Activities

The cytotoxic activities of the synthesized derivatives against ovarian cancer cell lines (SKOV-3) were evaluated using standard MTT assay [26,27]. SKOV-3 cells cultivated on DMEM medium supplemented with 10% FBS, 100×, 1% antibiotic/antimycotic solution and 3.6 g/L $NaHCO_3$ were used. Cells were incubated under standard laboratory conditions [28,29]. Before testing compounds, cells were trypsinized, centrifuged and prepared as per our developed protocol [30,31]. MTT assay relies on the enzymatic conversion of the MTT substrate into purple formazan by living cells mitochondrial enzymes. Shortly, 96 well plates were seeded (10,000 cells/100 μL/well), then incubated for 24 h at standard conditions. Afterwards, cells were exposed to different concentrations from prepared compounds and incubated for another 24 h. Thereafter, MTT (10 μL, 5 mg/mL, PBS) were added to each well, and plates were incubated for 4 h. Supernatants were then replaced discarded with 200 μL of DMSO to dissolve the precipitated formazan crystals. Formazan absorbance, proportional to living cell number, was read at 550 nm using a microplate reader. Viability percentages were calculated and the corresponding IC_{50} values were obtained from the linear regression of the calibration curve. For comparison, doxorubicin (DOX) and resveratrol (RES) were used as positive controls. Furthermore, the effect of the newly synthesized derivatives was tested against normal fibroblast cell line to assess their toxicities.

3.2.2. In Vitro Anti-Ovarian Xenograft Model

Anti-ovarian cancer xenograft animal model was developed in nude mouse using SKOV-3 cells according to McCauley et al. [32]. Treatment protocol was approved by the University of South Dakota, Institutional Animal Care and Use Committee (study protocol 50-01-05-08B). Immunodeficient (athymic nude-Foxn1nu) female mice were inoculated (1×10^6 cells/site). Upon tumor development, (av. volume ~50 mm^3), 10-mice groups were implanted s.c. with constant release pellets containing tested compound (1 μM/gm) or placebo. Animal and tumor development were monitored measured every 5 days after pellet implantation, using standardized Caliper in two perpendicular diameters of the implant according to our previous work [2]. Due to large tumor volumes, (5-fold difference between largest and smallest tumor), relative tumor volumes were used for comparison. Relative tumor volume = $Vt_{\text{volume at time t}}/V0_{\text{initial volume}}$.

3.2.3. Topoisomerase II Inhibition

The inhibitory effects of the synthesized compounds against topoisomerase II were investigated using relaxation assay according to Goyeneche, et al. [33]. Topoisomerase II was purified from P388 cells, where enzyme unit corresponds to the activity required complete relaxation of 0.125 g of supercoiled pBR-322 DNA at 30 °C for 1 h. The assay was performed as per protocol and samples were subjected to electrophoresis (0.7% agarose gels, TBE buffer. Ethidium bromide-stained DNA was examined under UV light.

3.2.4. In Vitro Kinase Inhibition

Protein Expression and Purification

BRAF wild-type and V600E mutant kinase domains were expressed and purified according to Nakamura et al. [34]. Shortly, Sf 9 cells infected with BRAF kinase domain containing baculovirus were resuspended, sonicated, and then cleared using ultracentrifugation. Afterwards, the cleared lysate with mixed with equilibrated Talon resin, and the resin then washed with 10 column volumes of wash buffer and then eluted with buffer (25 mM Tris, pH 7.0, 250 mM NaCl, 160 mM imidazole, 10% glycerol). The eluant was then diluted, concentrated using Superdex 200 gel filtration column, purified as previously described and finally stored at –80 °C until use.

In Vitro ELISA-Based Kinase Assay

"This method was adopted from Nakamura et al. [34] and Qin et al. [35]. The previously prepared GST MEK-His protein was diluted in TTBS buffer (100 μL, 50 μg/mL), and then bound to 96-plate wells coated with glutathione (Pierce Biotechnology). Two DMSO-dilutions of each compound (1 μL) were added to 50 μL (50mM HEPES, pH7.0, 0.7 pmol of $BRAF^{V600E}$ kinase). Tubes were incubated at ambient temperature for 1 h, then added to GST-MEK-His-plate wells. Afterwards, 50 μL of phosphorylation buffer were added to start kinase reaction (37 °C/30 min/shaking). Reaction was stopped, then substrate was added, and the signal was recorded. The high throughput inhibitor screening was carried out according to standard assay conditions at different concentrations, to generate a sigmoidal dose response curve, a four-parameter logistic model using GraphPad Prism, for BRAF proteins, which was used to obtain corresponding IC_{50} values".

3.2.5. Statistical Analysis

"Measurements were carried out in thrice and data are represented as means ± SEM. Significance was calculated by Student's t-test using SPSS software (SPSS Inc., Paris, France). * $p <0.05$, ** $p < 0.01$, *** $p < 0.001$. IC_{50} values were calculated using GraphPad Prism software, GraphPad Software, San Diego, CA, USA [36]".

4. Conclusions

During the current investigation, we synthesized a series of 17-hydrazino- and 17,16-c-pyrazoline estrone derivatives. Prepared compounds exhibited potential in vitro and in vivo anti-ovarian cancer activity against SKOV-3 cells. Compound **3a** was found to be the most potent with an IC_{50} value of 4.23 ± 0.12 nM. Additionally, in vivo xenograft ovarian cancer model showed that Cpd. **3a** was able to reduce tumor growth by 93.61 ± 0.7% after 40 days of treatment. Furthermore, the newly synthesized compounds were able to interfere with tumor proliferation through inhibiting the activity of topoisomerase II and ^{V600E}BRAF, where the obtained IC_{50} values for both enzymes were 3.45 ± 0.13 nM and 0.041 ± 0.0016 μM, respectively.

Author Contributions: M.E.-N., A.E.-G.E.A., A.A.F. performed most of the experiments; A.E.-G.E.A., M.A.A.-O., A.A.F. analyzed the data; E.A.E. and M.M.A. the contributed to the anticancer activity assays; All authors read and approved the final manuscript.

Acknowledgments: The authors are grateful to the Deanship of Scientific Research, king Saud University for funding through Vice Deanship of Scientific Research Chairs.

References

1. Gupta, A.; Kumar, B.S.; Negi, A.S. Current status on development of steroids as anticancer agents. *J. Steroid Biochem. Mol. Boil.* **2013**, *137*, 242–270. [CrossRef] [PubMed]
2. Amr, A.E.-G.E.; El-Naggar, M.; Al-Omar, M.A.; Elsayed, E.A.; Abdalla, M.M. In vitro and in vivo anti-breast cancer activities of some synthesized pyrazolinyl-estran-17-one candidates. *Molecules* **2018**, *23*, 1572. [CrossRef] [PubMed]
3. Afzal, M.; Al-Awadi, S.; Oommen, S. Antioxidant activity of biotransformed sex hormones facilitated by Bacillus stearothermophilus. In *Advanced Protocols in Oxidative Stress II, Methods in Molecular Biology*; Armstrong, D., Ed.; Springer: Basel, Switzerland, 2010.
4. Schönecker, B.; Lange, C.; Kötteritzsch, M.; Günther, W.; Weston, J.; Anders, E.; Görls, H. Conformational design for 13α-Steroids. *J. Org. Chem.* **2000**, *65*, 5487–5497. [CrossRef]
5. Jovanovic-Santa, S.; Petrović, J.; Andrić, S.; Kovačević, R.; Đurendić, E.; Sakač, M.; Lazar, D.; Stanković, S. Synthesis, structure, and screening of estrogenic and antiestrogenic activity of new 3,17-substituted-16,17-seco-estratriene derivatives. *Bioorg. Chem.* **2003**, *31*, 475–484. [CrossRef]
6. Minorics, R.; Bózsity, N.; Wölfling, J.; Mernyák, E.; Schneider, G.; Márki, A.; Falkay, G.; Ocsovszki, I.; Zupkó, I. Antiproliferative effect of normal and 13-epi-D-homoestrone and their 3-methyl ethers on human reproductive cancer cell lines. *J. Steroid Biochem. Mol. Biol.* **2013**, *132*, 168–175. [CrossRef] [PubMed]
7. Ayan, D.P.; Maltais, R.; Roy, J.; Poirier, D. Impact of estradiol structural modifications (18-methyl and/or 17-hydroxy inversion of configuration) on the in vitro and in vivo estrogenic activity. In Proceedings of the Endocrine Society's 93rd Annual Meeting & Expo, Boston, MA, USA, 4–7 June 2011; Volume 127.
8. Szabó, J.; Bacsa, I.; Wölfling, J.; Schneider, G.; Zupkó, I.; Varga, M.; Herman, B.E.; Kalmár, L.; Szécsi, M.; Mernyák, E. Synthesis and in vitro pharmacological evaluation of N-[(1-benzyl-1,2,3-triazol-4-yl)methyl]-

carboxamides on D-secoestrone scaffolds. *J. Enzyme Inhib. Med. Chem.* **2016**, *31*, 574–579. [CrossRef] [PubMed]

9. Szabó, J.; Jerkovics, N.; Schneider, G.; Wölfling, J.; Bózsity, N.; Minorics, R.; Zupkó, I.; Mernyák, E.; De Sousa, M.E. Synthesis and in vitro antiproliferative evaluation of c-13 epimers of triazolyl-d-secoestrone alcohols: the first potent 13α-d-secoestrone derivative. *Molecules* **2016**, *21*, 611. [CrossRef] [PubMed]
10. Szabó, J.; Pataki, Z.; Wölfling, J.; Schneider, G.; Bózsity, N.; Minorics, R.; Zupkó, I.; Mernyák, E. Synthesis and biological evaluation of 13α-estrone derivatives as potential antiproliferative agents. *Steroids* **2016**, *113*, 14–21. [CrossRef]
11. Mernyák, E.; Kovács, I.; Minorics, R.; Sere, P.; Czégány, D.; Sinka, I.; Wölfling, J.; Schneider, G.; Újfaludi, Z.; Boros, I.; et al. Synthesis of trans-16-triazolyl-13α-methyl-17-estradiol diastereomers and the effects of structural modifications on their in vitro antiproliferative activities. *J. Steroid Biochem. Mol. Boil.* **2015**, *150*, 123–134. [CrossRef]
12. Rao, P.N.; Cessac, J.W.; Tinley, T.L.; Mooberry, S.L. Synthesis and antimitotic activity of novel 2-methoxyestradiol analogs. *Steroids* **2002**, *67*, 1079–1089. [CrossRef]
13. Sundov, D.; Čarić, A.; Mrklić, I.; Gugic, D.; Čapkun, V.; Hofman, I.D.; Mise, B.P.; Tomic, S. P53, MAPK, topoisomerase II alpha and Ki67 immunohistochemical expression and KRAS/BRAF mutation in ovarian serous carcinomas. *Diagn. Pathol.* **2013**, *8*, 21. [CrossRef]
14. Kaur, P.V.; Kaur, S. DNA Topoisomerase II: promising target for anticancer drugs. In *Multi-Targeted Approach to Treatment of Cancer*; Gandhi, V., Ed.; Springer: Basel, Switzerland, 2015; pp. 323–338.
15. Nijenhuis, C.; Lucas, L.; Rosing, H.; Huitema, A.; Mergui-Roelvink, M.; Jamieson, G.C.; Fox, J.; Mould, D.; Schellens, J.; Beijnen, J. Metabolism and disposition of the anticancer quinolone derivative vosaroxin, a novel inhibitor of topoisomerase II. *Investig. New Drugs* **2017**, *35*, 478–490. [CrossRef]
16. Rahman, M.A.; Salajegheh, A.; Smith, R.A.; Lam, A.K.-Y.; Ariana, A. Inhibition of BRAF kinase suppresses cellular proliferation, but not enough for complete growth arrest in BRAF V600E mutated papillary and undifferentiated thyroid carcinomas. *Endocrine* **2016**, *54*, 129–138. [CrossRef]
17. Rahman, M.A.; Salajegheh, A.; Smith, R.A.; Lam, A.K.-Y.; Ariana, A. Multiple proliferation-survival signalling pathways are simultaneously active in BRAF V600E mutated thyroid carcinomas. *Exp. Mol. Pathol.* **2015**, *99*, 492–497. [CrossRef]
18. McCubrey, J.A.; Steelman, L.S.; Abrams, S.L.; Lee, J.T.; Chang, F.; Bertrand, F.E.; Navolanic, P.M.; Terrian, D.M.; Franklin, R.A.; D'Assoro, A.B.; et al. Roles of the RAF/MEK/ERK and PI3K/PTEN/AKT pathways in malignant transformation and drug resistance. *Adv. Enzym. Regul.* **2006**, *46*, 249–279. [CrossRef]
19. Ouf, N.H.; Amr, A.E. Synthesis and anti-inflammatory activity of some pyrimidines and thieno- pyrimidines using 1-(2-benzo[d][1,3]dioxol-5-yl)vinyl)-4-mercapto-6-methyl-pyrimidine-5-yl)-ethan-2- one as a starting material. *Monatsh. fur Chem.* **2008**, *139*, 579–585. [CrossRef]
20. Amr, A.E.; Abdulla, M.M. Synthesis and anti-inflammatory activities of new cynopyrane derivatives fused with steroidal nuclei. *Archiv. der Pharm.* **2008**, *339*, 88–95. [CrossRef]
21. Khalifa, N.M.; Al-Omar, M.A.; Amr, A.E.; Haiba, M.E. Antiviral activity of some new polycyclic nucleoside pyrene candidate against HIV-1 and HSV-1 virus. *Int. J. Biol. Macromol.* **2013**, *54*, 51. [CrossRef]
22. Abdel-Wahab, B.F.; Mohamed, S.F.; Amr, A.E.-G.E.; Abdalla, M.M. Synthesis and reactions of thiosemicarbazides, triazoles, and Schiff bases as antihypertensive α-blocking agents. *Monatsh. Chem.* **2008**, *139*, 1083–1090. [CrossRef]
23. Amr, A.E.-G.E.; Elsayed, E.A.; Al-Omar, M.A.; Eldin, H.O.B.; Nossier, E.S.; Abdallah, M.M.; Eldin, H.B. Design, synthesis, anticancer evaluation and molecular modeling of novel estrogen derivatives. *Molecules* **2019**, *24*, 416. [CrossRef]
24. Day, J.M.; Foster, P.A.; Tutill, H.J.; Schmidlin, F.; Sharland, C.M.; Hargrave, J.D.; Vicker, N.; Potter, B.V.L.; Reed, M.J.; Purohit, A. STX2171, a 17-hydroxysteroid dehydrogenase type 3 inhibitor, is efficacious in vivo in a novel hormone-dependent prostate cancer model. *Endocr. Relat. Cancer* **2013**, *20*, 53–64. [CrossRef]
25. Donald, P.; Ho-Jin, C.; Arezki, A.; Roch, P.B.; Sheng-Xiang, L. Estrone and estradiol C-16 derivatives as inhibitors of type 1 17β-hydroxysteroid dehydrogenase. *Mol. Cell. Endocrinol.* **2006**, *248*, 236–238.
26. Elsayed, E.A.; Sharaf-Eldin, M.; Wadaan, M. In vitro evaluation of cytotoxic activities of essential oil from moringa oleifera seeds on HeLa, HepG2, MCF-7, CACO-2 and L929 Cell Lines. *Asian Pac. J. Cancer Prev.* **2015**, *16*, 4671–4675. [CrossRef]

27. Elsayed, E.A.; Farooq, M.; Dailin, D.; El-Enshasy, H.A.; Othman, N.Z.; Malek, R.; Danial, E.; Wadaan, M. In vitro and in vivo biological screening of kefiran polysaccharide produced by Lactobacillus kefiranofaciens. *Biomed. Res.* **2017**, *28*, 594–600.
28. Al-Salahi, R.; Elsayed, E.A.; El Dib, R.A.; Wadaan, M.; Ezzeldin, E.; Marzouk, M. Synthesis, characterization and cytotoxicity evaluation of 5-hydrazono-[1,2,4]triazolo[1,5-a]quinazolines (Part I). *Lat. Am. J. Pharm.* **2016**, *35*, 58–65.
29. Al-Salahi, R.; Elsayed, E.A.; El Dib, R.A.; Wadaan, M.; Ezzeldin, E.; Marzouk, M. Cytotoxicity of new 5-hydrazono-[1,2,4]triazolo[1,5-a]quinazolines (Part II). *Lat. Am. J. Pharm.* **2016**, *35*, 66–73.
30. Elsayed, E.A.; Sharaf-Eldin, M.A.; El-Enshasy, H.A.; Wadaan, M. In vitro assessment of anticancer properties of Moringa peregrina essential seed oil on different cell lines. *Pak. J. Zool.* **2016**, *48*, 853–859.
31. Farooq, M.; Abu Taha, N.; Butorac, R.R.; Evans, D.A.; Elzatahry, A.A.; Elsayed, E.A.; Wadaan, M.A.M.; Al-Deyab, S.S.; Cowley, A.H.; Li, J. Biological screening of newly synthesized BIAN N-heterocyclic gold carbene complexes in zebrafish embryos. *Int. J. Mol. Sci.* **2015**, *16*, 24718–24731. [CrossRef]
32. McCauley, J.; Zivanovic, A.; Skropeta, D. Bioassays for anticancer activities. *Methods Mol. Biol.* **2013**, *1055*, 191–205.
33. Goyeneche, A.A.; Carón, R.W.; Telleria, C.M. Mifepristone inhibits ovarian cancer cancer cell growth in vitro and in vivo. *Clin. Cancer Res.* **2007**, *13*, 3370–3379. [CrossRef]
34. Nakamura, K.; Sugumi, H.; Yamaguchi, A.; Uenaka, T.; Kotake, Y.; Okada, T.; Kamata, J.; Niijima, J.; Nagasu, T.; Koyanagi, N.; et al. Antitumor activity of ER-37328, a novel carbazole topoisomerase II inhibitor. *Mol. Cancer Ther.* **2002**, *1*, 169–75.
35. Qin, J.; Xie, P.; Ventocilla, C.; Zhou, G.; Vultur, A.; Chen, Q.; Liu, Q.; Herlyn, M.; Winkler, J.; Marmorstein, R. Identification of a novel family of BRAF(V600E) inhibitors. *J. Med. Chem.* **2012**, *55*, 5220–5230. [CrossRef]
36. Stones, C.J.; Kim, J.E.; Joseph, W.R.; Leung, E.; Marshall, E.S.; Finlay, G.J.; Shelling, A.N.; Baguley, B.C. Comparison of responses of human melanoma cell lines to MEK and BRAF inhibitors. *Front. Genet.* **2013**, *4*, 66. [CrossRef]

2

Synthesis, Characterization and Biological Evaluation of Novel Dihydropyranoindoles Improving the Anticancer Effects of HDAC Inhibitors

Murat Bingul [1,2,3], Greg M. Arndt [2,4], Glenn M. Marshall [2,5], Belamy B. Cheung [2,6,*], Naresh Kumar [1,*] and David StC. Black [1,*]

1 School of Chemistry, UNSW Sydney, Sydney, NSW 2052, Australia; muratbingul1983@gmail.com
2 Children's Cancer Institute, Lowy Cancer Research Centre, UNSW Sydney, Sydney, NSW 2052, Australia; garndt@ccia.unsw.edu.au (G.M.A.); gmarshall@ccia.unsw.edu.au (G.M.M.)
3 School of Pharmacy, Dicle University, 21280 Diyarbakır, Turkey
4 ACRF Drug Discovery Centre for Childhood Cancer, Children's Cancer Institute, Lowy Cancer Research Centre, UNSW Sydney, Sydney, NSW 2052, Australia
5 Kids Cancer Centre, Sydney Children's Hospital, Randwick, NSW 2031, Australia
6 School of Women's and Children's Health, UNSW Sydney, Sydney, NSW 2052, Australia
* Correspondence: bcheung@ccia.unsw.edu.au (B.B.C.); n.kumar@unsw.edu.au (N.K.); d.black@unsw.edu.au (D.S.B.);

Academic Editor: Qiao-Hong Chen

Abstract: The dihydropyranoindole scaffold was identified as a promising target for improving the anti-cancer activity of HDAC inhibitors from the preliminary screening of a library of compounds. A suitable methodology has been developed for the preparation of novel dihydropyranoindoles via the Hemetsberger indole synthesis using azido-phenylacrylates, derived from the reaction of corresponding alkynyl-benzaldehydes with methyl azidoacetate, followed by thermal cyclization in high boiling solvents. Anti-cancer activity of all the newly synthesized compounds was evaluated against the SH-SY5Y and Kelly neuroblastoma cells as well as the MDA-MB-231 and MCF-7 breast adenocarcinoma cell lines. Biological studies showed that the tetracyclic systems had significant cytotoxic activity at higher concentration against the neuroblastoma cancer cells. More importantly, these systems, at the lower concentration, considerably enhanced the SAHA toxicity. In addition to that, the toxicity of designated systems on the healthy human cells was found to be significantly less than the cancer cells.

Keywords: dihydropyranoindole; anticancer; HDAC inhibitors; neuroblastoma; breast cancer

1. Introduction

Chemotherapy is one of the most widely used treatments for high-risk cancer patients [1,2]. A range of well-known agents, namely Doxorubicin, Cyclophosphamide, Etoposide have been used to combat various cancers in modern chemotherapeutic therapy [3,4]. However, a major problem faced in chemotherapy is resistance to commonly-used anti-cancer drugs [5]. Therefore, development of novel anti-cancer chemotherapeutic agents is of utmost importance in the area of drug discovery and development.

The histone deacetylase (HDAC) inhibitors are a class of chemotherapeutic agents that hold promise in cancer therapy [6,7]. HDAC inhibitors have been reported to suppress cell proliferation and angiogenesis, induce cell differentiation and promote apoptosis in a number of cancer cell types [8,9]. Suberoylanilide hydroxamic acid (SAHA) is the first HDAC inhibitor to obtain meet FDA approval [10], and has been considered to be a highly promising anticancer therapeutic agent due to its potent cytotoxic effect on a number of tumor cell types as well as low toxicity towards healthy normal cells [11–13]. However, single agent treatment with SAHA has been found to be ineffective against several cancers [14,15]. On the other hand, the combination of SAHA with other chemotherapeutic agents with different mechanisms of action has been considered to be more promising as the drug resistance caused by single agent therapies may be overcome [14,16]. Due to the significant cytotoxic effects observed during clinical trials of SAHA in combination with a variety of chemotherapeutic agents, many synthetic compounds have been produced and screened to identify molecules capable of enhancing the cytotoxic activity of SAHA, while producing fewer side effects.

In order to provide a basis for this study, a subset (10,560 compounds) of the Walter & Eliza Hall Institute (WEHI) compound library was screened to identify molecules that can act synergistically with a clinical dose of SAHA to overcome drug resistance in SAHA-resistant MDA-MB-231 breast cancer cell lines [17]. The compounds that reduced viability to $<40\%$ in the presence of SAHA but to $>70\%$ in the absence of SAHA, with a difference of at least 55% between the two conditions have been identified as hit molecules for their SAHA enhancing capability [17]. A structural analysis of the hit molecules demonstrated that the main structural feature to be the presence of 5- or 6-membered fused heterocyclic systems, most commonly containing one or more nitrogen atoms. Furthermore, these fused systems typically involved 3 or 4 conjoined rings. Due to the ongoing experiments regarding the hit molecules, the structures of these compounds are not discussed in this manuscript.

Identification of New Target Molecules

The starting point of the current work was the selection of a range of compounds exhibiting structural similarity to the hits from compound library in order to expand the structural diversity of the screening set. The six related monomeric dihydropyranoindoles **1–3** and dimeric furoquinolines **4–6** were selected in order to understand the effect of the indole and quinoline structures, as well as the fused dihydropyran and furan rings, on biological activities (Figure 1). The molecules were tested against SH-SY5Y neuroblastoma and MDA-MB-231 breast cancer cell lines, using the Alamar blue (Resazurin) assay [18] to measure the cell viability. The same screening conditions were used with WEHI screening. Briefly, the designated cells were exposed to 1 μM SAHA, 10 μM compound and the combination of SAHA and compound for 72 h.

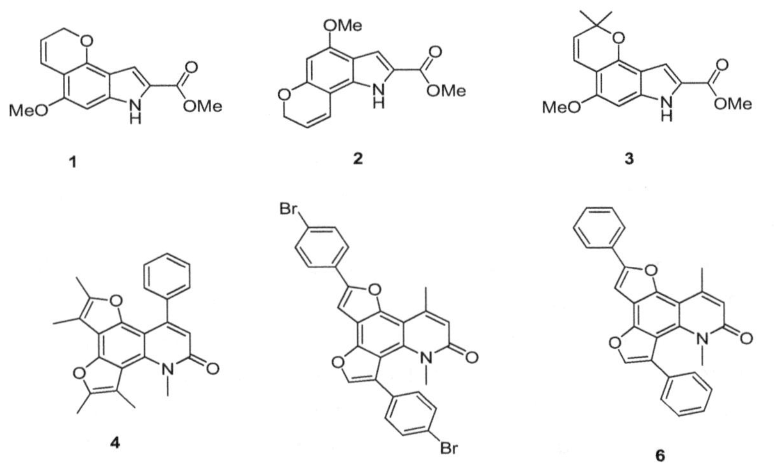

Figure 1. Six compounds from the NK library.

The in vitro assays revealed that the MDA-MB-231 were the more resistant cell lines than the SH-SY5Y cell lines for the single and combination treatments of all compounds. The compounds **5** and **6**, analogues of quinolines, displayed the lowest reduction on SH-SY5Y cell viability and also no SAHA enhancement was found by the combination with SAHA (Figure S1A, see Supplementary

Materials). In the case of compound **6**, the single and combination treatments showed no inhibition of MDA-MB-231 cell viability, while the 20% and 5% of inhibitions were obtained with the treatment of compound **5** alone and combination with 1 μM SAHA (Figure S1B, see Supplementary Materials). The compound **4** was the most active ligand among the quinoline candidates, with 30% inhibition of SH-SY5Y cell viability in the absence of SAHA and 20% additional cytotoxic effect in the presence of SAHA (Figure S1A, see Supplementary Materials). The designated compound displayed 25% reduction on MDA-MB-231 cells, while no SAHA enhancement effect was obtained against the same cell line (Figure S1B, see Supplementary Materials).

Overall, **1**, **3** and **4** were determined as the most promising compounds as SAHA enhancer and it was concluded that the indole heterocyclic systems **1** and **3** were found to be a potential target for the SAHA enhancement with the higher differential values between in the absence and presence of SAHA In order to further validate these compounds **1**, **3** and **4** as viable lead structures, it was essential to determine their toxicity towards normal and non-malignant cells. The most effective ligands were screened against the MRC-5 normal human lung fibroblast cells, as described for cytotoxic assay. This screen showed that the toxicity of **3** was found to be greater than **1** and **4** proposing that specificity of **3** against the normal and cancer cells was not different (Figure S2, see Supplementary Materials). The single treatment of compound **3** showed the cytotoxic activity with the values of 33% and 28% reduction against the SH-SY5Y and MDA-MB-231 cells respectively, while the toxicity of this compound against the MRC-5 cells was 26% and 30% greater than the SH-SY5Y and MDA-MB-231 cancer cells. However, compounds **1** and **4** displayed non-toxic behavior on the MRC-5 healthy human cells with values of 103% and 98% viable cells.

Based on the results of screening against the cancer cells and toxicity study on normal cells, the indole heterocyclic system **1** was identified as promising leads for further development on the enhancement of SAHA activity and compound **1** was also determined to be non-toxic across the healthy human cells. The main work described in this manuscript focused on the synthesis, characterization and in vitro biological evaluation of a series of targeted compounds based on tricyclic and tetracyclic dihydropyrano derivatives. The effectiveness of the novel compounds as single agents and in combination with a clinical dose of SAHA was determined against neuroblastoma and breast cancer cells.

2. Results and Discussion

The preparation of dihydropyranoindole systems was achieved by two synthetic methods, and the generality of these pathways were discussed in this paper. 3,4-Dihydroxybenzaldehyde **7** has been given as an example for the representation of two possible methods which could be used for the preparation of the desired pyranoindole methyl 5,10-dihydro-7*H*-dipyrano [3,2-*e*:2′,3′-*g*]indole-6-carboxylate **10** (Figure 2). The first method was to prepare the compound **10** via methyl hydroxyindole-2-carboxylate **8** which could be prepared by the Hemetsberger indole synthesis [19]. Methyl hydroxyindole-2-carboxylate **8** on reacting with haloalkynes would give the alkyne indole-ether **9** which upon Claisen cyclization would afford the desired dihydropyranoindole **10**. As an alternative pathway, aryl ether benzaldehyde **11** would be prepared via simple alkylation of phenol **7** with haloalkynes and the Hemetsberger indole synthesis would then be applied to build the indole moiety. It is anticipated that thermal cyclization would yield the desired compound **10** in one step.

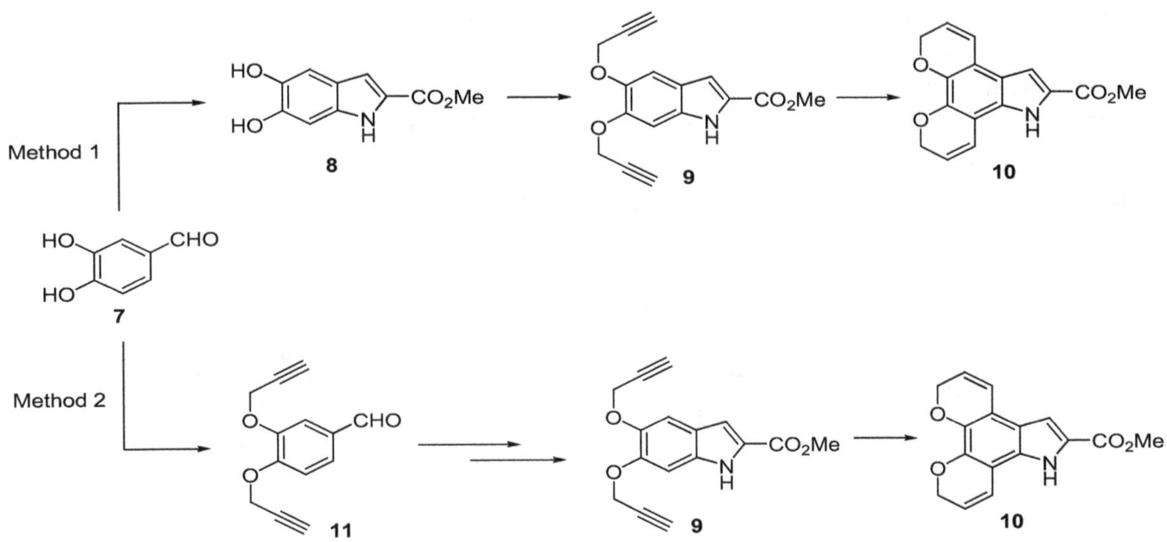

Figure 2. Two methods for the preparation of pyranoindole systems.

2.1. *Preparation of Tetracyclic Dihydropyranoindole 10 Via (Method 1)*

In the first synthetic method, methyl 5,6-dihydroxyindole-2-carboxylate **8** was generated via the Hemetsberger indole synthesis by benzyl-protected benzaldehydes and the subsequent deprotection afforded the corresponding hydroxyindoles. The 3,4-dihydroxybenzaldehyde **7** was reacted with benzyl bromide in the presence of potassium carbonate in acetone to afford the protected carbaldehydes **12** [20] in 88% yield (Scheme 1). Treatment of 3,4-dibenzyloxy benzaldehyde **12** with methyl azidoacetate in methanol, in the presence of strong basic environment (sodium methoxide) gave the vinyl azido intermediate **13** in 59% yield. Thermal decomposition of the arylazido **13** was performed by heating at reflux in xylene, generating the methyl 5,6-dibenzyloxyindole-2-carboxylate **14** in 71% yield. Hydrogenolysis of the benzyl group was carried out by treating the compound **14** with 5% *w/w* palladium on carbon under hydrogen atmosphere at room temperature for 2 h, to yield the desired methyl 5,6-dihydroxyindole-2-carboxylate **8** [21] in 77% yield. The dihydroxyindole **8** was reacted with propargyl bromide in the presence of potassium carbonate in acetone (Scheme 1). The desired dipropargyloxyindole intermediate **9** was prepared in 61% yield. The Claisen cyclization of **9** was explored in xylene, 1,2-dichlorobenzene and toluene. It was found that heating at reflux in chlorobenzene gave the optimum result in terms of the completion of the reaction as well as the yield and purity of the product. Using this approach, the desired tetracyclic dihydropyranoindole **10** was isolated in 51% yield.

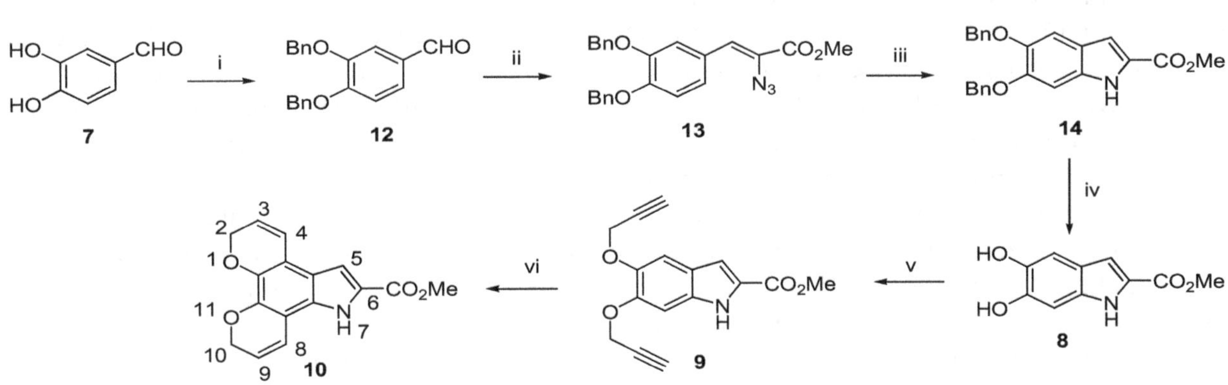

Scheme 1. Reagents and conditions: (i) Benzyl bromide, K_2CO_3, DMF, reflux, overnight; (ii) Methyl azidoacetate, NaOMe, anhyd. MeOH, <−10 °C, 4 h; (iii) Xylene, reflux, 2 h, (iv) 5% Pd/C, H_2, MeOH/THF, 2h, rt, (v) Propargyl bromide, K_2CO_3, acetone, reflux, 4 h, 61%, (vi) Chlorobenzene, reflux 2 h, 52%.

The possible reaction mechanism could be explained as in Figure 3. Methyl 5,6-bis(prop-2-yn-1-yloxy)-1*H*-indole-2-carboxylate **9** undergoes an initial Claisen rearrangement to generate intermediate **A**, which subsequently enolizes to produce 5,6-dihydroxyindole derivative (intermediate **B**). A double hydride shift in intermediate **B** gives the keto intermediate **C**, which undergoes an electrocyclic ring closing reaction to form methyl 5,10-dihydro-2*H*-dipyrano[3,2-*e*:2′,3′-*g*]indole-6-carboxylate **10**.

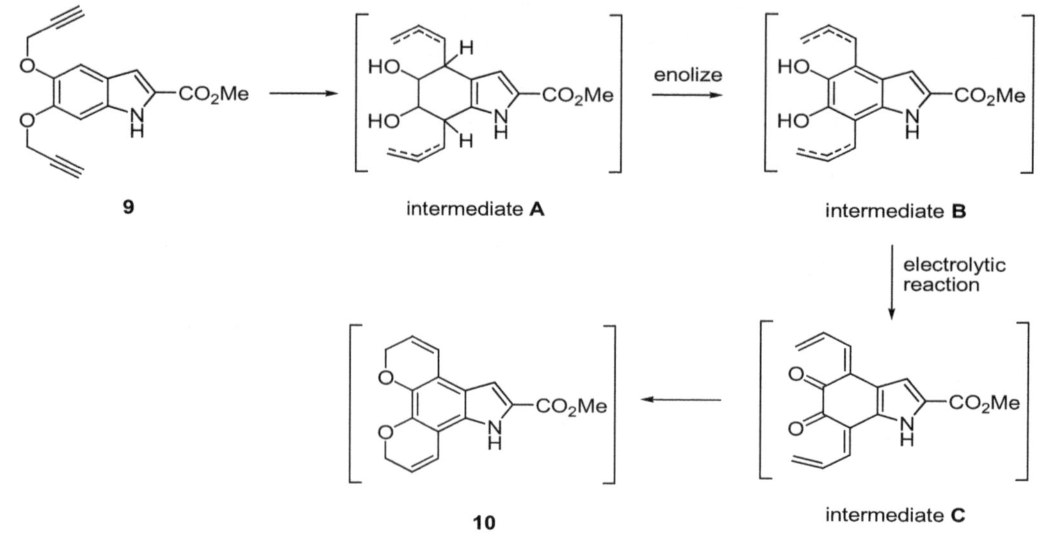

Figure 3. Possible reaction mechanism.

The ^{1}H-NMR spectrum of compound **10** in $CDCl_3$ showed a singlet at 3.96 ppm corresponding to the methyl ester protons, and two doublets of doublets at 4.91 and 4.96 ppm assigned to the two CH_2 groups. A multiplet at 5.87–5.97 ppm corresponded to H3 and H9, while another multiplet at 6.72–6.80 ppm corresponded to H4 and H8. Furthermore, H3 appeared as a doublet at 7.19 ppm and the NH proton appeared as a broad singlet at δ 8.85 ppm. The DEPT 135 spectrum of compound **10** confirmed the structure of the molecule, displaying the loss of two CH carbon signals as a result of cyclization of the alkyne group as well as the appearance of two negative signals at 64.68 and 64.72 ppm corresponding to the methylene carbon atoms in the product.

2.2. *Alternative Pathway for the Preparation of Tetracyclic Dihydropyranoindole 10 (Method 2)*

The alternative approach began with the reaction of 3,4-dihydroxybenzaldehyde **7** with propargyl bromide under basic conditions (potassium carbonate), which afforded the propargyloxy benzaldehyde **11** [22] in 87% yield. At this point, two synthetic strategies using benzaldehyde **11** as a key intermediate were envisioned (Scheme 2). The first route involved Claisen cyclization to build the dihydropyrano rings **15**, followed by the application of the Hemetsberger indole synthesis to construct the indole scaffold via the unsaturated azido intermediate **16** (Route 1). The cyclization of the aryl ether intermediate **11** was attempted by refluxing in high-boiling solvents such as xylene, toluene, 1,2-dichlorobenzene and chlorobenzene (Scheme 2). In all cases, the novel compound **15** was afforded in low yields, with unreacted starting material being recovered as the major product. The highest yield (35%) was obtained by the use of chlorobenzene. In order to synthesize the desired tetracyclic dihydropyranoindole **10**, the standard Hemetsberger indole synthesis was applied to new intermediate **15**. The condensation of benzaldehyde **15** with methyl azidoacetate was carried out at low temperature (ice-salt bath) in the presence of sodium methoxide. The addition of a small amount of crushed ice to the reaction mixture resulted in the isolation of azido ester **16** as an oily compound which was found to be unstable at room temperature, and was hence used in the next step without further purification. It was postulated that the presence of the dihydropyran ring caused the generation of an unstable azido ester intermediate.

Thermal cyclization of the azido ester **16** was performed by heating at reflux in xylene, which afforded the desired dihydropyranoindole **10** in 62% yield.

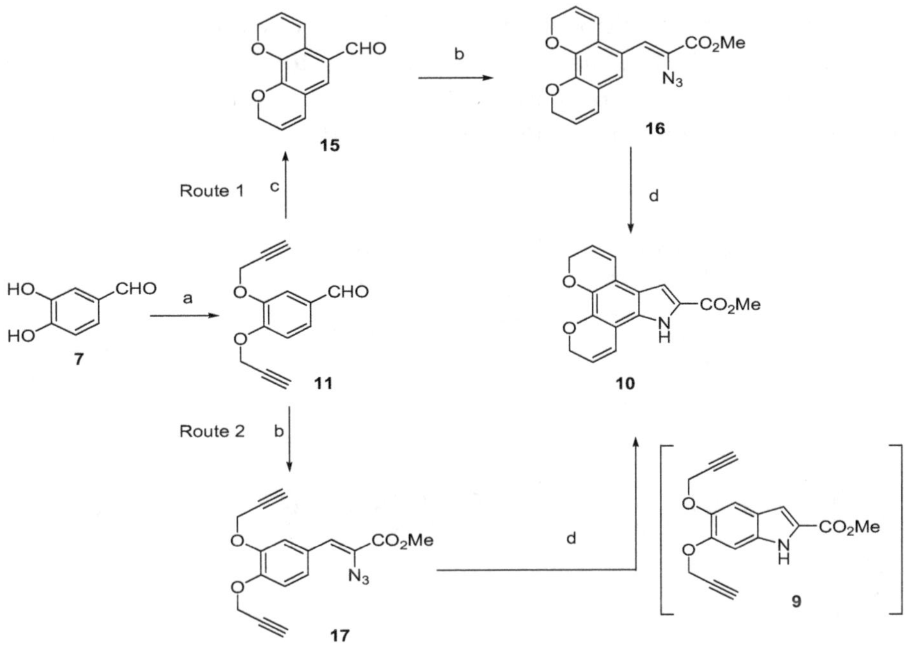

Scheme 2. Reagents and conditions: (a) Propargyl bromide, K_2CO_3, acetone, reflux, 4 h, (b) Methyl azidoacetate, metallic Na, anhyd. MeOH, <−10 °C, 2 h (c) Chlorobenzene, reflux, 2 h, (d) Xylene, reflux, 4 h.

In the second route, it was anticipated that the indole heterocyclic system could be constructed first, followed by the installation of dihydropyrano rings onto the indole moiety. Since the cyclization of both aryl ether and unsaturated azide ester moieties require refluxing conditions in a high-boiling solvent, it was predicted that the indole and dihydropyran rings could be prepared in one step from the key azide intermediate **17** (Route 2). The benzaldehyde **11** was condensed with methyl azidoacetate under strongly basic conditions at low temperature to generate the novel unsaturated stable azide intermediate **17** in 63% yield (Scheme 2). Since xylene was the common solvent for the generation of the indole moiety from the azido ester intermediate, the cyclization reaction was first carried out in refluxing xylene. As anticipated, the thermal cyclization of intermediate **17** resulted in both the decomposition of the azidocinnamate moiety and formation of the indole heterocyclic system, as well as the cyclization of the propargyloxy moiety to furnish the fused pyran ring in a single step. Hence, the desired tetracyclic dihydropyranoindole **10** was obtained in a yield of 72%.

Taken altogether, it was concluded that the first method is a less favorable synthetic pathway consisting of six steps to prepare the desired dihydropyranoindole and also generating the lowest of yield (51%) at the final step. In the case of the second method, route 1 was also found to be an unfavorable synthetic method for further synthesis due to the low-yielding cyclization step to generate the new tricyclic aldehyde **15**, the formation of the unstable azido intermediate **16** from the Hemestberger indole synthesis and the four step pathway for the desired dihydropyranoindole **10**. On the other hand, route 2 of the second strategy was deemed to be the most favorable synthetic route towards dihydropyranoindoles, as it contained three steps to afford the desired dihydropyranoindole and gave the highest yield of 72%. Thus, route 2 of the second method was chosen for further studies in this study.

2.3. The Preparation of Monomeric Hydropyrano System

The synthetic strategy (Route 2) was extended to the synthesis of indole systems containing a single fused dihydropyran ring. Hence, 4-hydroxy-3-methoxy benzaldehyde **18** was reacted with propargyl bromide in the presence of potassium carbonate to give aryl ether **19a** [23] in 84% yield, which was then reacted with methyl azidoacetate under basic conditions to give azidocinnamate **20a** in 76% yield (Scheme 3). Interestingly, thermal cyclization of the **20a** in xylene afforded the corresponding propargyloxy indole **21a** in the yield of 68% instead of the expected dihydropyranoindole system **22a**. Further heating of indole **21a** in refluxing chlorobenzene afforded the desired dihydropyranoindole **22a** in 77% yield.

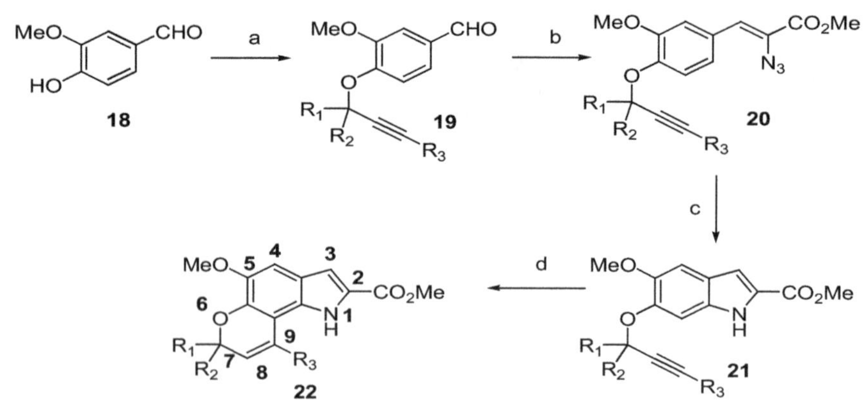

Compound	R1	R2	R3
22a	H	H	H
22b	H	H	Me
22c	Me	Me	H

Scheme 3. Reagents and conditions: (a) Propargyl bromide or 3-chloro-3-methylbut-1-yne or 1-bromobut-2-yne, K_2CO_3, acetone, reflux, 4 h, (b) Methyl azidoacetate, metallic Na, anhyd. MeOH, <−10 °C, 2 h (c) Xylene, reflux, 4 h, (d) Chlorobenzene, reflux, 2 h.

The ^{1}H-NMR spectrum of compound **22a** in $CDCl_3$ showed the presence of two singlets at 3.94 ppm and 3.96 ppm corresponding to the methoxy and methyl ester protons, and doublets of doublets at 4.96 ppm corresponding to the CH_2 protons. Protons H8 and H9 appeared as multiplets in a range of 5.89–5.95 ppm and 6.73–6.79 ppm respectively. Furthermore, H4 appeared as a singlet at 7.02 ppm, while H3 was appeared as a doublet at 7.13 ppm (J = 2.1 Hz) due to its coupling with the NH proton, which resonated as a broad singlet at 8.94 ppm. The DEPT 135 spectrum showed the presence of a negative peak at 65.79 ppm corresponding to a methylene carbon atom. Furthermore, the spectrum revealed the absence of the alkyne CH signal due to cyclization of the alkyne moiety in indole **21a**.

The synthesis of tricyclic dihydropyranoindole systems containing methyl substituents on the fused dihydropyran ring at different positions was also investigated. To achieve this, 4-hydroxy-3-methoxybenzaldehyde **18** was reacted with 1-bromobut-2-yne and 3-chloro-3-methylbut-1-yne in the presence of potassium carbonate to give the aryl ether aldehydes **19b** [24] and **19c** [25] in 92% and 84% yields, respectively (Scheme 3). The aldehydes **19b** and **19c** were treated with methyl azidoacetate in the presence of sodium methoxide to give azidocinnamates **20b** and **20c** in yields of 61% and 62%. Finally, the thermal cyclization of the unsaturated azide **20b** and **20c** in refluxing xylene generated the desired product **22c** in 74% yields, while the indole ether **21b** was isolated in 67% yield. The desired dihydropyranoindole **22b** was obtained in 49% yield, by the further cyclization of **21b** in refluxing chlorobenzene.

In the ^{1}H-NMR spectrum of methyl 5-methoxy-7,7-dimethyl-1,7-dihydropyrano[2,3-*g*]indole-2-carboxylate **22c**,the two methyl groups appeared as a singlet at 1.55 ppm, while H8 and H9 appeared as doublet signals at 5.71 and 6.66 ppm (J = 9.7 Hz). Furthermore, H4 appeared as a singlet at 7.01 ppm and H3 appeared as a doublet at 7.13 ppm (J = 2.1 Hz), confirming that cyclization occurred at C7. In the ^{1}H-NMR spectrum of the cyclization product **22b**, the olefinic proton on the dihydropyran ring appeared as multiplet signals in the ranges of 5.65–5.68 ppm, due to coupling with the neighboring

CH_2 and CH_3 groups. For compound **22b**, the O-CH_2 protons resonated as a multiplet at 4.77 ppm and the methyl protons of the dihydropyran ring appeared as a quartet at 1.71 ppm.

The same synthetic route was applied to 3-hydroxy-4-methoxy benzaldehyde **23** in order to generate an analogue with the dihydropyran ring fused at a different position. Thus, hydroxybenzaldehyde **23** was reacted with propargyl bromide in the presence of potassium carbonate to generate the intermediate ether **24a** [26] in 87% yield, which upon reaction with methyl azidoacetate in strongly basic conditions gave the azidocinnamate **25a** in 72% yield (Scheme 4). Heating the azidocinnamate **25a** in refluxing xylene gave the propargyloxy indole **26a** in 73% yield, which was then cyclized in chlorobenzene to afford the desired dihydropyranoindole **27a** in 74% yield.

The ^{1}H-NMR spectrum of compound **27a** in $CDCl_3$ showed two singlet signals at 3.92 and 3.93 ppm corresponding to the methoxy and methyl ester protons, and doublets of doublets at 4.90 ppm corresponding to the CH_2 protons. H8 and H9 appeared as multiplets at 5.89–5.95 and 6.76–6.79 ppm respectively. The H4 appeared as a singlet at 6.77 ppm, while H1 appeared as a doublet at 7.17 ppm (J = 2.1 Hz). Moreover, the NH proton resonated as a broad singlet at δ 8.96 ppm. The formation of the desired dihydropyranoindole was further confirmed by DEPT 135 spectroscopy which revealed the presence of a negative peak at 65.71 ppm corresponding to the CH_2 group accompanied by the disappearance of the signal corresponding to the CH group of the starting alkyne **26a**.

3-Hydroxy-4-methoxybenzaldehyde **23** was further treated with 1-bromobut-2-yne and 3-chloro-3-methylbut-1-yne under basic conditions to generate the corresponding intermediates **24b** [24] and **24c** [27] 89% and 82% yields, respectively (Scheme 4). The aryl ethers **24b** and **24c** were condensed with methyl azidoacetate in the presence of sodium methoxide to generate the azidoacrylates **25b** and **25c** in 64% and 62% yields respectively. Thermal decomposition of the unsaturated azides **25b** gave the indole ethers **26b** in 71%, while the desired hydropyrano compound **27c** was directly isolated in 68% yield. The desired dihydropyranoindoles **27b** was obtained in 54% yields respectively, by the cyclization of **26b** and in refluxing chlorobenzene. It was also of interest to construct new dihydropyranoindole systems containing substituents other than a methyl group on a pyran ring. The haloalkyne, 3-phenylprop-2-yn-1-ol, was treated with 3-hydroxy-4-methoxybenzaldehyde **23** in the presence of potassium carbonate to produce the alkylated carbaldehyde **24d** in 92% yield (Scheme 4). The reaction between the aryl ether **24d** with methyl azidoacetate afforded the unsaturated azido ester **25d** in 64% yield. Finally, heating compound **25d** in refluxing xylene afforded the corresponding indole ether **26d** in 74% yield, which further underwent thermal cyclization in chlorobenzene to furnish the desired dihydropyranoindole **27d** in 81% yield.

In the ^{1}H-NMR spectrum of methyl 5-methoxy-7,7-dimethyl-3,7-dihydropyrano[3,2-*e*]indole-2-carboxylate **27c**, the two methyl groups appeared as a sharp singlet at 1.53 ppm. The H8 and H9 of the dihydropyran ring appeared as two doublets at 5.73 and 6.68 ppm that coupled to each other with a coupling constant of 9.7 Hz. H1 appeared as a doublet (J = 2.1 Hz) at 7.20 ppm while H4 was assigned as a singlet at 6.79 ppm. In the ^{1}H-NMR spectrum of the cyclization product **27b** the olefinic protons on the dihydropyran ring appeared as multiplet signals in range of 5.69–5.72, due to coupling with the neighboring CH_2 and CH_3 groups. The characteristic O-CH_2 protons resonated as a multiplet at 4.77 ppm, while the methyl group of the dihydropyran ring appeared at as a quartet 1.63 ppm. The ^{1}H-NMR spectrum of compound **27d** displayed the O-CH_2 protons as a doublet at 4.85 ppm with a coupling constant of 4.4 Hz, and the olefinic proton as a multiplet at 5.94–5.97 ppm. The aromatic protons of phenyl ring appeared as multiplet in the range of 7.34–7.44 ppm. The H4 and H1 appeared as two singlets at 5.98 and 6.88 ppm.

Similar attempts were made to the prepare methyl substituted tetracyclic dihydropyranoindole compounds from the 3,4-dihydroxybenzaldehyde **7**, 1-bromobut-2-yne and 3-chloro-3-methylbut-1-yne. The benzaldehyde **7** was alkylated with 2 equivalents of 1-bromobut-2-yne in the presence of potassium carbonate to generate the novel aryl ether **29** in 87% yield (Scheme 5). The benzaldehyde **29** was then treated with methyl azidoacetate under strongly basic conditions to generate the azido compound **30** in 63% yield, which subsequently underwent thermal decomposition in refluxing xylene to afford the indole ether **31** in 65% yield. However, the cyclization of **31** could not be achieved in a number of solvents, including chlorobenzene, toluene, xylene and 1,2-dichlorobenzene which resulted in the formation of decomposed reaction mixture. The reaction between 3,4-dihydroxybenzaldehyde **7** and 3-chloro-3-methylbut-1-yne was investigated in an attempt to produce the dipropargyloxybenzaldehyde intermediate **28** (Scheme 5). However, this reaction resulted in a black reaction mixture, presumably due to decomposition.

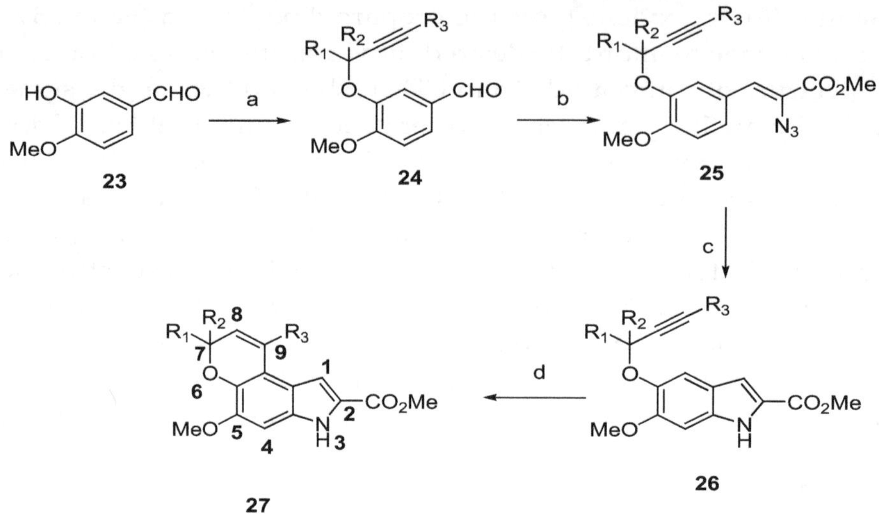

Compound	R_1	R_2	R_3
27a	H	H	H
27b	H	H	Me
27c	Me	Me	H
27d	H	H	Ph

Scheme 4. Reagents and conditions: (a) Propargyl bromide or 3-chloro-3-methylbut-1-yne or1-bromobut-2-yne or 3-phenylprop-2-yn-1-ol, K_2CO_3, acetone, reflux, 4 h, (b) Methyl azidoacetate, metallic Na, anhyd. MeOH, <−10 °C, 2 h (c) Xylene, reflux, 4 h, (d) Chlorobenzene, reflux, 2 h.

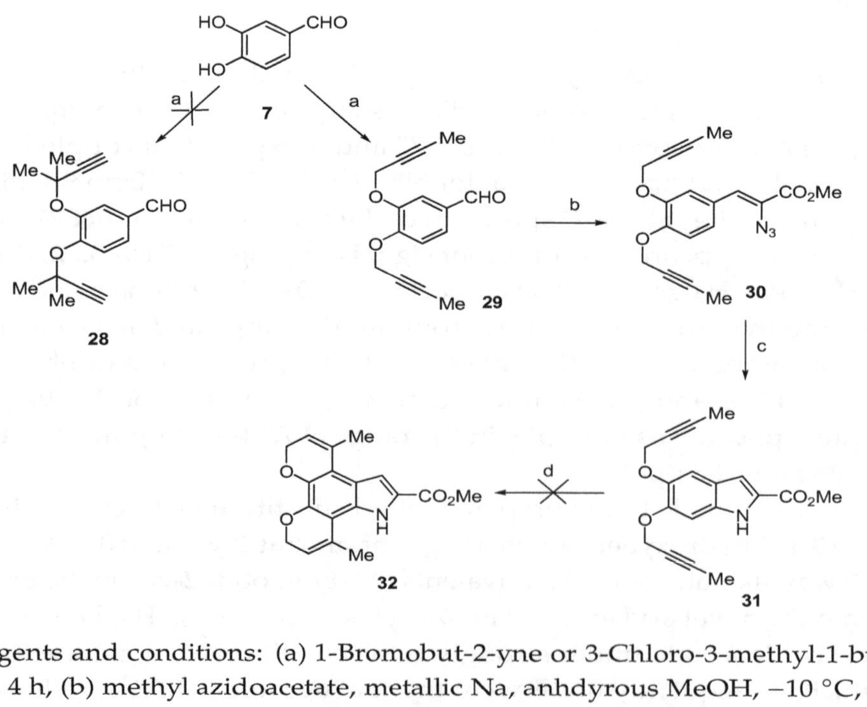

Scheme 5. Reagents and conditions: (a) 1-Bromobut-2-yne or 3-Chloro-3-methyl-1-butyne, K_2CO_3, acetone, reflux, 4 h, (b) methyl azidoacetate, metallic Na, anhdyrous MeOH, −10 °C, 2 h (c) Xylene, reflux, 2 h, (d) Xylene, chlorobenzene, toluene, 1,2-dichlorobenzene reflux, overnight.

2.4. *Biological Study*

2.4.1. Preliminary Biological Screening of Dihydropyranoindoles for SAHA Enhancement Activity

Novel dihydropyranoindole analogues were screened to determine the levels of SAHA enhancement activity as well as their own cytotoxic profile against the SH-SY5Y and Kelly neuroblastoma cells and the MDA-MB-231 and MCF-7 breast adenocarcinoma cell lines using the Alamar blue (Resazurin) assay [18]. Briefly, the cells were allowed to attach for 24 h in a 96-well culture plate before being exposed to the ligands at a concentration of 10 μM in DMSO for 72 h, either in the presence or absence of SAHA. Comparative values for cell viability in each well were determined by a Wallac 1420 Victor III spectrophotometer, which measured light absorbance in each well at 570 nm. The mean and standard deviation (SD) values for each compound were calculated from at least three replicate experiments. The anticancer activity of the compounds was evaluated by comparison to a negative (DMSO) control. Figure 4 shows the tested novel dihydropyranoindoles synthesized in this study and the compound **33** was selected from the NK library. In this assay, the cell lines were exposed to SAHA, 10 μM of the compounds as well as the combination of SAHA with the compounds for 72 h.

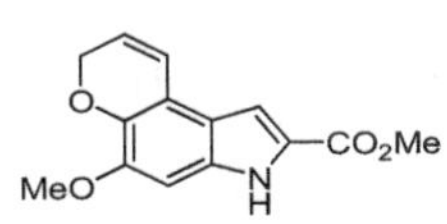

27a

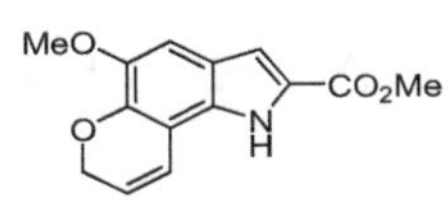

22a

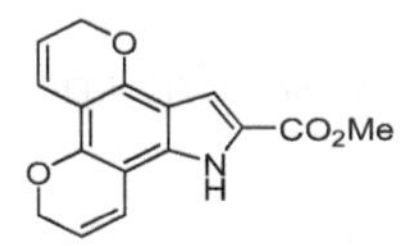

33

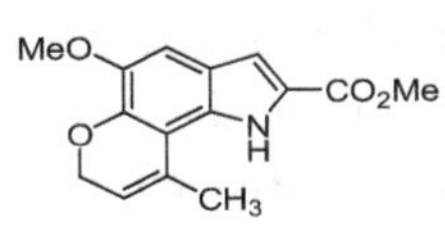

22b

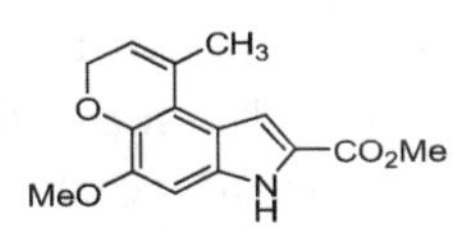

27b

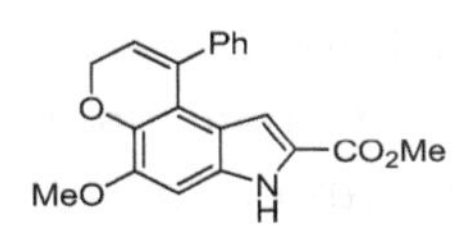

27d

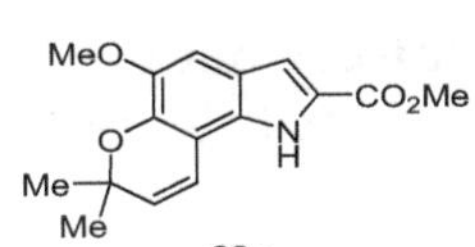

22c

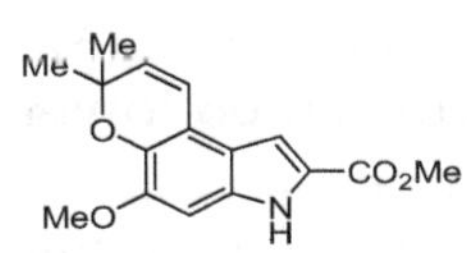

27c

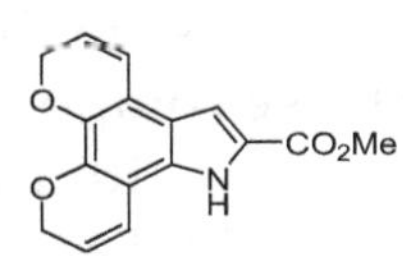

10

Figure 4. Synthesized and selected compounds.

According to the results from the screening, the neuroblastoma cells were found to be the more sensitive cells towards the treatment of new pyranoindoles, while these compounds showed a moderate effect on the breast cancer cell lines (Figures S3A,B and S4A,B, see Supplementary Materials). MDA-MB-231 cells were determined as the most resistant cell line for the single as well as the combination treatments (Figure S3A, see Supplementary Materials). The dihydropyranoindole **27c** exhibited the greatest cell viability inhibition with the values of 34% and 35% in the absence and presence of SAHA against the MDA-MB-231 cells. The SAHA enhancement was achieved by the additional reduction value of 20% across MDA-MB-231 viability. MCF-7 cells showed an identical pattern of sensitivity. However, most of the dihydropyranoindoles were able to reduce the viability by the value of 20% (Figure S3, see Supplementary Materials).

Compound **33** displayed the highest reduction with the 35% inhibition, while compounds **27c** and **22c** generated similar reductions with the values of 20% and 22% on the same cell line. Unfortunately the combination of pyranoindoles with 1 μM SAHA had very low SAHA enhancement by the average values of 5% across the MCF-7 cell lines.

It was observed that dihydropyranoindoles had a variety of impact on the viability of neuroblastoma cells (Kelly and SH-SY5Y) with the single and combination treatments (Figure S4A,B, see Supplementary Materials). Out of all the novel ligands synthesized, ligand **33** had the strongest cytotoxic activity with the reduction value of 50% at 10 μM, while ligands **27c** and **10** showed similar inhibition behaviors by the average reduction value of 32% against Kelly cells for the single treatment. The dihydropyranoindoles **27c** and **33** displayed the enhancement of SAHA cytotoxicity with the values of 24 and 22% respectively (Figure S4A, see Supplementary Materials). The value of 40% SAHA enhancement was obtained by the combination of compound **33**. However, the ligand **33** was considered as self-toxic compound due to the reduction value for the single treatment. The levels of individual cytotoxic efficiency against the SH-SY5Y were found to be higher than those observed on the Kelly cells (Figure S4B, see Supplementary Materials). The compounds **27d** and **10** showed the greatest cytotoxic activity reducing 44% and 56% of the cells respectively. Most importantly, the enhancement of SAHA activity was achieved by the treatment of almost all of the novel dihydropyranoindole analogues showing at least 20% additional reduction to SAHA cytotoxicity. Although the highest SAHA enhancement was obtained in the case of compound **10** with the value of 55%, it was not considered as a promising enhancer since the single treatment also generated the greatest reduction (56%) on the SH-SY5Y cell. The best enhancers were assigned as compounds **22a, 27a, 27c** and **33** with the reduction values of 25%, 29%, 30% and 31%respectively due to the lower toxicity but the higher enhancement effects on SAHA cytotoxicity.

2.4.2. Determination of SAHA Enhancement Activity of Selected Dihydropyranoindoles at Lower Concentrations

Since the levels of SAHA enhancement were found to be promising, further investigations were carried out using five different concentrations (0.01, 0.1, 1, 10, 20 μM), using the Alamar blue (Resazurin) assay [18] to determine whether the lower concentrations would provide higher enhancement of the SAHA cytotoxicity or the cytotoxic manner would be dependent on the dose usage. The initial screening revealed that the single treatment of dihydropyranoindoles **33, 27c** and **10** at a concentration of 10 μM showed the highest cytotoxic efficiency against the Kelly cells. The designated compounds were treated with the Kelly cells by the combinations of 0.5 μM SAHA with the five different concentrations (0.01, 0.1, 1, 10, 20 μM) and the results are shown at Figure S5A,C (see Supplementary Materials). In general, the single treatment of these compounds provided lower cytotoxic activity at the concentrations of 0.01, 0.1 and 1 μM compared with the values at 10 μM and the cell viability differentials between the absence and presence of SAHA were greater than those at 10 μM concentrations, suggesting that the designated compounds behave as suitable SAHA enhancers (Figure S5A,C, see Supplementary Materials). Similar SAHA enhancement pattern was observed at the concentrations of 0.01, 0.1 and 1 μM for all three compounds, while the combination of 1 μM compound **27c** or **10** with the 0.5 μM SAHA revealed the best SAHA enhancement with the values of 24% and 25% additional inhibition (Figure S5B,C, see Supplementary Materials).

In addition to those two compounds, compound **33** showed the greatest viability differentials with the values of 61%, 63% and 65% at the concentrations of 0.01, 0.1 and 1 μM and the desired SAHA enhancement was observed for all the concentrations. The lowest concentration of compound **33** (0.01 μM) revealed a remarkable reduction with the value of 25%, while the best combination for the highest SAHA enhancement was determined as a 10:0.5 ratio of compound and SAHA with the additional reduction value of 55% (Figure S5 A, see Supplementary Materials). It was concluded that the highest cell viability differentials was achieved by the use of nanomolar concentrations in the case of all three compounds and the best SAHA enhancer was determined as compound **33**.

Similarly, in the case of the SH-SY5Y cell line, further investigations were undertaken with **27a, 33** and **27c** which were chosen due to their highest additional effects on the SAHA cytotoxicity with the lower toxicity behavior in the absence of SAHA. Compound **10** was also explored to determine its cytotoxic behavior as well as the SAHA enhancement potential at lower concentrations. The combinations of 1 μM SAHA with the five different concentrations (0.01, 0.1, 1, 10, 20 μM) of designated compounds were treated with the SH-SY5Y cells and the results are shown at Figure S6A–D (see Supplementary Materials).

The SAHA enhancement pattern was found to be identical on SH-SY5Y value for all cases of combinations of **27a** with SAHA. The highest viability differential was obtained in the ratio 1:10 of SAHA to compound with the reduction value of 35% (Figure S6A, see Supplementary Materials). The dose-dependent pattern of single treatments of **33** and **27c** suggested that these compounds displayed higher toxicity at 20 μM with the values of 45% and 55% reductions. Furthermore, the combinations of these compounds at the concentrations of 0.01, 0.1 and 1 μM with SAHA enhanced the SAHA cytotoxicity in a similar manner and the best combinations were found to be as the ratio 1:10 of SAHA to compound with the additional reduction values of 28% and 33% (Figure S6B,C, see Supplementary Materials). The greatest cytotoxicity was obtained at a concentration of 20 μM of **10** alone with the reduction values of 88% on SH-SY5Y cell viability and the ratio of 1:20 SAHA to compound combination provided 94% cell death (Figure S6D, see Supplementary Materials).

More importantly, at the lower concentrations (0.01, 0.1 and 1 μM) of **10**, the cytotoxicity was found to be lower with the average reduction value of 25%. Encouragingly, the biggest cell viability differential was obtained at the ratio of 1:10 SAHA to compound with the value of 44%, and the greatest SAHA enhancement was also found as 37% at the same combination. It was concluded that **10** was the most cytotoxic compound at higher concentration (20 μM, 88% reduction) and also it was found to be the best SAHA enhancer at the ratio of 1:10 SAHA to compound combination.

2.4.3. SAR Study of Selected Dihydropyranoindoles

These observations suggested an important structure-activity relationship among **27a, 33, 27c** and **10**. That is, the incorporation of tetracyclic dihydropyranoindoles **33** and **10** resulted in lower cell viability reductions at higher concentrations (20 μM) and also this system was found to offer the best enhancement with the ratio of 1:10 SAHA to compound combinations against both neuroblastoma cancer cells (Kelly and SH-SY5Y). The SAR analysis revealed that the location of dihydropyran ring on the benzene ring was important for the cytotoxic efficiency of tricyclic dihydropyranoindoles, The compounds **27c**, an example of dihydropyrano[3,2-*e*]indole system, was found to be more potent than the dihydropyranoindole **22c** which is a member of dihydropyrano[2,3-*g*]indole scaffold against both neuroblastoma cells (Kelly and SH-SY5Y). In comparison of two tricyclic dihydropyranoindoles **27c** and **22c** at 20 μM, it was found that the compound **27c** reduced 20% more SH-SY5Y cell with the combination of 1 μM SAHA than compound **22c**, while the 20% SAHA enhancement was achieved using the combination of compound **27c** and SAHA but no SAHA enhancement was found with the compound **22c** in the case of Kelly cells. Furthermore, the dihydropyrano[2,3-*g*]indole analogues **22a** and **22b** displayed the lowest reduction on Kelly cells in the presence and absence of SAHA. Similar results were observed in the case of SH-SY5Y cells with the exception of 21% additional reduction on SAHA enhancement obtained by the use of **22a**.

2.4.4. Toxicity Study Against Normal Cells

While selected dihydropyranoindoles showed potent SAHA enhancement activity against Kelly and SH-SY5Y neuroblastoma and MCF-7 and MDA-MB-231 breast cancer cells, they must be markedly less toxic against the healthy cells in order to be considered as potential SAHA enhancers. Thus, the dihydropyranoindoles **27a, 33, 27c** and **10** were also examined for their toxicity effects on the MRC-5 and WI-38 lung fibroblasts in order to determine whether these compounds exhibited selectivity for tumor cells (Figure S7A–D, see Supplementary Materials). Comparison of the cytotoxic activity and toxicity levels of the dihydropyranoindoles against cancer cells and the healthy cells revealed that the cancer cells were more sensitive to the dihydropyranoindoles compared to the normal cells. The toxicity of 1 μM of SAHA reduced the viability of MRC-5 and WI-38 cells with the value of 9% and 24% respectively, while **27a** alone displayed a similar pattern of toxicity against normal cells with values of 10% for MRC-5 and 22% for WI-38 at a concentration of 10 μM (Figure S7A, see Supplementary Materials). The viability of MRC-5 and WI-38 were reduced 21% and 16%, 3% and 26% by the use of **33** and **10** alone (Figure S7B,C, see Supplementary Materials), while the highest toxicity levels were obtained in the case of **27c** with the reduction values of 20% and 43% (Figure S7D, see Supplementary Materials). The combination treatments were found to be quite identical to the reduction values of single treatments of each compound. These observations demonstrated that **27a, 33** and **10** were either less toxic or slightly less toxic than SAHA, while **27c** displayed more toxicity than SAHA for both normal cells.

3. Materials and Methods

3.1. General Information

Commercially available reagents were purchased from Fluka (Sydney, NSW, Australia), Aldrich (Sydney, NSW, Australia), Acros Organics (Morris Plains, NJ, USA), Alfa Aesar (Lancashire, UK) and Lancaster (Lancashire, UK) and purified if necessary. The synthetic procedures have been reported for all compounds as general methods and appropriate references have been given for known compounds. ^{1}H (300 MHz) and ^{13}C-NMR (75 MHz) spectra were obtained in the designated solvents on a DPX 300 spectrometer (Bruker, Sydney, NSW, Australia). Melting points were measured using a Mel-Temp melting point apparatus and are uncorrected. Infrared spectra were recorded on Avatar Series FT-IR spectrophotometer as KBr disks (Thermo Nicolet, Waltham, MA, USA). Ultraviolet spectra were measured using a Cary 100 spectrophotometer (Varian, Santa Clara, CA, USA) in the designated solvents and data reported as wavelength (λ) in nm and adsorption coefficient (ε) in $cm^{-1}M^{-1}$. High-resolution [ESI] mass spectra were recorded by the UNSW Bioanalytical Mass Spectrometry Facility, on an Orbitrap LTQ XL (Thermo Scientific, Waltham, MA, USA) ion trap mass spectrometer using a nanospray (nano-electrospray) ionization source.

3.1.1. GP-1: General Procedure for the Benzylation of Dihydroxybenzaldehydes

A solution of hydroxybenzaldehyde (1 equiv.), anhydrous potassium carbonate (per hydroxyl group, 1 equiv.) and benzyl bromide (per hydroxyl group, 1 equiv.) in anhydrous DMF (100 mL) was heated at reflux until TLC analysis showed consumption of the starting aldehyde (9 h). Upon cooling to room temperature, the reaction mixture was diluted with water (300 mL) and the resulting precipitate was collected via filtration and washed with water (2 × 250 mL). Upon drying, the residue was recrystallized from dichloromethane and *n*-hexane to give the title compound.

3.1.2. GP-2: General Procedure for the Preparation of Vinyl-Azido Intermediates

A solution of sodium methoxide was prepared via the portion-wise addition of metallic sodium (17 equiv.) to anhydrous methanol (30 mL) with stirring under nitrogen. A dropping funnel was attached to the reaction flask and charged with the corresponding aldehyde (1 equiv.) and methyl azidoacetate (10 equiv.) in methanol (15 mL). The contents of the funnel were added dropwise to the sodium methoxide solution over 1.5 h under a nitrogen atmosphere. Once the addition was completed, the reaction mixture was warmed to 5 °C, where it remained for 4 h. The heterogeneous mixture was poured into crushed ice. The resulting precipitate was filtered, washed with water and dried to give the title compound. The crude product was used in the next step without further purification.

3.1.3. GP-3: General Procedure for the Preparation of Methyl Benzyloxyindole-2-carboxylates

The vinyl azido intermediate (6.66 mmol) was dissolved in xylene (50 mL) and the reaction mixture was heated under reflux for 6 h. After refluxing, the solvent was evaporated under reduced pressure and the remaining residue was extracted with boiling hexane. Upon cooling, the resulting solid was filtered to give crude product which was recrystallized from dichloromethane and *n*-hexane to give the title compound.

3.1.4. GP-4: General Procedure for the Hydrogenolysis of Methyl Dibenzyloxyindole-2-carboxylate

After vacuum/H_2 cycles to remove air from the reaction flask, a stirred mixture of benzyloxyindole (1 mmol) and 5% Pd/C (10% *w/w*) in THF/MeOH (1:1, 15 mL) was exposed to a hydrogen atmosphere (1 atm) and stirred at room temperature for 2 h. The reaction mixture was filtered through a pad of Celite® and the filtrate was then concentrated under reduced pressure. The crude product was purified by flash column chromatography (SiO_2), eluted with dichloromethane to give the title compounds.

3.1.5. GP-5: General Procedure for the Synthesis of Propargyloxybenzaldehydes:

Propargyl bromide (per hydroxyl group, 1.2 equiv.) was added to a mixture of potassium carbonate (per hydroxyl group, 1 equiv.) and hydroxybenzaldehyde (1 equiv.) in acetone. The reaction mixture was heated under reflux with stirring until no more starting material remained (~30 h). The reaction mixture was cooled to room temperature and Et_2O (100 mL) was added. The ethereal solution was washed with NaOH (1 N, 3 × 50 mL). The organic layer was dried over $MgSO_4$, concentrated under reduced pressure and recrystallized from dichloromethane/*n*-hexane to give the compound.

3.1.6. GP-6 General Procedure for the Synthesis of Dihydropyranoindoles:

A solution of alkyne indole ethers (1.04 mmol) in chlorobenzene (20 mL) was heated under reflux until TLC analysis showed consumption of the starting indole (12 h). The heating was discontinued and the solvent was evaporated under reduced pressure. The crude product was purified using flash column chromatography (SiO_2), eluted with 30% dichloromethane/*n*-hexane, to give the dihydropyranoindole.

Methyl 2-azido-3-(3,4-dibenzyloxyphenyl)-propenoate (**13**) The *title* compound was prepared as described in GP-2 from 3,4-dibenzyloxybenzaldehyde (**12**) (2.95 g, 9.3 mmol) and methyl azidoacetate (10.69 g, 93 mmol) in anhydrous methanol (30 mL) to give the product (2.27 g, 59%) as a pale yellow granular solid; m.p. 114–116 °C; IR (KBr): υ_{max} 2917, 2119, 1701, 1683, 1590, 1508, 1432, 1379, 1233, 1201, 1130, 999, 802, 728 cm^{-1}; UV-vis (CH_3CN): λ_{max}325 (24,500); ^{1}H-NMR: (300 MHz, $CDCl_3$): δ 3.91 (s, 3H, CO_2Me), 5.25 (s, 4H, 2 × O-CH_2), 6.83 (s, 1H, CH=C), 7.35–7.52 (m, 12H, ArH), 7.64 (d, *J* = 2.2 Hz, 1H, H2′); ^{13}C-NMR: (75.6 MHz, $CDCl_3$): δ 52.7 ($CO_2\underline{Me}$), 70.9 (CH_2), 71.3 (CH_2), 113.8 (C2′), 116.6 (C5′), 123.3 ($\underline{C}$H=C), 125.4 (C6′), 125.7 (ArC), 126.6 (ArC), 127.1 (2 × ArC), 127.2 (2 × ArC), 127.8 (ArC), 127.9 (ArC), 128.5 (2 × ArC), 128.6 (2 × ArC), 136.8 (C1′), 137.1 (CH=$\underline{C}$), 148.3 (C4′), 150.1 (C3′), 164.1 ($\underline{C}O_2Me$); HRMS (+ESI): Found *m/z* 438.1439 $[M + Na]^+$, $C_{24}H_{21}N_3O_4Na$ requires 438.1439.

Methyl 5,6-dibenzyloxyindole-2-carboxylate (**14**) The *title* compound was prepared as described in GP-3 from methyl 2-azido-3-(3′,4′-dibenzyloxyphenyl)propenoate (**13**) (2.76 g, 6.66 mmol) in xylene (50 mL) to give the product (1.84 g, 71%) as a yellow granular solid; m.p. 148–150 °C; IR (KBr): υ_{max} 3309, 2942, 2871, 2113, 1680, 1627, 1519, 1488, 1452, 1353, 1288, 1246, 1208, 1144, 1000, 918, 905, 839, 794 cm^{-1}; UV-vis (CH_3CN): λ_{max} 208 nm (ε 72,400 cm^{-1} M^{-1}), 320 (31,700); ^{1}H-NMR (300 MHz, $CDCl_3$): δ 3.93 (s, 3H, CO_2Me), 5.21 (s, 2H, O-CH_2), 5.24 (s, 2H, O-CH_2), 7.00 (s, 1H, H4), 7.01 (s, 1H, H7), 7.23 (d, *J* = 2.1 Hz, 1H, H3), 7.33–7.51 (m, 10H, ArH), 8.73 (bs, 1H, NH); ^{13}C-NMR (75.6 MHz, $CDCl_3$): 51.8 ($CO_2\underline{Me}$), 71.3 (CH_2), 72.0 (CH_2), 97.0 (C7), 107.0 (C4), 108.8 (C3), 121.0 (ArC), 126.0 (C2), 127.0 (ArC), 127.2 (2 × ArC), 127.3 (ArC), 127.7 (2 × ArC), 127.8 (ArC), 128.4 (ArC), 128.5 (ArC), 132.4 (ArC), 137.0 (ArC), 137.4 (2 × ArC), 145.8 (C5), 149.9 (C6), 162.1 ($\underline{C}O_2Me$); HRMS (+ESI): Found *m/z* 410.1364 $[M + Na]^+$, $C_{24}H_{21}NO_4Na$ requires 410.1363.

Methyl 5,6-dihydroxyindole-2-carboxylate (**8**) The *title* compound was prepared as described in GP-4 from methyl 5,6-dibenzyloxyindole-2-carboxylate (**14**) (0.387 g, 1.0 mmol) and 5% Pd/C catalyst (40 mg) in methanol/THF mixture (15 mL) to give the product (159 mg, 77%) as yellow solid; m.p. 256–258 °C; IR (KBr): υ_{max} 3437, 3315, 2953, 2107, 1653, 1632, 1531, 1506, 1437, 1311, 1283, 1230, 1198, 1139, 992, 937, 849, 825, 767 cm^{-1}; UV-vis (CH_3CN): λ_{max} 203 nm (ε 42,100 cm^{-1} M^{-1}), 318 (27,000);^{1}H-NMR (300MHz, d_6-DMSO): δ 3.82 (s, 3H, CO_2Me), 6.79 (d, *J* = 0.8 Hz, 1H, H4), 6.88 (s, 1H, H3), 6.90 (d, *J* = 0.8 Hz, 1H, H7), 8.84 and 9.17 (bs, each 1H, OH), 11.28 (bs, 1H, NH); ^{13}C-NMR (75.6 MHz, $CDCl_3$): 52.0

(CO_2Me), 97.3 (C7), 105.4 (C4), 108.4 (C3), 120.3 (ArC), 125.0 (C2), 133.2 (ArC), 142.3 (C5), 146.7 (C6), 162.5 (CO_2Me); HRMS (+ESI): Found *m/z* 230.0423 $[M + Na]^+$, $C_{10}H_9NO_4Na$ requires 230.0424.

Methyl 5,6-bis(prop-2-yn-1-yloxy)-1H-indole-2-carboxylate (**9**) The *title* compound was prepared as described in GP-5 from methyl 5,6-dihydroxyindole-2-carboxylate (**8**) (993 mg, 4.8 mmol), potassium carbonate (1.32 g, 9.6 mmol) and propargyl bromide (1.36 g, 10.6 mmol) in acetone to give the product (828 mg, 61%) as a yellow solid;m.p. 170–172 °C; IR (KBr): ν_{max} 3332, 3285, 2939, 2925, 2865, 2292, 2108, 1720, 1684, 1625, 1520, 1480, 1435, 1380, 1365, 1280, 1247, 1203, 1150 1024, 986, 892, 819, 805, 759, 720, 672 cm^{-1}; UV-vis (CH_3CN): λ_{max} 209 nm (ε 28,300 cm^{-1} M^{-1}), 313 (18,000); ^{1}H-NMR (300 MHz, $CDCl_3$): δ 2.55 (t, *J* = 1.6 Hz, 1H, CH≡C), 2.57 (t, *J* = 1.6 Hz, 1H, CH≡C), 3.95 (s, 3H, CO_2Me), 4.82 (d, *J* = 2.4 Hz, 2H, O-CH_2), 4.85 (d, *J* = 2.4 Hz, 2H, O-CH_2), 7.10 (d, *J* = 0.7 Hz, 1H, H7), 7.16 (q, *J* = 0.9 Hz, 1H, H3), 7.31 (s, 1H, H4), 8.86 (bs, 1H, NH), ^{13}C-NMR (75.6 MHz, $CDCl_3$): δ51.8 (CO_2Me), 57.0 (O-CH_2), 57.5 (O-CH_2), 75.7 (C≡CH), 75.7 (C≡CH), 78.6 (C≡CH), 79.1 (C≡CH), 97.2 (C7), 107.2 (C4), 108.9 (C3), 121.3 (aryl C), 126.4 (C2), 132.4 (aryl C), 144.2 (C4), 148.2 (C5), 162.1 (CO_2Me); HRMS (+ESI): Found *m/z* 306.0736 $[M + Na]^+$, $C_{16}H_{13}NO_4Na$ requires 306.0737.

2,9-Dihydropyrano[3,2-h]chromene-5-carbaldehyde (**15**) The *title* compound was prepared as described in GP-6 from 3,4-bis(prop-2-yn-1-yloxy)benzaldehyde (**11**) (214 mg, 1.04 mmol) in chlorobenzene (20 mL) to give the product (77 mg, 35%) as a white solid; m.p. 102–104 °C; IR (KBr): ν_{max} 1680, 1570, 1490, 1440, 1340, 1301, 1205, 1102, 995, 945, 900, 898, 861, 745 cm^{-1}; UV-vis (CH_3CN): λ_{max} 225 nm (ε 27,400 cm^{-1} M^{-1}), 268 (18,800), 305 (17,500); ^{1}H-NMR (300 MHz, $CDCl_3$): δ 4.40 (dd, *J* = 3.0, 1.4 Hz, 2H, O-CH_2), 4.79 (dd, *J* = 3.0, 1.4 Hz, 2H, O-CH_2), 6.97 (d, *J* = 8.7 Hz, 2H, H4 and H7), 7.37 (s, 1H, H6), 7.40–7.42 (m, 2H, H3 and H8), 9.80 (s, 1H, CHO); ^{13}C-NMR (75.6 MHz, $CDCl_3$): δ71.3 (O-CH_2), 71.5 (O-CH_2), 119.6 (C6), 120.6 (aryl C), 121.6 (C4), 121.8 (C7), 125.3 (aryl C), 126.5 (C3), 126.9 (C8), 127.1 (C5), 147.9 (aryl C), 154.3 (aryl C), 190.7 (CHO); HRMS (+ESI): Found *m/z* 237.0533 $[M + Na]^+$, $C_{13}H_{10}O_3Na$ requires 237.0528.

3,4-Bis(but-2-yn-1-yloxy)benzaldehyde (**29**) The *title* compound was prepared as described in GP-5 from 3,4-dihydroxybenzaldehyde (7) (660 mg, 4.8 mmol), potassium carbonate (1.32 g, 9.6 mmol) and 1-bromobut-2-yne (1.40 g, 10.6 mmol) in acetone to give the product (1.01 g, 87%) as a white solid; m.p. 86–88 °C; IR (KBr): ν_{max} 1688, 1582, 1499, 1431, 1375, 1248, 1201, 1125, 987, 920, 857, 797, 729 cm^{-1}; UV-vis (CH_3CN): λ_{max} 228 nm (ε 31,500 cm^{-1} M^{-1}), 272 (22,200), 303 (14,800); ^{1}H-NMR (300 MHz, $CDCl_3$): δ 1.85–1.87 (m, 6H, 2 × C-CH_3), 4.79 (q, *J* = 2.3 Hz, 2H, O-CH2), 4.82 (q, *J* = 2.3 Hz, 2H, O-CH2), 7.17 (d, *J* = 8.2 Hz, 1H, H5), 7.52 (dd, *J* = 8.2, 1.9 Hz, 1H, H6), 7.57 (d, *J* = 1.9 Hz, 1H, H2), 9.89 (s, 1H, CHO); ^{13}C-NMR (75.6 MHz, $CDCl_3$): δ 3.6 (C-CH_3), 3.7 (C-CH_3), 57.2 (2 × O-CH_2), 73.1 (C-CH_3), 73.3 (C-CH_3), 84.6 (C≡C(CH_3)), 84.9 (C≡C(CH_3)), 112.0 (C5), 112.7 (C2), 126.4 (C6), 130.3 (aryl C), 147.9 (C4′), 152.9 (C3′), 190.8 (CHO); HRMS (+ESI): Found *m/z* 265.0840 $[M + Na]^+$, $C_{15}H_{14}O_3Na$ requires 265.0835.

4-Methoxy-3-((3-phenylprop-2-yn-1-yl)oxy)benzaldehyde (**24d**) The *title* compound was prepared as described in GP-5 from 3-hydroxy-4-methoxybenzaldehyde **23** (730 mg, 4.8 mmol), potassium carbonate (662 mg, 4.8 mmol) and 3-phenylprop-2-yn-1-yl-4-methylbenzenesulfonate (1.66 g, 5.8 mmol) in acetone to give the product (1.17 g, 92%) as a white solid; m.p. 112–114 °C; IR (KBr): ν_{max} 1673, 1579, 1506, 1430, 1378, 1256, 1221, 1165, 1130, 1012, 931, 874, 810, 754, 686 cm^{-1}; UV-vis (CH_3CN): λ_{max} 232 nm (ε 45,500 cm^{-1} M^{-1}), 272 (21,500), 302 (14,800); ^{1}H-NMR (300 MHz, $CDCl_3$): δ 4.00 (s, 3H, OMe), 5.08 (s, 2H, O-CH2), 7.03 (d, *J* = 8.2 Hz, 1H, H5), 7.30–7.33 (m, 3H, ArH), 7.34–7.45 (m, 2H, ArH), 7.54 (dd, *J* = 8.2, 1.9 Hz, 1H, H6), 7.68 (d, *J* = 1.9 Hz, 1H, H2), 9.90 (s, 1H, CHO); ^{13}C-NMR (75.6 MHz, $CDCl_3$): δ 56.2 (OMe), 57.5 (O-CH_2), 83.0 (C≡C(Ph)), 88.0 (C-Ph), 110.9 (C5), 112.1 (C2), 122.1 (aryl C), 127.1 (2 × aryl CH), 127.8 (aryl CH), 128.8 (C6), 130.0 (aryl C), 131.9 (2 × aryl CH), 147.5 (C4), 155.0 (C3), 190.7 (CHO); HRMS (+ESI): Found *m/z* 289.0837 $[M + Na]^+$, $C_{17}H_{14}O_3Na$ requires 289.0835.

Methyl (Z)-2-azido-3-(3,4-bis(prop-2-yn-1-yloxy)phenyl) acrylate (**17**) The *title* compound was prepared as described in GP-2 from 3,4-bis(prop-2-yn-1-yloxy)benzaldehyde (**11**) (558 mg, 2.6 mmol) and methyl azidoacetate (2.99 g, 26.0 mmol) in anhydrous methanol (30 mL) to give the product (582 mg, 63%) as a pale yellow granular solid; m.p. 114–116 °C; IR (KBr): ν_{max} 2954, 2123, 1709, 1594, 1506, 1433, 1378, 1239, 1133, 1081, 1009, 793, 745, 683 cm^{-1}; UV-vis (CH_3CN): λ_{max} 327 nm (ε 19,100 cm^{-1} M^{-1}); ^{1}H-NMR (300 MHz,$CDCl_3$): δ 2.57 (t, J = 2.4 Hz, 1H, CH≡C), 2.59 (t, J = 2.4 Hz, 1H, CH≡C), 3.92 (s, 3H, CO_2Me), 4.83 (d, J = 2.4 Hz, 4H, 2 × O-CH2), 6.91 (s, 1H, CH=C), 7.09 (d, J = 8.5 Hz, 1H, H5′), 7.44 (dd, J = 8.5, 2.0 Hz, 1H, H6′), 7.77 (d, J = 2.0 Hz, 1H, H2′), ^{13}C-NMR (75.6 MHz, $CDCl_3$): δ 52.8 ($CO_2\underline{Me}$), 56.6 (OMe), 57.0 (2 × O-CH_2), 76.1 (C≡$\underline{C}$H), 76.2 (C≡$\underline{C}$H), 77.2 ($\underline{C}$≡CH), 77.4 ($\underline{C}$≡CH), 113.8 (C5′), 116.6 (C2′), 123.9 ($\underline{C}$H=C), 125.3 (C6′), 125.6 (aryl C), 146.9 (aryl C), 148.5 (aryl C), 164.1 ($\underline{C}O_2Me$); HRMS could not be determined due to the unstable properties of the compound

Methyl (Z)-2-azido-3-(4-methoxy-3-(prop-2-yn-1-yloxy)phenyl)acrylate (**25a**) The *title* compound was prepared as described in GP-2 from 4-methoxy-3-(prop-2-yn-1-yloxy)benzaldehyde (24a) (494 mg, 2.6 mmol) and methyl azidoacetate (2.99 g, 26.0 mmol) in anhydrous methanol (30 mL) to give the product (537 mg, 72%) as a pale yellow granular solid; m.p. 116–118 °C; IR (KBr): ν_{max} 2951, 2101, 1698, 1592, 1507, 1432, 1379, 1254, 1214, 1139, 1084, 1016, 809, 745 cm^{-1}; UV-vis (CH_3CN): λ_{max} 235 nm (ε 16,600 cm^{-1} M^{-1}), 330 (27,100); ^{1}H-NMR (300 MHz, $CDCl_3$): δ 2.58 (t, J = 2.4 Hz, 1H, CH≡C), 3.94 (s, 3H, OMe), 3.94 (s, 3H, CO_2Me), 4.83 (d, J = 2.4 Hz, 2H, O-CH2), 6.90 (s, 1H, CH=C), 6.93 (d, J = 8.5 Hz, 1H, H5′), 7.43 (dd, J = 8.5, 2.0 Hz, 1H, H6′), 7.76 (d, J = 2.0 Hz, 1H, H2′); ^{13}C-NMR (75.6 MHz, $CDCl_3$): δ 52.8 ($CO_2\underline{Me}$), 55.9 (OMe), 56.8 (O-CH_2), 76.0 (C≡$\underline{C}$H), 77.4 ($\underline{C}$≡CH), 111.2 (C5′), 116.1 (C2′), 123.4 ($\underline{C}$H=C), 125.6 (C6′), 125.0 (aryl C), 126.1 (CH=$\underline{C}$), 146.3 (C4′), 150.8 (C3′), 164.1 ($\underline{C}O_2Me$); HRMS (+ESI): Found m/z 310.0800 $[M + Na]^+$, $C_{14}H_{13}N_3O_4Na$ requires 310.0798.

Methyl (Z)-2-azido-3-(3-methoxy-4-(prop-2-yn-1-yloxy) phenyl)acrylate (**20a**) The *title* compound was prepared as described in GP-2 from 3-methoxy-4-(prop-2-yn-1-yloxy)benzaldehyde (**19a**) (494 mg, 2.6 mmol) and methyl azidoacetate (2.99 g, 26.0 mmol) in anhydrous methanol (30 mL) to give the product (567 mg, 76%) as a pale yellow granular solid; m.p. 120–122 °C; IR (KBr): ν_{max} 2920, 2122, 1704, 1592, 1509, 1450, 1345, 1243, 1206, 1141, 1008, 922, 804, 764 cm^{-1}; UV-vis (CH_3CN): λ_{max} 323 nm (ε 17,500 cm^{-1} M^{-1}); ^{1}H-NMR (300 MHz, $CDCl_3$): δ 2.56 (t, J = 2.4 Hz, 1H, CH≡C), 3.94 (s, 3H, OMe), 3.95 (s, 3H, CO_2Me), 4.83 (d, J = 2.4 Hz, 2H, O-CH2), 6.91 (s, 1H, CH=C), 7.06 (d, J = 8.5 Hz, 1H, H5′), 7.43 (dd, J = 8.5, 1.9 Hz, 1H, H6′), 7.56 (d, J = 1.9 Hz, 1H, H2′); ^{13}C-NMR (75.6 MHz, $CDCl_3$): δ 52.8 ($CO_2\underline{Me}$), 55.9 (OMe), 56.5 (O-CH_2), 76.2 (C≡$\underline{C}$H), 77.4 ($\underline{C}$≡CH), 113.3 (C5′), 113.5 (C2′), 123.7 ($\underline{C}$H=C), 124.4 (C6′), 125.5 (aryl C), 127.3 (CH=$\underline{C}$), 147.9 (C3′), 149.1 (C4′), 164.1 ($\underline{C}O_2Me$); HRMS could not be determined due to the unstable properties of the compound.

Methyl (Z)-2-azido-3-(3,4-bis(but-2-yn-1-yl)oxy)phenyl) acrylate (**30**) The *title* compound was prepared as described in GP-2 from 3,4-bis(but-2-yn-1-yloxy)benzaldehyde (**29**) (629 mg, 2.6 mmol) and methyl azidoacetate (2.99 g, 26.0 mmol) in anhydrous methanol (30 mL) to give the product (555 mg, 63%) as a pale yellow granular solid; m.p. 124–126 °C; IR (KBr): ν_{max} 2918, 2119, 1712, 1687, 1590, 1506, 1432, 1373, 1314, 1243, 1128, 992, 804, 745 cm^{-1}; UV-vis (CH_3CN): λ_{max} 307 nm (ε 14,500 cm^{-1} M^{-1}); ^{1}H-NMR (300 MHz, $CDCl_3$): δ 1.87 (t, J = 2.3 Hz, 6H, 2 × C-CH_3), 3.93 (s, 3H, $CO_2\underline{Me}$), 4.79 (q, J = 2.3 Hz, 2H, O-CH_2), 4.82 (q, J = 2.3 Hz, 2H, O-CH_2), 6.91 (s, 1H CH=C), 7.05 (d, J = 8.5 Hz, 1H, H5′), 7.44 (dd, J = 8.5, 1.8 Hz, 1H, H6′), 7.73 (d, J = 2.0 Hz, 1H, H2′); ^{13}C-NMR (75.6 MHz, $CDCl_3$): δ 3.7 (2×C-$\underline{C}H_3$), 52.8 ($CO_2\underline{Me}$), 57.1 (OMe), 57.2 (O-CH_2), 57.5 (O-CH_2), 73.9 (2×$\underline{C}$-CH_3), 84.2 ($\underline{C}$≡C(CH_3)), 84.9 ($\underline{C}$≡C(CH_3)), 113.2 (C5′), 116.0 (C2′), 125.3 ($\underline{C}$H=C), 125.8 (C6′), 126.5 (aryl C), 126.6 (CH=$\underline{C}$), 147.9 (C4′), 148.8 (C3), 164.2 ($\underline{C}O_2Me$); HRMS could not be determined due to the unstable properties of the compound.

Methyl (Z)-2-azido-3-(3-(but-2-yn-1-yloxy)-4-methoxyphenyl) acrylate (**25b**) The *title* compound was prepared as described in GP-2 from 3-(but-2-yn-1-yloxy)-4-methoxybenzaldehyde (**24b**) (530 mg, 2.6 mmol) and methyl azidoacetate (2.9 g, 26.0 mmol) in anhydrous methanol (30 mL) to give the product (500 mg, 64%) as a pale yellow granular solid; m.p. 96–98 °C; IR (KBr): ν_{max} 2951, 2101, 1698, 1592,

1507, 1431, 1379, 1254, 1139, 1016, 810, 745 cm^{-1}; UV-vis (CH_3CN): λ_{max} 327 nm (ε 25,700 cm^{-1} M^{-1}); ^{1}H-NMR (300 MHz, $CDCl_3$): δ 1.89 (t, J = 2.3 Hz, 3H, CH_3), 3.93 (s, 3H, OMe), 3.94 (s, 3H, CO_2Me), 4.78 (q, J = 2.3 Hz, 2H, O-CH_2), 6.91 (d, J = 8.5 Hz, 1H, H5′), 6.92 (s, 1H, CH=C), 7.41 (dd, J = 8.5, 2.0 Hz, 1H, H6′), 7.73 (d, J = 2.0 Hz, 1H, H2′); ^{13}C-NMR (75.6 MHz, $CDCl_3$): δ 3.7 (C-$\underline{C}H_3$), 52.8 ($CO_2\underline{Me}$), 55.9 (OMe), 57.4 (O-CH_2), 73.7 ($\underline{C}$-CH_3), 84.3 ($\underline{C}$≡C(CH_3)), 111.0 (C5′), 115.6 (C2′), 123.3 ($\underline{C}$H=C), 125.6 (C6′), 125.9 (aryl C), 126.0 (CH=$\underline{C}$), 146.7 (C4′), 150.7 (C3′), 164.2 ($\underline{C}O_2Me$); HRMS (+ESI): Found *m/z* 324.0944 $[M + Na]^+$, $C_{15}H_{15}N_3O_4Na$ requires 324.0955.

Methyl (Z)-2-azido-3-(4-(but-2-yn-1-yloxy)-3-methoxyphenyl)acrylate (**20b**) The *title* compound was prepared as described in GP-2 from 4-(but-2-yn-1-yloxy)-3-methoxybenzaldehyde (19b)(530 mg, 2.6 mmol) and methyl azidoacetate (2.99 g, 26.0 mmol) in anhydrous methanol (30 mL) to give the product (477 mg, 61%) as a pale yellow granular solid; m.p. 94–96 °C; IR (KBr): ν_{max} 2920, 2120, 1702, 1592, 1509, 1434, 1377, 1244, 1140, 1011, 801, 763 cm^{-1}; UV-vis (CH_3CN): λ_{max} 324 nm (ε 14,900 cm^{-1} M^{-1}); ^{1}H-NMR (300 MHz, $CDCl_3$): δ 1.87 (t, J = 2.3 Hz, 3H, CH_3), 3.94 (s, 3H, OMe), 3.94 (s, 3H, $CO_2\underline{Me}$), 4.77 (q, J = 2.3 Hz, 2H, O-CH2), 6.90 (s, 1H, CH=C), 7.05 (d, J = 8.5 Hz, 1H, H5′), 7.38 (dd, J = 8.5, 1.8, Hz, 1H, H6′), 7.53 (d, J = 1.8 Hz, 1H, H2′); ^{13}CNMR (75.6 MHz, $CDCl_3$): δ 3.7 (C-$\underline{C}H_3$), 52.8 ($CO_2\underline{Me}$), 55.9 (OMe), 57.1 (O-CH_2), 73.5 ($\underline{C}$-CH_3), 84.4 ($\underline{C}$≡C(CH_3)), 112.9 (C5′), 113.3 (C2′), 123.4 (aryl C), 124.5 ($\underline{C}$H=C), 125.8 (C6′), 126.8 (CH=$\underline{C}$), 14.34 (C3′), 149.0 (C4′), 164.2 ($\underline{C}O_2Me$); HRMS (+ESI): Found *m/z* 324.0955 $[M + Na]^+$, $C_{15}H_{15}N_3O_4Na$ requires 324.0955.

Methyl (Z)-2-azido-3-(4-methoxy-3-((3-phenylprop-2-yn-1-yl) oxy)phenyl)acrylate (**25d**) The *title* compound was prepared as described in GP-2 from 4-methoxy-3-((3-phenylprop-2-yn-1-yl)oxy)benzaldehyde (**24d**) (692 mg, 2.6 mmol) and methyl azidoacetate (2.99 g, 26.0 mmol) in anhydrous methanol (30 mL) to give the product (632 mg, 67%) as a pale yellow granular solid; m.p. 118–120 °C; IR (KBr): ν_{max} 2921, 2827, 2119, 1674, 1612, 1580, 1506, 1431, 1378, 1275, 1232, 1129, 1008, 966. 873, 809, 753, 686 cm^{-1}; UV-vis (CH_3CN): λ_{max} 234 nm (ε 57,700 cm^{-1} M^{-1}), 272 (22,600), 306 (21,800); ^{1}H-NMR (300 MHz, $CDCl_3$): δ 3.93 (s, 3H, OMe), 3.96 (s, 3H, CO_2Me), 5.04 (d, J = 6.0 Hz, 2H, O-CH2), 6.91 (s, 1H, CH≡C), 6.92 (d, J = 8.0 Hz, 1H, H5′), 7.09 (dd, J = 8.0, 1.8 Hz, 1H, H6′), 7.27–7.33 (m, 3H, ArH), 7.43–7.46 (m, 2H, ArH), 7.85 (d, J = 1.8 Hz, 1H, H2′); ^{13}C-NMR (75.6 MHz, $CDCl_3$): δ 52.6 ($CO_2\underline{Me}$), 55.9 (OMe), 57.5 (O-CH_2), 83.9 ($\underline{C}$-Ph), 87.5 ($\underline{C}$≡C(Ph)), 111.1 (C5′), 116.0 (C2′), 120.4 (aryl C), 125.7 ($\underline{C}$H=C), 126.0 (C6′), 126.1 (aryl C), 128.3 (2×aryl CH), 128.6 (CH=$\underline{C}$), 130.6 (aryl CH), 131.9 (2×aryl CH), 146.7 (C4′), 150.9 (C3′), 164.2 ($\underline{C}O_2Me$); HRMS (+ESI): Found *m/z* 386.1099 $[M + Na]^+$, $C_{20}H_{17}N_3O_4Na$ requires 386.1117.

Methyl (Z)-2-azido-3-(4-methoxy-3-((2-methylbut-3-yn-2-yl) oxy)phenyl)acrylate (**25c**) The *title* compound was prepared as described in GP-2 from 4-methoxy-3-((2-methylbut-3-yn-2-yl)oxy)benzaldehyde (**24c**) (567 mg, 2.6 mmol) and methyl azidoacetate (2.99 g, 26.0 mmol) in anhydrous methanol (30 mL) to give the product (507 mg, 62%) as a pale yellow granular solid; m.p. 122–124 °C; IR (KBr): ν_{max} 2988, 2835, 2094, 1691, 1619, 1565, 1506, 1425, 1374, 1253, 1138, 1084, 1027, 962. 891, 799, 756, 687 cm^{-1}; UV-vis (CH_3CN): λ_{max} 238 nm (ε 16,800 cm^{-1} M^{-1}), 328 (35,400); ^{1}H-NMR (300 MHz, $CDCl_3$): δ 1.70 (s, 6H, 2 × C-CH_3), 2.59 (d, J = 0.9 Hz, 1H, CH≡C), 3.87 (s, 3H, OMe), 3.92 (s, 3H, CO_2Me), 6.91 (s, 1H, CH=C), 6.90 (d, J = 8.5 Hz, 1H, H5′), 7.45 (dd, J = 1.9, 8.5 Hz, 1H, H6′), 8.16 (d, J = 2.0 Hz, 1H, H2′);^{13}C-NMR (75.6 MHz, $CDCl_3$): δ 29.3 (2×C-$\underline{C}H_3$), 52.7 ($CO_2\underline{Me}$), 55.7 (OMe), 73.6 (C≡$\underline{C}$H), 74.1 ($\underline{C}$-(CH_3)$_2$), 86.1 ($\underline{C}$≡CH), 111.5 (C5′), 123.2 (C2′), 124.8 ($\underline{C}$H=C), 125.7 (C6′), 125.9 (aryl C), 127.4 (CH=$\underline{C}$), 144.2 (C4′), 153.9 (C3′), 164.2 ($\underline{C}O_2Me$); HRMS (+ESI): Found *m/z* 338.1099 $[M + Na]^+$, $C_{16}H_{17}N_3O_4Na$ requires 338.1117.

Methyl (Z)-2-azido-3-(3-methoxy-4-((2-methylbut-3-yn-2-yl)oxy)phenyl)acrylate (**20c**) The *title* compound was prepared as described in GP-2 from 3-methoxy-4-((2-methylbut-3-yn-2-yl)oxy)benzaldehyde (**19c**) (567 mg, 2.6 mmol) and methyl azidoacetate (2.1 g, 26. mmol) in anhydrous methanol (30 mL) to give the product (524 mg, 62%) as a pale yellow granular solid; m.p. 116–118 °C; IR (KBr): ν_{max} 2975, 2802, 2112, 1703, 1635, 1565, 1512, 1400, 1387, 1212, 1100, 1052, 998, 957, 888, 765, 745, 677 cm^{-1}; UV-vis (CH_3CN): λ_{max} 328 nm (ε 17,100 cm^{-1} M^{-1}); ^{1}H-NMR (300 MHz, $CDCl_3$): δ 1.72 (s, 6H, 2 × C-CH_3),

2.60 (d, J = 0.9 Hz, 1H, CH≡C), 3.89 (s, 3H, OMe), 3.93 (s, 3H, CO_2Me), 6.91 (s, 1H, CH=C), 7.33 (dd, J = 8.5, 1.9 Hz, 1H, H6′), 7.45 (d, J = 8.5 Hz, 1H, H5′), 7.52 (d, J = 1.9 Hz, 1H, H2′); ^{13}C-NMR (75.6 MHz, $CDCl_3$): δ 29.4 (2 × C-$\underline{C}H_3$), 52.8 ($CO_2\underline{Me}$), 55.9 (OMe), 73.9 (C≡$\underline{C}$H), 73.9 ($\underline{C}$-$(CH_3)_2$) 85.8 ($\underline{C}$≡CH), 113.9 (C5′), 121.5 (C2′), 123.8 ($\underline{C}$H=C), 123.9 (C6′), 125.7 (aryl C), 128.5 (CH=$\underline{C}$), 146.1 (C3′), 152.0 (C4′), 164.1 ($\underline{C}O_2Me$); HRMS (+ESI): Found m/z 338.1104 $[M + Na]^+$, $C_{16}H_{17}N_3O_4Na$ requires 338.1117.

Methyl 6-methoxy-5-(prop-2-yn-1-yloxy)-1H-indole-2-carboxylate (**26a**) The *title* compound was prepared as described in GP-3 from methyl (Z)-2-azido-3-(3-(but-2-yn-1-yloxy)-4-methoxyphenyl)acrylate (**25a**) (596 mg, 2.08 mmol) in xylene (20 mL) to give the product (196 mg, 73%) as a yellow solid; m.p. 164–166 °C; IR (KBr): ν_{max} 3325, 3259, 2953, 2925, 2123, 1671, 1624, 1520, 1480, 1440, 1367, 1320, 1249, 1208, 1185, 1146, 1005, 890, 833, 766, 694 cm^{-1}; UV-vis (CH_3CN): λ_{max} 208 nm (ε 40,600 cm^{-1} M^{-1}), 318 (28,700); ^{1}H-NMR (300 MHz, $CDCl_3$): δ 2.55 (t, J = 2.4 Hz, 1H, CH≡C), 3.95 (s, 3H, OMe), 3.96 (s, 3H, CO_2Me), 4.82 (d, J = 2.4 Hz, 2H, O-CH_2), 6.90 (d, J = 0.8 Hz, 1H, H4), 7.16 (q, J = 0.9 Hz, 1H, H3), 7.28 (s, 1H, H7), 8.91 (bs, 1H, NH), ^{13}C-NMR (75.6 MHz, $CDCl_3$): δ 51.8 ($CO_2\underline{Me}$), 56.0 (OMe), 57.3 (O-CH_2), 75.7 (C≡$\underline{C}$H), 78.7 ($\underline{C}$≡CH), 94.0 (C7), 106.6 (C4), 109.0 (C3), 120.2 (aryl C), 125.9 (C2), 132.9 (aryl C), 143.7 (C6), 150.6 (C5), 162.3 ($\underline{C}O_2Me$); HRMS (+ESI): Found m/z 282.0725 $[M + Na]^+$, $C_{14}H_{13}NO_3Na$ requires 282.0742.

Methyl 5-methoxy-6-(prop-2-yn-1-yloxy)-1H-indole-2-carboxylate (**21a**) The *title* compound was prepared as described in GP-3 from methyl (Z)-2-azido-3-(4-(but-2-yn-1-yloxy)-3-methoxyphenyl)acrylate (**20a**) (596 mg, 2.08 mmol) in xylene (20 mL) to give the product (183 mg, 68%) as a yellow solid; m.p. 152–154 °C; IR (KBr): ν_{max} 3325, 3241, 2999, 2937, 2113, 1681, 1638, 1522, 1475, 1452, 1360, 1280, 1237, 1211, 1195, 1143, 1003, 924, 843, 819, 761, 675 cm^{-1}; UV-vis (CH_3CN): λ_{max} 209 nm (ε 35,800 cm^{-1} M^{-1}), 308 (21,400); ^{1}H-NMR (300 MHz, $CDCl_3$): δ 2.57 (t, J = 2.4 Hz, 1H, CH≡C), 3.95 (s, 3H, OMe), 3.96 (s, 3H, CO_2Me), 4.85 (d, J = 2.4 Hz, 2H, O-CH_2), 7.08 (d, J = 0.8 Hz, 1H, H4), 7.11 (s, 1H, H7), 7.15 (q, J = 0.9 Hz, 1H, H3), 8.87 (bs, 1H, NH); ^{13}C-NMR (75.6 MHz, $CDCl_3$): δ 51.8 ($CO_2\underline{Me}$), 56.2 (OMe), 56.9 (O-CH_2), 76.1 (C≡$\underline{C}$H), 77.4 ($\underline{C}$≡CH), 96.8 (C7), 103.0 (C4), 108.7 (C3), 121.4 (aryl C), 126.1 (C2), 131.6 (aryl C), 146.6 (C5), 147.6 (C6), 162.2 ($\underline{C}O_2Me$); HRMS (+ESI): Found m/z 282.0726 $[M + Na]^+$, $C_{14}H_{13}NO_3Na$ requires 282.0742.

Methyl 5,6-bis(but-2-yn-1-yloxy)-1H-indole-2-carboxylate (**31**) The *title* compound was prepared as described in GP-3 from methyl (Z)-2-azido-3-(3,4-bis(but-2-yn-1-yloxy)phenyl)acrylate (**30**) (704 mg, 2.08 mmol) in xylene (20 mL) to give the product 210 mg, 65%) as a yellow solid; m.p. 146–148 °C; IR (KBr): ν_{max} 3332, 2912, 2294, 2120, 1682, 1644, 1519, 1434, 1379, 1244, 1204, 1145, 984, 891, 819, 765 cm^{-1}; UV-vis (CH_3CN): λ_{max} 210 nm (ε 39,600 cm^{-1} M^{-1}), 317 (24,900); ^{1}H-NMR (300 MHz, $CDCl_3$): δ 1.87 (q, J = 2.4 Hz, 6H, 2 × C-CH_3), 3.96 (s, 3H, CO_2Me), 4.76 (q, J = 2.4 Hz, 2H, O-CH2), 4.79 (q, J = 2.4 Hz, 2H, O-CH2), 7.08 (d, J = 0.7 Hz, 1H, H4), 7.16 (q, J = 0.9 Hz, 1H, H3), 7.25 (s, 1H, H7), 9.03 (bs, 1H, NH); ^{13}C-NMR (75.6 MHz, $CDCl_3$): δ 3.7 (2 × C-$\underline{C}H_3$), 51.8 ($CO_2\underline{Me}$), 57.4 and 57.8 (O-CH_2), 73.9 ($\underline{C}$-CH_3), 74.2 ($\underline{C}$-CH_3), 83.8 ($\underline{C}$≡C(CH_3)), 84.2 ($\underline{C}$≡C(CH_3)), 96.5 (C7), 106.1 (C4), 108.9 (C3), 120.9 (aryl C), 126.0 (C2), 132.5 (aryl C), 144.4 (C5), 148.5 (C6), 162.3 ($\underline{C}O_2Me$); HRMS (+ESI): Found m/z 334.1046 $[M + Na]^+$, $C_{18}H_{17}NO_4Na$ requires 334.1050.

Methyl 5-(but-2-yn-1-yloxy)-6-methoxy-1H-indole-2-carboxylate (**26b**) The *title* compound was prepared as described in GP-3 from methyl (Z)-2-azido-3-(3-(but-2-yn-1-yloxy)-4-methoxyphenyl)acrylate (**25b**) (626 mg, 2.08 mmol) in xylene (20 mL) to give the product (201 mg, 71%) as a yellow solid; m.p. 160–162 °C; IR (KBr): ν_{max} 3324, 3258, 3009, 2918, 2795, 2123, 2108, 1672, 1600, 1520, 1490, 1425, 1400, 1385, 1346, 1249, 1208, 1185, 1146, 1005, 980, 890, 833, 766 cm^{-1}; UV-vis (CH_3CN): λ_{max} 208 nm (ε 27,700 cm^{-1} M^{-1}), 319 (18,900);^{1}H-NMR (300 MHz, $CDCl_3$): δ 1.88 (q, J = 2.4 Hz, 3H, C-CH_3), 3.95 (s, 3H, OMe), 3.96 (s, 3H, CO_2Me), 4.77 (q, J = 2.4 Hz, 2H, O-CH_2), 6.88 (d, J = 0.7 Hz, 1H, H4), 7.16 (q, J = 0.9 Hz, 1H, H3), 7.23 (s, 1H, H7), 8.82 (bs, 1H, NH); ^{13}C-NMR (75.6 MHz, $CDCl_3$): δ 5.2 (C-$\underline{C}H_3$), 53.2 ($CO_2\underline{Me}$), 57.4 (OMe), 59.1 (O-CH_2), 75.5 ($\underline{C}$-CH_3), 85.3 ($\underline{C}$≡C), 95.2 (C7), 107.1 (C4), 110.4 (C3), 121.7 (aryl C),

127.1 (C2), 134.0 (aryl C), 145.5 (C6), 151.9 (C5), 163.7 ($\underline{C}O_2Me$); HRMS (+ESI): Found *m/z* 296.0884 $[M + Na]^+$, $C_{15}H_{15}NO_4Na$ requires 296.0899.

Methyl 6-(but-2-yn-1-yloxy)-5-methoxy-1H-indole-2-carboxylate (**21b**) The *title* compound was prepared as described in GP-3 from methyl (Z)-2-azido-3-(4-(but-2-yn-1-yloxy)-3-methoxyphenyl)acrylate (**20b**) (626 mg, 2.08 mmol) in xylene (20 mL) to give the product (190 mg, 67%) as a yellow solid; m.p. 164–166 °C; IR (KBr): ν_{max} 3324, 3224, 3005, 2936, 2835, 2215, 2108, 1680, 1584, 1495, 1455, 1433, 1362, 1285, 1243, 1228, 1146, 1045, 988, 946, 846, 819, 760, 672 cm^{-1}; UV-vis (CH_3CN): λ_{max} 210 nm (ε 37,100 cm^{-1} M^{-1}), 319 (22,300); ^{1}H-NMR (300 MHz, $CDCl_3$): δ 1.87 (q, *J* = 2.4 Hz, 3H, C-CH_3), 3.94 (s, 3H, OMe), 3.96 (s, 3H, CO_2Me), 4.80 (q, *J* = 2.4 Hz, 2H, O-CH2), 7.06 (d, *J* = 0.7 Hz, 1H, H4), 7.08 (s, 1H, H7), 7.14 (q, *J* = 0.9 Hz, 1H, H3), 9.01 (bs, 1H, NH); ^{13}C-NMR (75.6 MHz, $CDCl_3$): δ 3.7 (C-$\underline{C}H_3$), 51.8 ($CO_2\underline{Me}$), 56.1 (OMe), 57.4 (O-CH_2), 73.8 ($\underline{C}$-CH_3), 84.3 ($\underline{C}$≡C(CH_3)), 96.2 (C7), 102.7 (C4), 108.7 (C3), 121.0 (aryl C), 125.8 (C2), 131.8 (aryl C), 146.1 (C5), 148.0 (C6), 162.3 ($\underline{C}O_2Me$); HRMS (+ESI): Found *m/z* 296.0883 $[M + Na]^+$, $C_{15}H_{15}NO_4Na$ requires 296.0889.

Methyl 6-methoxy-5-((3-phenylprop-2-yn-1-yl)oxy)-1H-indole-2-carboxylate (**26d**) The *title* compound was prepared as described in GP-3 from methyl (Z)-2-azido-3-(4-methoxy-3-((3-phenylprop-2-yn-1-yl)oxy)phenyl)acrylate (**25d**) (754 mg, 2.08 mmol) in xylene (20 mL) to give the product (257 mg, 74%) as a yellow solid; m.p. 138–140 °C; IR (KBr): ν_{max} 3326, 2984, 2924, 2740, 2113, 1675, 1645, 1520, 1480, 1439, 1381, 1247, 1195, 1145, 996, 845, 823, 761, 672 cm^{-1}; UV-vis (CH_3CN): λ_{max} 203 nm (ε 58,900 cm^{-1} M^{-1}), 318 (22,200); ^{1}H-NMR (300 MHz, $CDCl_3$): δ 3.95 (s, 3H, OMe), 3.98 (s, 3H, CO_2Me), 5.04 (s, 2H, O-CH2), 6.90 (s, 1H, H4), 7.17 (q, *J* = 0.9 Hz, 1H, H3), 7.31 (s, 1H, H7), 7.32–7.36 (m, 3H, ArCH), 7.44–7.47 (m, 2H, ArCH), 8.84 (bs, 1H, NH); ^{13}C-NMR (75.6 MHz, $CDCl_3$): δ 51.8 ($CO_2\underline{Me}$), 56.0 (OMe), 58.2 (O-CH_2), 84.1 ($\underline{C}$≡C(Ph)), 87.4 ($\underline{C}$-Ph), 93.9 (C7), 106.6 (C4), 109.0 (C3), 120.3 (aryl C), 122.4 (aryl C), 125.8 (C2), 128.2 (2 × aryl CH), 128.5 (aryl CH), 131.8 (2 × aryl CH), 132.8 (aryl C), 144.0 (C6), 150.7 (C5), 162.2 ($\underline{C}O_2Me$); HRMS (+ESI): Found *m/z* 336.1221 $[M + H]^+$, $C_{20}H_{18}NO_4$ requires 336.1236.

Methyl 5,10-dihydro-7H-dipyrano[3,2-e:2′,3′-g]indole-6-carboxylate (**10**) *Method 2: Route* 2 The title compound was prepared as described in GP-3 from methyl (Z)-2-azido-3-(3,4-bis(prop-2-yn-1-yloxy)phenyl) acrylate (**9**) (646 mg, 2.08 mmol) in xylene (20 mL) to give the product (61.4 mg, 72%) as a yellow solid; m.p. 168–170 °C; IR (KBr): ν_{max} 3415, 3328, 2947, 2831, 2341, 2116, 1674, 1640, 1575, 1524, 1486, 1441, 1400, 1274, 1213, 1158, 1135, 1025, 1000, 920, 813, 755 cm^{-1}; UV-vis (CH_3CN): λ_{max} 225 nm (ε 24,100 cm^{-1} M^{-1}), 269 (13,800), 360 (13,000); ^{1}H-NMR (300 MHz, $CDCl_3$): δ 3.96 (s, 3H, CO_2Me), 4.91 (dd, J = 3.8, 1.8 Hz, 2H, O-CH_2), 4.94 (dd, *J* = 3.8, 1.8 Hz, 2H, O-CH_2), 5.87–5.97 (m, 2H, H3 and H9), 6.72–6.80 (m, 2H, H4 and H8), 7.19 (d, *J* = 2.1 Hz, 1H, H5), 8.85 (s, 1H, NH); ^{13}C-NMR (75.6 MHz, $CDCl_3$): δ52.0 ($CO_2\underline{Me}$), 65.7 (O-CH_2), 65.8 (O-CH_2), 106.5 (C5), 107.0 (aryl C), 115.3 (aryl C), 118.8 (C4), 119.3 (C8), 120.8 (aryl C), 121.8 (C3), 121.9 (C9), 126.5 (C6), 128.8 (aryl C), 138.1 (aryl C), 141.7 (aryl C), 162.3 ($\underline{C}O_2Me$); HRMS (+ESI): Found *m/z* 306.0736 $[M + Na]^+$, $C_{16}H_{13}NO_4Na$ requires 306.0737.

This compound was also prepared by the methods described below. Method 1: The title compound was prepared as described in GP-6 from methyl 5,6-bis(prop-2-yn-1-yloxy)-1*H*-indole-2-carboxylate (**16**) (118 mg, 0.42 mmol) in chlorobenzene (30 mL) to give the product (43.5 mg, 51%) as a yellow solid.

Method 2: Route 1 The title compound was prepared as described in GP-6 from methyl (Z)-2-azido-3-(2*H*,10*H*-pyrano[4,3-h]chromen-5-yl)acrylate (**17**) (646 mg, 2.08 mmol) in xylene (20 mL) to give the product (52.9 mg, 62%) as a yellow solid.

Methyl 5-methoxy-3,7-dihydropyrano[3,2-e]indole-2-carboxylate (**27a**) The title compound was prepared as described in GP-6 from methyl 6-methoxy-5-(prop-2-yn-1-yloxy)-1H-indole-2-carboxylate (**26a**) (108 mg, 0.42 mmol) in chlorobenzene (30 mL) to give the product (80 mg, 74%) as a yellow solid; m.p. 166–168 °C; IR (KBr): ν_{max} 3325, 2948, 2839, 2340, 2110, 1677, 1637, 1515, 1439, 1271, 1193, 1143, 1098,

998, 931, 883, 808, 752 cm^{-1}; UV-vis (CH_3CN): λ_{max} 212 nm (ε 37,400 cm^{-1} M^{-1}), 271 (13,300), 322 (30,600); ^{1}H-NMR (300 MHz, $CDCl_3$): δ 3.92 (s, 3H, OMe), 3.93 (s, 3H, CO_2Me), 4.90 (dd, *J* = 3.7, 1.7 Hz, 2H, O-CH2), 5.89–5.95 (m, 1H, H8), 6.76–6.79 (m, 1H, H9), 6.79 (s, 1H, H4), 7.17 (d, *J* = 2.1 Hz, 1H, H1), 8.96 (s, 1H, NH); ^{13}C-NMR (75.6 MHz, $CDCl_3$): δ 51.8 ($CO_2\underline{Me}$), 56.0 (OMe), 65.7 (O-CH_2), 93.8 (C4), 106.1 (C1), 114.9 (aryl C), 118.3 (aryl C), 121.6 (C9), 121.8 (C8), 126.0 (C2), 132.2 (aryl C), 139.3 (aryl C), 148.8 (C5), 162.2 ($\underline{C}O_2Me$); HRMS (+ESI): Found *m/z* 282.0731 [M + Na]$^+$, $C_{14}H_{13}NO_4Na$ requires 282.0737.

Methyl 5-methoxy-1,7-dihydropyrano[2,3-g]indole-2-carboxylate (**22a**) The *title* compound was prepared as described in GP-6 from methyl 5-methoxy-6-(prop-2-yn-1-yloxy)-1*H*-indole-2-carboxylate (**21a**) (108 mg, 0.42 mmol) in chlorobenzene (30 mL) to give the product (83 mg, 77%) as a yellow solid; m.p. 188–190 °C; IR (KBr): ν_{max} 3327, 2944, 2827, 2366, 2106, 1677, 1528, 1444, 1306, 1221, 1148, 1101, 989, 955, 831, 755 cm^{-1}; UV-vis (CH_3CN): λ_{max} 226 nm (ε 28,100 cm^{-1} M^{-1}), 290 (16,700), 339 (18,400); ^{1}H-NMR (300 MHz, $CDCl_3$): δ 3.94 (s, 3H, OMe), 3.96 (s, 3H, CO_2Me), 4.96 (dd, *J* = 3.8, 1.8 Hz, 2H, O CH_2), 5.89–5.95 (m, 1H, H8), 6.75–6.79 (m, 1H, H9), 7.02 (s, 1H, H4), 7.13 (d, *J* = 2.1 Hz, 1H, H3), 8.94 (s, 1H NH); ^{13}C-NMR (75.6 MHz, $CDCl_3$): δ51.9 ($CO_2\underline{Me}$), 56.2 (OMe), 65.7 (O-CH_2), 103.1 (C4), 107.1 (aryl C), 109.2 (C3), 119.3 (aryl C), 120.8 (C8), 121.0 (C9), 126.0 (C2), 128.7 (aryl C), 137.6 (aryl C), 145.2 (C5), 162.3 ($\underline{C}O_2Me$); HRMS (+ESI): Found *m/z* 282.0738 [M + Na]$^+$, $C_{14}H_{13}NO_4Na$ requires 282.0737.

Methyl 5-methoxy-9-methyl-3,7-dihydropyrano[3,2-e]indole-2-carboxylate (**27b**) The *title* compound was prepared as described in GP-6 from methyl 5-(but-2-yn-1-yloxy)-6-methoxy-1*H*-indole-2-carboxylate (**26b**) (114 mg, 0.42 mmol) in chlorobenzene (30 mL) to give the product (62 mg, 54%) as a yellow solid; m.p. 196–198 °C; IR (KBr): ν_{max} 3310, 2948, 2925, 2833, 2106, 1675, 1640, 1517, 1495, 1439, 1366, 1274, 1265, 1194, 1146, 1080, 1004, 960, 880, 815, 765, 672 cm^{-1}; UV-vis (CH_3CN): λ_{max} 213 nm (ε 28,900 cm^{-1} M^{-1}), 267 (9,500), 322 (24,200); ^{1}H-NMR (300 MHz, $CDCl_3$): δ 1.63 (s, 3H, C-CH_3), 3.94 (s, 3H, OMe), 3.95 (s, 3H, CO_2Me), 4.77 (q, *J* = 2.4 Hz, 2H, O-CH_2), 5.69–5.72 (m, 1H, H8), 6.87 (s, 1H, H1), 7.23 (s, 1H, H4), 8.82 (bs, 1H, NH); ^{13}C-NMR (75.6 MHz, $CDCl_3$): δ 22.6 (C-$\underline{C}H_3$), 51.8 ($CO_2\underline{Me}$), 56.1 (OMe), 65.2 (O-CH_2), 93.8 (C4), 109.3 (C1), 117.4 (aryl C), 117.9 (aryl C), 118.3 (C8), 126.5 (C2), 132.0 ($\underline{C}$-CH_3), 132.9 (aryl C), 140.4 (aryl C), 149.0 (C5), 162.2 ($\underline{C}O_2Me$); HRMS (+ESI): Found *m/z* 296.0887 [M + Na]$^+$, $C_{15}H_{15}NO_4Na$ requires 296.0893.

Methyl 5-methoxy-9-methyl-1,7-dihydropyrano[2,3-g]indole-2-carboxylate (**22b**) The *title* compound was prepared as described in GP-6 from methyl 6-(but-2-yn-1-yloxy)-5-methoxy-1*H*-indole-2-carboxylate (**21b**) (114 mg, 0.42 mmol) in chlorobenzene (30 mL) to give the product (56 mg, 49%) as a yellow solid; m.p. 176–178 °C; IR (KBr): ν_{max} 3410, 2980, 2930, 2845, 1695, 1645, 1606, 1534, 1445, 1430, 1385, 1375, 1232, 1189, 1139, 1096, 1040, 998, 981, 927, 857, 744, 712cm^{-1}; UV-vis (CH_3CN): λ_{max} 224 nm (ε 32,500 cm^{-1} M^{-1}), 286 (22,200), 337 (23,500); ^{1}H-NMR (300 MHz, $CDCl_3$): δ 1.71 (s, 3H, C-CH_3), 3.94 (s, 3H, OMe), 3.96 (s, 3H, CO_2Me), 4.77 (q, *J* = 1.6 Hz, 2H, O-CH_2), 5.65–5.68 (m, 1H, H8), 7.05 (s, 1H, H4), 7.14 (d, *J* = 2.1 Hz, 1H, H3), 8.81 (bs, 1H, NH), ^{13}C-NMR (75.6 MHz, $CDCl_3$): δ 20.8 (C-$\underline{C}H_3$), 51.8 ($CO_2\underline{Me}$), 56.2 (OMe), 65.4 (O-CH_2), 103.2 (C4), 108.9 (C3), 109.9 (aryl C), 117.7 (C8), 121.9 (aryl C), 126.0 (C2), 128.7 ($\underline{C}$-CH_3), 129.3 (aryl C), 144.2 (aryl C), 145.4 (C5), 162.1 ($\underline{C}O_2Me$); HRMS (+ESI): Found *m/z* 296.0886 [M + Na]$^+$, $C_{15}H_{15}NO_4Na$ requires 296.0893.

Methyl 5-methoxy-9-phenyl-3,7-dihydropyrano[3,2-e]indole-2-carboxylate (**27d**) The *title* compound was prepared as described in GP-6 from methyl 6-methoxy-5-((3-phenylprop-2-yn-1-yl)oxy)-1*H*-indole-2-carboxylate (**26d**) (140 mg, 0.42 mmol) in chlorobenzene (30 mL) to give the product (113 mg, 81%) as a yellow solid; m.p. 188–190 °C; IR (KBr): ν_{max} 3311, 2949, 2816, 2114, 1684, 1639, 1598, 1515, 1500, 1438, 1400, 1360, 1260, 1241, 1193, 1141, 1042, 1011, 995, 920, 823, 759, 703 cm^{-1}; UV-vis (CH_3CN): λ_{max} 274 nm (ε 11,600 cm^{-1} M^{-1}), 326 (26,400); ^{1}H-NMR (300 MHz, $CDCl_3$): δ 3.82 (s, 3H, OMe), 4.00 (s, 3H, CO_2Me), 4.85 (d, *J* = 4.4 Hz, 2H, O-CH_2), 5.94–5.97 (m, 1H, H8), 5.98 (s, 1H, H4), 6.88 (s, 1H, H1), 7.30–7.34 (m, 2H, ArH), 7.41–7.44 (m, 3H, ArH), 8.76 (bs, 1H, NH), ^{13}C-NMR (75.6 MHz, $CDCl_3$): δ 51.7 ($CO_2\underline{Me}$), 58.1 (OMe), 65.1 (O-CH_2), 94.2 (C4),

109.4 (C1), 117.0 (aryl C), 117.5 (aryl C), 125.0 (C2), 120.4 (C8), 127.9 (aryl CH), 128.3 (2 × arylCH), 128.5 (2 × aryl CH), 132.8 (aryl C), 139.4 (C-Ph), 139.4 (aryl C), 141.1 (aryl C), 149.0 (C5), 162.1 ($\underline{C}O_2Me$); HRMS (+ESI): Found *m/z* 358.1057 $[M + Na]^+$, $C_{20}H_{17}NO_4Na$ requires 358.1055.

Methyl 5-methoxy-7,7-dimethyl-3,7-dihydropyrano[3,2-e] indole-2-carboxylate (**27c**)
The title compound was prepared as described in GP-3 from methyl (Z)-2-azido-3-(4-methoxy-3-((2-methylbut-3-yn-2-yl)oxy)phenyl)acrylate (**25c**) (654 mg, 2.08 mmol) in xylene (20 mL) to give the product (220 mg, 68%) as a yellow solid; m.p. 144–146 °C; IR (KBr): ν_{max} 3316, 2962, 2975, 2111, 1681, 1625, 1600, 1510, 1439, 1400, 1366, 1270, 1230, 1192, 1131, 1075, 999, 934, 887, 818, 754, 728 cm^{-1}; UV-vis (CH_3CN): λ_{max} 219 nm (ε 40,000 cm^{-1} M^{-1}), 271 (13,500), 323 (31,100); ^1H-NMR (300 MHz, $CDCl_3$): δ 1.53 (s, 6H, 2 × CH_3), 3.92 (s, 3H, OMe), 3.95 (s, 3H, CO_2Me), 5.73 (d, *J* = 9.7 Hz, 1H, H8), 6.68 (d, *J* = 9.7 Hz, 1H, H9), 6.79 (s, 1H, H4), 7.19 (d, *J* = 2.1 Hz, 1H, H1), 9.00 (bs, 1H, NH); ^{13}C-NMR (75.6 MHz, $CDCl_3$): δ 27.3 (2 × C-$\underline{C}H_3$), 51.7 ($CO_2\underline{Me}$), 58.1 (OMe), 76.2 ($\underline{C}$-$(CH_3)_2$), 93.1 (C4), 106.1 (C1), 113.4 (aryl C), 118.2 (aryl C), 119.3 (C9), 125.7 (C2), 130.6 (C8), 132.0 (aryl C), 138.1 (aryl C), 149.5 (C5), 162.3 ($\underline{C}O_2Me$); HRMS (+ESI): Found *m/z* 310.1044 $[M + Na]^+$, $C_{16}H_{17}NO_4Na$ requires 310.1050.

Methyl 5-methoxy-7,7-dimethyl-1,7-dihydropyrano[2,3-g] indole-2-carboxylate (**22c**)
The title compound was prepared as described in GP-3 from methyl (Z)-2-azido-3-(3-methoxy-4-((2-methylbut-3-yn-2-yl)oxy)phenyl)acrylate (**20c**) (654 mg, 2.08 mmol) in xylene (20 mL) to give the product (203 mg, 74%) as a yellow solid; m.p. 158–160 °C; IR (KBr): ν_{max} 3338, 2955, 2919, 2845, 2111, 1676, 1640, 1595, 1534, 1444, 1370, 1350, 1310, 1265, 1217, 1195, 1134, 1099, 1050, 985, 960, 880, 826, 760, 714 cm^{-1}; UV-vis (CH_3CN): λ_{max} 226 nm (ε 29,600 cm^{-1} M^{-1}), 262 (15,200), 341 (19,000); ^1H-NMR (300 MHz, $CDCl_3$): δ 1.55 (s, 6H, 2 × CH_3), 3.93 (s, 3H, OMe), 3.96 (s, 3H, CO_2Me), 5.71 (d, *J* = 9.7 Hz, 1H, H8), 6.66 (d, *J* = 9.7 Hz, 1H, H9), 7.02 (s, 1H, H4), 7.13 (d, *J* = 2.1 Hz, 1H, H3), 8.95 (bs, 1H, NH); ^{13}C-NMR (75.6 MHz, $CDCl_3$): δ 27.4 (2 × C-$\underline{C}H_3$), 51.8 ($CO_2\underline{Me}$), 56.5 (OMe), 76.6 ($\underline{C}$-$(CH_3)_2$), 103.3 (C4), 105.8 (aryl C), 109.3 (C3), 116.8 (C9), 120.6 (aryl C), 125.7 (C2), 128.9 (aryl C), 129.8 (C8), 142.3 (aryl C), 149.9 (C5), 162.4 ($\underline{C}O_2Me$); HRMS (+ESI): Found *m/z* 288.1228 $[M + H]^+$, $C_{16}H_{18}NO_4$ requires 288.1236.

3.2. Cell Biology Techniques

The SH-SY5Y and Kelly human neuroblastoma cell lines were generously donated by Dr. J. Biedler (Memorial Sloan-Kettering Cancer Center, New York, NY, USA). The MDA-MB-231 and MCF-7 breast cancer cell lines were purchased from the American Type Culture Collection. All cell lines were cultured under standard conditions at 37 °C in 5% CO_2 as an adherent monolayer in Dulbecco's modified Eagle's medium supplemented with L-glutamine (DMEM) (Invitrogen, Waltham, MA, USA) and 10% fetal calf serum (FCS) (Thermo Fisher Scientific, Waltham, MA, USA).

Method for Cell Viability Assays

Cell viability was measured by the standard Alamar blue assay, as previously described [18]. Briefly, cells were allowed to attach for 24 h in 96-well culture plates. The cells were then continuously exposed to serial dilutions of the hydrazide-hydrazone derivatives for 72 h, either in the presence or absence of SAHA (0.5 or 1 μM), with five replicate wells for each determination. Cell viability was determined by the addition of 22 μL of Alamar blue reagent, recorded at comparative 0 h and 5 h values, using a Wallac 1420 Victor III spectrophotometer (GMI, Ramsey, MN, USA), which measured light absorbance in each well at 570 nm. The cell viability of each plate was calculated as a percentage compared to matched DMSO controls (0.5%). The mean (+/'SEM) is shown for three independent experiments.

3.3. *Statistical Analysis*

Results of the cell viability studies were statistically analyzed using the two-tailed, unpaired Student's t-test. Results are expressed as mean values with 95% confidence intervals.

4. Conclusions

The studies presented in this study have contributed to the investigation of the potential of dihydropyranoindoles to act as SAHA enhancers for the treatment of neuroblastoma and breast cancer cells. To the best of our knowledge, this is the first study which was carried out on the combination of SAHA with dihydropyranoindoles. The desired tricyclic and tetracyclic dihydropyranoindoles was achieved by the reaction of corresponding hydroxybenzaldehydes with haloalkynes followed by the application of the Hemetsberger indole synthesis to yield the related indoles. Claisen cyclization in the presence of chlorobenzene afforded the desired compounds in good yields. Some of the dihydropyranoindoles were successfully synthesized from the corresponding azido intermediates in one step by the thermal decomposition step of the Hemetsberger indole synthesis. The biological studies revealed that the breast cancer cells displayed significant resistance towards the combination treatments of the dihydropyranoindoles compared to the neurobalstoma cells. It was also found that tetracyclic analogues of dihydropyranoindoles **33** and **10** were found to be more favorable for the enhancement of SAHA activity, while only dihydropyrano[3,2-*e*]indole tricyclic systems **27a** and **27c** resulted in the additional reduction of the SAHA cytotoxicity against the neuroblastoma cell lines. Taken altogether, the tetracyclic dihydropyranoindole **10** was determined as the most cytotoxic compound at the concentration 20 μM, while the lower concentration of the designated compound displayed the best enhancement on SAHA activity with the value of 44% additional reduction at the ratio of 1:10 SAHA to compound.

Supplementary Materials: Figure S1 Cell viability of A) SH-SY5Y, B) MDA-MB-231 cancer cells treated with the selected six compounds **1–6** (10 μM) over 72 h. Error bars represent mean values (±S.D.) for three independent determinations. **Figure S2**. Comparative toxicity of compounds **1, 3** and **4** (10 μM) against SH-SY5Y, MDA-MB-231 and MRC-5 cell lines after 72 h exposure. Error bars represent mean values (±S.D.) for three independent determinations. **Figure S3**. Cell viability of A) MCF-7 $p < 0.01$ B) MDA-MB-231 $p < 0.05$ breast cancer cells treated with 10 μM compounds over 72 h, in the presence or absence of 1 μM of SAHA. Error bars represent mean values (±S.D.) for three independent determinations **Figure S4**. Cell viability of A) Kelly $p \geq 0.05$ (ns) B) SH-SY5Y $p < 0.0005$ neuroblastoma cancer cellstreated with 10 μM compounds over 72 h, in the presence or absence of 1 μM of SAHA. Error bars represent mean values (±S.D.) for three independent determinations. **Figure S5**. Cell viability of KELLY neuroblastoma cancer cells treated with compounds A) **33** $p < 0.01$ B) **27c** $p < 0.05$ and C) **10** $p < 0.05$ at different concentrations (0.01, 0.1, 1, 10, 20 μM) over 72 h in the absence and presence of SAHA. Error bars represent mean values (±S.D.) for three independent determinations. **Figure S6**. Cell viability of SH-SY5Y neuroblastoma cancer cells treated with compounds A) **27a**, $p < 0.0005$ B) **33**, $p < 0.0005$ C) **10**, $p < 0.01$ and D) **27c**, $p < 0.01$ at different concentrations (0.01, 0.1, 1, 10, 20 μM) over 72 h in the absence and presence of SAHA. Error bars represent mean values (±S.D.) for three independent determinations. **Figure S7**. Comparative toxicity of compounds A) **27a**, $p < 0.05$ B) **33**, $p < 0.05$ C) **10**, $p < 0.05$ and D) **27c**, $p < 0.0005$ (10 μM) against cancer cells (Kelly, SH-SY5Y, MCF-7 and MDA-MB-231) and human lung fibroblasts (WI-38 and MRC-5) cell lines after 72 h exposure. Error bars represent mean values (±S.D.) for three independent determinations.

Author Contributions: N.K., D.S.B., G.M.M. and B.B.C. conceived and designed the experiments, G.M.A. provided the data from library screening, M.B. performed the experiments, analyzed, interpreted the data and wrote the paper, N.K. and G.M.M. supported financially. All authors have read and agree to the published version of the manuscript.

Acknowledgments: We thank the University of New South Wales, and the Australian Research Council (ARC) for funding to N.K. and D.S.B. Mass spectrometric analysis for this work was carried out at the Bioanalytical Mass Spectrometry Facility, UNSW and was supported in part by infrastructure funding from the New South Wales Government as part of its co-investment in the National Collaborative Research Infrastructure Strategy. This research was supported by Australian Postgraduate Research Scholarships, University of NSW, Program Grants from the NHMRC Australia, Cancer Institute NSW Australia and Cancer Council NSW Australia. The Children's Cancer Institute Australia for Medical Research is affiliated with the University of NSW and Sydney Children's Hospital.

References

1. Matthay, K.K.; Yanik, G.; Messina, J.; Quach, A.; Huberty, J.; Cheng, S.C.; Veatch, J.; Goldsby, R.; Brophy, P.; Kersun, L.S.; et al. Phase II study on the effect of disease sites, age, and prior therapy on response to iodine-131-metaiodobenzylguanidine therapy in refractory neuroblastoma. *J. Clin. Oncol.* **2007**, *25*, 1054–1060. [CrossRef]
2. DuBois, S.G.; Kalika, Y.; Lukens, J.N.; Brodeur, G.M.; Seeger, R.C.; Atkinson, J.B.; Haase, G.M.; Black, C.T.; Perez, C.; Shimada, H.; et al. Metastatic sites in stage IV and IVS neuroblastoma correlate with age, tumor biology, and survival. *J. Pediat Hematol Onc.* **1999**, *21*, 181–189. [CrossRef] [PubMed]
3. Matthay, K.K.; Reynolds, C.P.; Seeger, R.C.; Shimada, H.; Adkins, E.S.; Haas-Kogan, D.; Gerbing, R.B.; London, W.B.; Villablanca, J.G. Iodine-131- metaiodobenzylguanidine double infusion with autologous stem-cellrescue for neuroblastoma: A new approaches to neuroblastoma therapyphase I study. *J. Clin Oncol.* **2009**, *27*, 1020–1025. [CrossRef] [PubMed]
4. Smith, M.A.; Seibel, N.L.; Altekruse, S.F.; Ries, L.A.G.; Melbert, D.L.; O'Leary, M.; Smith, F.O.; Reaman, G.H. Outcomes for children and adolescents with cancer: Challenges for the twenty-first century. *J. Clin. Oncol.* **2010**, *28*, 2625–2634. [CrossRef]
5. Lautz, T.B.; Jie, C.; Clark, S.; Naiditch, J.A.; Jafari, N.; Qiu, Y.Y.; Zheng, X.; Chu, F.; Madonna, M.B. The effect of vorinostat on the development of resistance to doxorubicin in neuroblastoma. *PLoS ONE* **2012**, *7*, 40816. [CrossRef] [PubMed]
6. Huang, J.M.; Sheard, M.A.; Ji, L.Y.; Sposto, R.; Keshelava, N. Combination of Vorinostat and Flavopiridol Is Selectively Cytotoxic to Multidrug-Resistant Neuroblastoma Cell Lines with Mutant *TP53*. *Mol. Cancer Ther.* **2010**, *9*, 3289–3301. [CrossRef]
7. Ozaki, K.; Kishikawa, F.; Tanaka, M.; Sakamoto, T.; Tanimura, S.; Kohno, M. Histone deacetylase inhibitors enhance the chemosensitivity of tumor cells with cross-resistance to a wide range of DNA-damaging drugs. *Cancer Sci.* **2008**, *99*, 376–384. [CrossRef] [PubMed]
8. Basu, H.S.; Mahlum, A.; Mehraein-Ghomi, F.; Kegel, S.J.; Guo, S.; Peters, N.R.; Wilding, G. Pre-treatment with anti-oxidants sensitizes oxidatively stressed human cancer cells to growth inhibitory effect of suberoylanilide hydroxamic acid (SAHA). *Cancer Chemoth. Pharm.* **2011**, *67*, 705–715. [CrossRef]
9. Richon, V.M. Cancer biology: Mechanism of antitumour action of vorinostat (suberoylanilide hydroxamic acid), a novel histone deacetylase inhibitor. *Brit. J. Cancer* **2006**, *95*, 2–6. [CrossRef]
10. Duvic, M.; Zhang, C. Clinical and laboratory experience of vorinostat (suberoylanilide hydroxamic acid) in the treatment of cutaneous T-cell lymphoma. *Brit. J. Cancer.* **2006**, *95*, 13–19. [CrossRef]
11. Mann, B.S.; Johnson, J.R.; He, K.; Sridhara, R.; Abraham, S.; Booth, B.P.; Verbois, L.; Morse, D.E.; Jee, J.M.; Pope, S.; et al. Vorinostat for treatment of cutaneous manifestations of advanced primary cutaneous T-cell lymphoma. *Clin. Cancer Res.* **2007**, *13*, 2318–2322. [CrossRef] [PubMed]
12. Kelly, W.K.; O'Connor, O.A.; Krug, L.M.; Chiao, J.H.; Heaney, M.; Curley, T.; MacGregore-Cortelli, B.; Tong, W.; Secrist, J.P.; Schwartz, L.; et al. Phase I study of an oral histone deacetylase inhibitor, suberoylanilide hydroxamic acid, in patients with advanced cancer. *J. Clin. Oncol.* **2005**, *23*, 3923–3931. [CrossRef] [PubMed]
13. Krug, L.M.; Curley, T.; Schwartz, L.; Richardson, S.; Marks, P.; Chiao, J.; Kelly, W.K. Potential role of histone deacetylase inhibitors in mesothelioma: Clinical experience with suberoylanilide hydroxamic acid. *Clin. Lung. Cancer* **2006**, *7*, 257–261. [CrossRef] [PubMed]
14. Rundall, B.K.; Denlinger, C.E.; Jones, D.R. Suberoylanilide hydroxamic acid combined with gemcitabine enhances apoptosis in non-small cell lung cancer. *Surgery.* **2005**, *138*, 360–367. [CrossRef] [PubMed]
15. Sonnemann, J.; Gange, J.; Kumar, K.S.; Muller, C.; Bader, P.; Beck, J.F. Histone deacetylase inhibitors interact synergistically with tumor necrosis factor-related apoptosis-inducing ligand (TRAIL) to induce apoptosis in carcinoma cell lines. *Investig. New Drug.* **2005**, *23*, 99–109. [CrossRef] [PubMed]
16. Denlinger, C.E.; Rundall, B.K.; Jones, D.R. Proteasome inhibition sensitizes non-small cell lung cancer to histone deacetylase inhibitor-induced apoptosis through the generation of reactive oxygen species. *J. Thorac Cardiov Sur.* **2004**, *128*, 740–748. [CrossRef]
17. Arndt, G.; Children's Cancer Institute, Sydney, Australia. Personal Communication, 2009.
18. Marks, P. Discovery and development of SAHA as an anticancer agent. *Oncogene.* **2007**, *26*, 1351–1356. [CrossRef]

19. Hemetsberger, H.; Knittel, D.; Weidmann, H. Synthese und Thermolyse von α-Azidoacrylestern. *Monatsh. Chem.* **1972**, *103*, 149. [CrossRef]
20. McElhanon, J.R.; Wu, M.J.; Escobar, M.; Chaudhry, U.; Hu, C.L.; McGrath, D.V. Asymmetric Synthesis of a Series of Chiral AB2 Monomers for Dendrimer Construction. *J. Org. Chem.* **1997**, *62*, 908–915. [CrossRef]
21. Büchi, G.; Kamikawa, T. An alternative synthesis of 5,6-dihydroxy-2,3-hydroindole-2-carboxylates (Cyclodopa). *J. Org. Chem.* **1977**, *42*, 4153–4154. [CrossRef]
22. Li, J.; Zhang, D.M.; Zhu, X.; He, Z.J.; Liu, S.; Li, M.F.; Pang, J.Y.; Lin, Y.C. Studies on synthesis and structure-activity relationship (SAR) of derivatives of a new natural product from marine fungi as inhibitors of influenza virus neuraminidase. *Mar. Drugs.* **2011**, *9*, 1887–1901. [CrossRef] [PubMed]
23. Guantai, E.M.; Ncokazi, K.; Egan, T.J.; Gut, J.; Rosenthal, P.J.; Smith, P.J.; Chibale, K. Design, synthesis and in vitro antimalarial evaluation of triazole-linked chalcone and dienone hybrid compounds. *Bioorg. Med. Chem.* **2010**, *18*, 8243–8256. [CrossRef] [PubMed]
24. Elomri, A.; Michel, S.; Tillequin, F.; Koch, M. A novel synthesis of 6-demethoxyacronycine. *Heterocycles* **1992**, *34*, 799–806.
25. Suresh, T.; Kumar, R.N.; Mohan, P.S. A Facile approach to dibenzo [bf| [1,6] naphthyridines using Vilsmeier Conditions. *Heterocycl Commun.* **2003**, *9*, 83–88. [CrossRef]
26. Zammit, S.C.; Cox, A.J.; Gow, R.M.; Zhang, Y.; Gilbert, R.E.; Krum, H.; Kelly, D.J.; Williams, S.J. Evaluation and optimization of antifibrotic activity of cinnamoyl anthranilates. *Bioorg. Med. Chem. Lett.* **2009**, *19*, 7003–7006. [CrossRef]
27. Crombie, L.; Jamieson, S.V. Dihydrostilbenes of cannabis. Synthesis of canniprene. *J. Chem. Soc. Perkin Trans. 1* **1982**, 1467–1475. [CrossRef]

3

Improved Anticancer Activity of the Malloapelta B-Nanoliposomal Complex against Lung Carcinoma

Thi Thao Do [1,2,*], Thi Nga Nguyen [1], Thi Phuong Do [1], Thi Cuc Nguyen [1], Ha Phuong Trieu [1], Phuong Thi Thu Vu [1] and Tuan Anh Hoang Le [3]

1. Institute of Biotechnology, Vietnam Academy of Science and Technology, 18 Hoang Quoc Viet Road, Hanoi 10000, Vietnam; nguyenngaibt@gmail.com (T.N.N.); dothiphuong74@yahoo.com.vn (T.P.D.); nguyencuc125@gmail.com (T.C.N.); trieuhaphuong95@gmail.com (H.P.T.); vuthuphuong9x@gmail.com (P.T.T.V.)
2. Graduate University of Science and Technology, Vietnam Academy of Science and Technology, 18 Hoang Quoc Viet Road, Hanoi 10000, Vietnam
3. Center for Research and Technology Transfer, Vietnam Academy of Science and Technology, 18 Hoang Quoc Viet Road, Hanoi 10000, Vietnam; hoangletuananh.cretech@gmail.com

* Correspondence: thaodo@ibt.ac.vn

Featured Application: Anticancer Drug Activity and Underlying Mechanisms.

Abstract: Previous studies regarding malloapelta B (malB), a natural compound isolated from the Vietnamese medicinal plant, showed a strong NF-κB inhibitory effect, making it a promising source for the development of novel anticancer drugs. However, similar to many other natural compounds from plants, malB has several disadvantages for clinical applications, including high toxicity and low solubility. To improve its bioavailability, malB was conjugated into nanoliposomes, which are ideal drug carriers. The formulations with 1,2-dipalmitoyl-sn-glycero-3-phosphocholine, mPEG-cholesterol, malB, with or without cholesterol exhibited nanoliposomes with an average diameter of approximately 76.98 nm, PDI of 0.28, zeta potential of −5.53 mV, and the highest encapsulation efficiency of 78.73% ± 9.5%. These malB-nanoliposomes inhibited the survival of all lung cancer cell lines examined with IC_{50} values ranging from 11.86 to 13.12 μM. Moreover, malB-nanoliposomes showed stronger inhibition of A549 colony-forming activity compared to that of the free compound. The effects of malB and its nanoliposomal formulation may be mediated through activation of apoptosis by the significant induction of caspase 3 activity. The nanoliposomal formulations also showed potential to inhibit tumor growth (37.03%) and prolong survival (32.20 days) of tumor-bearing mice compared with the unloaded drug ($p < 0.05$). The improved antitumor activity of malB-nanoliposomes suggests their promising clinical applications.

Keywords: apoptosis; caspase 3; Lewis lung carcinoma; malloapelta B; nanoliposome

1. Introduction

Lung cancer is the leading cause of cancer-related death worldwide (18.4%), and is especially prevalent in male smokers [1]. The most common type of lung cancer is non-small cell lung cancer (NSCLC), accounting for 85% of cases of lung cancer [2]. Approximately 40% of lung cancers are adenocarcinomas, and most cases of lung cancer in smokers are of this type. Several therapeutic methods are available for treatment of lung adenocarcinomas, including surgery, radiofrequency ablation, radioactive therapy, chemotherapy, and immunotherapy, alone or in various combinations. However, these therapeutic options are not only expensive but also insufficiently effective. Therefore, there is an increasing need for new, safer, and more effective clinical treatments. Our previous study showed that 1-(5,7-dimetoxy-2,2dimetyl-2H-cromen-8-yl)-but-2-en-1-on (malloapelta B), isolated from *Mallotus apelta*, is a potential active anticancer compound [3]. This compound, malloapelta B (malB), inhibits the activation of nuclear factor kappa B (NF-κB) with an IC_{50} value of 5.0 μM. This IC_{50} value is much lower than that of parthenolide (PTN, 6.66 ± 0.07 μM) [4,5]. The compound was also shown to downregulate genes that contribute to inflammatory mechanisms, such as tumor necrosis factor (TNF)-α, interleukin (IL)-6, and Il-1β [6]. Additionally, as reported, the enone side chain may play an important role in the activity of this molecule [4]. However, the potential effects of malB against lung carcinomas in vitro and in vivo have not been studied in detail. In addition, its high toxicity and low solubility represent barriers to the development of malB as an anticancer drug for use in chemotherapy. Nanoliposomes have recently emerged as ideal drug carriers with a number of beneficial characteristics, including minimal immune response, biocompatibility, biodegradability, reduction of drug toxicity, etc. [7]. Nanoliposomes can be used to encapsulate hydrophobic drugs as a means of improving their solubility in water. Due to these advantages, a number of nanoliposomal formulations incorporating different anticancer drugs are available commercially, including daunorubicin (DaunoXome), doxorubicin in PEG-liposomes (Doxil), vincristine (Marqibo), topotecan (INX-0076), nystatin (Nyotran), and paclitaxel (LEP-ET) [8]. Therefore, in the present study, malB was entrapped in nanoliposomes at different concentrations, and anticancer activities of these malB-nanoliposomal formulations against lung carcinomas were examined as well as their anti-malignant potential in Lewis lung carcinoma (LLC) tumor-bearing mice.

2. Materials and Methods

2.1. Chemicals

1,2-Dipalmitoyl-sn-glycero-3-phosphocholine (DPPC) was purchased from Avanti Polar Lipids (Alabaster, AL, USA); cholesterol was produced at Acros Organics, a part of Thermo Fisher Scientific, (Merelbeke, Belgium), and mPEG-cholesterol was provided by Dr. Chun-Liang Lo, National Yang-Ming National University, Taipei, Taiwan. The compound malloapelta B (malB) was provided by the MienTrung Institute for Scientific Research, Vietnam Academy of Science and Technology (Hue, Vietnam). Other chemicals and cell culture reagents were from Sigma Chemical Co. (St. Louis, MO, USA) and Invitrogen (Carlsbad, CA, USA).

2.2. Animals

Male and female albino BALB/c mice (8–10 weeks old) were received from the Institute of Biotechnology, Vietnam Academy of Science and Technology (VAST, Hanoi, Vietnam). All mice were caged in a temperature-controlled room on a 12-h light/12-h dark cycle with food and water ad libitum. Experiments were performed in accordance with Vietnamese Ethical Laws, European Communities Council Directives of 24 November 1986 (86/609/EEC) guidelines and Approval from the Scientific Council of Institute of Biotechnology, Vietnam Academy of Science and Technology, for the care and use of laboratory animals.

2.3. MalB-Nanoliposome Preparation

2.3.1. Bangham Thin Film Method

Liposome production was carried out according to the Bangham thin film method [9] with some modifications. Briefly, a complex including lipids and malB was diluted in dichloromethane (DCM) solvent (Table 1). A magnetic stirrer was used to dissolve the complex at 200 rpm, room temperature (RT) for 20 min. DCM was then removed by a rotary evaporator for the formation of thin film. The solvent was thoroughly dispatched by nitrogen gas flushing. Subsequently, the thin film was hydrated with PBS (pH = 7.2) at 60 °C. To obtain nanoliposomes, the hydrated complex was then immediately subjected to a probe sonicator that directly inserted the probed head into the solution with an ultrasonic frequency of 2 atm, 20 s of ultrasound and 10 s of rest, repeated five times. The ultrasonic solution was shaken at 60 °C and 500 rpm for one hour before large size nanoliposomes were removed by filtering with a 0.22 μm polyvinylidene difluoride (PVDF) membrane. The filtered nanoliposomes were washed three times with PBS (pH = 7.2).

Table 1. Lipid components including 1,2-Dipalmitoyl-sn-glycero-3-phosphocholine (DPPC), mPEG-cholesterol, with/without cholesterol and malloapelta B (malB) compound ratio.

Types	DPPC (mg)	mPEG-Cholesterol (mg)	Cholesterol (mg)	malB (mg)	DCM (mL)
Formulation A	4	1	0.50	0.50	10
Formulation B	4	1	0.75	0.25	10
Formulation C	4	1	0	0.25	10
Formulation D	4	1	0	0.50	10
Blank	4	1	0.75	-	10

2.3.2. Nanoliposomal Characterization

The size (z-average), polydispersity indexes (PDIs), and zeta potential of the nanoparticles were measured using a dynamic light scattering instrument (DLS, Horiba Instruments Inc., Irvine, CA, USA). The malB-nanoliposomes were also stained with 4% uranyl acetate (UR 4%) dye on the surface of a thin carbon-coated copper plate to a thickness of 200–500 A° and dried at RT. Then, the plates were magnified 200× to capture the morphology of the prepared nanoparticles using high-solution transmission electronic microscopy (TEM) (Jeol 1200EX TEM, Jeol Company, Tokyo, Japan).

2.3.3. Encapsulated Efficiency

The encapsulated efficiency (EE) of the loaded malB was calculated by UV–spectrophotometry method. The pure malB compound was dissolved in DMSO (100%) as a standard curve with a two time diluted concentration range which was started from0.25 mg/mL. The malB-nanoliposomes were re-diluted in DMSO (100%) to release all packed malB. Then, 100 μL of both the standard curve and the nanoliposomal samples were placed into a 96-well plate, repeated three times to ensure accuracy. The optical density values (ODs) were measured at 280 nm on a ThermoScientific™ Varioskan™ Flash Multimode Reader. The standard curve drawn using Microsoft Office Excel 2016 software was used to calculate the amount of active ingredient that was packed into the nanoliposomes. The encapsulated efficiency (EE) of the process was determined using the following equation:

$$EE(\%) = 100 \times (\text{weight of conjugated malB})/(\text{weight of initial malB})$$

2.4. Cell Lines and Cell Culture

A549, SK-LU-1, CL-141, and LLC lung cancer cell lines were provided by Prof. Chi-Ying Huang, Institute of Biopharmaceutical Sciences, National Yang Ming University, Taipei, Taiwan and Prof. J Meier, Milan University, Milan, Italy. Cells were cultured in DMEM medium supplemented with 10% fetal bovine serum (FBS), 100 μg/mL streptomycin, 100 IU/mL penicillin, and 2mM L-glutamine. All cells were maintained in a humidified incubator with 5% CO_2 at 37 °C, and harvested with trypsin-EDTA.

2.5. Cytotoxic Activities of malB-Conjugated Nanoliposomes

Cells were seeded in 96-well plates at a density of 2000 cells per well in triplicate for 24 h before sample exposure. Cells were then treated with different unloaded malB concentrations and corresponding malB-nanoliposomes of indicated treatments for 48 h. Cytotoxicity was assessed by using the sulforhodamine B (SRB) assay [10]. Briefly, the medium was discarded, and adherent cells were fixed by 100 μL/well of cold 10% trichloroacetic acid (*w/v*) for 1 h at 4 °C. After fixation, cells were stained with 0.4% SRB solution (*w/v* in 1% acetic acid) for 30 min at RT, and then washed twice with 1% acetic acid. After air-drying, 100 µL of 20 mM Tris-base were added to each well and the absorbance was measured at 540 nm. Cytotoxicity is expressed as the percent of cells relative to the number of cells in the solvent only as control (set to 100%). Each experiment was performed independently at least 3 times.

2.6. *Clonogenic Inhibition of malB-Conjugated Nanoliposomes*

Clonogenic assay was performed to determine the ability of a single cell to grow into a colony under the compound treatment. In detail, 800 cells were seeded in each well of 6-well plates at 37 °C, 5% CO_2. The addition of drugs was manipulated after 24 h of seeding and triplication of experiments was carried out. The medium including drugs was changed each 3 days. The cells were harvested after 8 days of treatment. After the treatment, the cells were washed with 1 mL phosphate-buffered saline (PBS), and fixed with 1mL mixture of methanol and acetic acid (3:1) in 15 min at RT. Subsequently, the colonies were stained with 0.5 mL of 0.5% crystal violet in methanol for 15 min. Then, crystal violet was discarded and the plate were rinsed under tap water. Only colonies consisting of approximately 50 cells were counted. The percentage of cell survival after drug treatment was expressed as a percentage of the control-colony efficiency.

2.7. *Caspase 3 Inducible Activities of malB-Conjugated Nanoliposome*

Caspase 3 activity was performed using a Caspase-3 Colorimetric Assay Kit (BioVision Inc., USA). According to the assaying protocol of the kit manufacturer, 1×10^6 cells treated with malB or malB-nanoliposome at different concentrations for 24h were lysed with chilled lysis buffer. The lysates were then centrifuged to collect the supernatant. After measurement of protein content using Bradford reagent, caspase 3 activity was specified by mixing 50 µL of cell lysis supernatant with 50 µL of 10 mM dithiothrcitol (DTT) and 5 µL of the 4 mM DEVD-p-nitroaniline (DEVD-pNA) substrate (from the kit). The caspase 3 activity, which corresponds with the presence of the chromophore pNA, a product formed from the cleavage of the DEVD-pNA substrate in enzyme reaction, can be detected by using a spectrophotometer at 405 nm.

2.8. *In Vivo Antitumor Activity*

The experiment was carried out using 36 healthy BALB/c mice at 20–25 g weight. Mice were subcutaneously injected with 1×10^6 LLC cells to induce tumors. After 5 days, tumorized mice were randomly distributed to 6 groups (n = 6). Group 1 served as the negative control that received normal saline. Group 2 was treated with blank nanoliposome (with lipid components only). Groups 3 and 4 received malB-nanoliposome at doses of 5 mg/kg and 2.5 mg/kg body weight (b.w.) by intraperitoneal injection (i.p.) every 2 days for 14 days continuously. Group 5 was i.p. injected with unconjugated malB compound at a dose of 5 mg/kg b.w. every 2 days for the same duration. Group 6 was treated with the reference control (doxorubicin 5 mg/kg b.w. i.p. injection). The tumor size of each mouse was measured every 7 days for 28 days and tumor volume was calculated by the following equation:

$$V = (W^2 \times L)/2,$$

where V is the volume of the tumor, W is the width of the tumor, and L is the length of the tumor.

The survival time of tumorized mice in all experimental groups was also determined. It was calculated from the day of LLC cell inoculation to the day of death and percentage increase in average life span (ILS) was calculated by the following equation:

$$\%\ ILS = (A/B - 1) \times 100,$$

where A is the survival time of the treated group, B is the mean survival time of the control group, and ILS is the increase in the average life span group.

2.9. Statistical Analyses

All data were expressed as means ± standard error of the mean (SEM). Statistical differences were analyzed by two-tailed paired Student's *t*-test or one-way analysis of variance (one-way ANOVA). A value of $p < 0.05$ was considered a statistically significant difference.

3. Results

3.1. Preparation and Morphology of malB-Encapsulated Nanoliposomes

The main components used to produce drug-encapsulating nanoliposomes included malB compound at different concentrations, DPPC, mPEG-cholesterol, with or without cholesterol. The physicochemical characteristics of the nanoliposomes thus formed were assessed by determining the mean diameter (nm), polydispersity index (PDI), zeta potential, and encapsulation efficiency (EE).

Based on the results shown in Table 2, all of the nanoliposomal formulations had not only a mean diameter <200 nm, but also PDI <0.3, and carried a low negative charge. However, the formulations without cholesterol as a component showed significantly higher packing efficiency ($p < 0.01$). The EE of formulations A and B containing cholesterol were only about 10%, whereas the EEs of the cholesterol-free structures were >50%. The EE was also dependent on the malB concentration; a lower malB concentration of 0.25 mg was associated with higher EE (78.73%), whereas a higher concentration of 0.5 mg showed a lower EE (51.33%). Due to the highest efficient effect, structure C was selected for further studies.

Table 2. Characteristics of obtained malB-loaded nanoliposomes.

Types	Size (nm)	PDI	Zeta Potential (mV)	EE (%)
Formulation A	130.53 ± 4.38	0.26 ± 0.04	−2.02 ± 0.95	12.80 ± 1.55
Formulation B	101.53 ± 3.89	0.28 ± 0.03	−0.52 ± 0.04	9.85 ± 0.21
Formulation C	76.98 ± 13.18	0.28 ± 0.04	−5.53 ± 0.21	78.73 ** ± 9.52
Formulation D	124.41 ± 35.41	0.30 ± 0.03	−2.70 ± 0.13	51.33 ** ± 6.53
Blank	119.70 ± 22.17	0.22 ± 0.02	−2.80 ± 0.24	-

Note: ** $p < 0.01$ compared to the formulation without cholesterol; blank liposome including DPPC, cholesterol, and mPEG-cholesterol.

The morphology of the malB-nanoliposomal formulation C was examined by transmission electron microscopy (TEM) (Figure 1). The malB-nanoliposomes were small unilamellar vesicles, likely spherical in shape, and fairly homogeneous in size with an average diameter of 76.98 ± 9.57 nm (Table 2). Based on morphological assessment, the mal B-nanoliposomal formulation C was suitable to manipulate in the further experiments for anticancer activities.

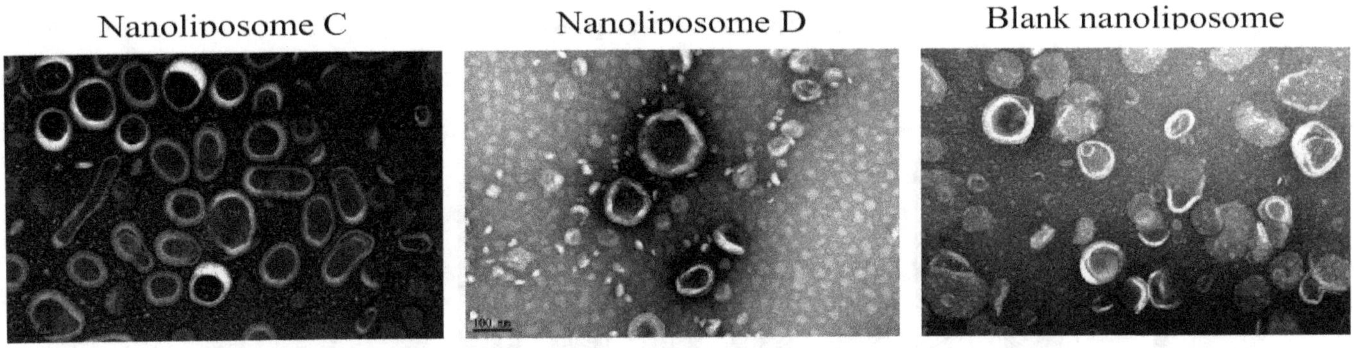

Figure 1. TEM morphological images of malB-loaded nanoliposomes: nanoliposome C (malB entrapped in nanoliposomes at 0.25 mg, EE = 78.73% ± 9.52%); nanoliposome D (malB entrapped in nanoliposomes at 0.50 mg, EE = 51.33% ± 16.53%). Blank nanoliposomal particles.

3.2. Compound Encapsulation by Nanoliposomes and Their Cytotoxicity

To determine the cytotoxicity of free malB and malB-nanoliposomes on non-small cell lung cancer cell lines, the viability of different cell lines was examined by sulforhodamine B (SRB) assay with malB treatment at several concentrations. As shown in Figure 2 and Table 3, both free compound and malB-nanoliposomes inhibited cell growth in a dose-dependent manner and significantly compared with the control ($p < 0.005$). High doses of malB and malB-nanoliposomes (7.5 µM and 15 µM) remarkably inhibited viability of all tested lung cancer cell lines. However, the cytotoxic effects of malB and malB-nanoliposomes on all cell lines were decreased at a dose of 3.75 µM, and minimal effects were observed at a dose of 1.875 µM. Based on the IC_{50} values, malB-nanoliposomes exhibited the strongest cytotoxicity against the A549 cell line. Free malB showed stronger cytotoxic activity than that of the malB-nanoliposomal formulation on all examined cell lines. However, the difference was insignificant ($p > 0.05$). Blank nanoliposomes showed no significant effects on cell growth (cell survival >90%). Therefore, the IC_{50} value of blank liposomes could not be determined.

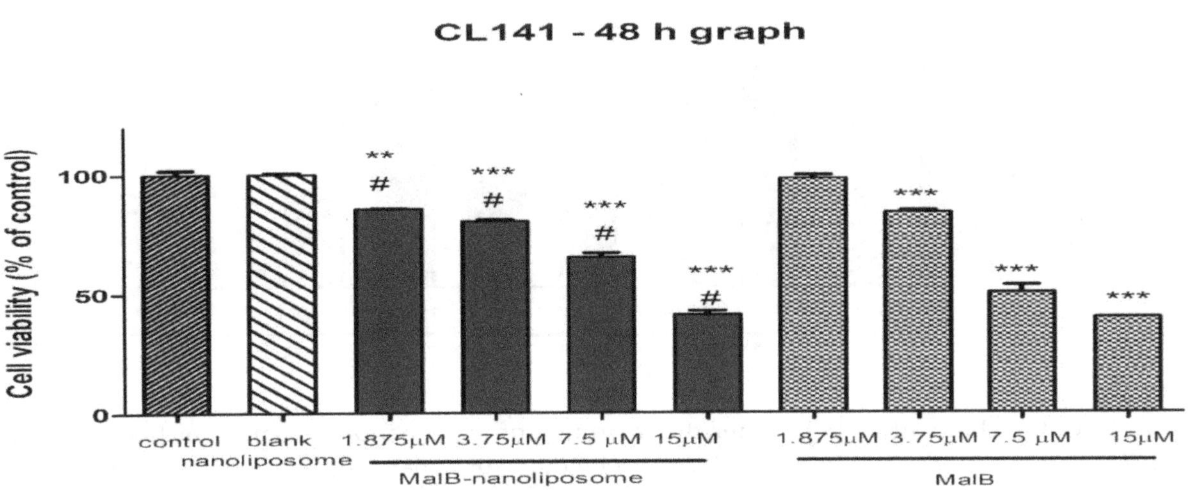

Figure 2. *Cont.*

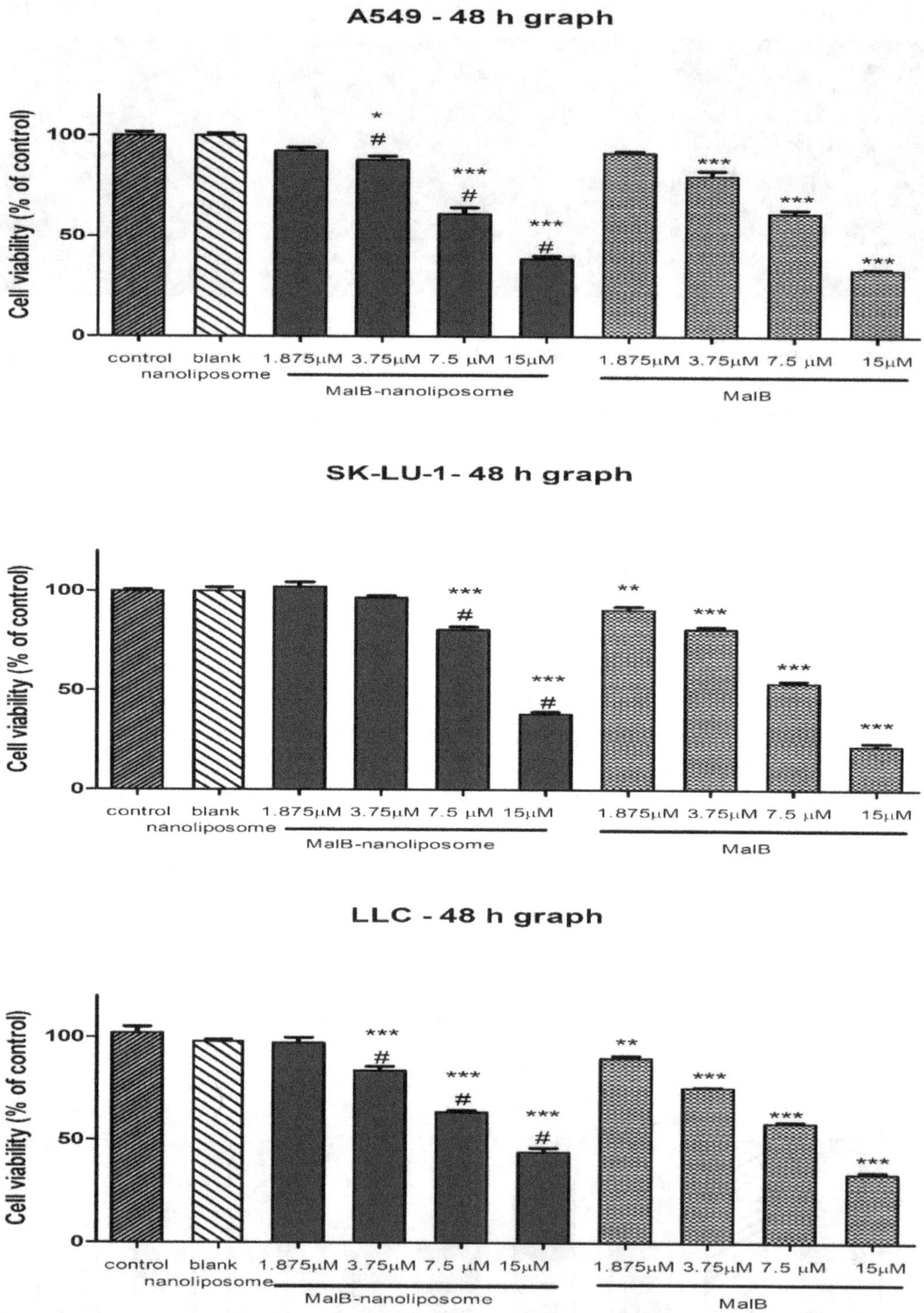

Figure 2. Cell viability after 48 h under the treatment of malB-nanoliposome C or free compound on different lung cancer cell lines. Cultured cells (2×10^3 cells/well) were treated with different concentrations of either malB-nanoliposomal or free malB. Normal saline served as the negative control. Each value represents the mean ± SEM. One-way ANOVA was used for analyzing statistical differences between groups. * $p < 0.05$, ** $p < 0.01$, *** $p < 0.001$ when compared with negative control. # $p < 0.01$ when compared with blank liposome.

Table 3. Cytotoxic activities of malB-nanoliposomes and untrapped compound malB on different lung cancer cell lines.

Samples	IC_{50} Values (μM)			
	SK-LU-1	**LLC**	**CL141**	**A549**
MalB compound	8.67 ± 0.89	9.59 ± 0.52	9.81 ± 0.81	10.35 ± 0.32
MalB-nanoliposomes	13.12 ± 1.47	12.35 ± 1.45	12.24 ± 1.38	11.86 ± 0.99
Blank nanoliposomes	NA	NA	NA	NA

Note: NA means not available.

3.3. *Inhibition of Colony Formation malB–Nanoliposome Complex*

One of the most important characteristics of cancer is self-renewal ability, which allows tumor cells to proliferate and grow from a single cancer stem cell (CSC). To evaluate the effects of malB and malB-nanoliposomes on cellular self-renewal, a colony-forming assay was performed on the A549 cell line, cells of which were able to form colonies in vitro. The outcome after 8 days of treatment showed that both malB-liposomes and free malB decreased the numbers of colonies derived from A549 cells (Figure 3). The number of colonies decreased markedly at 5 μM and 2.5 μM malB in comparison to the controls. However, a lower concentration of malB had a minimal effect on the number of colonies. In addition, malB-nanoliposome C also inhibited colony formation by >50% at concentrations of 5 μM and 2.5 μM. The IC_{50} values of malB and malB-nanoliposomes were calculated as 2.28 μM and 1.75 μM, respectively. These inhibitory activities of the compound in both forms were significant compared to the control ($p < 0.001$). The results suggested that malB encapsulated in nanoliposomes had a stronger inhibitory effect on the formation of A549 lung adenocarcinomas than the free form. In addition, the effects of free malB and malB-nanoliposomes were different as the concentration increased. In detail, at the same dose of 0.75 μM, malB-nanoliposomes inhibited the formation of A549 colonies by up to 40.66%, whereas the free malB showed only 17.21% inhibition of A549 colony formation. The same was also true at a dose of 1.25 μM.

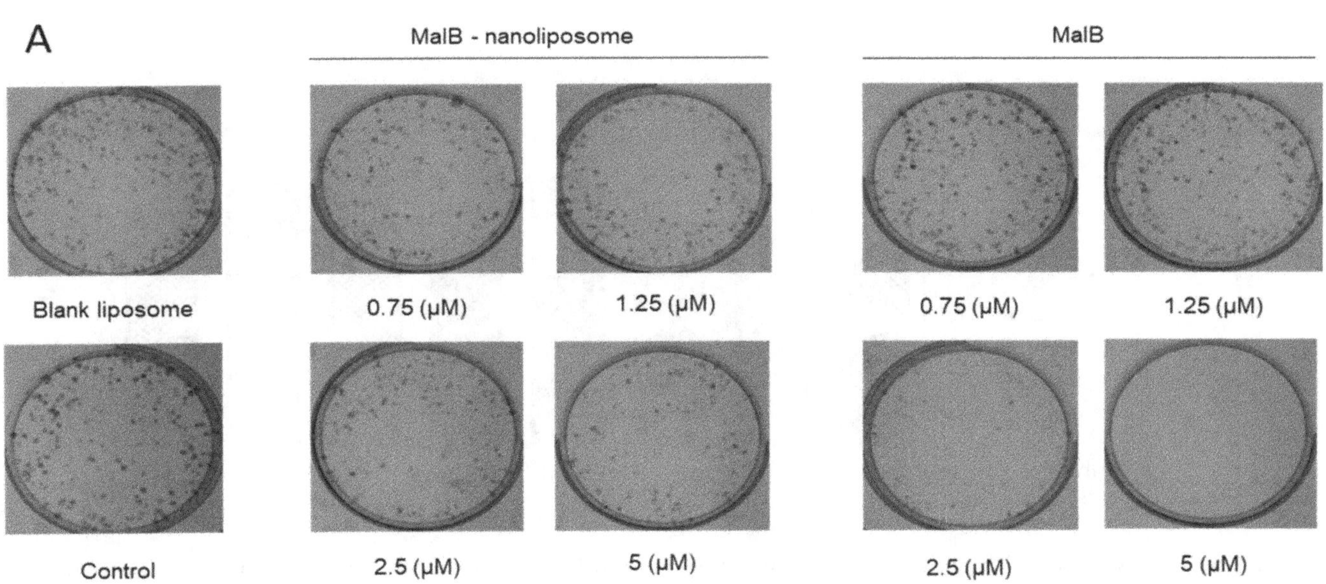

Figure 3. *Cont.*

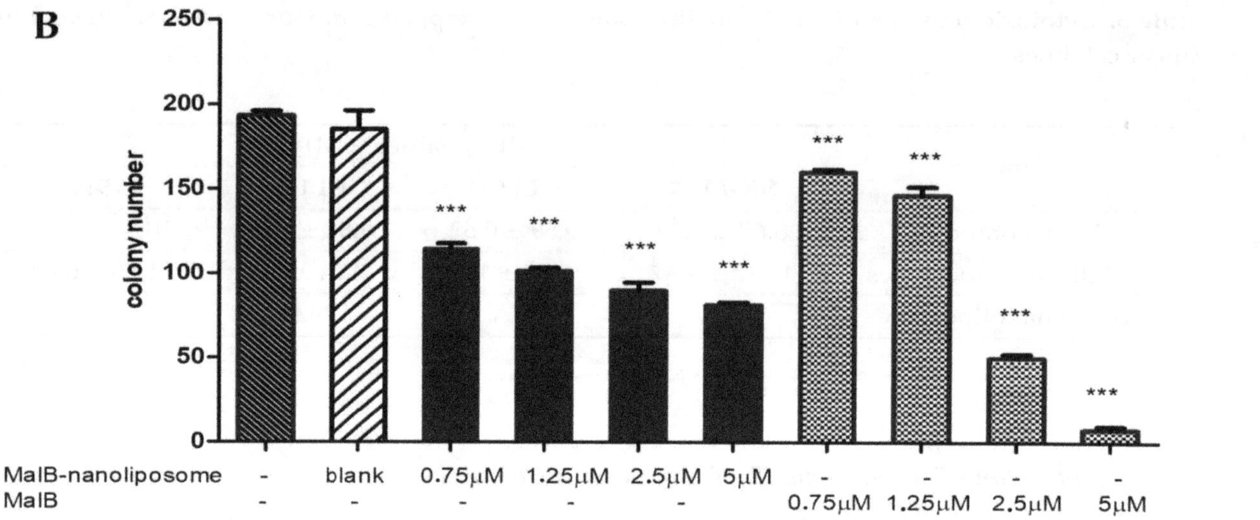

Figure 3. Antitumorigenic activity of malB-nanoliposome and free compound on A549 cells. (**A**) Colony images after treatment of malB-nanoliposome and free-compound at different concentrations compared to the negative control (normal saline) and blank liposome on day 8. (**B**) Colony number after treated with blank nanoliposome, malB-nanoliposome, and malB compared to the negative control. Each value represents the mean ± SEM. *** $p < 0.001$.

3.4. Caspase 3 Inductive Activities of malB and malB-Nanoliposome

Caspase 3 is a typical enzyme related to the apoptosis of mammalian cells. To determine the apoptosis-inducing activity of malB and malB-liposomes, caspase 3 activity was measured under conditions of treatment with the free compound or its nanoliposomes using a caspase 3 colorimetric kit. As shown in Figure 4, malB and structure C malB-nanoliposomes significantly increased the changes in caspase 3 activity at doses of 10 μM and 5 μM in comparison with the control ($p < 0.01$ and $p < 0.05$, respectively). However, no significant differences in caspase 3 induction were observed between malB and malB-nanoliposomes.

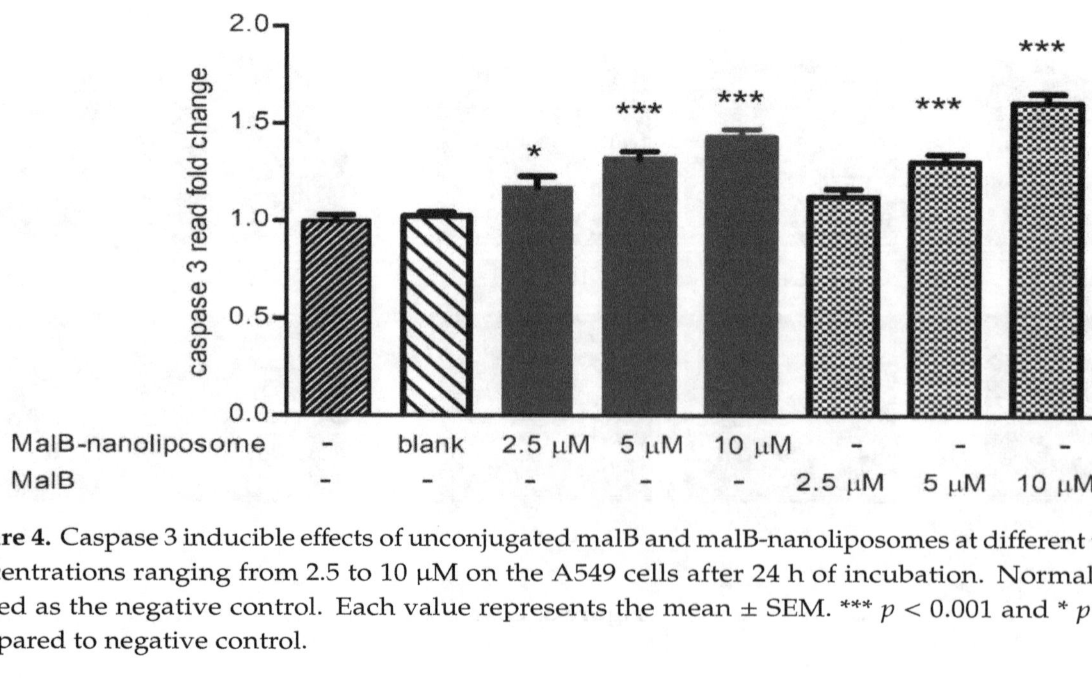

Figure 4. Caspase 3 inducible effects of unconjugated malB and malB-nanoliposomes at different treated concentrations ranging from 2.5 to 10 μM on the A549 cells after 24 h of incubation. Normal saline served as the negative control. Each value represents the mean ± SEM. *** $p < 0.001$ and * $p < 0.05$ compared to negative control.

3.5. Tumor Inhibition Activity

The antitumor activity of malB-liposomes was examined in the LLC tumor model in BALB/c mice. MalB and malB-liposome had no significant change in body weight of mice at both initial time and the end time of treatment (Figure 5). As shown in Figure 6, animals treated with free malB at a concentration of 5 mg/kg body weight (b.w.) did not show a significant reduction in tumor size compared to negative controls. However, malB-nanoliposomes significantly inhibited tumor growth at the same concentration (5 mg/kg b.w.) ($p < 0.05$). After 28 days of treatment with malB-nanoliposomes, the tumor size was decreased by 37.03% compared to the saline-treated negative control, whereas the free form reduced the tumor size by only 13.09%. When the concentration was decreased, the tumor suppression effect of malB-nanoliposomes was markedly reduced and was not significant compared with the control. Moreover, blank liposome did not affect the tumors' growth at any tested time points.

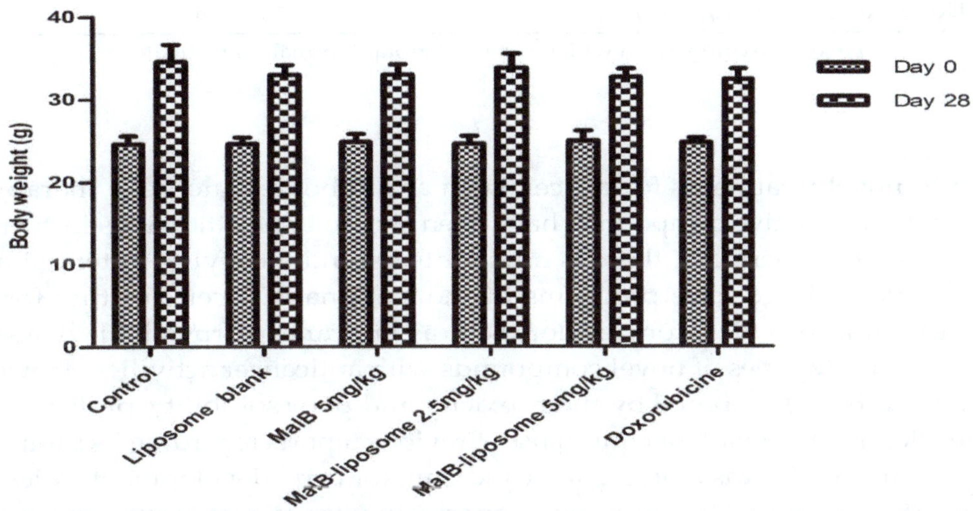

Figure 5. Effects of malB or malB-nanoliposomes on body weight of BALB/c mice harboring a malignant tumor induced by LLC cells ($n = 6$). Error bars represent standard error of the mean (SEM).

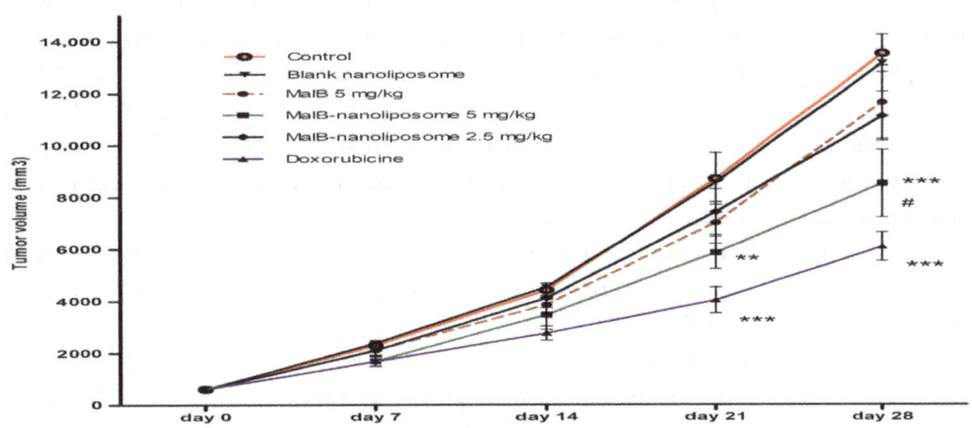

Figure 6. Anti-tumor effects of malB or malB-nanoliposomes on BALB/c mice harboring a malignant tumor induced by LLC cells ($n = 6$). Liposome-conjugated malB at the dose 5.0 mg/kg b.w. significantly inhibited tumor growth after 21 and 28 days compared with the negative control (normal saline treated) (** $p < 0.01$ and *** $p < 0.005$, respectively). # $p < 0.05$ compared to the free malB at the same dose. Error bars represent standard error of the mean (SEM).

In addition, the administration of malB-nanoliposomes prolonged the survival of the mice but still insignificantly ($p > 0.05$) (Table 4). The median survival of mice treated with the malB-nanoliposomal formulation was 32.20 ± 0.97 days, which was 6.62% longer than that of control mice. Survival was also increased slightly (31.00 ± 0.84 days) in the free malB-treated group at the treated dose.

Table 4. Effect of malB-nanoliposome and free malB on survival time of LLC-induced tumor-bearing mice from different experimented groups (mean ± SEM) ($n = 6$).

Groups	Mean Survival Time (Days)	% ILS
Control group (normal saline)	30.20 ± 0.86	-
Blank nanoliposome	30.67 ± 0.80	1.56
malB free (5 mg/kg b.w.)	31.00 ± 0.84	2.65
malB-nanoliposomes (2.5 mg/kg b.w.)	31.20 ± 0.86	3.31
malB-nanoliposomes (5 mg/kg b.w.)	32.20 ± 0.97	6.62
Doxorubicin (5 mg/kg b.w.)	36.20 * ± 0.86	19.86

* $p < 0.05$ in comparison with the control group (normal saline treated).

4. Discussion

In addition to novel treatments for cancer, such as antibodies and gene therapy, a number of drugs based on natural bioactive compounds have been shown to be efficacious in chemotherapy and the prevention of cancer. Therefore, there is much interest in identifying potential new anticancer compounds, such as the large-scale programs of the National Cancer Institute for the discovery and screening of natural products for development as anticancer drugs [11]. These studies have identified a number of categories of novel compounds with anticancer activities. However, the use of these compounds has been hampered by their toxicity and poor solubility, problems that have also prevented the development of malB for clinical use. Previous reports regarding its promising anticancer activities suggested that malB was a promising candidate for drug development. Microarray analysis demonstrated that this compound has anticancer capacity in vitro by regulating gene expression similar to the commercial anticancer drug, withanolide A [12]. This compound was also shown to inhibit the activation of NF-κB with an IC_{50} value in the range of 3.5–5.0 μM [3,5]. The compound affected NF-κB activation by inhibiting the activation of IκB kinase (IKK) [6]. However, malB shows high toxicity and is insoluble, which has limited its pharmaceutical applications. The use of nanoliposomal carriers for drug design to reduce toxicity and enhance the bioavailability of natural compounds is appropriate for anticancer drug development. Drugs packed into liposomes show improved blood circulation activity, promotion of deposition in tumors, protection from metabolism, direct distribution of the drug into tumors, as well as enhanced uptake in adenocarcinoma, mononuclear macrophages, and the intracellular lattice system (liver, spleen, bone marrow). Furthermore, liposomal-encapsulated drugs show reduced uptake in the kidneys, myocardium, and brain tissues [13,14].

In the present study, malB was experimentally incorporated into liposomal nanocarriers. The nanoliposomes containing malB were small unilamellar vesicles <200 nm in diameter with a slight negative charge and low PDI. Magin reported that nanoliposomes in the size range of 50–200 nm would be the most suitable for liposomal stability in the body [15–17]. However, liposomes containing cholesterol had much lower EE in comparison with the non-cholesterol formulations. Similar results were reported previously for some lipophilic drugs, such as ciprofloxacin [18] and dexamethasone [19], as well as natural compounds, such as ascorbic acid [20]. Cholesterol molecules are normally located in the space between lipid bilayer membranes. Therefore, it was supposed that cholesterol competed out malB molecules and some positions in the bilayers were occupied, preventing successful incorporation of the test compound. Furthermore, cholesterol makes the bilayer more rigid, which would make the incorporation of malB molecules difficult. In this study, the addition of cholesterol caused a noticeable decrease in EE, which was taken to indicate that EE depends on the normal structure of the liposomal bilayer [21].

The investigation of liposomal stability in this study showed that malB-nanoliposomes were stable at 4 °C in PBS for approximately 30 days, as the average size of the liposomes was still <200 nm and they had a slight negative charge. However, the PDI of liposomes was significantly increased at around 30 days to almost twice that on day 1 (data not shown). The PDI parameter is an indicator of whether the formed liposomes are monodispersed and have an average size distribution. The PDI should be as low as possible, as higher PDI indicates a broader size distribution of nanoparticles. Thus, the results of the present study suggested that malB-liposomes exhibited an appropriate PDI and this characteristic seems to change after 30 days of storage at 4 °C in PBS.

With regard to assessment of bioactivity, malB encapsulated in nanoliposomes still showed strong anticancer activities in vitro that were comparable to those of the free form. Indeed, the nanoliposomal formulation inhibited cancer cell survival after 48 h with IC_{50} values ranging from 11.86 to 13.12 μM, which was slightly higher than that of free malB (8.67 – 10.35 μM). However, the anti-clonogenic activity of malB-nanoliposomes was more obvious than that of the free compound in the A549 colony-forming assay. In addition, malB and malB-nanoliposomes affected the activity of caspase 3, a crucial protease that mediates apoptosis. This caspase catalyzes the specific cleavage of many key cellular proteins, and plays an important role in apoptotic chromatin condensation and DNA fragmentation [22,23]. The significant caspase 3 induction and activation by malB and malB-nanoliposomes, which contributed to both intrinsic and extrinsic apoptotic pathways, were reported here for the first time.

Furthermore, the improved cytotoxic and antitumorigenic effects of malB-nanoliposomes were also verified in tumor-bearing mice. The malB-nanoliposomes showed the ability to effectively inhibit tumor growth in comparison with negative controls as well as with free malB at the same concentration of 5 mg/kg. There have been many studies on loading of potential anticancer agents into nanoliposomes to improve their activities. Those studies showed that the encapsulation of drugs into liposomes reduces toxicity, improves bioactivity, and increases the circulation time of drugs in the body, leading to increased effectiveness of these drugs in clinical treatment [24]. The intraperitoneal (i.p.) administration of liposomes also has advantages, such as reduction of local toxicity [25]. In addition, when administered by the i.p. route, the drug is absorbed into the organs through the peritoneum or the lymphatic system [26]. Drugs packaged in liposomes could be stable for longer period in the abdominal cavity or in the lymph vessels, thus improving the effectiveness of treatment for peritoneal carcinomas, such as ovarian cancer and liver cancer [27]. However, the uptake of the drug into the blood via the abdominal cavity also depends on the size of the liposomes. Feng reported that liposomes approximately 100 nm in diameter show a high concentration in blood equivalent to intravenous (i.v.) administration, and could therefore be used to treat cancer far from the peritoneum [28]. On the other hand, PEGylation of liposomes plays a central role in prolonging their circulation in the blood. PEGylation helps protect drug-nanoliposomes from mononuclear phagocytes by impeding the absorption of opsonin protein in the circulation on the liposome surface, which would minimize clearance of the drug by these cells [29,30]. The characteristics of PEGylated liposomes allow them to circulate longer in the bloodstream than free drugs, leading to increased effectiveness in cancer treatment. In the present study, the PEG-cholesterol components in the malB-nanoliposome complex may have enhanced the antitumor activity in comparison with the free drug.

5. Conclusions

The results of this study confirmed that malB has the potential for development as an anticancer drug after nanoliposomal encapsulation. The malB-encapsulated formulation had typical characteristics of nanoliposomes, such as size <200 nm, negative charge, and PDI <0.3. The free form of malB and malB-nanoliposomes showed activities against all lung cancer cell lines examined. Both malB forms significantly inhibited colony formation and increased caspase 3 activity of A549 cancer cells. The malB-nanoliposomes showed significantly stronger tumor growth inhibition compared with the free form. The malB-nanoliposomes could slightly prolong the survival period of tumor-bearing mice in comparison with the untreated group.

Author Contributions: Conceptualization, T.T.D.; Methodology, T.N.N., T.P.D., T.C.N., H.P.T., P.T.T.V., and T.A.H.L.; Software, validation, formal analysis, investigation, resources, and data curation, T.N.N. and P.T.T.V.; Writing—original draft preparation: P.T.T.V. and T.N.N.; Writing—review and editing, T.T.D. All authors have read and agreed to the published version of the manuscript.

Acknowledgments: The authors wish to thank Chi-Ying Huang, Lu-Yi Yu, Chun-Liang Lo, Department of Biomedical Engineering, National Yang-Ming University, Taipei, Taiwan, for their kind guidance and their support with all equipment, especially the Jeol 1200EX Transmission Electronic Microscope (TEM system) (Jeol Ltd., Japan).

References

1. Bray, F.; Ferlay, J.; Soerjomataram, I.; Siegel, R.L.; Torre, L.A.; Jemal, A. Global cancer statistics 2018: GLOBOCAN estimates of incidence and mortality worldwide for 36 cancers in 185 countries. *CA Cancer J. Clin.* **2018**, *68*, 394–424. [CrossRef]
2. Kim, J.S.; Cho, M.S.; Nam, J.H.; Kim, H.-J.; Choi, K.-W.; Ryu, J.-S. Prognostic impact of EGFR mutation in non-small-cell lung cancer patients with family history of lung cancer. *PLoS ONE* **2017**, *12*, e0177015. [CrossRef]
3. Van Kiem, P.; Dang, N.H.; Bao, H.V.; Huong, H.T.; Van Minh, C.; Lee, J.J.; Kim, Y.H. New cytotoxic benzopyrans from the leaves ofMallotus apelta. *Arch. Pharm. Res.* **2005**, *28*, 1131–1134. [CrossRef]
4. Van Luu, C.; Van Chau, M.; Lee, J.-J.; Jung, S.-H. Exploration of essential structure of malloapelta B for the inhibitory activity against TNF induced NF-κB activation. *Arch. Pharmacal Res.* **2006**, *29*, 840–844. [CrossRef]
5. Nam, N.H.; Dang, N.H.; Van Kiem, P.; Van Chinh, L.; Binh, P.T.; La Dinh, M.; Van Minh, C. Study on benzopyrans and other isolated compounds from *Mallotus apelta*. *J. Chem.* **2007**, *45*, 111–121.
6. Ma, J.; Shi, H.; Mi, C.; Li, H.L.; Lee, J.J.; Jin, X. Malloapelta B suppresses LPS-induced NF-κB activation and NF-κB-regulated target gene products. *Int. J. Immunopharmacol.* **2015**, *24*, 147–152. [CrossRef] [PubMed]
7. Gurunathan, S.; Kang, M.-H.; Qasim, M.; Kim, J.-H. Nanoparticle-mediated combination therapy: Two-in-one approach for cancer. *Int. J. Mol. Sci.* **2018**, *19*, 3264. [CrossRef] [PubMed]
8. ElBayoumi, T.A.; Torchilin, V.P. Current trends in liposome research. *Methods Mol. Biol.* **2010**, *605*, 1–27.
9. Bangham, A.D.; Horne, R. Negative staining of phospholipids and their structural modification by surface-active agents as observed in the electron microscope. *Adv. Drug Deliv. Rev.* **1964**, *8*, 660-IN10. [CrossRef]
10. Skehan, P.; Storeng, R.; Scudiero, D.; Monks, A.; McMahon, J.; Vistica, D.; Warren, J.T.; Bokesch, H.; Kenney, S.; Boyd, M.R. New colorimetric cytotoxicity assay for anticancer-drug screening. *J. Natl. Cancer Inst.* **1990**, *82*, 1107–1112. [CrossRef]
11. Nobili, S.; Lippi, D.; Witort, E.; Donnini, M.; Bausi, L.; Mini, E.; Capaccioli, S. Natural compounds for cancer treatment and prevention. *Pharmacol. Res.* **2009**, *59*, 365–378. [CrossRef] [PubMed]
12. Thao, D.T.; Phuong, D.T.; Trang, N.T.; Nga, N.T.; Chi, H.Y. Study the anticancer mechanism of the promissing compound 2B2D by using microarray technique. *Vietnam J. Sci. Technol.* **2012**, *50*, 267.
13. Lomis, N.; Westfall, S.; Farahdel, L.; Malhotra, M.; Shum-Tim, D.; Prakash, S. Human serum albumin nanoparticles for use in cancer drug delivery: Process optimization and in vitro characterization. *J. Nanomater.* **2016**, *6*, 116. [CrossRef] [PubMed]
14. Prathyusha, K.; Muthukumaran, M.; Krishnamoorthy, B. Liposomes as targetted drug delivery systems present and future prospectives: A review. *J. Drug Deliv. Ther.* **2013**, *3*, 195–201. [CrossRef]
15. Lin, C.-M.; Li, C.-S.; Sheng, Y.-J.; Wu, D.T.; Tsao, H.-K. Size-dependent properties of small unilamellar vesicles formed by model lipids. *Langmuir* **2012**, *28*, 689–700. [CrossRef] [PubMed]
16. Olusanya, T.O.; Haj Ahmad, R.R.; Ibegbu, D.M.; Smith, J.R.; Elkordy, A.A.J.M. Liposomal drug delivery systems and anticancer drugs. *Molecules* **2018**, *23*, 907. [CrossRef]
17. Magin, R.L.; Hunter, J.M.; Niesman, M.R.; Bark, G.A. Effect of vesicle size on the clearance, distribution, and tumor uptake of temperature-sensitive liposomes. *Cancer Drug Deliv.* **1986**, *3*, 223–237. [CrossRef]
18. Hosny, K.M. Ciprofloxacin as ocular liposomal hydrogel. *AASP PharmSciTech* **2010**, *11*, 241–246. [CrossRef]
19. Tsotas, V.-A.; Mourtas, S.; Antimisiaris, S.G. Dexamethasone incorporating liposomes: Effect of lipid composition on drug trapping efficiency and vesicle stability. *Drug Deliv.* **2007**, *14*, 441–445. [CrossRef]

20. Tabandeh, H.; Mortazavi, S.A. An investigation into some effective factors on encapsulation efficiency of alpha-tocopherol in MLVs and the release profile from the corresponding liposomal gel. *Iran J. Pharm. Res.* **2013**, *12*, 21.
21. Epand, R.M.; Epand, R.F.; Maekawa, S. The arrangement of cholesterol in membranes and binding of NAP-22. *Chem. Phys. Lipids* **2003**, *122*, 33–39. [CrossRef]
22. Porter, A.G.; Jänicke, R.U. Emerging roles of caspase-3 in apoptosis. *Cell Death Differ.* **1999**, *6*, 99–104. [CrossRef] [PubMed]
23. Chang, H.Y.; Yang, X. Proteases for Cell Suicide: Functions and Regulation of Caspases. *Microbiol. Mol. Biol. Rev.* **2000**, *64*, 821–846. [CrossRef]
24. Allen, T.M.; Cullis, P.R. Liposomal drug delivery systems: From concept to clinical applications. *Adv. Drug Deliv. Rev.* **2013**, *65*, 36–48. [CrossRef] [PubMed]
25. De Smet, L.; Ceelen, W.; Remon, J.P.; Vervaet, C. Optimization of drug delivery systems for intraperitoneal therapy to extend the residence time of the chemotherapeutic agent. *Sci. World J.* **2013**, *2013*, 720858. [CrossRef] [PubMed]
26. Al Shoyaib, A.; Archie, S.R.; Karamyan, V.T. Intraperitoneal Route of Drug Administration: Should it Be Used in Experimental Animal Studies? *J. Pharm. Res.* **2020**, *37*, 12. [CrossRef] [PubMed]
27. Mirahmadi, N.; Babaei, M.; Vali, A.; Dadashzadeh, S. Effect of liposome size on peritoneal retention and organ distribution after intraperitoneal injection in mice. *Int. J. Pharm.* **2010**, *383*, 7–13. [CrossRef] [PubMed]
28. Feng, J.; Iyer, A.; Seo, Y.; Broaddus, C.; Liu, B.; VanBrocklin, H.; He, J. Effects of size and targeting ligand on biodistribution of liposome nanoparticles in tumor mice. *J. Nucl. Med.* **2013**, *54*, 1339.
29. Singhania, A.; Wu, S.Y.; McMillan, N.A. Effective delivery of PEGylated siRNA-containing lipoplexes to extraperitoneal tumours following intraperitoneal administration. *J. Drug Deliv.* **2011**, *2011*, 192562. [CrossRef]
30. Mohamed, M.; Abu Lila, A.S.; Shimizu, T.; Alaaeldin, E.; Hussein, A.; Sarhan, H.A.; Szebeni, J.; Ishida, T. PEGylated liposomes: Immunological responses. *Sci. Technol. Adv. Mater.* **2019**, *20*, 710–724. [CrossRef]

4

Novel Homo-Bivalent and Polyvalent Compounds Based on Ligustrazine and Heterocyclic Ring as Anticancer Agents

Jiawen Wang [1,†], Ge Hong [2,3,†], Guoliang Li [2], Wenzhi Wang [2] and Tianjun Liu [1,2,3,*]

1 Graduate Institute, Tianjin University of Traditional Chinese Medicine, Tianjin 301617, China; m13260192393@163.com

2 Tianjin Key Laboratory of Biomedical Materials, Institute of Biomedical Engineering, Chinese Academy of Medical Sciences & Peking Union Medical College, Tianjin 300192, China; hongge6688@aliyun.com (G.H.); liguoliangsx@163.com (G.L.); wxwnx123@163.com (W.W.)

3 State Key Laboratory of Bioactive Substances and Functions of Natural Medicines, Institute of Materia Medica, Chinese Academy of Medical Sciences and Peking Union Medical College, Beijing 100050, China

* Correspondence: Liutj@bme.org.cn

† These authors contributed equally to this work.

Academic Editor: Qiao-Hong Chen

Abstract: Bivalent and polyvalent inhibitors can be used as antitumor agents. In this experiment, eight ligustrazine dimers and seven ligustrazine tetramers linked by alkane diamine with different lengths of carbon chain lengths were synthesized. After screening their antiproliferation activities against five cancer cell lines, most ligustrazine derivatives showed better cytotoxicity than the ligustrazine monomer. In particular, ligustrazine dimer **8e** linked with decane-1,10-diamine exhibited the highest cytotoxicity in FaDu cells with an IC_{50} (50% inhibiting concentration) value of 1.36 nM. Further mechanism studies suggested that **8e** could induce apoptosis of FaDu cells through the depolarization of mitochondrial membrane potential and S-phase cell cycle arrest. Inspired by these results, twenty-seven additional small molecule heterocyclic dimers linked with decane-1,10-diamine and nine cinnamic acid dimers bearing ether chain were synthesized and screened. Most monocyclic and bicyclic aromatic systems showed highly selective anti-proliferation activity to FaDu cells and low toxicity to normal MCF 10A cells. The structure-activity relationship revealed that the two terminal amide bonds and the alkyl linker with a chain length of 8–12 carbon were two important factors to maintain its antitumor activity. In addition, the ADMET calculation predicted that most of the potent compounds had good oral bioavailability.

Keywords: bivalency; polyvalency; antitumor; apoptosis; cell cycle

1. Introduction

Natural products play a vital role in the development of the drug, especially anticancer drugs [1]. Ligustrazine (2,3,5,6-tetramethylpyrazine, TMP), an important component of the Chinese traditional medicinal herb Chuanxiong (*Ligusticum chuanxiong Hort)*, has been of wide clinical use for cardiovascular and cerebrovascular diseases [2]. Recently, TMP has been reported to possess anticancer activity in vitro and in vivo, inducing cancer cell apoptosis and cell cycle modulation [3,4]. More importantly, the introduction of different substituted groups into ligustrazine has helped to improve the antitumor activity. Many ligustrazine derivatives with potent antitumor activity have been developed in the past few years, like monocarbonyl ligustrazine-curcumin hybrids [5], ligustrazine-betulinic acid hybrids [6], and ligustrazine-rhein derivatives [7]. This advancement stimulated our interest in using TMP as the scaffold to synthesize new antitumor agents.

In the interaction between host and guest molecules, both bivalency and polyvalency could enhance the affinity and activity of monovalent ligand [8,9]. This phenomenon has attracted attention in drug design. Many effective bivalent anti-cancer drugs have been found, such as artemisinin-derivative dimers [10], jesterone dimer [11], indole-3-carbinol dimer [12], bis-daunorubicin [13]. Previous work in this field has designed and synthesized several ligustrazine dimers linked by cyclohexanone and oxime [14], curcumin [15], or triterpenes [16], which had a good cytotoxic effect on human cancer cells. The result showed that the dimerization of ligustrazine could obviously improve the antitumor potency of its monomer.

With an effort to developing new antitumor agents, we designed and synthesized a series of novel TMP dimers and tetramers linked with different alkyl diamines and screened their anti-proliferation potential on a panel of human cancer cell lines, including HeLa, Hep G2, MCF-7, FaDu, and A549. Based on these experimental results, according to the importance of small molecular heterocyclic rings in drug discovery [17], additional dimers series of aromatic rings instead of ligustrazine, a total of 51 new compounds were synthesized, screened, and their structure-activity relationship was briefly discussed. Meanwhile, through morphological observation and flow cytometric analysis, the antitumor mechanisms of the most potent one were preliminarily discussed in this study. ADMET properties of all compounds were also evaluated to explore the drug-likeness.

2. Results and Discussion

2.1. Chemistry

In this study, 51 novel designed compounds were synthesized. Series **6a–g** and **8a–f** were obtained according to the synthetic method described in Schemes 1 and 2. The important intermediate 2-chloromethyl-3,5,6-trimethyl-pyrazine **5** was prepared from ligustrazine by the tandem reaction: Boekelheide reaction [18] and deprotection and the chlorination reaction [19]. The key intermediate 2-carboxylic acid-3,5,6-trimethyl-pyrazine **7** was synthesized by the one-pot reaction, as previously reported [20]. To explore the length effect, the TMP moieties, with 2–12 methylene alkyl chain as a linker, were synthesized.

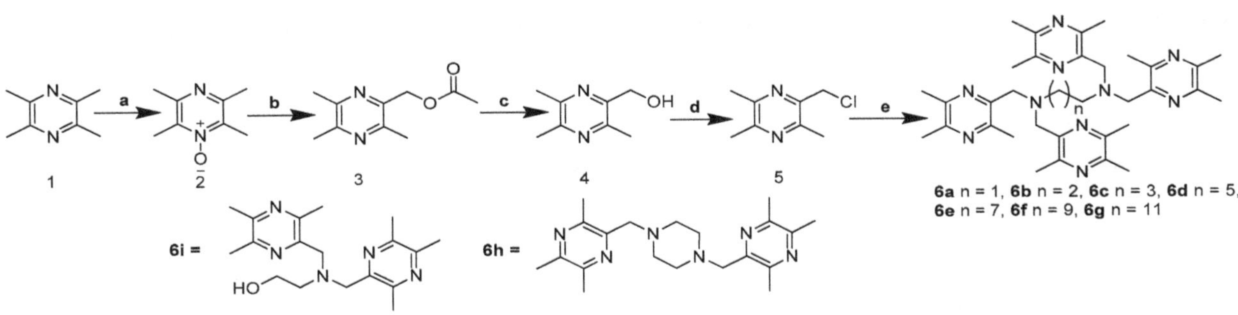

Scheme 1. Synthesis of the TMP complexes **6a–6i**. *Reagents and conditions*: (a) 30% H_2O_2, CH_3COOH, 95 °C, 2 h; (b) $(CH_3CO)_2O$, 140 °C, 2.5 h; (c) CH_3ONa, CH_3OH, r.t., 0.5 h; (d) $SOCl_2$, CH_2Cl_2, r.t., 2.5 h; (e) n-diaminoalkane (piperazine and monoethanolamine), K_2CO_3, CH_3CN, 95 °C, 2 h.

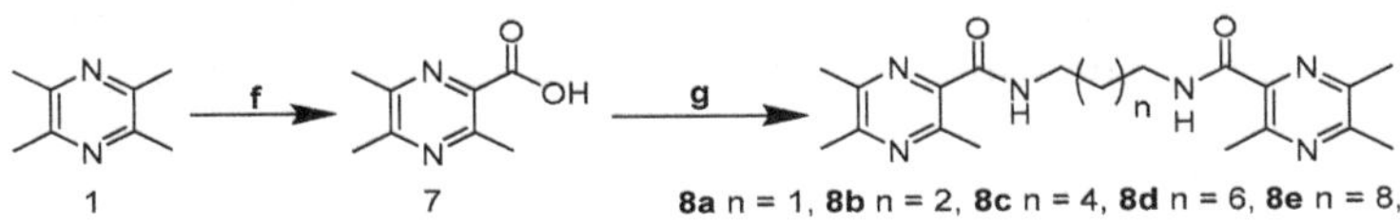

Scheme 2. Synthesis of the Bis-TMP hybrids **8a–8f**. *Reagents and conditions*: (f) $KMnO_4$, H_2O, 37 °C, 24 h; (g) n-diamino-alkane, EDCI/DMAP, r.t., 12 h.

Using heteroaromatic acids with decane-1,10-diamine as raw materials, the target compounds **9e–35e** (outlined in Scheme 3) linked by amide chain were synthesized with EDCI (1-(3-Dimethylaminopropyl)-3-ethylcarbodiimide hydrochloride) and DMAP

(4-Dimethylaminopyridine) in anhydrous CH_2Cl_2 at room temperature. Series **9d**, **9f–l** (shown in Scheme 4) linked by ether chain or amide chain were synthesized by the above method. All the newly synthesized compounds were characterized by ^{1}H-NMR, ^{13}C-NMR, and high-resolution mass spectra (HRMS). Details were provided in the experimental part. The purity of the compounds was over 95% measured by HPLC (Figure 1).

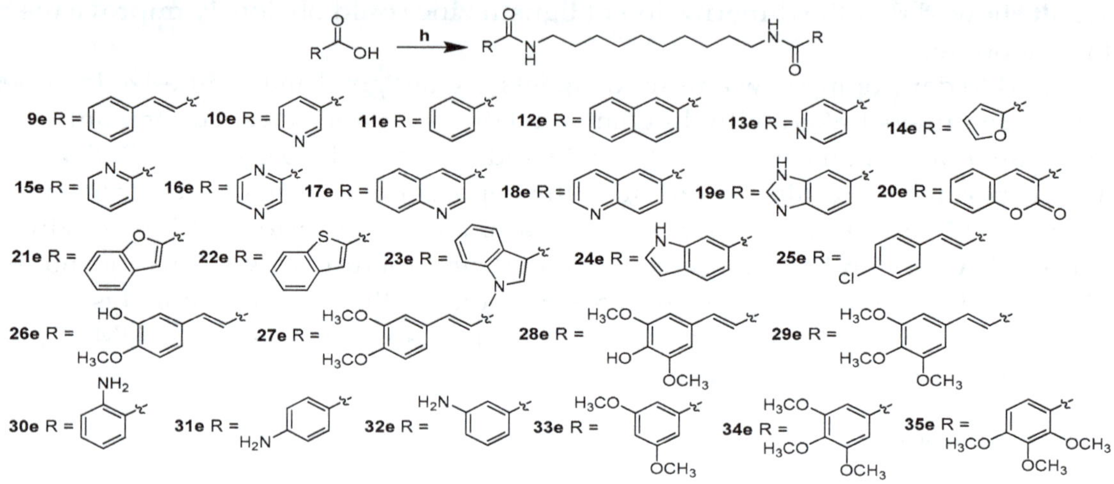

Scheme 3. Synthesis of compounds **9e–35e**. *Reagents and conditions*: (h) decane-1,10-diamine, EDCI/DMAP, r.t., 12 h.

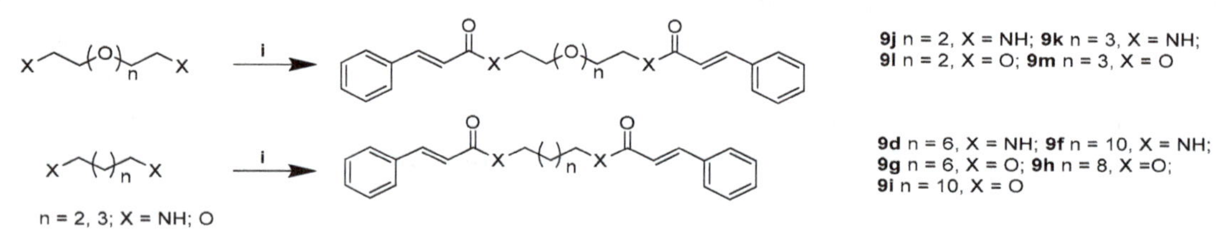

Scheme 4. Synthesis of compounds **9d**, **9f–9m**. *Reagents and conditions*: (i) cinnamic acid, EDCI/DMAP, r.t., 12 h.

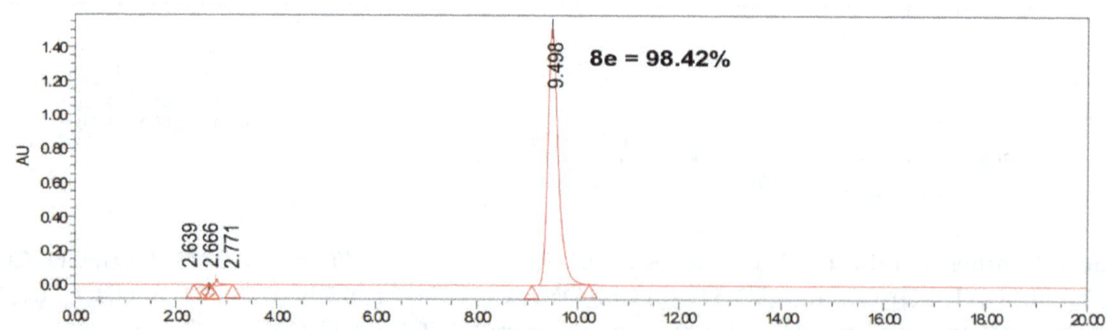

Figure 1. The purity of compound **8e** as a representative analyzed by HPLC (Kromasil C18 column, eluted by methanol/water (80/20) containing 0.1% trifluoroacetic acid at a flow rate of 1 mL/min).

2.2. *Anti-Proliferative Activity In Vitro*

For the newly synthesized compounds, their anti-proliferative activity on human cancer cell lines, HeLa (cervical carcinoma), Hep G2 (hepatoma carcinoma), MCF-7 (breast carcinoma), FaDu (head and neck carcinoma), A549 (lung carcinoma), and normal mammary epithelial cell line MCF 10A, was screened by MTT assay [21] with doxorubicin (DOX) as the positive control. The IC_{50} values of these compounds are summarized in Table 1. Among the ligustrazine derivatives, **6a–g** and **8a–f**, the tetramers **6f** and **6g** had broad-spectrum cytotoxic activities in all cell lines (IC_{50}

6.57–20.83 μM), and the cytotoxicity activities increased with the increase of carbon chain length. The dimeric ligustrazine **8d, 8e, 8f** showed the most promising anticancer activity in most tested tumor cell lines with IC_{50} values between 0.00136 and 6.35 μM, a much better result than DOX and TMP. In particular, compound **8e**, two ligustrazine rings linked with decane-1,10-diamine, exhibited the best anti-proliferative ability in cells (except Hep G2), and compared with other linkers, its IC_{50} values were 1.42 ± 0.71 μM, 0.037 ± 0.001 μM, 0.00136 ± 0.00035 μM, 1.05 ± 0.05 μM, and 0.047 ± 0.008 μM against HeLa, MCF-7, FaDu, A549, and MCF 10A, respectively. In light of these results, we replaced TMP with aromatic heterocycles similar to ligustrazine in electronic space. The novel small aromatic molecule and heterocyclic dimers **9e–35e** were synthesized, and their anti-proliferative ability was evaluated. Compounds **9e, 10e, 11e, 17e, 18e, 21e, 22e, 23e,** and **25e,** aromatic acid dimers (cinnamoyl, nicotinoyl, benzoyl, quinoline-3-carboxyl, quinoline-6-carboxyl, benzofuran-2-carboxyl, benzothiophene-2-carboxyl, indol-3-carboxyl, chlorinated cinnamoyl), were linked by decane-1,10-diamine, which had potent anti-proliferative ability in FaDu or A549 cell lines. Their IC_{50} in FaDu cell lines were less than 1 μM, in the range of 20 nM (benzothiophene-2-carboxyl) and 697 nM (benzofuran-2-carboxyl). Also, they had nearly no toxicity in normal cells like MCF 10A. In series **9d–n**, compounds **9d–f** (IC_{50} < 1 μM), two cinnamic acids linked by C8, C10, C12 chain with two terminal amide bonds, were more effective than compounds **9g–i** (IC_{50} > 20 μM), two cinnamic acids linked by the same alkyl chain with two terminal ester bonds instead of amide bonds. This demonstrated the vital role of two-terminal amide bonds in antitumor activity. Compared with compounds **9d–f**, the inhibition of compounds **9j–m**, two cinnamic acids linked by the similar length ether chain instead of alky chain, was weaker in tumor cells (IC_{50} > 20 μM), which confirmed that the alkyl chain played an important role in the structure. Then, we evaluated the position effect of the substitution at the ortho, meta, or para positions of the same aromatic ring. Compounds **25–35e** and the unsubstituted compounds **9e** and **11e** were all derivatives of cinnamic acid or benzoic acid with different substituents and electronic effects. The results of the compounds **26–27e** or **28–29e** confirmed that the substituents had a general effect on the activity, -OH, $-OCH_3$, $-NH_2$, and other electron donor groups could significantly reduce the activity, with the influence of -OH greater than that of $-OCH_3$. However, the electron attraction group like -Cl (**25e**) had no obvious effect. The compounds with para-substituted analogs (**31e**, para position, IC_{50} = 5.594 μM) exhibited better cell growth inhibitory activities in FaDu cells than ortho- and meta- substituted analogs (**30e**, **32e**, ortho and meta position, IC_{50} > 20 μM). It is worth noting that para $-OCH_3$ substitution could enhance anticancer activity. The IC_{50} value of compound **34e** was 5.853 ± 0.408 μM, the IC_{50} value of para- OCH_3 was half that of the parent compound **33e**, and the IC_{50} value of compound **33e** was 10.393 ± 0.949 μM. Generally, there were three crucial elements in the structure-activity relationship of these systems: alkyl chain linker, two-terminal amide bonds, and heteroaromatic substituents. This SAR (structure-activity relationship) study would help to discover more effective compounds in the future.

To study the selective antiproliferative activities of bivalent and polyvalent inhibitors in normal cells and cancer cell lines, the cytotoxicity of compounds in FaDu cells and normal mammary epithelial MCF 10A cells was measured. The results listed in Table 1 showed that although the ligustrazine dimers **8d** and **8e** had high cytotoxicity in MCF 10A, their IC_{50} values were 2.69 ± 0.46 and 0.047 ± 0.008 μM, while the IC_{50} values in FaDu cells were 110 ± 30 and 1.36 ± 0.035 nM, respectively, which were far lower than that in MCF 10A. The selective index (SI) between MCF10A and Fadu ($IC_{50}^{MCF\ 10A}/IC_{50}^{FaDu}$) was 24.45 and 34.56, respectively. In addition, the heteroaromatic acid dimers **9e–12e, 21e–23e,** and **25e** had the similar activity, which was stronger than doxorubicin in FaDu cells, and had high selectivity in FaDu cells and MCF 10A cells with SI ($IC_{50}^{MCF\ 10A}/IC_{50}^{FaDu}$) values over 28.69. In contrast, the SI ($IC_{50}^{MCF\ 10A}/IC_{50}^{FaDu}$) value of doxorubicin was 0.43. These results encouraged us to further investigate the possible cellular mechanisms.

Table 1. Inhibitory effects of synthetic compounds on the growth of different types of human cancer cells and normal mammary epithelial cells.

Comp.	Antiproliferative Activity $IC_{50} \pm SEM$ (μM)						
	HeLa[a]	**Hep G2[b]**	**MCF-7[c]**	**FaDu[d]**	**A549[e]**	**MCF 10A[f]**	**SI[g]**
6a	>100	>100	>100	>100	>100	90.29 ± 3.41	NC[h]
6b	>100	>100	>100	>100	>100	>100	NC[h]
6c	>100	>100	>100	>100	>100	>100	NC[h]
6d	>100	>100	>100	>100	>100	>100	NC[h]
6e	62.67 ± 4.19	50.77 ± 1.35	66.36 ± 0.05	49.50 ± 1.61	>100	85.44 ± 2.28	1.73
6f	10.16 ± 0.55	10.72 ± 0.22	20.83 ± 0.14	10.94 ± 0.12	20.05 ± 0.41	12.97 ± 0.55	1.19
6g	7.89 ± 0.86	9.62 ± 0.11	9.83 ± 0.17	6.80 ± 0.05	9.23 ± 0.16	6.57 ± 0.30	0.97
6h	>100	>100	>100	>100	>100	>100	NC[h]
6i	>100	>100	>100	>100	>100	>100	NC[h]
8a	>100	>100	>100	>100	>100	>100	NC[h]
8b	>100	>100	>100	>100	>100	>100	NC[h]
8c	>100	>100	>100	80.41 ± 1.36	>100	46.59 ± 0.65	NC[h]
8d	3.31 ± 0.14	>20	0.480 ± 0.003	0.11 ± 0.03	6.35 ± 0.05	2.69 ± 0.46	24.45
8e	1.42 ± 0.71	>20	0.037 ± 0.001	0.00136 ± 0.00035	1.05 ± 0.05	0.047 ± 0.008	34.56
8f	4.96 ± 1.62	>20	0.158 ± 0.009	0.174 ± 0.010	2.46 ± 0.05	0.051 ± 0.021	0.29
9e	>100	>100	>100	0.054 ± 0.002	11.27 ± 0.81	>100	>1851.85
10e	>100	>100	>100	0.25 ± 0.02	2.94 ± 0.25	38.60 ± 2.48	154.40
11e	>100	>100	>100	0.50 ± 0.06	64.30 ± 3.46	80.54 ± 7.60	161.08
12e	>100	>100	>100	1.33 ± 0.07	8.77 ± 0.47	>100	>75.19
13e	>100	>100	>100	48.31 ± 3.17	>100	>100	>2.07
14e	>100	97.75 ± 1.55	>100	6.33 ± 0.65	44.37 ± 0.29	19.82 ± 1.41	3.13
15e	37.74 ± 4.32	26.34 ± 5.36	21.48 ± 1.47	8.85 ± 0.45	23.08 ± 0.12	54.65 ± 5.92	6.18
16e	>100	>100	>100	88.11 ± 1.37	>100	>100	NC[h]
17e	>20	>20	>20	0.236 ± 0.005	>20	>20	>84.75
18e	>20	>20	>20	0.697 ± 0.021	>20	>20	>28.69
19e	>20	>20	>20	8.74 ± 0.44	>20	>20	>2.29
20e	>20	>20	>20	>20	>20	>20	NC[h]
21e	>20	>20	>20	0.665 ± 0.028	>20	>20	>30.08
22e	>20	>20	>20	0.020 ± 0.002	>20	>20	>1000
23e	>20	>20	>20	0.638 ± 0.089	>20	>20	>31.35
24e	>20	>20	>20	5.296 ± 0.366	>20	>20	>3.78
25e	>20	>20	>20	0.056 ± 0.016	>20	>20	>357.14
26e	>20	>20	>20	>20	>20	>20	NC[h]
27e	>20	>20	>20	4.621 ± 0.539	>20	>20	>4.33
28e	>20	>20	>20	>20	>20	>20	NC[h]
29e	>20	>20	>20	5.067 ± 0.461	>20	>20	>3.95
30e	>20	>20	>20	>20	>20	>20	NC[h]
31e	>20	>20	>20	5.594 ± 0.628	>20	>20	>3.58
32e	>20	>20	>20	>20	>20	>20	NC[h]
33e	>20	>20	>20	10.393 ± 0.949	>20	>20	>1.92
34e	>20	>20	>20	5.853 ± 0.408	>20	>20	>3.42
35e	>20	>20	>20	>20	>20	>20	NC[h]
9d	>20	>20	>20	1.054 ± 0.091	>20	>20	>18.98
9f	>20	>20	>20	0.027 ± 0.002	>20	>20	>740.74
9g	>20	>20	>20	>20	>20	>20	NC[h]
9h	>20	>20	>20	>20	>20	>20	NC[h]
9i	>20	>20	>20	>20	>20	>20	NC[h]
9j	>20	>20	>20	>20	>20	>20	NC[h]
9k	>20	>20	>20	4.447 ± 0.208	>20	>20	>4.50
9l	>20	>20	>20	>20	>20	>20	NC[h]
9m	>20	>20	>20	>20	>20	>20	NC[h]
TMP	>100	>100	>100	>100	>100	>100	NC[h]
DOX	11.39 ± 0.48	28.04 ± 1.09	6 ± 0.07	1.27 ± 0.13	>100	0.55 ± 0.03	0.43

[a] HeLa (cervical cancer cell line); [b] Hep G2 (hepatocarcinoma cell line); [c] MCF-7 (breast cancer cell line); [d] FaDu (head and neck squamous carcinoma cell line); [e] A549 (epithelial cancer cell line); [f] MCF 10A (normal mammary epithelial cell); [g] SI: selectivity index. It was calculated as: SI = $IC_{50\ (MCF\ 10A)}/IC_{50\ (FaDu)}$; [h] NC: not calculated.

2.3. *Colony Formation Assay*

As ligustrazine dimer **8e** had the most potent antiproliferative activity in all synthesized compounds, the colony formation assay in FaDu cells was conducted. As shown in Figure 2, FaDu cells treated with compound **8e** at concentrations 0.75 nM, 1.50 nM, 3 nM, 6 nM for 10 days formed smaller and fewer colonies compared to untreated control group, indicating that compound **8e** had a dose-dependent inhibition on the proliferation of FaDu cells, and the colony inhibition rate reached around 85.4% at 6 nM.

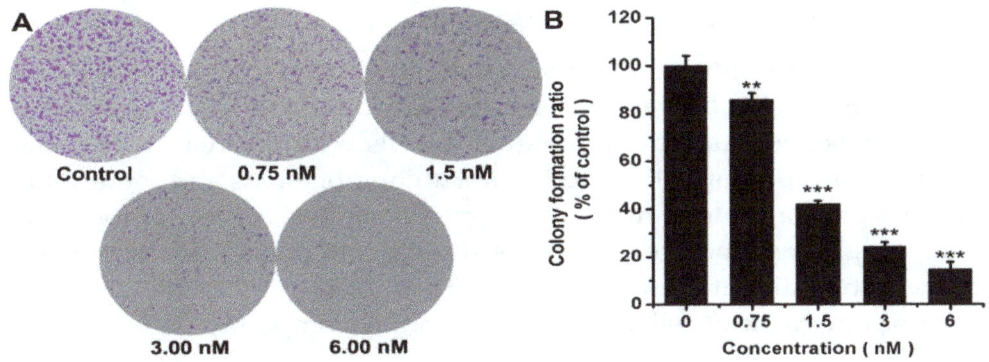

Figure 2. Effect of **8e** on the colony formation in FaDu cells. (**A**) Representative images of FaDu colonies after treatment at the indicated concentrations for 10 days; (**B**) The percentage of colonies compared with control group, $n = 3$. **: $p < 0.01$; ***: $p < 0.001$ versus control.

2.4. Live/Dead Staining

Live-dead double staining experiment was conducted to visually evaluate the cell toxicity of compound **8e**, the most potent one obtained by MTT assay. Propidium iodide (PI)-stained dead cells in red and calcein AM-stained living cells in green. The number of dead cells increased with the dose of **8e** while living cells decreased. Simultaneously, the densities of **8e**-treated cells were much lower than that of the control group. The concentration-dependent loss of FaDu cell viability was consistent with the MTT results (Figure 3).

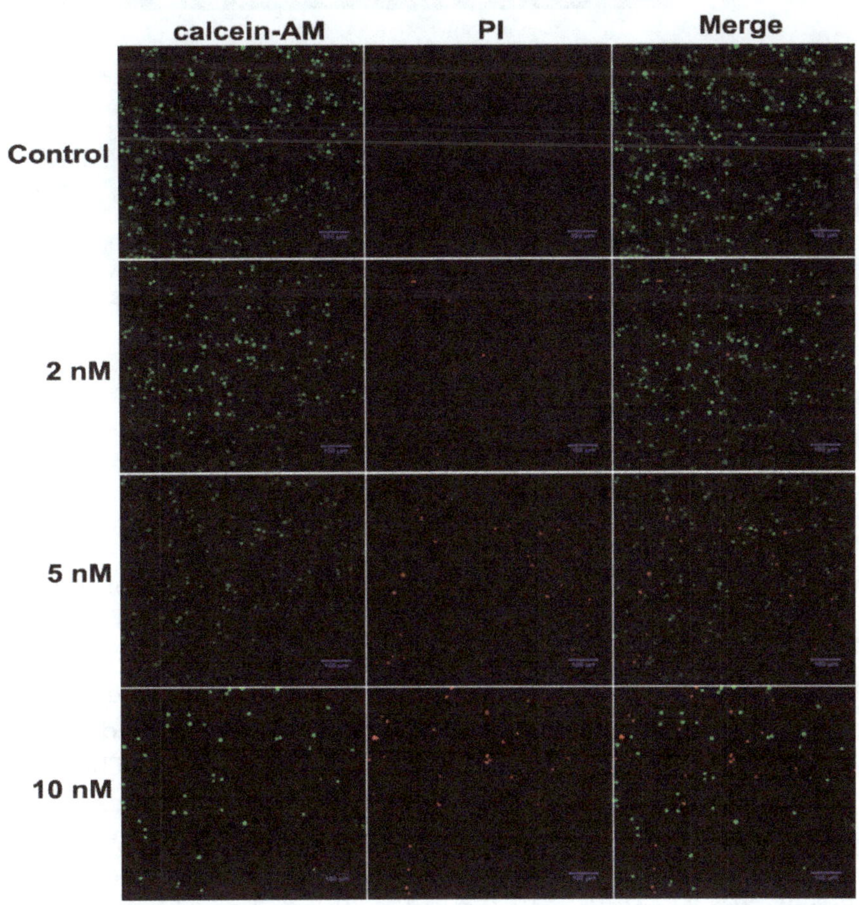

Figure 3. The confocal images of FaDu cells after incubation with compound **8e** at concentrations of 0, 2, 5, and 10 nM for 24 h, respectively. Viable cells were stained in green with Calcein-AM, and dead cells were stained in red with PI. The scale bar was 100 μm.

2.5. Morphological Observation by Hoechst 33,342 Staining

To investigate whether the anti-proliferation behavior of **8e** was related to the apoptosis pathway, the interaction between **8e**- and FaDu cells was analyzed through Hoechst 33,342 staining with a laser scanning confocal microscope. As shown in Figure 4, cells without treatment as the control group exhibited almost negligible apoptotic characteristics with homogenous and round blue-stained nuclei. On the contrary, the typical apoptotic nuclei with irregular nuclear morphology and condensation of chromatin (much brighter stained cells) were observed, and most FaDu cells were shrunken and rounded up from the culture dish after exposure to **8e**. The result demonstrated that inducing apoptosis in FaDu cells might be one cause of cell growth inhibition by compound **8e**.

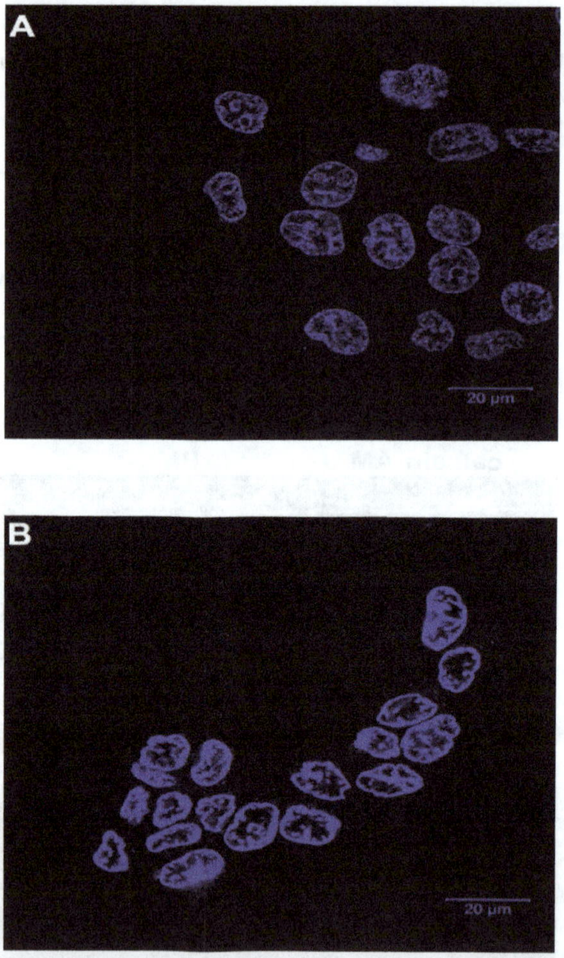

Figure 4. Hoechst staining of FaDu cells treated with compound **8e,** (**A**) Control group; (**B**) 20 nM group.

2.6. Apoptosis Analysis by Annexin V-FITC/PI Staining

To substantiate whether the cell death induced by the ligustrazine dimer **8e** was associated with apoptosis, the interaction of FaDu cells with **8e** was further analyzed by an annexin V-FITC/PI staining, and the apoptosis ratios were quantitated by flow cytometry. The cells were divided into four quadrants: Q1 represented necrotic cells (annexin V^-/PI^+), Q2 represented late apoptotic cells (annexin V^+/PI^+), Q3 represented early apoptotic cells (annexin V^+/PI^-), Q4 represented living cells (annexin V^-/PI^-). As shown in Figure 5, after being exposed to different concentrations of **8e** (2, 5, 10 nM) for 24 h in FaDu cells, the apoptotic cells (including the early and late apoptosis ratios) increased gradually from 8.23% of the control to 34.2%, 57.7%, 79.5%, respectively. The results revealed that **8e** could induce FaDu cells' apoptosis in a dose-dependent manner. This was consistent with other reports showing TMP and its derivatives could induce apoptosis of cancer cells [22–24].

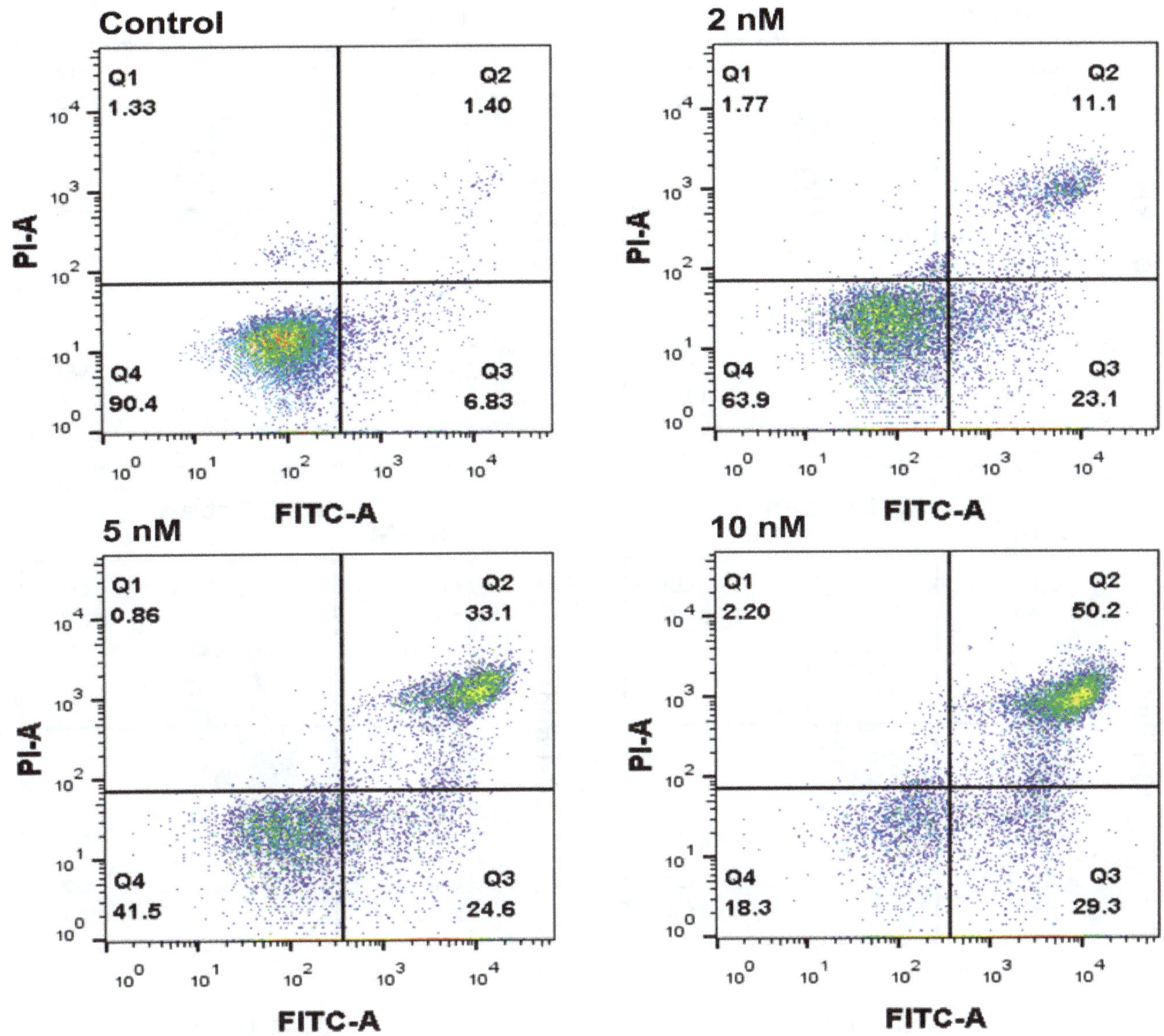

Figure 5. Flow cytometry analysis of apoptosis using annexin V-FITC/PI double staining in FaDu cells treated with compound **8e** at the indicated concentrations for 24 h. The percentage of cells was given in the respective quadrants.

2.7. Mitochondrial Membrane Potential (ΔΨm) Analysis

Mitochondria play an essential role in cell apoptotic progression by regulating mitochondrial membrane potential (ΔΨm). Depolarization of ΔΨm is considered an indicator of cell apoptosis [25]. To better understand the mechanism of **8e**-induced FaDu cells apoptosis, the depolarization of ΔΨm was quantitated by JC-1 (tetraethylbenzimidazolylcarbocyanine iodide) dye. As a mitochondrial-specific dual-fluorescence probe, JC-1 selectively entered the mitochondria. In healthy cells with high ΔΨm, it accumulated in the mitochondrial matrix as J-aggregates with red fluorescence, while in the reduced ΔΨm cells, it remained in the cytoplasm as a monomer with green fluorescence. The change of ΔΨm could be easily detected by the change of fluorescence color. Flow cytometric analysis of FaDu cells treated with different concentrations of **8e** (2, 5, 10 nM) for 24 h revealed that the ratio of green to red fluorescence was significantly higher than that of the control group in a concentration-dependent manner, indicating that the number of lower ΔΨm cells increased (Figure 6). These results suggested that **8e** could induce apoptosis of FaDu cells by decreasing ΔΨm.

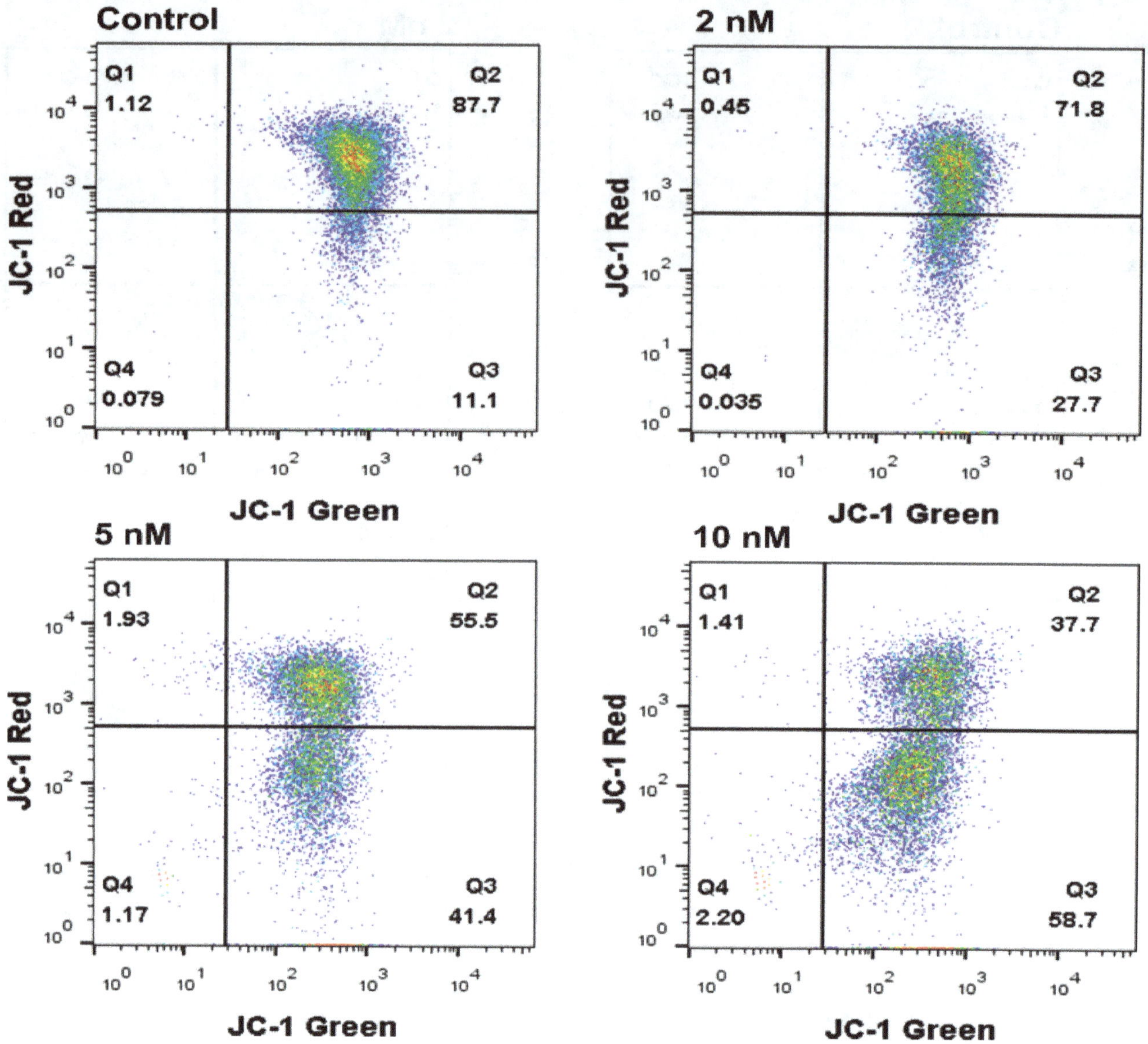

Figure 6. Flow cytometry analysis of the mitochondrial membrane potential using the JC-1 (tetraethylbenzimidazolylcarbocyanine iodide) dye in FaDu cells treated with compound **8e** at the indicated concentrations for 24 h. The percentage of cells was given in the respective quadrants.

2.8. Cell Cycle Analysis

In order to investigate whether **8e** induced cell cycle disturbances in FaDu cells, the flow cytometric analysis was performed with PI staining. The fluorescence intensity was proportional to the content of double-stranded DNA. The separation of cells in G0/G1, S, and G2/M was based upon the distribution of DNA content. Cytometric profiles of the PI-stained DNA showed that after being treated with **8e** at different concentrations (2, 5, 10 nM) for 24 h, the cell cycle of FaDu cells was arrested. As shown in Figure 7, the percentage of cells in the S phase (33.7%, 44.3%, and 54.7%) was markedly improved compared with the control group (28.1%), and this effect was concentration-dependent in FaDu cells. The population of the G0/G1 phase decreased from 51.9% to 41.8%, 44.2%, and 32.4%, respectively. These data indicated that **8e** significantly arrested cell cycle at S phase. This was different from the previously reported cell cycle arrest in the G0/G1 phase induced by TMP [4], which revealed that the dimerization of TMP could change the modulation of the cell cycle of its monomer.

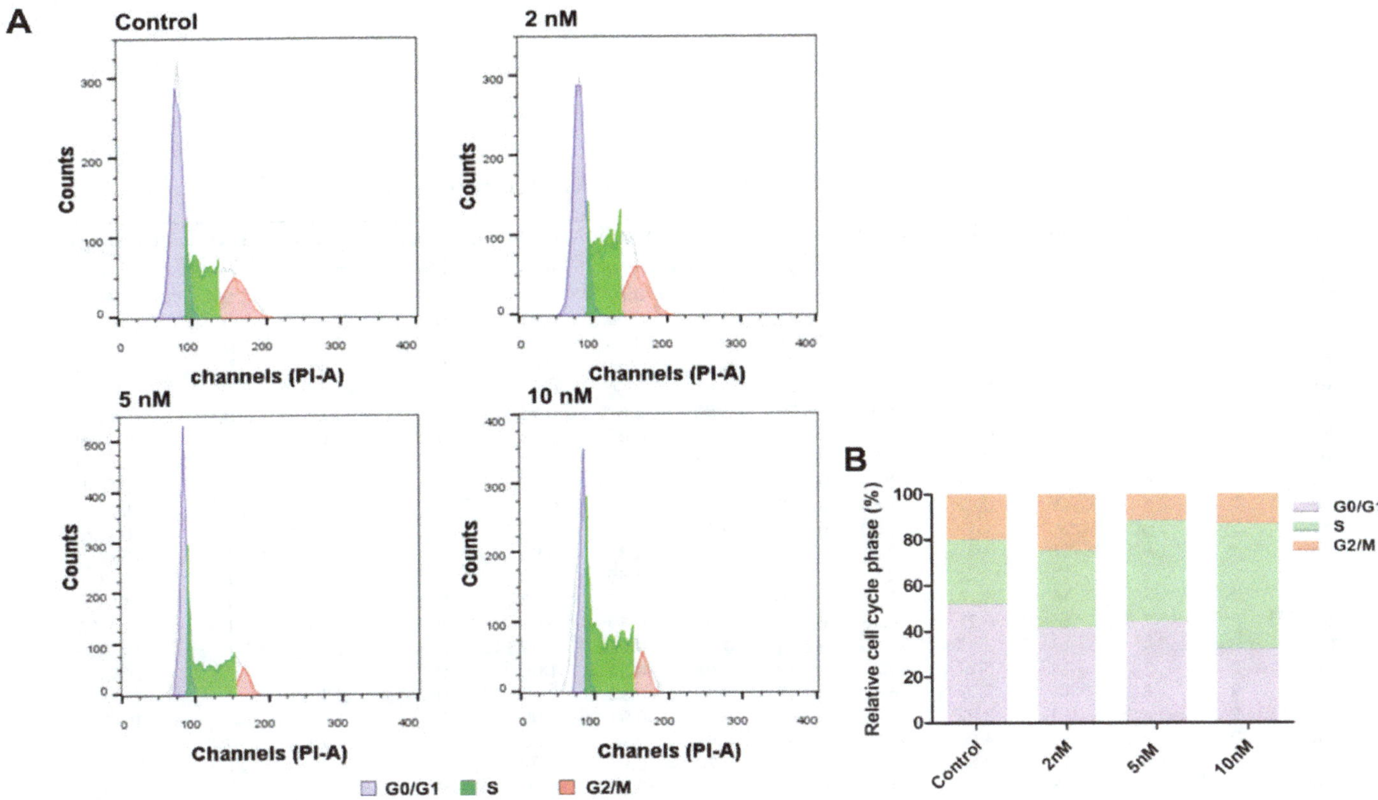

Figure 7. Flow cytometry analysis for cell cycle distribution of FaDu cells. (**A**) Representative cell cycle distribution of FaDu cells with compound 8e treatment (0, 2, 5, and 10 nM) for 24 h. The tall peak (**left**) represents cells in the G0/G1 phase, the small peak (**right**) represents cells in the G2/M phase, and the middle area represents cells in the S phase. (**B**) Quantification of the percentage of cell cycle distribution.

2.9. *In Silico ADMET Prediction*

ADMET prediction is becoming increasingly crucial as most drugs fail in clinical trials owing to poor pharmacokinetic parameters [26,27]. Table 2 shows the ADMET calculated descriptors for our synthesized compounds and two biplots shown in Figure 8. All compounds had 0–4 HBD (hydrogen bond donor) and 4–10 HBA (hydrogen bond acceptor), which were under Lipinski's rule of five (HBD < 5, HBA < 10). PPB (plasma protein binding) was one of the key properties related to drug efficacy. Except for compounds **10–15e**, **17–24e**, and **9d**, most of the compounds had weak (<90%) binding with plasma proteins in the blood, which were predicted to be non-inhibitors of cytochrome P450 2D6, and participated in the good- metabolism of phase I metabolism. $T_{1/2}$ of the target molecules was in the range of 1.63–2.29 h, showing the characteristic of rapid metabolism. The HT (hepatotoxicity) values estimated the hepatoxicity of the chemical compounds. HT values for series **6a–i**, **13–14e**, **20e**, **29e**, **31–35e**, **9f**, **9i**, **9k**, and **9m** were zero, and there was no hepatoxicity, while other compounds might be hepatotoxic. Moreover, the LD_{50} (median lethal dose) predicted that series **8a–f**, **9–35e**, and **9d–m** were over 500 mg/kg, implying they were less toxic. In addition, an ADMET model formed with descriptors 2D polar surface area (PSA) and AlogP98 could predict human intestinal absorption and the blood-brain barrier penetration (BBB) at 95% and 99% confidence level. In the absorption plot, compounds **6a–f**, **6h–i**, **8a–f**, **9–11e**, **13–19e**, **23e**, **30–33e**, **9d**, **9g**, and **9j–m** were predicted to be easily absorbed by the intestine at 99% confidence level. While in the BBB plot, the most potent compounds **8e** and **8f** were fallen out of the 99% ellipse (undefined), suggesting its poor blood-brain barrier penetration ability. Therefore, these molecules might possess low or no side effects of the central nervous system (CNS). In conclusion, ADMET prediction of the compounds might be helpful for further designing new drugs with favorable oral bioavailability.

Table 2. The ADMET properties of all synthetic compounds.

Comp.	HBD[a]	HBA[b]	RBN[c]	logP[d]	logS[e]	PSA[f]	HIA[g]	PPB[h]	BBB[i]	CYP3A4[j]	$T_{1/2}$ (h)[k]	HT[l]	LD_{50}(mg/kg)[m]
6a	0	10	11	1.84	−2.23	96.79	0.81	0.68	0.94	0	2.02	0	459.04
6b	0	10	12	1.90	−1.93	96.79	0.80	0.67	0.91	0	2.13	0	429.48
6c	0	10	13	2.48	−2.05	96.79	0.80	0.68	0.91	0	2.14	0	462.17
6d	0	10	15	3.39	−2.02	96.79	0.80	0.65	0.91	0	2.12	0	447.58
6e	0	10	17	4.31	−1.90	96.79	0.80	0.65	0.91	0	2.14	0	425.74
6f	0	10	19	5.22	−1.67	96.79	0.80	0.66	0.91	0	2.18	0	460.97
6g	0	10	21	6.13	−1.35	96.79	0.80	0.67	0.91	0	2.23	0	508.77
6h	0	6	4	0.97	−2.49	51.75	0.79	0.67	0.98	0	2.00	0	664.69
6i	1	6	6	0.47	−1.52	69.21	0.78	0.70	0.75	0	1.77	0	1011.08
8a	2	6	6	−0.09	−1.53	105.27	0.69	0.78	0.98	0	1.81	1	1027.40
8b	2	6	7	0.49	−1.87	105.27	0.72	0.79	0.98	0	1.88	1	988.28
8c	2	6	9	1.40	−2.30	105.27	0.72	0.80	0.98	0	1.89	1	1033.87
8d	2	6	11	2.31	−2.67	105.27	0.72	0.83	0.98	0	1.92	1	1099.10
8e	2	6	13	3.22	−2.97	105.27	0.72	0.85	0.98	0	2.03	1	1278.93
8f	2	6	15	4.14	−3.21	105.27	0.72	0.85	0.98	0	2.01	1	1318.54
9e	2	2	15	6.21	−4.45	60.22	0.69	0.89	0.99	0	1.93	1	961.82
10e	2	4	13	2.97	−2.60	82.74	0.70	0.91	0.99	0	1.85	1	1075.58
11e	2	2	13	5.27	−4.27	60.22	0.68	0.91	1.00	0	1.96	1	1653.45
12e	2	2	13	7.09	−6.11	60.22	0.69	0.92	0.99	0	2.12	1	1818.99
13e	2	4	13	2.97	−2.60	82.74	0.72	0.91	0.99	0	1.89	0	1070.63
14e	2	2	13	4.06	−3.66	85.33	0.41	0.90	1.00	0	1.78	0	1145.12
15e	2	4	13	3.83	−3.35	82.74	0.70	0.91	0.99	0	1.89	1	1128.86
16e	2	6	13	1.53	−1.68	105.27	0.68	0.85	0.99	0	1.82	1	1461.77
17e	2	4	13	5.65	−5.10	82.74	0.70	0.95	0.98	0	2.22	1	1217.90
18e	2	4	13	5.65	−5.10	82.74	0.72	0.96	0.95	0	1.99	1	1254.91
19e	4	4	13	4.31	−4.38	112.85	0.69	0.90	0.94	0	1.91	1	1167.64
20e	2	6	13	5.33	−4.57	112.68	0.43	0.93	0.98	0	2.29	0	973.08
21e	2	2	13	6.46	−6.02	85.33	0.47	0.94	0.99	0	2.00	1	966.72
22e	2	2	13	7.40	−6.99	60.22	0.69	0.91	0.99	0	2.07	1	904.88
23e	2	2	13	6.27	−5.55	70.92	0.75	0.95	0.99	0	2.27	1	995.92
24e	4	2	13	5.86	−5.15	90.33	0.72	0.95	0.96	0	2.01	1	1072.61
25e	2	2	15	7.54	−5.78	60.22	0.67	0.89	0.99	0	1.98	1	1322.11
26e	4	6	17	5.69	−3.28	119.71	0.45	0.87	0.85	0	1.93	1	1249.90
27e	2	6	19	6.14	−3.64	95.94	0.54	0.82	0.98	0	1.82	1	1217.58
28e	4	8	19	5.66	−3.13	137.57	0.46	0.77	0.94	0	2.02	1	1163.97
29e	2	8	21	6.11	−3.08	113.80	0.54	0.73	0.96	0	1.95	0	927.46
30e	4	4	13	3.78	−2.74	113.30	0.59	0.90	0.99	0	1.96	1	849.92
31e	4	4	13	3.78	−2.69	113.30	0.64	0.90	0.97	0	1.93	0	951.43
32e	4	4	13	3.78	−2.72	113.30	0.64	0.90	0.98	0	1.94	0	853.84
33e	2	6	17	5.21	−3.97	95.94	0.53	0.81	0.99	0	1.76	0	1184.47
34e	2	8	19	5.18	−3.62	113.80	0.54	0.76	0.98	0	1.63	0	1073.30
35e	2	8	19	5.18	−3.67	113.80	0.53	0.76	0.97	0	1.72	0	1061.01
9d	2	2	13	5.30	−4.11	60.22	0.69	0.91	0.99	0	1.92	1	1523.97
9f	2	2	17	7.12	−4.73	60.22	0.69	0.87	0.99	0	1.95	0	1003.19
9g	0	4	15	6.59	−5.34	52.46	0.55	0.88	0.98	0	1.96	1	6181.36
9h	0	4	17	7.50	−5.69	52.46	0.55	0.86	0.98	0	1.96	1	4624.51
9i	0	4	19	8.42	−5.96	52.46	0.55	0.85	0.98	0	1.96	0	3127.76
9j	2	4	13	2.57	−2.06	78.08	0.37	0.86	0.99	0	1.97	1	1574.67
9k	2	5	16	2.44	−1.41	87.01	0.37	0.85	0.99	0	1.90	0	1693.04
9l	0	6	15	3.86	−2.96	70.32	0.50	0.88	0.98	0	1.89	1	4511.05
9m	0	7	18	3.73	−2.14	79.25	0.50	0.86	0.98	0	1.83	0	4493.16
DOX	6	12	5	−0.04	−4.80	209.31	0.02	0.78	0.02	0	2.71	1	324.50
TMP	0	2	0	0.66	−1.51	22.52	0.93	0.49	0.99	0	1.77	0	1194.46

[a] HBD (hydrogen bond donor), [b] HBA (hydrogen bond acceptor), [c] RBN (number of rotatable bonds), [d] logP (log of the octanol/water partition coefficient), [e] log S (log of the aqueous solubility), and [f] PSA (polar surface area) were predicted using Discovery Studio 2.0 software. [g] HIA (human intestinal absorption), [h] PPB (plasma protein binding), [I] CYP3D4 (CYP3D4 inhibition), [j] T1/2 (half lifetime), [k] HT (human hepatoxicity), and [l] LD50 (median lethal dose) were calculated via http://admet.scbdd.com/home/index/

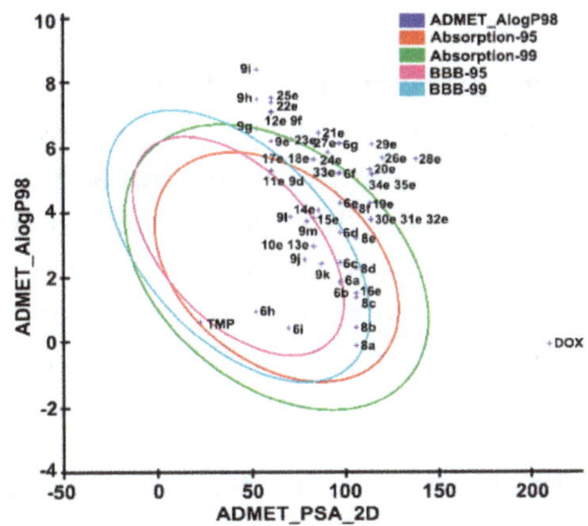

Figure 8. The plot of PSA (polar surface area) versus AlogP98 for the newly synthesized compounds showing the 95% and 99% confidence limit ellipses corresponding to the intestinal absorption and blood-brain barrier models.

3. Conclusions

Using ligustrazine, aromatic, or heteroaromatic acids as the main raw materials and linked by alkyl or ether chain, bivalent antitumor agents were synthesized and screened from five different human cancer cell lines and one normal mammary epithelial cell line. SAR revealed that the two terminal amide bonds and the alky chain were the dominant factors with 10 C atom chain showing the most potent antitumor effect. Among different aromatic moieties, the ligustrazine dimer **8e** was the best candidate; its IC_{50} was 1.36 nM in FaDu cell, it showed a broad-spectrum antitumor activity with IC_{50} in the range of 0.00136–1.42 μM, and the selective ratio MCF 10A/FaDu was 34.56. The subsequent fluorescence staining and flow cytometry analysis indicated that **8e** could induce apoptosis through depolarization of the mitochondrial membrane potential in FaDu cells. Further mechanism investigation showed that **8e** could arrest cell cycle at the S phase in FaDu cells. Furthermore, ADMET predicted that most of the potent compounds followed Lipinski's law and became 'drug-like' molecules, further confirming that the dimerization of ligustrazine could improve the antitumor activity of its monomer. The highly selective inhibition of these dimers on the proliferation of FaDu cells might be related to the effect on a specific target in FaDu cells. Based on the characteristics of FaDu cells, further targeted screening would give insight into the selectivity of such potent compounds.

4. Materials and Methods

4.1. Chemistry

^{1}H-NMR and ^{13}C-NMR spectra were recorded on a Mercury Vx-300 (300 MHz) or AVANCE III (400 MHz). Chemical shifts were reported in ppm (δ) using the residue solvent line as the internal standard (for TMS: 0 ppm, ^{1}H and ^{13}C; for $CHCl_3$-*d*: 7.26 ppm, ^{1}H and 77.16 ppm, ^{13}C). Coupling constants were given in Hertz (*J*). High-resolution MS (HRMS) were recorded on an Agilent 6520 Q-TOF LC/MS. Melting points were uncorrected and were determined on a digital melting point apparatus (Shenguang WRS-1B, shanghai, China). Flash column chromatography was carried out by using silica gel (200–300 mesh). Reactions were monitored by thin-layer chromatography (TLC) on silica gel GF254 plates (Qingdao Haiyang Chemical Plant, Qingdao, China). Reagents and solvents were used as purchased from commercial sources without further purification. The purity of the synthesized compounds was over 95% analyzed by HPLC (Waters 2695 Alliance system, Waters Corp., Milford, MA, USA), with the Kromasil C18 column eluted by methanol/water (80/20) containing 0.1% trifluoroacetic acid at a flow rate of 1 mL/min. Compounds **4** and **5** were prepared, as reported previously [19]. ^{1}H-NMR, ^{13}C-NMR and HR-MS spectra of compounds **6a–9m** can be seen in supplementary materials.

4.2. *General Synthetic Procedure for* **6a–g**

A mixture of alkane-diamine (10 mmol), TMP-Cl (50 mmol), KOH (60 mmol), and dimethylformamide (35 mL) was heated to reflux. The reaction progress was monitored via TLC. After 2 h, the reaction mixture was cooled to room temperature. Subsequently, the solid was filtered off, and the filtrate was added with H_2O (100 mL) and extracted with ethyl acetic acid three times. The organic layers were combined and washed with H_2O and brine, and then separated and dried over anhydrous Na_2SO_4 for 8 h. The solvent was removed under reduced pressure; the resulting residue was separated on flash column chromatography eluted by a mixture of petroleum ether/acetone in a volume ratio of 7:1–3:1, and further recrystallized from acetone to give pale white solid.

4.2.1. N^1,N^1,N^2,N^2-Tetrakis((3,5,6-Trimethylpyrazin-2-yl)Methyl)Ethane-1,2-Diamine (**6a**)

Pale white solid, yield 28%, m.p. 207.6–208.3 °C; ^{1}H-NMR (300 MHz, $CDCl_3$) δ: 3.60 (s, 8H), 2.67 (s, 4H), 2.43 (s, 12H), 2.41 (s, 12H), 2.23 (s, 12H); ^{13}C-NMR (101 MHz, DMSO) δ: 149.91, 149.63, 148.37, 147.85, 58.75, 52.14, 50.83, 21.61, 21.42, 20.65; HRMS (ESI) *m/z*: 597.4134 $[M + H]^+$, calcd. for $[C_{34}H_{49}N_{10}]^+$ 597.4142.

4.2.2. N^1,N^1,N^3,N^3-Tetrakis((3,5,6-Trimethylpyrazin-2-yl)Methyl)Propane-1,3-Diamine (**6b**)

Pale white solid, yield 27%, m.p. 113–114.3 °C; ^{1}H-NMR (300 MHz, $CDCl_3$) δ: 3.65 (s, 8H), 2.46 (s, 12H), 2.43 (s, 12H), 2.41–2.38 (m, 4H), 2.32 (s, 12H), 1.81–1.71 (m, 2H). ^{13}C-NMR (101 MHz, DMSO) δ: 149.93, 149.53, 148.51, 147.82, 58.63, 53.36, 21.61, 21.44, 20.70; HRMS (ESI) *m/z*: 611.4286 $[M + H]^+$, calcd. for $[C_{35}H_{51}N_{10}]^+$ 611.4298.

4.2.3. N^1,N^1,N^4,N^4-Tetrakis((3,5,6-Trimethylpyrazin-2-yl)Methyl)Butane-1,4-Diamine (**6c**)

Pale white solid, yield 37%, m.p. 129.2–129.5 °C; ^{1}H-NMR (300 MHz, $CDCl_3$) δ: 3.62 (s, 8H), 2.44 (s, 24H), 2.40–2.37 (m, 4H), 2.30 (s, 12H), 1.37 (s, 4H); ^{13}C-NMR (101 MHz, DMSO) δ: 150, 149.53, 148.60, 147.79, 58.54, 54.85, 24.39, 21.64, 21.47, 20.71; HRMS (ESI) *m/z*: 625.4451 $[M + H]^+$, calcd. for $[C_{36}H_{53}N_{10}]^+$ 625.4455.

4.2.4. N^1,N^1,N^6,N^6-Tetrakis((3,5,6-Trimethylpyrazin-2-yl)Methyl)Hexane-1,6-Diamine (**6d**)

Pale white solid, yield 43%, m.p. 146.7–147.9 °C; ^{1}H-NMR (300 MHz, $CDCl_3$) δ: 3.67 (s, 8H), 2.46–2.45 (m, 24H), 2.43–2.40 (m, 4H), 2.34 (s, 12H), 1.43 (br, 4H), 1.04 (br, 4H); ^{13}C-NMR (101 MHz, DMSO) δ: 150.05, 149.48, 148.71, 147.77, 58.64, 54.93, 27.34, 26.56, 21.65, 21.48, 20.74; HRMS (ESI) *m/z*: 653.4765 $[M + H]^+$, calcd. for $[C_{38}H_{57}N_{10}]^+$ 653.4768.

4.2.5. N^1,N^1,N^8,N^8-Tetrakis((3,5,6-Trimethylpyrazin-2-yl)Methyl)Octane-1,8-Diamine (**6e**)

Pale white solid, yield 48%, m.p. 107.8–108.6 °C; ^{1}H-NMR (300 MHz, $CDCl_3$) δ: 3.67 (s, 8H), 2.45 (br, 24H), 2.42–2.38 (m, 4H), 2.34 (s, 12H), 1.48–1.40 (m, 4H), 1.05 (br, 8H); ^{13}C-NMR (101 MHz, $CDCl_3$) δ: 150.09, 149.47, 148.75, 147.76, 58.69, 54.90, 29.52, 27.46, 26.55, 21.65, 21.47, 20.73; HRMS (ESI) *m/z*: 681.5076 $[M + H]^+$, calcd. for $[C_{40}H_{61}N_{10}]^+$ 681.5081.

4.2.6. N^1,N^1,N^{10},N^{10}-Tetrakis((3,5,6-Trimethylpyrazin-2-yl)Methyl)Decane-1,10-Diamine (**6f**)

Pale white solid, yield 76%, m.p. 67.4–68 °C; ^{1}H-NMR (300 MHz, $CDCl_3$) δ: 3.69 (s, 8H), 2.46 (br, 24H), 2.41–2.39 (m, 4H), 2.35 (s, 12H), 1.47 (br, 4H), 1.11 (br, 12H); ^{13}C-NMR (101 MHz, DMSO) δ: 150.10, 149.45, 148.78, 147.76, 58.71, 54.92, 29.73, 29.52, 27.48, 26.57, 21.64, 21.47, 20.74; HRMS (ESI) *m/z*: 709.5378 $[M + H]^+$, calcd. for $[C_{42}H_{65}N_{10}]^+$ 709.5394.

4.2.7. N^1,N^1,N^{12},N^{12}-Tetrakis((3,5,6-Trimethylpyrazin-2-yl)Methyl)Dodecane-1,12-Diamine (**6g**)

Pale white solid, yield 76%, m.p. 84.7–85.3 °C; ^{1}H-NMR (300 MHz, $CDCl_3$) δ: 3.69 (s, 8H), 2.46 (br, 24H), 2.44 (br, 4H), 2.35 (s, 12H), 1.47 (br, 4H), 1.15–1.12 (br, 16H); ^{13}C-NMR (101 MHz, DMSO) δ:

150.10, 149.44, 148.78, 147.74, 58.72, 54.89, 29.75, 29.53, 27.46, 26.56, 21.64, 21.47, 20.73; HRMS (ESI) *m/z*: 737.5689 $[M + H]^+$, calcd. for $[C_{44}H_{69}N_{10}]^+$ 737.5707.

4.3. *1,4-Bis((3,5,6-Trimethylpyrazin-2-yl)Methyl)Piperazine* (**6h**)

A mixture of piperazine (0.800 g, 9.29 mmol), TMP-Cl (3.80 g, 22.29 mmol), KOH (1.56 g, 27.66 mmol), and dimethylformamide (20 mL) was heated under reflux for 2 h. The reaction was monitored by TLC. The reaction was quenched, filtered, and the filtrate was added with 100 mL H_2O and extracted with ethyl acetate three times. The organic layers were combined, washed with H_2O and brine, and then dried over anhydrous Na_2SO_4 for 8 h. The solvent was evaporated in vacuo. The resulting residue was separated on flash column chromatography with a mixture of petroleum ether/acetone 7:1–3:1(volume ratio) as eluent, and then further recrystallized from acetone to afford compound **6h**.

Pale white solid, yield 62%, m.p. 155.8–156.3 °C; ^{1}H-NMR (300 MHz, $CDCl_3$) δ: 3.58 (s, 4H), 2.55 (s, 8H), 2.47 (br, 18H); ^{13}C-NMR (101 MHz, DMSO) δ: 150.01, 149.57, 148.10, 147.98, 61.88, 53.26, 50.70, 21.61, 21.51, 21.04; HRMS (ESI) *m/z*: 355.2610 $[M + H]^+$, calcd. for $[C_{20}H_{31}N_6]^+$ 355.2610.

4.4. *2-(Bis((3,5,6-Trimethylpyrazin-2-yl)Methyl)Amino)Ethanol* (**6i**)

A mixture of ethanolamine (0.500 g, 8.19 mmol), TMP-Cl (3.35 g, 19.65 mmol), K_2CO_3 (3.39 g, 24.56 mmol), and acetonitrile (20 mL) was heated under reflux for 3 h. The product formation was monitored via TLC. After cooling, the mixture was filtered, and the filtrate was evaporated in vacuo. The residue was purified by flash column chromatography with an eluent of petroleum ether/acetone = 10:1–3:1 to afford compound **6i**.

Light yellow oil, yield 72%; ^{1}H-NMR (300 MHz, $CDCl_3$) δ: 3.82 (13s, 4H), 3.66 (t, J = 5 Hz, 2H), 2.87 (t, J = 5.1 Hz, 2H), 2.41 (s, 6H), 2.37 (s, 6H), 2.35 (s, 6H); ^{13}C-NMR (101 MHz, DMSO) δ: 149.54, 148.94, 148.27, 147.87, 59.67, 58.15, 57.36, 21.41, 21.21, 20.52; HRMS (ESI) *m/z*: 330.2290 $[M + H]^+$, calcd. for $[C_{18}I\,I_{28}N_5O]^+$ 330.2294.

4.5. *General Synthetic Procedure for* **8a–f**

Compound **7** was gained according to the method described by Wu [20]. A mixture of tetramethylpyrazine acid (4.40 mmol), EDCI (4.72 mmol), triethylamine (12 mmol), DMAP (2.40 mmol), and anhydrous dichloromethane (10 mL) was stirred to dissolve, then diamino-alkane (2 mmol) was added and stirred at room temperature until the reaction was finished (monitored by TLC). The reaction mixture was washed with brine and water, extracted with dichloromethane (20 mL), dried over anhydrous sodium sulfate for 8 h, filtered, and the solvent was evaporated. The resulting residue was purified by flash column chromatography with an eluent of petroleum ether/acetone = 15:1–3:1(volume ratio) to give pale white solid.

4.5.1. N,N′-(Propane-1,3-Diyl)Bis(3,5,6-Trimethylpyrazine-2-Carboxamide) (**8a**)

Pale white solid, yield 16%, m.p. 125.4–126.4 °C; ^{1}H-NMR (300 MHz, $CDCl_3$) δ: 8.30 (t, J = 5.9 Hz, 2H), 3.58–3.52 (m, 4H), 2.92 (s, 6H), 2.56 (s, 6H), 2.50 (s, 6H), 1.99–1.90 (m, 2H); ^{13}C-NMR (101 MHz, CDC13) δ: 165.57, 154.09, 151.29, 147.80, 139.09, 36.89, 29.87, 22.94, 22.07, 21.47; HRMS (ESI) *m/z*: 371.2189 $[M + H]^+$, calcd. for $[C_{19}H_{27}N_6O_2]^+$ 371.2195.

4.5.2. N,N′-(Butane-1,4-Diyl)Bis(3,5,6-Trimethylpyrazine-2-Carboxamide) (**8b**)

Pale white solid, yield 30%, m.p. 168.4–168.6 °C; ^{1}H-NMR (300 MHz, $CDCl_3$) δ: 8.07 (t, J = 5.5 Hz, 2H), 3.50–3.48 (m, 4H), 2.91 (s, 6H), 2.56 (s, 6H), 2.52 (s, 6H), 1.75–1.73 (m, 4H); ^{13}C-NMR (101 MHz, $CDCl_3$) δ: 165.25, 154.15, 151.38, 147.75, 139.07, 50.90, 39.13, 27.49, 22.96, 22.06, 21.48; HRMS (ESI) *m/z*: 385.2352 $[M + H]^+$, calcd. for $[C_{20}H_{29}N_6O_2]^+$ 385.2352.

4.5.3. N,N′-(Hexane-1,6-Diyl)Bis(3,5,6-Trimethylpyrazine-2-Carboxamide) (**8c**)

Pale white solid, yield 47%, m.p. 114.2–114.7 °C; ^{1}H-NMR (300 MHz, $CDCl_3$) δ: 8.02 (t, *J* = 5.4 Hz, 2H), 3.45–3.38 (m, 4H), 2.90 (s, 6H), 2.55 (s, 6H), 2.51 (s, 6H), 1.67–1.63 (m, 4H), 1.47–1.43 (m, 4H); ^{13}C-NMR (101 MHz, $CDCl_3$) δ: 165.12, 154.03, 151.35, 147.63, 139.11, 39.33, 29.74, 26.82, 22.98, 22.06, 21.48; HRMS (ESI) *m/z*: 413.2662 [M + H]$^+$, calcd. for $[C_{22}H_{33}N_6O_2]^+$ 413.2665.

4.5.4. N,N′-(Octane-1,8-Diyl)Bis(3,5,6-Trimethylpyrazine-2-Carboxamide) (**8d**)

Pale white solid, yield 68%, m.p. 113.6–113.8 °C; ^{1}H-NMR (300 MHz, $CDCl_3$) δ: 8 (t, *J* = 5.3 Hz, 2H), 3.45–3.38 (m, 4H), 2.91 (s, 6H), 2.56 (s, 6H), 2.52 (s, 6H), 1.65–1.60 (m, 4H), 1.37–1.37 (m, 8H); ^{13}C-NMR (101 MHz, $CDCl_3$) δ: 165.10, 154.02, 151.40, 147.65, 139.20, 39.45, 29.81, 29.34, 27.11, 23.01, 22.08, 21.53; HRMS (ESI) *m/z*: 441.2975 [M + H]$^+$, calcd. for $[C_{24}H_{37}N_6O_2]^+$ 441.2978.

4.5.5. N,N′-(Decane-1,10-Diyl)Bis(3,5,6-Trimethylpyrazine-2-Carboxamide) (**8e**)

Pale white solid, yield 66%, m.p. 110.3–110.6 °C; ^{1}H-NMR (300 MHz, $CDCl_3$) δ: 8 (t, *J* = 5.2 Hz, 2H), 3.44–3.37 (m, 4H), 2.91 (s, 6H), 2.55 (s, 6H), 2.51 (s, 6H), 1.64–1.57 (m, 4H), 1.34–1.30 (m, 12H); ^{13}C-NMR (101 MHz, $CDCl_3$) δ: 165.07, 153.97, 151.33, 147.66, 139.21, 39.47, 29.80, 29.56, 29.39, 27.14, 22.94, 22.02, 21.49; HRMS (ESI) *m/z*: 469.3287 [M + H]$^+$, calcd. for $[C_{26}H_{41}N_6O_2]^+$ 469.3291.

4.5.6. N,N′-(Dodecane-1,12-Diyl)Bis(3,5,6-Trimethylpyrazine-2-Carboxamide) (**8f**)

Pale white solid, yield 72%, m.p. 98.3–99.1 °C; ^{1}H-NMR (300 MHz, $CDCl_3$) δ: 8 (t, *J* = 4.9 Hz, 2H), 3.45–3.38 (m, 4H), 2.91 (s, 6H), 2.56 (s, 6H), 2.52 (s, 6H), 1.67–1.57 (m, 4H), 1.34–1.27 (m, 16H); ^{13}C-NMR (101 MHz, $CDCl_3$) δ: 165.07, 153.98, 151.37, 147.62, 139.22, 39.49, 29.83, 29.66, 29.44, 27.18, 22.99, 22.07, 21.51; HRMS (ESI) *m/z*: 497.3602 [M + H]$^+$, calcd. for $[C_{28}H_{45}N_6O_2]^+$ 497.3604.

4.6. General Synthetic Procedure for **9e–35e**

Compounds **9e–35e** were obtained by using one-pot reaction. A mixture of aromatic acid (6.30 mmol), EDCI (7.50 mmol), DMAP (0.60 mmol), and anhydrous dichloromethane (20 mL) was stirred to dissolve, then decane-diamine (3 mmol) was added and stirred at room temperature for 12 h. The mixture solution was filtered under reduced pressure. After that, the residue was washed with little amount of CH_2Cl_2 and water successively, and dried to give the solid. Then, the residue was purified on preparative TLC eluted with chloroform/methanol = 40:1–7:1 to yield compounds **26e**, **28e, 30e,** and **31e**.

4.6.1. (2E,2′E)-N,N′-(Decane-1,10-Diyl)Bis(3-Phenylacrylamide) (**9e**)

Pale white solid, yield 62%, m.p. 169.8–170.5 °C; ^{1}H-NMR (300 MHz, $CDCl_3$+CD_3OD) δ: 7.54 (d, *J* = 15.7 Hz, 2H), 7.49–7.46 (m, 4H), 7.36–7.31 (m, 6H), 6.47 (d, *J* = 15.6 Hz, 2H), 3.33–3.28 (m, 4H), 1.57–1.54 (m, 4H), 1.52–1.28 (m, 12H); ^{13}C-NMR (101 MHz, $CDCl_3$+CD_3OD) δ: 150.10, 149.45, 148.78, 147.76, 58.71, 54.92, 29.73, 29.52, 27.48, 26.57, 21.64, 21.47, 20.74; HRMS (ESI) *m/z*: 433.2851 [M + H]$^+$, calcd. for $[C_{28}H_{45}N_6O_2]^+$ 433.2855

4.6.2. N,N′-(Decane-1,10-Diyl)Dinicotinamide (**10e**)

Pale white solid, yield 67%, m.p. 167.4–167.8 °C; ^{1}H-NMR (300 MHz, $CDCl_3$+CD_3OD) δ: 8.84 (s, 2H), 8.55 (d, *J* = 3.9 Hz, 2H), 8.11 (dt, *J* = 8, 1.7 Hz, 2H), 7.35 (dd, *J* = 7.9, 4.9 Hz, 2H), 3.34 (t, *J* = 7.2 Hz, 4H), 1.58–1.51 (m, 4H), 1.27–1.24 (m, 12H); ^{13}C-NMR (101 MHz, $CDCl_3$+CD_3OD) δ: 165.85, 151.29, 147.53, 135.93, 130.87, 123.79, 40.16, 29.28, 29.12, 26.86; HRMS (ESI) *m/z*: 383.2441 [M + H]$^+$, calcd. for $[C_{28}H_{45}N_6O_2]^+$ 383.2447.

4.6.3. N,N′-(Decane-1,10-Diyl)Dibenzamide (**11e**)

Pale white solid, yield 70%, m.p. 154.3–154.6 °C; ^{1}H-NMR (300 MHz, $CDCl_3$+CD_3OD) δ: 7.77–7.73 (m, 4H), 7.51–7.33 (m, 6H), 3.42–3.35 (m, 4H), 1.63–1.56 (m, 4H), 1.34–1.30 (m, 12H); ^{13}C-NMR (101 MHz, $CDCl_3$+CD_3OD) δ: 168.39, 134.55, 131.36, 128.45, 126.86, 40.02, 29.36, 29.27, 29.13, 26.84. HRMS (ESI) *m/z*: 381.2702 $[M + H]^+$, calcd. for $[C_{24}H_{33}N_2O_2]^+$ 381.2542.

4.6.4. N,N′-(Decane-1,10-Diyl)Bis(2-Naphthamide) (**12e**)

Pale white solid, yield 64%, m.p. 163.9–164 °C; ^{1}H-NMR (300 MHz, $CDCl_3$+CD_3OD) δ: 8.22–8.17 (m, 2H), 7.89–7.82 (m, 4H), 7.54–7.39 (m, 8H), 3.49–3.44 (m, 4H), 1.67–1.60 (m, 4H), 1.38–1.34 (m, 12H); ^{13}C-NMR (101 MHz, $CDCl_3$ + CD_3OD) δ: 170.38, 134.50, 133.56, 130.33, 129.96, 128.22, 126.89, 126.29, 125.10, 124.77, 124.65, 39.94, 29.36, 29.30, 29.11, 26.85. HRMS (ESI) *m/z*: 481.2853 [M + H]+, calcd. for $[C_{32}H_{37}N_2O_2]^+$ 481.2855.

4.6.5. N,N′-(Decane-1,10-Diyl)Diisonicotinamide (**13e**)

Pale white solid, yield 60%, m.p. 175.6–176.3 °C; ^{1}H-NMR (300 MHz, $CDCl_3$+CD_3OD) δ: 8.62 (d, *J* = 5.6 Hz, 4H), 7.71 (dd, *J* = 6.1, 2.8 Hz, 4H), 3.41–3.33 (m, 4H), 1.64–1.57 (m, 4H), 1.33–1.31 (m, 12H); ^{13}C-NMR (101 MHz, $CDCl_3$+CD_3OD) δ: 165.88, 149.48, 142.45, 121.46, 40.04, 29.16, 28.99, 26.71. HRMS (ESI) *m/z*: 383.2445 $[M + H]^+$, calcd. for $[C_{22}H_{31}N_4O_2]^+$ 383.2447.

4.6.6. N,N′-(Decane-1,10-Diyl)Bis(Furan-2-Carboxamide) (**14e**)

Pale white solid, yield 62%, m.p. 132.6–133.3 °C; ^{1}H-NMR (300 MHz, $CDCl_3$) δ: 7.41 (dd, *J* = 1.7, 0.8 Hz, 2H), 7.09 (dd, *J* = 3.5, 0.7 Hz, 2H), 6.48 (dd, *J* = 3.5, 1.7 Hz, 2H), 6.37 (br, 2H), 3.45–3.38 (m, 4H), 1.65–1.55 (m, 4H), 1.36–1.30 (m, 12H); ^{13}C-NMR (101 MHz, $CDCl_3$) δ: 158.53, 148.38, 143.77, 114.02, 112.22, 39.29, 29.80, 29.48, 29.33, 26.98. HRMS (ESI) *m/z*: 383.1944 $[M + Na]^+$, calcd. for $[C_{20}H_{28}N_2NaO_4]^+$ 383.1947.

4.6.7. N,N′-(Decane-1,10-Diyl)Dipicolinamide (**15e**)

Pale white solid, yield 68%, m.p. 156.6–156.9 °C; ^{1}H-NMR (300 MHz, $CDCl_3$) δ: 9.35 (d, *J* = 1.4 Hz, 2H), 8.69 (d, *J* = 2.5 Hz, 2H),.8.47–8.46 (m, 2H), 7.77 (br, 2H), 3.47–3.40 (m, 4H), 1.65–1.55 (m, 4H), 1.34–1.26 (m, 12H); ^{13}C-NMR (101 MHz, $CDCl_3$) δ: 163.01, 147.26, 144.76, 144.55, 142.58, 39.61, 29.68, 29.51, 29.34, 27.03. HRMS (ESI) *m/z*: 383.2441 $[M + H]^+$, calcd. for $[C_{22}H_{31}N_4O_2]^+$ 383.2447

4.6.8. N,N′-(Decane-1,10-Diyl)Bis(Pyrazine-2-Carboxamide) (**16e**)

Pale white solid, yield 70%, m.p. 77.6–80.1 °C; ^{1}H-NMR (300 MHz, $CDCl_3$) δ: 8.54–8.51 (m, 2H), 8.20–8.17 (m, 2H), 8.05 (br, 2H), 7.85–7.80 (m, 2H), 7.42–7.38 (m, 2H), 3.49–3.43 (m, 4H), 1.68–1.58 (m, 4H), 1.38–1.26 (m, 12H); ^{13}C-NMR (101 MHz, $CDCl_3$) δ: 164.31, 150.25, 148.09, 137.49, 126.13, 122.34, 39.61, 29.77, 29.56, 29.41, 27.11. HRMS (ESI) *m/z*: 385.2350 $[M + H]^+$, calcd. for $[C_{20}H_{29}N_6O_2]^+$ 385.2352.

4.6.9. N,N′-(Decane-1,10-Diyl)Bis(Quinoline-3-Carboxamide) (**17e**)

Pale white solid, yield 59%, m.p. 206.7–207.1 °C; ^{1}H-NMR (300 MHz, DMSO-d_6 + CD_3OD) δ: 8.57 (d, *J* = 1.8 Hz, 2H), 8.09 (s, 2H), 7.39 (dd, *J* = 8.3, 3.1 Hz, 4H), 7.17 (t, *J* = 7.6 Hz, 2H), 7 (t, *J* = 7.4 Hz, 2H), 2.68 (t, *J* = 7 Hz, 4H), 0.99–0.88 (m, 4H), 0.76–0.62 (m, 12H). ^{13}C-NMR (101 MHz, $CDCl_3$) δ: 165.92, 148.01, 136.52, 131.47, 128.81, 127.93, 127.56, 127.35, 127.06, 40.11, 29.20, 29.15, 29.04, 26.78. HRMS (ESI) *m/z*: 483.2756 $[M + H]^+$, calcd. for $[C_{30}H_{35}N_4O_2]^+$ 483.2760.

4.6.10. N,N′-(Decane-1,10-Diyl)Bis(Quinoline-6-Carboxamide) (**18e**)

Pale yellow solid, yield 73%, m.p. 197.7–198.3 °C; ^{1}H-NMR (300 MHz, $CDCl_3$ + CD_3OD) δ: 8.71 (dd, *J* = 4.3, 1.6 Hz, 2H), 8.19 (d, *J* = 1.6 Hz, 2H), 8.16 (dd, *J* = 8.3, 1.3 Hz, 2H), 7.95 (dd, *J* = 8.8, 1.9 Hz, 2H), 7.91 (s, 2H), 7.35 (dd, *J* = 8.3, 4.3 Hz, 2H), 3.28 (t, *J* = 7.2 Hz, 4H), 1.53–1.45 (m, 5H), 1.22–1.13

(m, 12H). ^{13}C-NMR (101 MHz, $CDCl_3$ + CD_3OD) δ: 167.43, 151.15, 148.21, 137.99, 132.82, 128.38, 127.79, 127.71, 127.64, 121.81, 40.14, 29.19, 29.04, 26.78. HRMS (ESI) *m/z*: 483.2758 $[M + H]^+$, calcd. for $[C_{30}H_{35}N_4O_2]^+$ 483.2760.

4.6.11. N,N′-(Decane-1,10-Diyl)Bis(1H-Benzo[d]Imidazole-6-Carboxamide) (**19e**)

Brick red solid, yield 75%, m.p. 229.7–230.3 °C; ^{1}H-NMR (300 MHz, $CDCl_3$+ CD_3OD) δ: 8.11 (s, 2H), 8.07 (s, 2H), 7.73 (dd, *J* = 8.5, 1.6 Hz, 2H), 7.61 (d, *J* = 8.5 Hz, 2H), 3.42 (t, *J* = 7.1 Hz, 4H), 1.70–1.56 (m, 4H), 1.42–1.25 (m, 12H). ^{13}C-NMR (101 MHz, $CDCl_3$+ CD_3OD) δ: 168.61, 142.46, 128.70, 121.15, 39.32, 28.66, 28.62, 28.50, 26.19. HRMS (ESI) *m/z*: 461.2662 $[M + H]^+$, calcd. for $[C_{26}H_{33}N_6O_2]^+$ 461.2665.

4.6.12. N,N′-(Decane-1,10-Diyl)Bis(2-Oxo-2H-Chromene-3-Carboxamide) (**20e**)

Pale white solid, yield 60%, m.p. 208.9–209.3 °C; ^{1}H-NMR (300 MHz, $CDCl_3$) δ: 8.90 (s, 2H), 8.80 (s, 2H), 7.71–7.61 (m, 4H), 7.43–7.32 (m, 4H), 3.45 (dd, *J* = 13, 7 Hz, 4H), 1.63 (dt, *J* = 14.4, 7.2 Hz, 4H), 1.44–1.26 (m, 12H). ^{13}C-NMR (101 MHz, $CDCl_3$ + CD_3OD) δ: 161.74, 161.44, 154.23, 148.38, 134.16, 129.80, 125.30, 118.46, 117.97, 116.38, 39.69, 29.20, 29.02, 29.01, 26.77. HRMS (ESI) *m/z*: 517.2338 $[M + H]^+$, calcd. for $[C_{30}H_{33}N_2O_6]^+$ 517.2339.

4.6.13. N,N′-(Decane-1,10-Diyl)Bis(Benzofuran-2-Carboxamide) (**21e**)

Pale white solid, yield 43%, m.p. 135.8–136.3 °C; ^{1}H-NMR (300 MHz, DMSO-d_6) δ: 8.64 (s, 2H), 7.74 (d, *J* = 7.7 Hz, 2H), 7.62 (d, *J* = 8.2 Hz, 2H), 7.49 (s, 2H), 7.43 (t, *J* = 7.5 Hz, 2H), 7.30 (t, *J* = 7.4 Hz, 2H), 3.25 (dd, *J* = 13.1, 6.6 Hz, 4H), 1.58–1.43 (m, 4H), 1.37–1.14 (m, 12H). ^{13}C-NMR (101 MHz, DMSO-d_6) δ: 157.94, 154.13, 149.37, 127.17, 126.61, 123.59, 122.63, 111.70, 109.02, 38.68, 29.01, 28.91, 28.71, 26.39. HRMS (ESI) *m/z*: 461.2438 $[M + H]^+$, calcd. for $[C_{28}H_{33}N_2O_4]^+$ 461.2430.

4.6.14. N,N′-(Decane-1,10-Diyl)Bis(Benzo[b]Thiophene-2-Carboxamide) (**22e**)

Pale yellow solid, yield 46%, m.p. 175–175.7 °C; ^{1}H-NMR (300 MHz, DMSO-d_6) δ: 8.68 (s, 2H), 8.04 (s, 2H), 8.01–7.95 (m, 2H), 7.93–7.87 (m, 2H), 7.41 (p, *J* = 7 Hz, 4H), 3.25 (dd, *J* = 12.8, 6.6 Hz, 4H), 1.58–1.44 (m, 4H), 1.37–1.21 (m, 12H). ^{13}C-NMR (101 MHz, DMSO-d_6) δ: 161.28, 140.28, 140.07, 139.16, 126, 125.02, 124.80, 124.33, 122.72, 28.99, 28.92, 28.72, 26.43. HRMS (ESI) *m/z*: 493.1976 $[M + H]^+$, calcd. for $[C_{28}H_{33}N_2O_2S_2]^+$ 493.1983.

4.6.15. N,N′-(Decane-1,10-Diyl)Bis(1-Methyl-1H-Indole-3-Carboxamide) (**23e**)

Pale white solid, yield 43%, m.p. 192.8–193.2 °C; ^{1}H-NMR (300 MHz, DMSO-d_6 + CD_3OD) δ: 8.08 (d, *J* = 7.7 Hz, 2H), 7.86 (s, 2H), 7.41 (d, *J* = 8 Hz, 2H), 7.20–7.13 (m, 2H), 7.13–7.06 (m, 2H), 3.78 (s, 6H), 3.22 (t, *J* = 7.1 Hz, 4H), 1.55–1.43 (m, 4H), 1.32–1.22 (m, 12H). ^{13}C-NMR (101 MHz, $CDCl_3$ + CD_3OD) δ: 166.26, 137.01, 131.75, 125.56, 122.27, 121.03, 120.13, 109.63, 39.26, 32.62, 29.33, 29.07, 28.94, 26.66. HRMS (ESI) *m/z:* 487.3064 $[M + H]^+$, calcd. for $[C_{30}H_{39}N_4O_2]^+$ 487.3073.

4.6.16. N,N′-(Decane-1,10-Diyl)Bis(1H-Indole-6-Carboxamide) (**24e**)

Pale white solid, yield 47%, m.p. 168.4–169.2 °C; ^{1}H-NMR (300 MHz, DMSO-d_6) δ: 11.32 (s, 2H), 8.30 (s, 2H), 7.92 (s, 2H), 7.59–7.41 (m, 6H), 6.46 (s, 2H), 3.25 (dd, *J* = 12.7, 6.4 Hz, 4H), 1.61–1.43 (m, 4H), 1.38–1.21 (m, 12H). ^{13}C-NMR (101 MHz, DMSO) δ: 167.04, 135.24, 129.61, 127.74, 127.66, 119.27, 117.90, 111.07, 101.14, 39.21, 29.27, 29, 28.83, 26.55. HRMS (ESI) *m/z*: 459.2760 $[M + H]^+$, calcd. for $[C_{28}H_{35}N_4O_2]^+$ 459.2760.

4.6.17. (2E,2′E)-N,N′-(Decane-1,10-Diyl)Bis(3-(4-Chlorophenyl)Acrylamide) (**25e**)

Pale white solid, yield 64%, m.p. 230.3–230.9 °C; ^{1}H-NMR (300 MHz, $CDCl_3$ +CF_3COOD) δ: 7.64 (d, *J* = 13 Hz, 2H), 7.54–7.38 (m, 8H), 6.51 (d, *J* = 11.9 Hz, 2H), 3.62–3.37 (m, 4H), 1.73–1.54 (m, 4H),

1.46–1.18 (m, 12H). ^{13}C-NMR (101 MHz, $CDCl_3$ + CF_3COOD) δ: 129.71, 118.78, 115.96, 113.13, 110.30, 29.22, 28.99, 26.64. HRMS (ESI) *m/z*: 501.2075 [M + H]$^+$, calcd. for $[C_{28}H_{35}Cl_2N_2O_2]^+$ 501.2076.

4.6.18. (2E,2′E)-N,N′-(Decane-1,10-Diyl)Bis(3-(3-Hydroxy-4-Methoxyphenyl)Acrylamide) (**26e**)

Pale yellow solid, yield 35%, m.p. 192.9–195.3 °C; ^{1}H-NMR (300 MHz, $CDCl_3$ + CD_3OD) δ: 7.42 (d, *J* = 15.3 Hz, 2H), 7.05 (s, 2H), 6.98 (d, *J* = 8.1 Hz, 2H), 6.83 (d, *J* = 8.3 Hz, 2H), 6.33 (d, *J* = 15.6 Hz, 2H), 3.89 (s, 6H), 3.29 (t, *J* = 7 Hz, 4H), 1.55–1.50 (m, 4H), 1.31–1.27 (m, 12H). ^{13}C-NMR (101 MHz, $CDCl_3$ + CD_3OD) δ: 167.37, 148.94, 146.05, 140.42, 128.11, 121.06, 118.25, 113.07, 111, 55.57, 39.50, 29.13, 28.98, 26.69. HRMS (ESI) *m/z*: 525.2951 [M + H]$^+$, calcd. for $[C_{30}H_{41}N_2O_6]^+$ 525.2965.

4.6.19. (2E,2′E)-N,N′-(Decane-1,10-Diyl)Bis(3-(3,4-Dimethoxyphenyl)Acrylamide) (**27e**)

Pale white solid, yield 59%, m.p. 168.9–169.9 °C; ^{1}H-NMR (300 MHz, DMSO-d_6) δ: 7.95 (br, 2H), 7.30 (br, 2H), 7.11 (br, 4H), 6.97 (br, 2H), 6.50 (br, 2H), 3.78 (br, 12H), 3.14 (br, 4H), 1.42 (br, 4H), 1.27 (br, 12H). ^{13}C-NMR (101 MHz, $CDCl_3$+ CD_3OD) δ: 167.15, 150.31, 148.90, 140.25, 127.89, 121.77, 118.56, 111.04, 109.74, 55.66, 55.58, 39.47, 29.16, 29.14, 28.99, 26.69. HRMS (ESI) *m/z:* 553.3272 [M + H]$^+$, calcd. for $[C_{32}H_{45}N_2O_6]^+$ 553.3278.

4.6.20. (2E,2′E)-N,N′-(Decane-1,10-Diyl)Bis(3-(4-Hydroxy-3,5-Dimethoxyphenyl)Acrylamide) (**28e**)

Pale yellow solid, yield 33%, m.p. 179.8–180.5 °C; ^{1}H-NMR (300 MHz, $CDCl_3$ + CD_3OD) δ: 7.44 (d, *J* = 15.5 Hz, 3H), 6.76 (s, 4H), 6.37 (d, *J* = 15.6 Hz, 2H), 3.88 (s, 12H), 3.30 (t, *J* = 7.1 Hz, 4H), 1.61–1.49 (m, 4H), 1.38–1.24 (m, 12H). ^{13}C-NMR (101 MHz, $CDCl_3$ + CD_3OD) δ: 166.94, 147.48, 141.03, 136.87, 126.16, 118.46, 104.99, 56.23, 39.63, 29.39, 29.21, 29.08, 26.79. HRMS (ESI) *m/z*: 585.3164 [M+H]$^+$, calcd. for $[C_{32}H_{45}N_2O_8]^+$ 585.3176

4.6.21. (2E,2′E)-N,N′-(Decane-1,10-Diyl)Bis(3-(3,4,5-Trimethoxyphenyl)Acrylamide) (**29e**)

Pale white solid, yield 67%, m.p. 193.4–194.3 °C; ^{1}H-NMR (300 MHz, $CDCl_3$ + CD_3OD) δ: 7.45 (d, *J* = 15.4 Hz, 2H), 6.76 (s, 4H), 6.44 (d, *J* = 15.6 Hz, 2H), 3.88 (s, 12H), 3.85 (s, 6H), 3.31 (t, *J* = 7.1 Hz, 4H), 1.63–1.47 (m, 4H), 1.40–1.23 (m, 12H). ^{13}C-NMR (101 MHz, $CDCl_3$ + CD_3OD) δ: 166.73, 153.26, 140.53, 139.33, 130.65, 120.18, 104.99, 60.81, 56, 39.63, 29.28, 29.21, 29.05, 26.76. HRMS (ESI) *m/z*:613.3472 [M + H]$^+$, calcd. for $[C_{34}H_{49}N_2O_8]^+$ 613.3489.

4.6.22. N,N′-(Decane-1,10-Diyl)Bis(2-Aminobenzamide) (**30e**)

Pale white solid, yield 67%, m.p. 90.2–91 °C; ^{1}H-NMR (300 MHz, $CDCl_3$ + CD_3OD) δ: 7.36 (dd, *J* = 7.8, 1.2 Hz, 2H), 7.22–7.15 (m, 2H), 6.79–6.60 (m, 4H), 3.35 (dt, *J* = 9.7, 5.5 Hz, 4H), 1.66–1.49 (m, 4H), 1.41–1.24 (m, 12H). ^{13}C-NMR (101 MHz, $CDCl_3$ + CD_3OD) δ: 173.92, 151.77, 135.96, 131.40, 121.48, 121.28, 120.96, 43.54, 33.31, 33.26, 33.11, 30.83. HRMS (ESI) *m/z*:411.2759 [M + H]$^+$, calcd. for $[C_{24}H_{35}N_4O_2]^+$ 411.2760.

4.6.23. N,N′-(Decane-1,10-Diyl)Bis(4-Aminobenzamide) (**31e**)

Pale yellow solid, yield 31%, m.p. 186.7–187.7 °C; ^{1}H-NMR (300 MHz, $CDCl_3$ + CD_3OD) δ: 7.57 (d, *J* = 8.6 Hz, 4H), 6.66 (d, *J* = 8.6 Hz, 4H), 3.34 (t, *J* = 7.2 Hz, 4H), 1.63–1.53 (m, 4H), 1.31–1.26 (m, 12H). ^{13}C-NMR (101 MHz, $CDCl_3$ + CD_3OD) δ: 168.44, 150.01, 128.49, 123.39, 114.04, 39.77, 29.33, 29.18, 29.06, 26.76. HRMS (ESI) *m/z*: 411.2755 [M + H]$^+$, calcd. for $[C_{24}H_{35}N_4O_2]^+$ 411.2760.

4.6.24. N,N′-(Decane-1,10-Diyl)bis(3-Aminobenzamide) (**32e**)

Pale white solid, yield 57%, m.p. 135.7–136.3 °C; ^{1}H-NMR (300 MHz, $CDCl_3$ + CD_3OD) δ: 7.30–6.97 (m, 6H), 6.83 (dd, *J* = 20.8, 7.2 Hz, 2H), 3.36 (t, *J* = 6.8 Hz, 4H), 1.67–1.47 (m, 4H), 1.46–1.06 (m, 12H). ^{13}C-NMR (101 MHz, $CDCl_3$ + CD_3OD) δ: 168.75, 146.84, 135.56, 129.27, 118.09, 116.55, 113.73,

77.48, 77.16, 76.84, 49.31, 49.09, 48.88, 48.67, 48.45, 39.93, 29.29, 29.22, 29.09, 26.79. HRMS (ESI) *m/z*: 411.2758 $[M + H]^+$, calcd. for $[C_{24}H_{35}N_4O_2]^+$ 411.2760

4.6.25. N,N′-(Decane-1,10-Diyl)Bis(3,5-Dimethoxybenzamide) (**33e**)

Pale white solid, yield 56%, m.p. 143.4–144.2 °C; ^{1}H-NMR (300 MHz, $CDCl_3$ + CD_3OD) δ: 6.79 (d, J = 2.1 Hz, 4H), 6.43 (t, J = 1.9 Hz, 2H), 3.69 (s, 12H), 3.25 (t, J = 7.2 Hz, 4H), 1.50–1.45 (m, 4H), 1.25–1.15 (m, 12H). ^{13}C-NMR (101 MHz, $CDCl_3$ + CD_3OD) δ: 168.01, 160.73, 136.74, 104.94, 103.34, 55.40, 40.03, 29.28, 29.26, 29.11, 26.82. HRMS (ESI) *m/z:* 501.2959 $[M + H]^+$, calcd. for $[C_{28}H_{41}N_2O_6]^+$ 501.2965.

4.6.26. N,N′-(Decane-1,10-Diyl)Bis(3,4,5-Trimethoxybenzamide) (**34e**)

Pale white solid, yield 63%, m.p. 194–194.9 °C; ^{1}H-NMR (300 MHz, $CDCl_3$ + CD_3OD) δ: 6.91 (s, 4H), 3.72 (s, 12H), 3.67 (s, 6H), 3.22–3.16 (m, 4H), 1.50–1.36 (m, 4H), 1.22–1.08 (m, 12H). ^{1}H-NMR (300 MHz, $CDCl_3$ + CD_3OD). δ: 6.91 (s, 4H), 3.72 (s, 12H), 3.67 (s, 6H), 3.22–3.16 (m, 4H), 1.50–1.36 (m, 4H), 1.22–1.08 (m, 12H). ^{13}C-NMR (101 MHz, $CDCl_3$ + CD_3OD) δ: 167.81, 152.77, 129.84, 104.42, 60.53, 55.85, 40.01, 29.17, 29.03, 26.73. HRMS (ESI) *m/z:* 561.3169 $[M + H]^+$, calcd. for $[C_{30}H_{45}N_2O_8]^+$ 561.3176.

4.6.27. N,N′-(Decane-1,10-Diyl)Bis(2,3,4-Trimethoxybenzamide) (**35e**)

Pale white solid, yield 26%, m.p. 112.3–112.5 °C; ^{1}H-NMR (300 MHz, $CDCl_3$) δ: 7.94 (s, 2H), 7.89 (d, J = 8.9 Hz, 2H), 6.76 (d, J = 9 Hz, 2H), 3.96 (s, 6H), 3.90 (s, 6H), 3.87 (s, 6H), 3.44 (dd, J = 12.7, 6.9 Hz, 4H), 1.62 (dt, J = 14.3, 7.1 Hz, 4H), 1.41–1.29 (m, 12H). ^{13}C-NMR (101 MHz, $CDCl_3$) δ: 164.90, 156.35, 152.42, 141.83, 126.76, 119.31, 107.67, 61.71, 61.08, 56.15, 39.71, 29.78, 29.65, 29.43, 27.24. HRMS (ESI) *m/z:* 561.3172 $[M + H]^+$, calcd. for $[C_{30}H_{45}N_2O_8]^+$ 561.3176.

4.7. *General Synthetic Procedure for* **9d**, **9f**

A mixture of cinnamic acid (6.30 mmol), EDCI (7.50 mmol), DMAP (0.60 mmol), and anhydrous dichloromethane (20 mL) was stirred to dissolve, then diamino-alkane (3 mmol) was added and stirred at room temperature for 12 h. The mixture solution was filtered under reduced pressure. After that, the residue was washed with dichloromethane and water successively, and then dried to give a pale white solid. TLC indicated that it was a single point.

4.7.1. (2E,2′E)-N,N′-(Octane-1,8-Diyl)Bis(3-Phenylacrylamide) (**9d**)

Pale white solid, yield 63%, m.p. 186–186.4 °C; ^{1}H-NMR (300 MHz, $CDCl_3$ + CD_3OD) δ: 7.58–7.29 (m, 12H), 6.53 (d, J = 15.7 Hz, 2H), 3.31 (t, J = 7.1 Hz, 4H), 1.59–1.55 (m, 4H), 1.35 (s, 8H). ^{13}C-NMR (101 MHz, $CDCl_3$ + CD_3OD) δ: 166.96, 140.39, 134.78, 129.42, 128.59, 127.54, 120.60, 39.43, 29.04, 28.85, 26.57. HRMS (ESI) *m/z:* 405.2537 $[M + H]^+$, calcd. for $[C_{26}H_{33}N_2O_2]^+$ 405.2542.

4.7.2. (2E,2′E)-N,N′-(Dodecane-1,12-Diyl)Bis(3-Phenylacrylamide) (**9f**)

Pale white solid, yield 49%, m.p. 164.7–165 °C; ^{1}H-NMR (300 MHz, $CDCl_3$ + CD_3OD) δ: 7.56–7.49 (m, 6H), 7.40–7.28 (m, 6H), 6.53 (d, J = 15.7 Hz, 2H), 3.30 (t, J = 7.1 Hz, 4H), 1.62–1.51 (m, 4H), 1.38–1.23 (m, 16H). ^{13}C-NMR (101 MHz, $CDCl_3$ + CD_3OD) δ: 166.94, 140.22, 134.73, 129.29, 128.47, 127.42, 120.54, 39.42, 29.19, 29.03, 28.99, 26.66. HRMS (ESI) *m/z:* 461.3166 $[M + H]^+$, calcd. for $[C_{30}H_{41}N_2O_2]^+$ 461.3168.

4.8. *General Synthetic Procedure for* **9g–9i**

A mixture of cinnamic acid (6.30 mmol), EDCI (7.50 mmol), DMAP (0.60 mmol), and anhydrous dichloromethane (20 mL) was stirred to dissolve, then alkane-diol (3 mmol) was added and stirred at room temperature for 12 h. The mixture solution was filtered under reduced pressure. After that, the residue was washed with dichloromethane and water successively, subsequently, purified by preparative TLC eluted with petroleum ether/ethyl acetate = 5:1 to give pale white solid.

4.8.1. Octane-1,8-Diyl (2E,2′E)-Bis(3-Phenylacrylate) (**9g**)

Pale white solid, yield 35%, m.p. 61.1–62.5 °C; ^{1}H-NMR (300 MHz, $CDCl_3$) δ: 7.68 (d, J = 16 Hz, 2H), 7.58–7.46 (m, 4H), 7.43–7.30 (m, 6H), 6.45 (d, J = 16 Hz, 2H), 4.21 (t, J = 6.7 Hz, 4H), 1.77–1.68 (m, 4H), 1.46–1.40 (m, 8H). ^{13}C-NMR (101 MHz, $CDCl_3$) δ: 167.22, 144.72, 134.62, 130.35, 129.01, 128.19, 118.43, 64.79, 29.31, 28.85, 26.05. HRMS (ESI) *m/z:* 407.2223 $[M + H]^+$, calcd. for $[C_{26}H_{31}O_4]^+$ 407.2222.

4.8.2. Decane-1,10-Diyl (2E,2′E)-Bis(3-Phenylacrylate) (**9h**)

Pale white solid, yield 33%, m.p. 118.6–119.2 °C; ^{1}H-NMR (300 MHz, $CDCl_3$) δ: 7.68 (d, J = 16 Hz, 2H), 7.57–7.48 (m, 4H), 7.38 (dd, J = 6.6, 3.6 Hz, 6H), 6.45 (d, J = 16 Hz, 2H), 4.21 (t, J = 6.7 Hz, 4H), 1.77–1.62 (m, 4H), 1.48–1.25 (m, 12H). ^{13}C-NMR (101 MHz, $CDCl_3$) δ: 167.23, 144.69, 134.64, 130.35, 129.01, 128.19, 118.46, 64.85, 29.58, 29.40, 28.88, 26.12. HRMS (ESI) *m/z:* 435.2534 $[M + H]^+$, calcd. for $[C_{28}H_{35}O_4]^+$ 435.2535.

4.8.3. Dodecane-1,12-Diyl (2E,2′E)-Bis(3-Phenylacrylate) (**9i**)

Pale white solid, yield 28%, m.p. 63.1–64 °C; ^{1}H-NMR (300 MHz, $CDCl_3$) δ: 7.68 (d, J = 16 Hz, 2H), 7.52 (dt, J = 4.6, 3.2 Hz, 4H), 7.42–7.33 (m, 6H), 6.45 (d, J = 16 Hz, 2H), 4.21 (t, J = 6.7 Hz, 4H), 1.77–1.65 (m, 4H), 1.43–1.25 (m, 16H). ^{13}C-NMR (101 MHz, $CDCl_3$) δ: 167.22, 144.68, 134.64, 130.34, 129.01, 128.18, 118.47, 64.87, 29.68, 29.66, 29.42, 28.87, 26.12. HRMS (ESI) *m/z:* 463.2851 $[M + H]^+$, calcd. for $[C_{30}H_{39}O_4]^+$ 463.2828.

4.9. General Synthetic Procedure for **9j–9m**

A mixture of cinnamic acid (6.30 mmol), EDCI (7.50 mmol), DMAP (0.60 mmol), and anhydrous dichloromethane (20 mL) was stirred to dissolve, then diamino-ether (3 mmol) was added and stirred at room temperature for 12 h. Then, the solid was filtered off, the filtrate was added with H_2O (50 mL) and extracted by dichloromethane three times. The combined organic layers were washed with H_2O and brine, dried with anhydrous sodium sulfate for 8 h, filtered, and evaporated. The resulting residue was purified by preparative TLC with petroleum ether/ethyl acetate = 2:1–1:1 to give pale white solid or light yellow oil.

4.9.1. (2E,2′E)-N,N′-((Ethane-1,2-Diylbis(Oxy))Bis(Ethane-2,1-Diyl))Bis(3-Phenylacrylamide) (**9j**)

Pale white solid, yield 78%, m.p. 117.9–118.5 °C; ^{1}H-NMR (300 MHz, $CDCl_3$) δ: 7.62 (d, J = 15.6 Hz, 2H), 7.51–7.41 (m, 4H), 7.37–7.27 (m, 6H), 6.48 (d, J = 15.6 Hz, 2H), 3.65–3.60 (m, 12H). ^{13}C-NMR (101 MHz, $CDCl_3$) δ: 166.26, 141.19, 134.95, 129.77, 128.92, 127.92, 120.82, 70.50, 70.05, 39.63. HRMS (ESI) *m/z*: 409.2121 $[M + H]^+$, calcd. for $[C_{24}H_{29}N_2O_4]^+$ 409.2127.

4.9.2. (2E,2′E)-N,N′-(((Oxybis(Ethane-2,1-Diyl))Bis(Oxy))Bis(Ethane-2,1-Diyl))Bis(3-Phenylacrylamide) (**9k**)

Light yellow oil, yield 28%; ^{1}H-NMR (300 MHz, $CDCl_3$) δ: 7.60 (d, J = 15.6 Hz, 2H), 7.45 (dd, J = 6.5, 3.1 Hz, 4H), 7.32–7.30 (m, 4H), 6.71 (t, J = 5.7 Hz, 2H), 6.47 (d, J = 15.6 Hz, 2H), 3.65 (s, 8H), 3.63–3.54 (m, 8H). ^{13}C-NMR (101 MHz, $CDCl_3$) δ: 166.17, 140.96, 134.98, 129.70, 128.89, 127.86, 120.93, 70.49, 70.27, 70, 39.59. HRMS (ESI) *m/z:* 453.2387 $[M + H]^+$, calcd. for $[C_{26}H_{33}N_2O_5]^+$ 453.2389.

4.9.3. (Ethane-1,2-Diylbis(Oxy))Bis(Ethane-2,1-Diyl) (2E,2′E)-Bis(3-Phenylacrylate) (**9l**)

Light yellow oil, yield 65%; ^{1}H-NMR (300 MHz, $CDCl_3$) δ: 7.70 (d, J = 16 Hz, 2H), 7.54–7.48 (m, 4H), 7.40–7.34 (m, 6H), 6.48 (d, J = 16 Hz, 2H), 4.42–4.36 (m, 4H), 3.84–3.77 (m, 4H), 3.73 (s, 4H). ^{13}C-NMR (101 MHz, $CDCl_3$) δ: 167.03, 145.21, 134.50, 130.44, 129.01, 128.23, 118, 70.79, 69.48, 63.78. HRMS (ESI) *m/z:* 411.1805 $[M + H]^+$, calcd. for $[C_{24}H_{27}O_6]^+$ 411.1808.

4.9.4. ((Oxybis(Ethane-2,1-Diyl))Bis(Oxy))Bis(Ethane-2,1-Diyl) (2E,2′E)-bis(3-Phenylacrylate) (**9m**)

Light yellow oil, yield 87%; ^{1}H-NMR (300 MHz, $CDCl_3$) δ: 7.70 (d, J = 16 Hz, 2H), 7.55–7.48 (m, 4H), 7.38 (dd, J = 3.8, 2.7 Hz, 6H), 6.48 (d, J = 16 Hz, 2H), 4.37 (dd, J = 5.5, 4.1 Hz, 4H), 3.81–3.74 (m, 4H), 3.70 (s, 8H). ^{13}C-NMR (101 MHz, $CDCl_3$) δ: 167.03, 145.19, 134.52, 130.45, 129.02, 128.23, 118.04, 77.48, 77.36, 77.16, 76.84, 70.82, 70.79, 69.42, 63.80. HRMS (ESI) *m/z*: 472.2337 $[M + NH_4]^+$, calcd. for $[C_{26}H_{34}NO_7]^+$ 472.2335.

4.10. Biological Assays

4.10.1. Cell Culture

The tested cells were obtained from Shanghai Institute of Biochemistry and Cell Biology of the Chinese Academy of Sciences (Shanghai, China). HeLa and Hep G2 cell lines were cultured in Dulbecco's modified Eagle's medium (DMEM; gibco, Life Technologies, Carlsbad, CA, USA) supplemented with 10% fetal bovine serum (FBS; Biological Industries), 100 U/mL penicillin-streptomycin (PS; gibco, Life Technologies, Carlsbad, CA, USA). MCF-7 and A549 cell lines were maintained in RPMI-1640 media (gibco, Life Technologies, Carlsbad, CA, USA) supplemented with 10% FBS and 100 U/mL PS. FaDu cell lines were cultured in minimum essential medium (MEM; Gibco, Life Technologies, Carlsbad, CA, USA) supplemented with 10% FBS and 100 U/mL PS. MCF 10A cell lines were maintained in Mammary MEGM kit (Lonza/Clonetics) supplemented with 100 ng/mL cholera toxin (Sigma, Shanghai, China). Cell lines were grown at 37 °C in a humidified atmosphere of 5% CO_2.

4.10.2. Cell Viability Assay

The growth-inhibitory effects against HeLa, Hep G2, MCF-7, FaDu, and A549 cancer cells and normal cell lines MCF 10A were determined by MTT assay [21]. All of the synthesized compounds and the positive control drug doxorubicin were dissolved in 0.1% DMSO. Cells were seeded in 96 well plates at a density of 1×10^4 cells per well and incubated for 24 h at 37 °C in a humidified atmosphere of 5% CO_2. The cells were then incubated with various concentrations of drugs for 48 h in a 5% CO_2 incubator at 37 °C. After treatment with 1 mg/mL 3-(4,5-dimethylthiazol-2-yl)-2,5-diphenyltetrazolium bromide (MTT) solution for 4 h, the formazan crystals were dissolved in 100 μL DMSO in each well. Plates were read on a microplate reader (Thermo Varioskan Flash 3001) at 490 nm. The experiment was performed in triplicate. The inhibitory concentration at 50% (IC_{50}) was calculated based on concentration-inhibition relationships via regression using SPSS software (Version 17.0).

4.10.3. Colony Formation Assay

FaDu cells were seeded in a 6-well plate with 500 cells per well and incubated for 24 h. Then, the cells were treated with compound **8e** at various final concentrations of 0, 0.75, 1.50, 3 nM. Following treatment for 10 days, the cells were washed with PBS twice and fixed with 4% paraformaldehyde for 10 min at room temperature. Then, the cell colonies were visualized by staining with 0.1% crystal violet for 10 min. The image was photographed with Handy camera, and the numbers of cell colonies were analyzed using the open Image J software (Developed by National Institutes of Health). A group of >50 cells was defined as one colony. Triplicate wells were set up for each concentration.

4.10.4. Live/Dead Staining

The Calcein AM/propidium iodide (PI) double staining was performed following the manufacturer's instructions (Dojindo Laboratory, Kumamoto, Japan). Briefly, FaDu cells were seeded in 6-well plates overnight. Then, the **8e** solutions at final concentrations of 2.5 nM, 5 nM, and 10 nM were added. After incubation for 24 h, the cells were collected, washed with PBS, and stained by a mixture of 2 μM Calcein-AM (live cells, green) and 4.5 μM PI (dead cells, red) solution in the dark for 30 min at 37 °C (excitation 490 nm). Then, the cells were rinsed with PBS twice and re-suspended in the cell medium. Confocal fluorescence images were acquired using a laser scanning confocal microscope (LSCM, Carl-Zeiss LSM 710).

4.10.5. Hoechst 33,342 Staining

For Hoechst staining, FaDu cells were seeded onto a glass-bottom of cell culture dish at a density of 1×10^5 cells. After incubation for 24 h, the media containing 20 nM of the compound **8e** was used to replace the culture medium. Then, the cells were stained with Hoechst 33,342 solution (10 μg/mL in the culture medium, Beyotime Institute of Biotechnology, Shanghai, China) at 37 °C in the dark for 20 min after treatment with **8e**. Then, the cells were washed with the serum-free medium to remove excess dye. LSCM (Carl-Zeiss LSM 710) was used to capture the images of nuclear morphological changes to find apoptotic cells.

4.10.6. Flow Cytometric Analysis of Apoptosis by Annexin V-FITC/PI Staining

Apoptosis in FaDu cells was evaluated by an annexin V-FITC/PI apoptosis detection kit (Beyotime Institute of Biotechnology, Shanghai, China). Briefly, FaDu cells were treated with various concentrations of compound **8e** (2, 5, 10 nM) or DMSO as vehicle control for 24 h at 37 °C; then, the cells were washed twice with cold 1× PBS and centrifuged at 1000 rpm for 5 min. The harvested cells were resuspended gently in 400 μL binding buffer, containing 5 μL annexin V-FITC and 10 μL PI. After incubating for 15 min in the dark at room temperature, the cells were analyzed with flow cytometry (CyFlow® Cube 6, Sysmex). Data were shown as pseudo color graphs and analyzed using FlowJo Software (Tree Star Inc, Ashland, OR).

4.10.7. Mitochondrial Membrane Potential (ΔΨm) Analysis

The mitochondrial membrane potential (ΔΨm) was detected by a mitochondrial membrane potential assay kit with JC-1 (Beyotime Institute of Biotechnology, Shanghai, China). Briefly, after treatment with various concentrations of compound **8e** (2, 5, 10 nM) for 24 h, FaDu cells were harvested and stained with 500 μL 1× JC-1 dye solution at 37 °C for 20 min in the dark. Then, the treated cells were washed twice and resuspended by 1× JC-1 staining buffer. The fluorescence of approximately 1×10^4 cells was analyzed using flow cytometry (CyFlow® Cube 6, Sysmex).

4.10.8. Cell Cycle Analysis

The cell cycle analysis was carried out by a cell cycle and apoptosis analysis kit with a propidium iodide (PI) staining method (Beyotime Institute of Biotechnology, Shanghai, China). Briefly, FaDu cells were incubated with the above-mentioned doses of compound **8e** for 24 h; all samples were collected, washed once with cold 1× PBS, and fixed by 70% ice-cold ethanol at 4 °C for 12 h. Then, the fixed cells were washed once with cold 1× PBS and stained with 500 μL 1× PI dye solution (containing 10 μL RNase A) at 37 °C for 30 min in the dark. The red fluorescence was detected using a flow cytometer (CyFlow® Cube 6, Sysmex). The data were analyzed using FlowJo Software (Tree Star Inc, Ashland, OR, USA).

4.10.9. In Silico ADMET Prediction

A computational study of all synthesized compounds was carried out for the prediction of ADMET (absorption, distribution, metabolism, excretion, and toxicity) properties. In this module, thirteen mathematical models, such as HBD (hydrogen bond donor), HBA (hydrogen bond acceptor), RBN (number of rotatable bonds), logP (log of the octanol/water partition coefficient), log S (log of the aqueous solubility), and PSA (polar surface area) were predicted via Discovery Studio 2.0 Software (Studio 2.5, Accelrys, Co. Ltd., San Diego, CA, USA) and HIA (human intestinal absorption), PPB (plasma protein binding), CYP3D4 (CYP3D4 inhibition), $T_{1/2}$ (half lifetime), HT (human hepatotoxicity), and LD_{50} (median lethal dose) were calculated using web-based applications and then analyzed to predict the drug likeliness profile (Xiangya School of Pharmaceutical Sciences and Central South University, http://admet.scbdd.com/home/index/) [28]. We also screened our novel derivatives through the prediction model by Egan et al. [29,30]. Two molecular descriptors, AlogP98 and PSA, were computed and plotted in a 2D plane to comprehensively evaluate the absorption and blood-brain penetration of the compounds.

Author Contributions: Ideas and experiment design: J.W., G.H., and T.L.; Chemistry and Biology: J.W., G.H., G.L., and W.W.; Analysis and interpretation of data: J.W., G.H., G.L., and W.W.; Writing and review of the manuscript: J.W., G.H., G.L., W.W., and T.L.; Study supervision: T.L. and G.H.

Acknowledgments: The authors gratefully acknowledge the Institute of Materia Medica, Chinese Academy of Medical Sciences and Peking Union Medical College and information technology center for affording the Discovery Studio 2.0 Software.

References

1. Cragg, G.M.; Newman, D.J. Natural products: A continuing source of novel drug leads. *Biochim. Et Biophys. Acta (Bba) - Gen. Subj.* **2013**, *1830*, 3670–3695. [CrossRef] [PubMed]
2. Chang, C.-Y.; Kao, T.-K.; Chen, W.-Y.; Ou, Y.-C.; Li, J.-R.; Liao, S.-L.; Raung, S.-L.; Chen, C.-J. Tetramethylpyrazine inhibits neutrophil activation following permanent cerebral ischemia in rats. *Biochem. Biophys. Res. Commun.* **2015**, *463*, 421–427. [CrossRef] [PubMed]
3. Cao, J.; Miao, Q.; Miao, S.; Bi, L.; Zhang, S.; Yang, Q.; Zhou, X.; Zhang, M.; Xie, Y.; Zhang, J.; et al. Tetramethylpyrazine (TMP) exerts antitumor effects by inducing apoptosis and autophagy in hepatocellular carcinoma. *Int. Immunopharmacol.* **2015**, *26*, 212–220. [CrossRef] [PubMed]
4. Bi, L.; Yan, X.; Chen, W.; Gao, J.; Qian, L.; Qiu, S. Antihepatocellular Carcinoma Potential of Tetramethylpyrazine Induces Cell Cycle Modulation and Mitochondrial-Dependent Apoptosis: Regulation of p53 Signaling Pathway in HepG2 Cells In Vitro. *Integr. Cancer Ther.* **2016**, *15*, 226–236. [CrossRef]
5. Ai, Y.; Zhu, B.; Ren, C.; Kang, F.; Li, J.; Huang, Z.; Lai, Y.; Peng, S.; Ding, K.; Tian, J.; et al. Discovery of New Monocarbonyl Ligustrazine–Curcumin Hybrids for Intervention of Drug-Sensitive and Drug-Resistant Lung Cancer. *J. Med. Chem.* **2016**, *59*, 1747–1760. [CrossRef]
6. Xu, B.; Yan, W.-Q.; Xu, X.; Wu, G.-R.; Zhang, C.-Z.; Han, Y.-T.; Chu, F.-H.; Zhao, R.; Wang, P.-L.; Lei, H.-M. Combination of amino acid/dipeptide with ligustrazine-betulinic acid as antitumor agents. *Eur. J. Med. Chem.* **2017**, *130*, 26–38. [CrossRef]
7. Wang, P.-L.; Cheng, Y.-T.; Xu, K.; An, Y.-W.; Wang, W.; Li, Q.-S.; Han, Q.-J.; Li, Q.; Zhang, H.-G.; Lei, H.-M. Synthesis and Antitumor Evaluation of One Novel Tetramethylpyrazine-Rhein Derivative. *Asian J. Chem.* **2013**, *25*, 4885–4888. [CrossRef]
8. Chow, L.M.C.; Chan, T.H. Novel Classes of Dimer Antitumour Drug Candidates. *Curr. Pharm. Des.* **2009**, *15*, 659–674. [CrossRef]
9. Joshi, A.; Vance, D.; Rai, P.; Thiyagarajan, A.; Kane, R.S. The Design of Polyvalent Therapeutics. *Chem. –A Eur. J.* **2008**, *14*, 7738–7747. [CrossRef]
10. Beekman, A.C.; Barentsen, A.R.W.; Woerdenbag, H.J.; Van Uden, W.; Pras, N.; Konings, A.W.T.; El-Feraly, F.S.; Galal, A.M.; Wikström, H.V. Stereochemistry-Dependent Cytotoxicity of Some Artemisinin Derivatives. *J. Nat. Prod.* **1997**, *60*, 325–330. [CrossRef]
11. Hu, Y.; Li, C.; Kulkarni, B.A.; Strobel, G.; Lobkovsky, E.; Torczynski, R.M.; Porco, J.A. Exploring Chemical Diversity of Epoxyquinoid Natural Products: Synthesis and Biological Activity of (−)-Jesterone and Related Molecules. *Org. Lett.* **2001**, *3*, 1649–1652. [CrossRef] [PubMed]
12. Verhoeven, D.T.; Goldbohm, R.A.; van Poppel, G.; Verhagen, H.; van den Brandt, P.A. Epidemiological studies on brassica vegetables and cancer risk. *Cancer Epidemiol. Biomark. Amp; Prev.* **1996**, *5*, 733–748.

13. Chaires, J.B.; Leng, F.; Przewloka, T.; Fokt, I.; Ling, Y.H.; Perezsoler, R.; Priebe, W. Structure-based design of a new bisintercalating anthracycline antibiotic. *J. Med. Chem.* **1997**, *40*, 261–266. [CrossRef] [PubMed]
14. Zha, G.-F.; Qin, H.-L.; Youssif, B.G.M.; Amjad, M.W.; Raja, M.A.G.; Abdelazeem, A.H.; Bukhari, S.N.A. Discovery of potential anticancer multi-targeted ligustrazine based cyclohexanone and oxime analogs overcoming the cancer multidrug resistance. *Eur. J. Med. Chem.* **2017**, *135*, 34–48. [CrossRef]
15. Wang, P.; She, G.; Yang, Y.; Li, Q.; Zhang, H.; Liu, J.; Cao, Y.; Xu, X.; Lei, H. Synthesis and Biological Evaluation of New Ligustrazine Derivatives as Anti-Tumor Agents. *Molecules* **2012**, *17*, 4972–4985. [CrossRef]
16. Xu, B.; Chu, F.; Zhang, Y.; Wang, X.; Li, Q.; Liu, W.; Xu, X.; Xing, Y.; Chen, J.; Wang, P.; et al. A Series of New Ligustrazine-Triterpenes Derivatives as Anti-Tumor Agents: Design, Synthesis, and Biological Evaluation. *Int. J. Mol. Sci.* **2015**, *16*, 21035–21055. [CrossRef]
17. Taylor, A.P.; Robinson, R.P.; Fobian, Y.M.; Blakemore, D.C.; Jones, L.H.; Fadeyi, O. Modern advances in heterocyclic chemistry in drug discovery. *Org. Biomol. Chem.* **2016**, *14*, 6611–6637. [CrossRef]
18. Klein, B.; Berkowitz, J. Pyrazines. I. Pyrazine-N-oxides. Preparation and Spectral Characteristics1. *J. Am. Chem. Soc.* **1959**, *81*, 5160–5166. [CrossRef]
19. Cheng, X.-C.; Liu, X.-Y.; Xu, W.-F.; Guo, X.-L.; Zhang, N.; Song, Y.-N. Ligustrazine derivatives. Part 3: Design, synthesis and evaluation of novel acylpiperazinyl derivatives as potential cerebrocardiac vascular agents. *Bioorganic Med. Chem.* **2009**, *17*, 3018–3024. [CrossRef]
20. Wu, G.-R.; Xu, B.; Yang, Y.-Q.; Zhang, X.-Y.; Fang, K.; Ma, T.; Wang, H.; Xue, N.-N.; Chen, M.; Guo, W.-B.; et al. Synthesis and biological evaluation of podophyllotoxin derivatives as selective antitumor agents. *Eur. J. Med. Chem.* **2018**, *155*, 183–196. [CrossRef]
21. van Meerloo, J.; Kaspers, G.J.L.; Cloos, J. Cell Sensitivity Assays: The MTT Assay. In *Cancer Cell Culture: Methods and Protocols*; Cree, I.A., Ed.; Humana Press: Totowa, NJ, USA, 2011; pp. 237–245.
22. Yi, B.; Liu, D.; He, M.; Li, Q.; Liu, T.; Shao, J. Role of the ROS/AMPK signaling pathway in tetramethylpyrazine-induced apoptosis in gastric cancer cells. *Oncol. Lett.* **2013**, *6*, 583–589. [CrossRef] [PubMed]
23. Shen, J.; Zeng, L.; Pan, L.; Yuan, S.; Wu, M.; Kong, X. Tetramethylpyrazine regulates breast cancer cell viability, migration, invasion and apoptosis by affecting the activity of Akt and caspase-3. *Oncol. Lett.* **2018**, *15*, 4557–4563. [CrossRef] [PubMed]
24. Chu, F.; Xu, X.; Li, G.; Gu, S.; Xu, K.; Gong, Y.; Xu, B.; Wang, M.; Zhang, H.; Zhang, Y.; et al. Amino acid derivatives of ligustrazine-oleanolic acid as new cytotoxic agents. *Molecules* **2014**, *19*, 18215–18231. [CrossRef] [PubMed]
25. Song, F.; Zhang, L.; Yu, H.-X.; Lu, R.-R.; Bao, J.-D.; Tan, C.; Sun, Z. The mechanism underlying proliferation-inhibitory and apoptosis-inducing effects of curcumin on papillary thyroid cancer cells. *Food Chem.* **2012**, *132*, 43–50. [CrossRef] [PubMed]
26. Lipinski, C.A.; Lombardo, F.; Dominy, B.W.; Feeney, P.J. Experimental and computational approaches to estimate solubility and permeability in drug discovery and development settings. *Adv. Drug Deliv. Rev.* **2012**, *64*, 4–17. [CrossRef]
27. Meena, A.; Yadav, D.K.; Srivastava, A.; Khan, F.; Chanda, D.; Chattopadhyay, S.K. In Silico Exploration of Anti-Inflammatory Activity of Natural Coumarinolignoids. *Chem. Biol. Drug Des.* **2011**, *78*, 567–579. [CrossRef]
28. Dong, J.; Wang, N.-N.; Yao, Z.-J.; Zhang, L.; Cheng, Y.; Ouyang, D.; Lu, A.-P.; Cao, D.-S. ADMETlab: A platform for systematic ADMET evaluation based on a comprehensively collected ADMET database. *J. Cheminformatics* **2018**, *10*, 29. [CrossRef]
29. Egan, W.J.; Lauri, G. Prediction of intestinal permeability. *Adv. Drug Deliv. Rev.* **2002**, *54*, 273–289. [CrossRef]
30. Egan, W.J.; Merz, K.M.; Baldwin, J.J. Prediction of Drug Absorption Using Multivariate Statistics. *J. Med. Chem.* **2000**, *43*, 3867–3877. [CrossRef]

5

P-MAPA and Interleukin-12 Reduce Cell Migration/Invasion and Attenuate the Toll-Like Receptor-Mediated Inflammatory Response in Ovarian Cancer SKOV-3 Cells

Luiz Antonio Lupi [1], Flávia Karina Delella [2], Maira Smaniotto Cucielo [1], Graziela Gorete Romagnoli [3], Ramon Kaneno [3], Iseu da Silva Nunes [4], Raquel Fantin Domeniconi [1], Marcelo Martinez [5], Francisco Eduardo Martinez [1], Wagner José Fávaro [6] and Luiz Gustavo de Almeida Chuffa [1,*]

1 Department of Anatomy, UNESP-São Paulo State University, Institute of Biosciences, Botucatu, 18618-689 São Paulo, Brazil; luiz.lupi@unesp.br (L.A.L.); maira.cucielo@gmail.com (M.S.C.); raquel.domeniconi@unesp.br (R.F.D.); fe.martinez@unesp.br (F.E.M.)

2 Department of Morphology, UNESP-São Paulo State University, Institute of Biosciences, Botucatu, 18618-689 São Paulo, Brazil; flavia.delella@unesp.br

3 Department of Microbiology and Immunology, UNESP-São Paulo State University, Institute of Biosciences, Botucatu, 18618-689 São Paulo, Brazil; graziela.romagnoli@unesp.br (G.G.R.); rskaneno@yahoo.com.br (R.K.)

4 Farmabrasilis R&D Division, Campinas, 13279-020 SP, Brazil; iseununes@gmail.com

5 Department of Morphology and Pathology, Federal University of São Carlos, 13565-905 São Paulo, Brazil; martinez@ufscar.br

6 Department of Structural and Functional Biology, UNICAMP-University of Campinas, Campinas, 13083-970 São Paulo, Brazil; favarowj@unicamp.br

* Correspondence: guchuffa@yahoo.com.br;

Academic Editor: Qiao-Hong Chen

Abstract: Immunotherapies have emerged as promising complementary treatments for ovarian cancer (OC), but its effective and direct role on OC cells is unclear. This study examined the combinatory effects of the protein aggregate magnesium–ammonium phospholinoleate–palmitoleate anhydride, known as P-MAPA, and the human recombinant interleukin-12 (hrIL-12) on cell migration/invasion, apoptosis, toll-like receptor (TLR)-mediated inflammation, and cytokine/chemokine profile in human OC cell line SKOV-3. P-MAPA and IL-12 showed cancer cell toxicity under low doses after 48 h. Although apoptosis/necrosis and the cell cycle were unchanged by the treatments, P-MAPA enhanced the sensitivity to paclitaxel (PTX) and P-MAPA associated with IL-12 significantly reduced the migratory potential and invasion capacity of SKOV-3 cells. P-MAPA therapy reduced TLR2 immunostaining and the myeloid differentiation factor 88 (MyD88), but not the TLR4 levels. Moreover, the combination of P-MAPA with IL-12 attenuated the levels of MyD88, interferon regulatory factor 3 (IRF3) and nuclear factor kappa B (NF-kB p65). The IL-12 levels were increased and P-MAPA stimulated the secretion of cytokines IL-3, IL-9, IL-10, and chemokines MDC/CCL22 and, regulated on activation, normal T cells expressed and secreted (RANTES)/CCL5. Conversely, combination therapy reduced the levels of IL-3, IL-9, IL-10, MDC/CCL22, and RANTES/CCL5. Collectively, P-MAPA and IL-12 reduce cell dynamics and effectively target the TLR-related downstream molecules, eliciting a protective effect against chemoresistance. P-MAPA also stimulates the secretion of anti-inflammatory molecules, possibly having an immune response in the OC microenvironment.

Keywords: ovarian cancer; P-MAPA; IL-12; TLR signaling; inflammation; chemoresistance

1. Introduction

Ovarian cancer (OC) is the fifth largest cause of cancer-related death in the United States and is the most lethal of all gynecological malignancies [1]. OC originates from the ovarian surface epithelium, fallopian tube (fimbriae region) or endometriosis-related tissue, and often exhibits a late diagnosis due to the lack of clear signs or symptoms in the early stages of development [2–5]. Unfortunately, there is no screening method for achieving the best curative result, and traditional chemotherapy and surgery are limited for patients with advanced OC [6]. After cisplatin and paclitaxel (PTX) resistance, several patients become susceptible to developing recurrent OC and metastasis [7]. Therefore, new therapeutic options that overcome chemoresistance and enhance drug sensitivity are promising for the treatment of OC.

Immunotherapies have demonstrated great efficiency by activating host immune responses into the OC microenvironment [8]; however, what is happening with the cancer cells as a direct result of immunostimulation requires further investigation. We recently reported the effect of the immunomodulatory agent termed protein aggregate magnesium-ammonium phospholinoleate-palmitoleate anhydride (P-MAPA), a natural biopolymer extracted from the *Aspergillus oryzae*, which exhibits a number of antitumor responses in different experimental models of cancer [9–11]. In association with cisplatin, P-MAPA showed a greater survival rate and a reduced OC volume in addition to the increased expression of proteins involved in toll-like receptor (TLR)-mediated inflammatory response (canonical and non-canonical pathways) in OC-bearing animals [11]. Recent studies also supported the immunological mechanism of action of P-MAPA through the activation of TLR2 and TLR4 signaling in both cancer and infections, in addition to regulating the activity of T cells (especially CD4+T and CD8+T cells) and natural killer (NK) cells [9,10]. Importantly, P-MAPA did not show toxicity in preclinical in vitro (V-79 Chinese hamster cell line) and in vivo models (Swiss mice, Wistar rats, and monkeys) nor in human clinical trial phase I [9]; its effects in cancer treatment have been tested in non-muscle invasive urinary bladder cancer [9,10] and in OC [11]. The directive role of P-MAPA on human OC cells, considering its feasibility, sensibility, resistance, and toxicity, has not been explored yet.

TLRs are transmembrane molecules that signal via myeloid differentiation factor 88 (MyD88) or TLR-associated activator of interferon (TRIF) to induce cell proliferation, chemoresistance, and cytokine/chemokine production [12]. Most importantly, TLRs can trigger a different response depending on the cell type (e.g., cancer cell or immune cell), and particularly, TLR4 has been reported to be a precursor of the immune escape of OC cells [13,14]. The crosstalk between the immunoadjuvant and the OC cells targeting the TLR signaling and related cytokine secretion has never been proposed as to their impact and specific response.

Interleukin-12 (IL-12) is a cytokine related to innate and adaptive immunity, being mainly produced by the antigen-presenting cells (APCs), such as B lymphocytes, dendritic cells (DCs), and others [15,16]. It acts on T and NK cells stimulating a cytotoxic CD8+ response and inducing cytokine production, especially interferon-γ (IFN-γ) [15,17]; IL-12 is involved in the differentiation of naïve T cells into a polarized T helper 1 (Th1) immune response. Patients with recurrent OC who underwent IL-12 treatment, in a well-established dosage regimen, showed significant tumor regression [18]; the major challenge involving the treatment with IL-12 is related to the adverse effects due to its high diffusion and toxicity (e.g., lymphopenia and irreversible elevation of transaminases at 600 ng/kg and neutropenia, fatigue, and headache at 300 ng/kg) [19], and a more precise and direct administration may limit their undesirable effects. Notably, a phase II study involving intraperitoneal infusions of recombinant IL-12 in patients with residual disease $\leq$1 cm showed to be well-tolerated after fist-line therapy for OC-related peritoneal carcinomatosis [19]. Recently, Cohen et al. [16] studied the relationship between membrane-bound IL-12 in tumor cells and the potential to disrupt protumorigenic signaling and tumor outgrowth within peritoneal cavities; IL-12 significantly led to a tumor refractory state, thereby delaying the onset of metastatic disease.

Because P-MAPA is thought to increase IFN-γ levels, which may potentiate the Thelper (Th1)-mediated immune response, and adjuvant therapies with IL-12 have long been proposed as beneficial for patients with OC, this study investigates the effects of P-MAPA and IL-12, alone or in combination, on cancer cell activities with focus to the TLR-mediated inflammatory process and cytokines/chemokines profiling in human SKOV-3 cell line.

2. Results

2.1. P-MAPA and IL-12 Reduce Cell Viability and Induce Apoptosis in the Presence of PTX in SKOV-3 Cells

An MTT assay was carried out using three biological and technical replicates to unravel the most suitable dose and period of treatment. Based on previous results, the SKOV-3 cells were challenged with P-MAPA at doses of 25 μg/mL, 50 μg/mL, and 100 μg/mL, and rhIL-12 at doses of 0.5 ng/mL, 1 ng/mL, and 2 ng/mL for 24 h, 48 h, and 72 h. Then, we tested three different cell concentrations to achieve the better treatment response (1×10^3 cells, 1×10^4 cells, and 5×10^4 cells; Supplementary Figure S1). The SKOV-3 cell viability was efficiently reduced after the low-dose P-MAPA treatment (25 μg/mL for 48 h; viability was reduced by ~27%), and then started to increase after 72 h exposure (Figure 1A). Treatment with rhIL-12 also showed reduction in cell viability at an intermediate dose of 1 ng/mL mainly after 48-h exposure (Figure 1B; viability reduction by ~25% after 48 h). Combinatory therapy with P-MAPA and IL-12 also reduced the cell viability by about 33% (Figure 1C), and the treatment doses were set at 25 μg/mL of P-MAPA and 1 ng/mL of IL-12. Annexin V- fluorescein isothiocyanate (FITC)/Propidium iodide (PI) staining was used to effectively determine the apoptosis/necrosis rate induced by P-MAPA and rhIL-12 immunotherapies. In this study, we set early apoptosis (Annexin V-FITC+/PI−) as apoptosis and late apoptosis (Annexin V+/PI+) and necrosis (Annexin V−/PI+) as necrosis. The apoptosis index was not influenced by P-MAPA, IL-12, or P-MAPA+IL-12 (Figure 1D,E), which pointed out that these agents are unable to induce cell death at this concentration. We also observed that P-MAPA and IL-12 did not alter the cell cycle significantly (Figure 1F,G). These data indicate that these immunotherapeutic agents do not have a direct and high toxic effect to the cell, which is, in fact, expected from immunotherapies. Because the treatments did not promote cell death or cell proliferation, the reduction of cell viability might have been a result of decreased cell metabolism, because the MTT test indirectly reflects the mitochondrial activity.

To better understand whether P-MAPA and IL-12 therapies potentially increase the effect of standard chemotherapy, they were tested in association with PTX (Figure 2A,B). After 48 h, P-MAPA decreased cell viability in association with different doses of PTX compared with cells treated with PTX only (~30% reduction with 5 μM PTX; ~30% reduction with 2.5 μM PTX; ~24% reduction with 1.25 μM PTX and ~34% reduction with 0.625 μM PTX). Because IL-12 had no effect on cell viability when associated with PTX, the decreased cell viability observed after combining P-MAPA with IL-12 in association with doses of PTX is probably due to the P-MAPA effect (~19% reduction with 5 μM PTX, ~30% reduction with 2.5 μM PTX, ~30% reduction with 1.25 μM PTX, and ~38% reduction with 0.625 μM PTX). To confirm these effects on SKOV-3 cell death, an Annexin V-FITC/PI assay was performed using the lowest dose of PTX (0.625 μM). Concordantly, with the MTT results, P-MAPA and P-MAPA+IL-12 increased cell death in association with PTX at dose of 0.625 μM. The apoptosis/necrosis ratio of PTX was 0.64 and became higher when associated with P-MAPA (1.18) or P-MAPA+IL-12 (0.88), thus enhancing the P-MAPA effect as apoptotic inductor. Finally, PTX significantly increased the number of cells in G0/G1 and decreased cells in G2/M phase of the cell cycle, thus inducing cell cycle arrest. In this case, the addition of P-MAPA and IL-12 did not potentiate the PTX effects in cell cycle (Figure 2D,E).

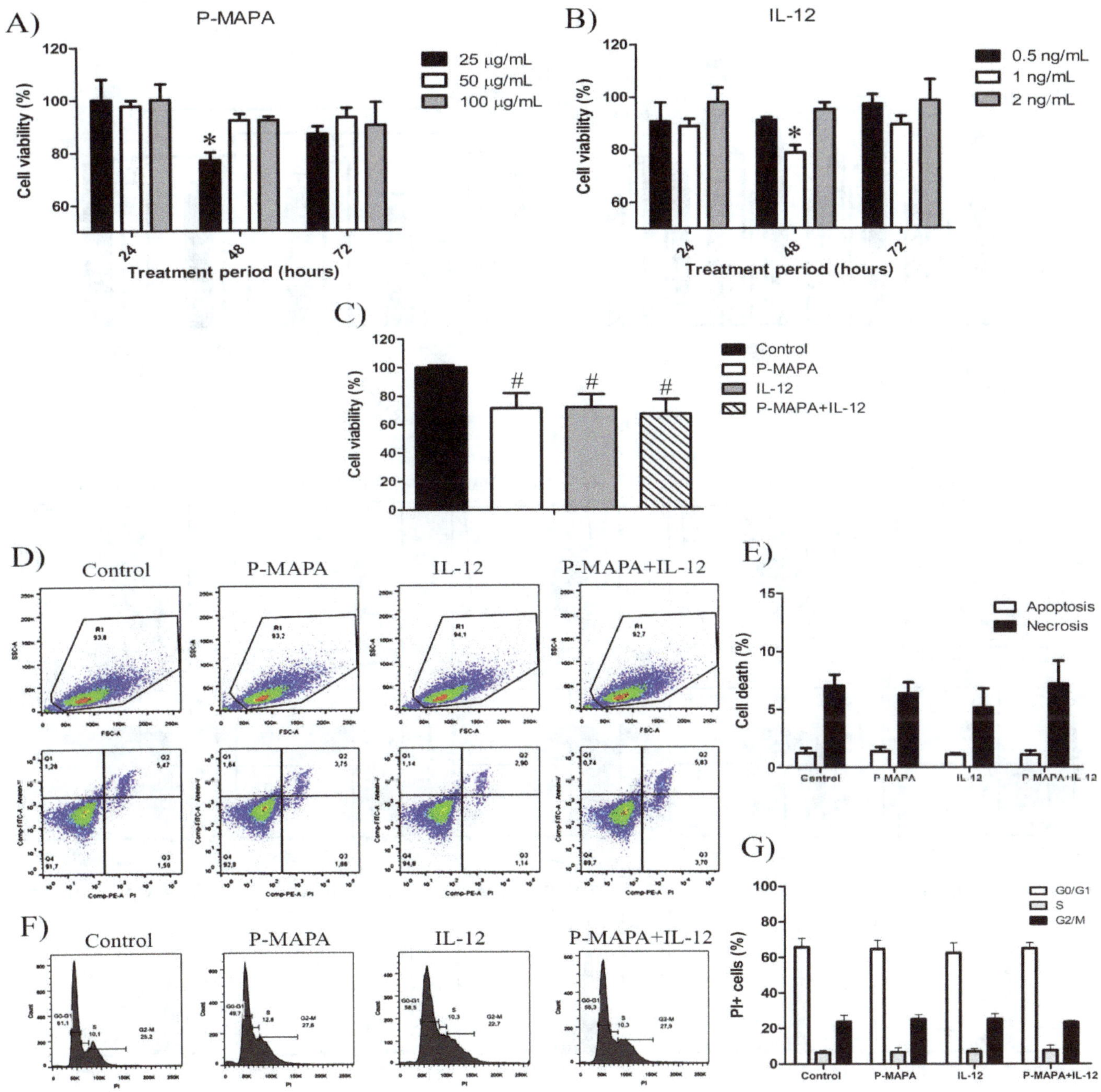

Figure 1. Protein aggregate magnesium–ammonium phospholinoleate–palmitoleate anhydride (P-MAPA) and interleukin-12 (IL-12) suppress cell viability without changing the apoptosis rate and cell cycle. SKOV-3 cells were treated with various concentrations of P-MAPA (**A**) and IL-12 (**B**) for 24, 48, and 72 h, and the cytotoxicity (expressed as percentage) was assayed by MTT; (**C**) Cell viability (%) after standardization of treatments (25 µg P-MAPA and 1 ng IL-12) after 48 h exposure; 1×10^3 SKOV-3 cells showed the best reproducibility. (**D**) Representative apoptotic index in SKOV-3 cells treated with P-MAPA and IL-12 for 48 h detected by annexin V/PI flow cytometry. (**E**) Percentage of cells in apoptosis and necrosis. (**F**) Representative cell cycle analysis in SKOV-3 cells treated with P-MAPA and IL-12 for 48 h detected by PI and RNAase flow cytometry. (**G**) Percentage of PI+ cells in G0/G1, S, and G2/M phases. The samples were assayed in three technical and biological replicates. Results are expressed as the mean ± SD and described as column chart. * $p < 0.05$ vs. different doses at 48 h; # $p < 0.05$ vs. control group.

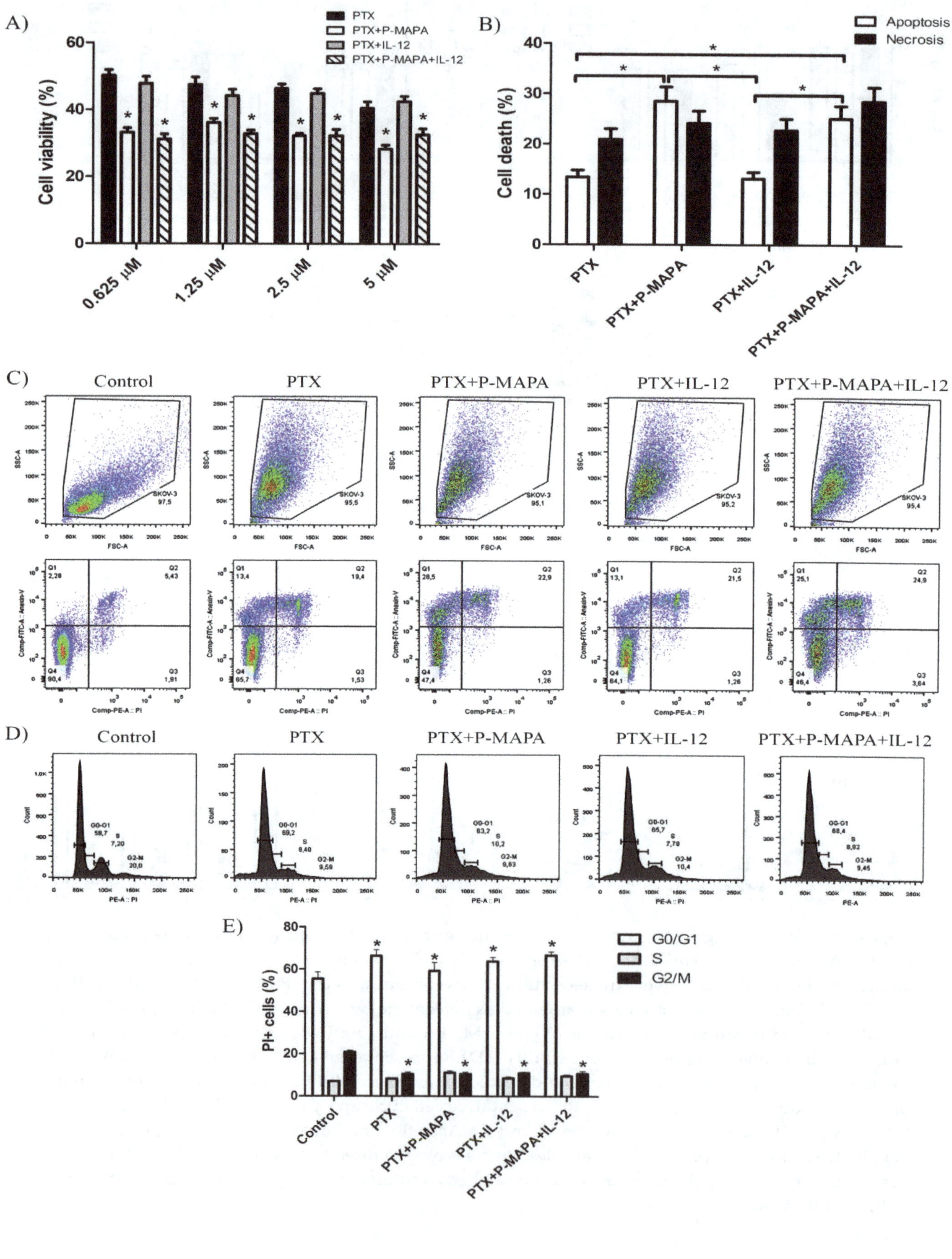
A)
PTX
PTX+P-MAPA
PTX+IL-12
PTX+P-MAPA+IL-12
Cell viability (%)
60
40
20
0
0.625 μM
1.25 μM
2.5 μM
5 μM
B)
Apoptosis
Necrosis
Cell death (%)
40
30
20
10
0
PTX
PTX+P-MAPA
PTX+IL-12
PTX+P-MAPA+IL-12
C)
Control
PTX
PTX+P-MAPA
PTX+IL-12
PTX+P-MAPA+IL-12
SSC-A
FSC-A
SKOV-3 97,5
SKOV-3 95,5
SKOV-3 95,1
SKOV-3 95,2
SKOV-3 95,4
Comp-FITC-A :: Anexin-V
Comp-PE-A :: PI
Q1 2,28
Q2 5,43
Q3 1,91
Q4 90,4
Q1 13,4
Q2 19,4
Q3 1,53
Q4 65,7
Q1 28,5
Q2 22,9
Q3 1,26
Q4 47,4
Q1 13,1
Q2 21,5
Q3 1,26
Q4 64,1
Q1 25,1
Q2 24,9
Q3 3,64
Q4 46,4
D)
Control
PTX
PTX+P-MAPA
PTX+IL-12
PTX+P-MAPA+IL-12
Count
PE-A :: PI
G0-G1 58,7
S 7,20
G2-M 20,0
G0-G1 69,2
S 8,40
G2-M 9,59
G0-G1 63,2
S 10,2
G2-M 9,83
G0-G1 65,7
S 7,79
G2-M 10,4
G0-G1 68,4
S 8,82
G2-M 9,45
E)
G0/G1
S
G2/M
PI+ cells (%)
80
60
40
20
0
Control
PTX
PTX+P-MAPA
PTX+IL-12
PTX+P-MAPA+IL-12

Figure 2. P-MAPA and P-MAPA+IL-12 reduce cell viability and apoptosis/necrosis rate in the presence of PTX. (**A**) Cell viability was assessed by an MTT assay; SKOV-3 cells were treated with various concentrations of PTX alone or in association with P-MAPA and IL-12 for 48 h. * $p < 0.05$ vs. PTX and PTX+IL-12 groups. (**B**) Percentage of cells in apoptosis and necrosis after exposure to 0.625 μM PTX plus P-MAPA, IL-12, or P-MAPA+IL-12. * $p < 0.05$. (**C**) Representative apoptotic index in SKOV-3 cells detected by Annexin V/PI flow cytometry. (**D**) Representative cell cycle analysis in SKOV-3 cells treated with PTX, P-MAPA and IL-12 for 48 h detected by PI and RNase flow cytometry. (**E**) Percentage of PI+ cells in the G0/G1, S, and G2/M phases. The samples were assayed in three technical and biological replicates.* $p < 0.05$ vs. control group. Results are expressed as the mean ± SD.

2.2. Combination of P-MAPA with IL-12 Is Essential to Reduce Cell Migration Whereas P-MAPA Alone Decreased The Invasive Potential of SKOV-3 Cells

To investigate the inhibitory effect of P-MAPA and IL-12 as a single or combinatory treatment on SKOV-3 cells, a wound-healing assay was performed in different periods. Although the treatment with IL-12 showed a reduced migration rate (~ 17%) after 36 h and 48 h exposure, cells treated with P-MAPA migrated significantly less (~ 13%) only at 48 h exposure (Figure 3A,B). Combination of P-MAPA and IL-12 reduced the migratory potential of cells after 36 h and 48 h treatment (>20%), being the most efficient after 36 h (Figure 3A,B); this overall analysis suggests that IL-12 was more effective than P-MAPA in delaying wound closure. SKOV-3 cells that were treated with 0.9% saline solution (control group) had an accelerated growth and migration rate when compared with all the treatments. Because the wound-healing assay might be biased by cell proliferation, transwell migration and invasion assays were performed and effectively showed that P-MAPA reduced cell migration when administered alone or in association with IL-12 (Figure 4A). When Geltrex® was added to the chambers, the number of invasive cells was reduced after P-MAPA treatment in comparison to IL-12 treatment or its association (Figure 4B).

2.3. Immunotherapy with P-MAPA and IL-12 Significantly Reduced the TLR-Mediated Downstream Molecules Involved in the Inflammatory Process of SKOV-3 Cells

One of the most important factors responsible for the acquisition of malignant phenotypes of OC cells is associated with chemoresistance to treatments and uncovering new agents that downregulate the inflammatory pathway(s) may be of significant interest. To evaluate whether P-MAPA or IL-12 play a role on OC-related inflammation, TLR2- and TLR4-mediated pathways were evaluated through canonical and non-canonical signaling. Although the expressions of TLR2 and TLR4 did not vary significantly, the downstream target molecules were affected by the treatments (Figure 5A,B). P-MAPA and IL-12 alone or in combination led to a profound reduction in the MyD88 levels (0.53-, 0.48-, and 0.61-fold reduction, respectively vs. the control group; Figure 5A,B). We also evaluated the NF-kB p65 expression in the extracts of SKOV-3 cells, and notably, IL-12 alone or combined with P-MAPA induced a significant reduction in the p65 levels (0.66- and 0.63-fold reduction, respectively vs. control group; Figure 5A,B). To explore the non-canonical pathway, the TRIF and IRF3 levels were measured. Although the TRIF levels were unchanged after the treatments ($p > 0.05$), P-MAPA, IL-12, and the combination of P-MAPA with IL-12 induced a significant decrease in the IRF3 levels (0.70-, 0.43-, and 0.71-fold reduction, respectively vs. the control group; Figure 5A,B). These findings provide evidence that P-MAPA and IL-12 potentially act on MyD88-dependent and MyD88-independent pathways, which also encourages the possibility that these immunomodulatory agents could even increase the chemosensitivity of other therapeutics.

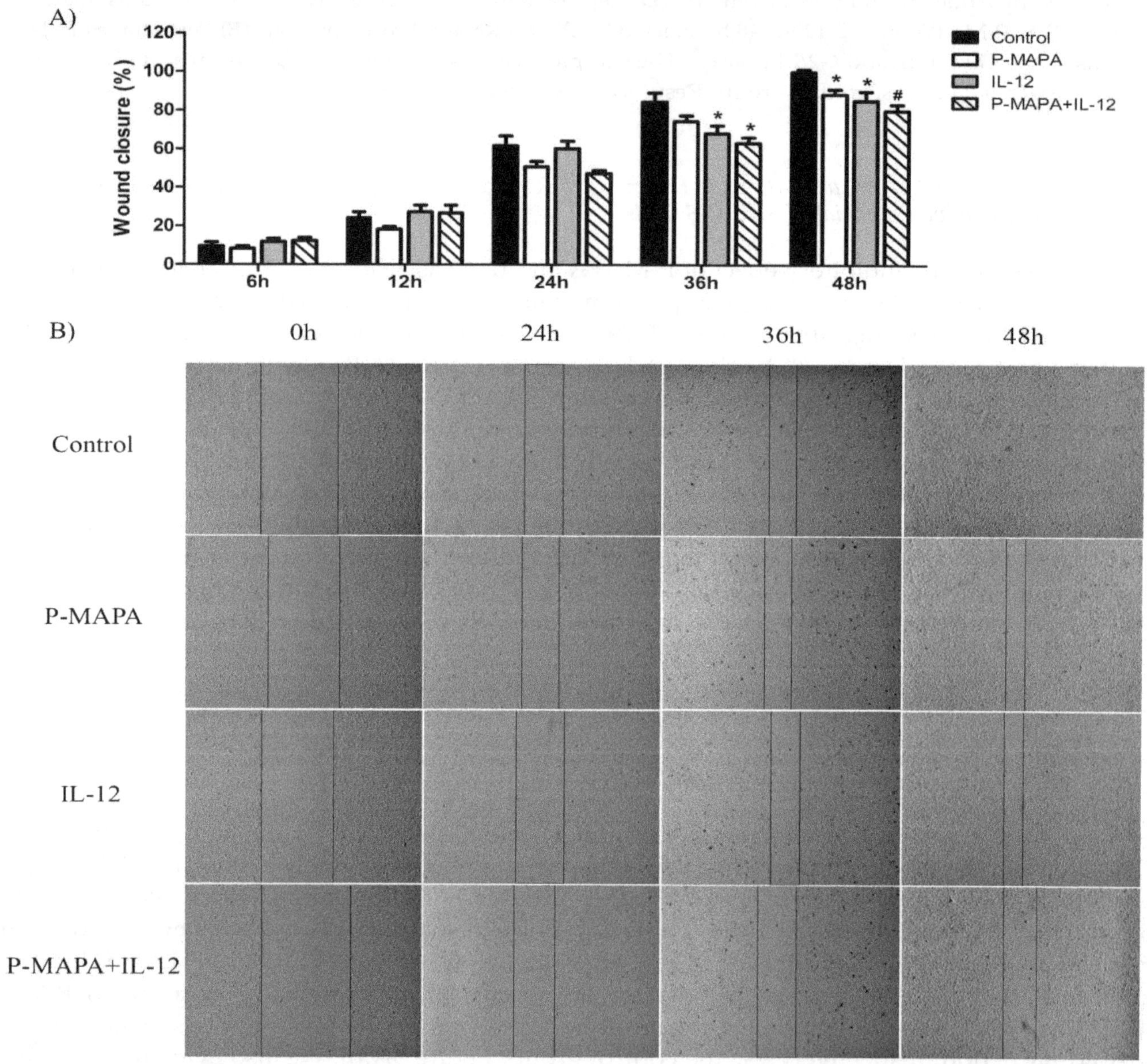

Figure 3. Migratory potential of SKOV-3 cells determined by wound-healing assay. (**A**) Percentage of wound closure after 0, 6, 12, 24, 36, and 48 h. * $p < 0.05$, # $p < 0.01$ vs. control group. (**B**) Photographs of each wound-healing analysis at 0, 24, 36, and 48 h which were representative for specific closing area; vertical black bars were used to show the incision edges (10× magnification). The samples were assayed in three technical and biological replicates.

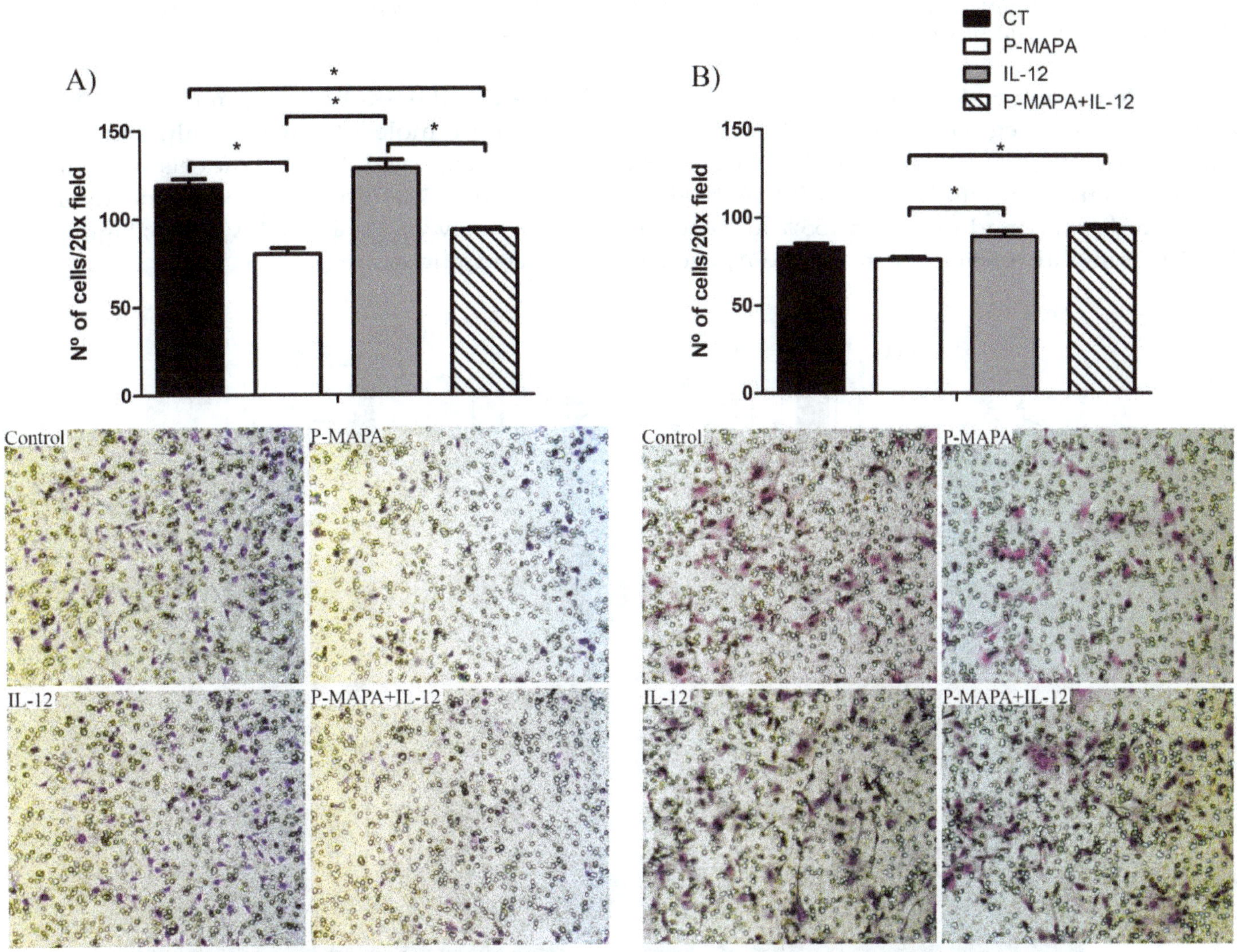

Figure 4. Effects of P-MAPA and IL-12 alone or in combination on the migration and invasion capacity of SKOV-3 cells. (**A**) Cell migration was measured by the amount of cells located in the lower part of the insert. (**B**) Cell invasion was determined by the amount of cells located in the lower part of the insert previously covered by Geltrex®. Representative images of the assay were obtained at 20× magnification. The samples were assayed in three technical and biological replicates. Results are expressed as the mean ± SD; * $p < 0.05$; CT, control group.

To further investigate and elucidate the location and the relative expression levels of the TLR2 and TLR4 receptors, an immunofluorescence assay was performed on SKOV-3 cells. As evidenced by the cellular fluorescence level, the P-MAPA treatment significantly decreased the expression level of cytoplasmic and nuclear TLR2 (48% fluorescence reduced vs. the control group; Figure 5C). On the contrary, IL-12 and the combination of P-MAPA and IL-12 promoted the highest TLR2 immunofluorescence intensity (135% and 151% fluorescence level, respectively vs. P-MAPA; Figure 5C), which suggests that IL-12 is responsible for restoring TLR2 activation after P-MAPA therapy in SKOV-3 cells. Lastly, the relative immunofluorescence of the TLR4 was unchanged after the treatments (Figure 5D).

2.4. P-MAPA Stimulates the Secretion of Pro- and Anti-Inflammatory Molecules, Whereas Its Association with IL-12 Induced the Synthesis of Inflammatory Cytokines in SKOV-3 Cells

To determine which cytokines/chemokines are secreted by the SKOV-3 cells and how P-MAPA and IL-12 act to regulate its production, a wide range of these molecules were evaluated in both supernatants (Figure 6A) and cellular extracts (Figure 6B). As expected, the IL-12 levels were higher in the cells treated with IL-12 and P-MAPA+IL-12 (244% and 243% fold-increased, respectively vs. the control group, and 154% and 155% fold-increased, respectively vs. the P-MAPA group; Figure 6A); IL-12 was slightly elevated with P-MAPA, even at low concentrations.

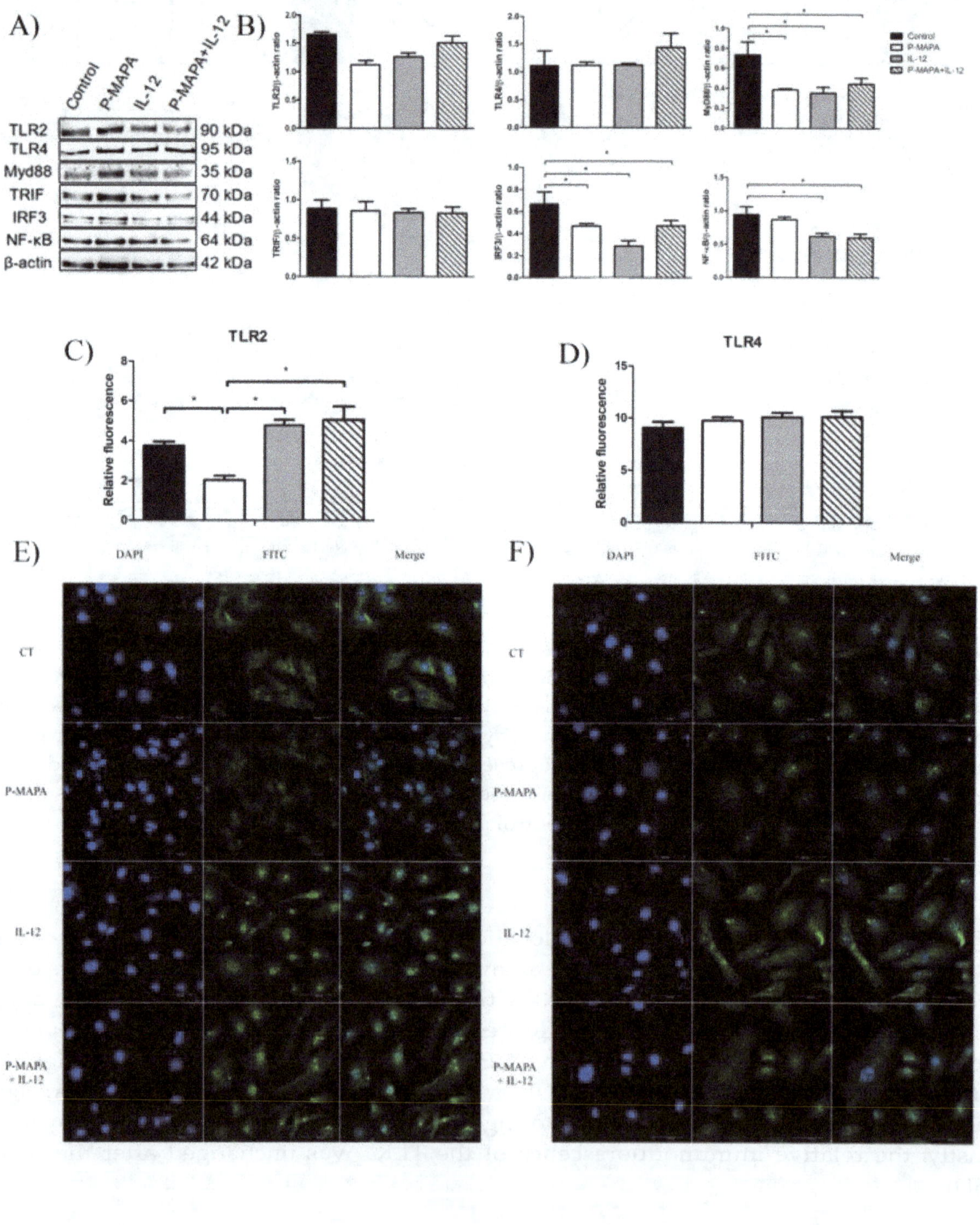

Figure 5. TLR2- and TLR4-mediated signaling pathways are involved with inflammatory process and chemoresistance in human OC. (**A**) Representative protein profiles of TLR2, TLR4, MyD88, TRIF, IRF3, and NF-kB; fractions containing 50 μg protein were pooled from 5 samples per group. (**B**) Individual blots were used for densitometric analysis of the TLR2 and TLR4 levels and related downstream molecules (MyD88, TRIF, IRF3, and NF-kB) after normalization to the β-actin. Data are expressed as the mean ± SD. * $p < 0.05$ vs. control group. Relative fluorescence intensity of TLR2 (**C**) and TLR4 (**D**) receptors. The values are expressed as the mean ± SD. The samples were assayed in three technical and biological replicates. * $p < 0.05$. Confocal imaging of TLR2 (**E**) and TLR4 (**F**) immunostaining using fluorescein isothiocyanate (FITC)-conjugated antibodies anti-TLR2 and anti-TLR4 was obtained in SKOV-3 cells (Alexafluor®488, bar = 50 μm). DAPI was used for nuclear staining and merged images were performed using Image J software. Negative controls were used. CT, control; DAPI, 4′,6-diamidino-2-phenylindole; FITC, fluorescein isothiocyanate.

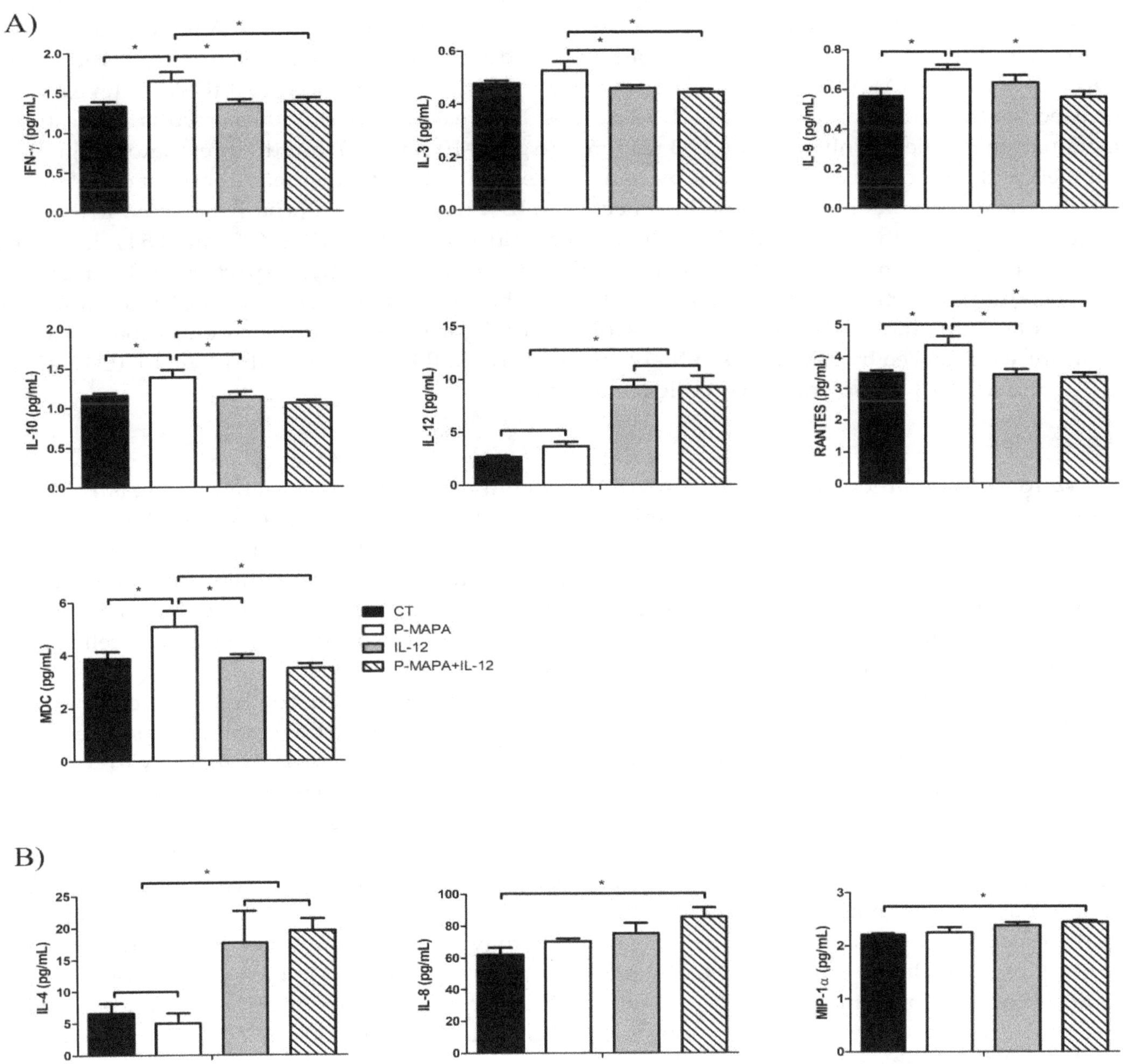

Figure 6. Multiplex analysis of cytokines and chemokines produced by SKOV-3 cells in response to P-MAPA and IL-12 treatments. (**A**) Concentrations of IFN-γ, IL-3, IL-9, IL-10, IL-12, RANTES, and MDC were altered in the supernatants of cell culture. (**B**) Levels of IL-4, IL-8, and MIP-1α were altered in SKOV-3 cell extracts. All data are expressed as the mean ± SD. * $p < 0.05$ as compared with the corresponding group; One-way ANOVA complemented by the Tukey test. The samples were assayed in three technical and biological replicates. CT, control; IFN-γ, interferon gamma; RANTES, regulated on activation, normal T cell expressed and secreted; MDC, macrophage-derived chemokine; MIP-1α, macrophage inflammatory protein 1-alpha.

Comparing the treatments, P-MAPA significantly stimulated the secretion of IFN-γ (24% vs. the control, IL-12 and P-MAPA+IL-12 groups; Figure 6A), which is probably related to the activation of the Th1 response. P-MAPA also stimulated IL-10 (21% vs. control, 23% vs. IL-12 and 32% vs. P-MAPA+IL-12 groups), MDC/CCL22 (31% vs. control and IL-12 groups, and 45% vs. P-MAPA+IL-12), and, regulated on activation, normal T cells expressed and secreted (RANTES)/CCL5 (25% vs. the control, 27% vs. the IL-12, and 30% vs. the P-MAPA+IL-12 groups). Furthermore, P-MAPA increased IL-3 and treatment with IL-12 or P-MAPA+IL-12 promoted a reduction in its levels (13% and 17% reduction, respectively vs. P-MAPA; Figure 6A). Treatment with P-MAPA also increased the IL-9 levels (25% increased vs. the control and P-MAPA+IL-12 groups; Figure 6A). A part of these results suggests the secretion of molecules involved in the Th2 response (e.g., IL-10, CCL22), but their regulatory signaling combined with other molecules released by immune cells into the OC microenvironment could not be proved to have a favorable or unfavorable effect. The IL-4 levels were internally elevated in SKOV-3 cells (Figure 6B) after therapies with IL-12 alone or combined with P-MAPA (169% and 254% increased vs. the control group and 198% and 293% increased vs. the P-MAPA group, respectively). Interestingly, the association of P-MAPA with IL-12 induced the highest production of intracellular IL-8 (37% vs. the control group) and MIP-1α (11% vs. control group; Figure 6B). In brief, cytokines that were not significantly influenced by P-MAPA and IL-12 included IL-1β, IL-2, IL-6, IL-7, IL-13, IL-15, IL-17, IP-10, MCP-1, and MIP-1β (Supplementary Tables S1 and S2).

3. Discussion

We reported that lower doses of P-MAPA efficiently reduce cell invasion, whereas P-MAPA in combination with IL-12 reduces cell migration in addition to attenuating the TLR-mediated inflammatory response in human SKOV-3 cells (Figure 7). Although these compounds have individually showed important effects in reducing OC volume and mass while enhancing overall survival and immunostimulation in animals and humans [11,16], this study is the first to describe a therapeutic rationale against human OC, thus revealing the mechanisms underlying cancer cell-related inflammatory aspects rather than those of immune cells.

P-MAPA and IL-12 elicited a decrease in cell metabolism, but no effect on cell apoptosis/necrosis and cell cycle was observed. Although an MTT assay is largely used as the viability/toxicity assay, it could be biased by decreased metabolism activity. This utilizes mitochondrial machinery to convert a colorless tetrazolium salt solution into purple formazan crystals [20]. Once we had pursued a treatment dose with low cell toxicity but considerable modulatory potential, we believed that either P-MAPA or IL-12 may be changing OC cell metabolism to a reduced activity (metabolomics could be of significant value to find the targets more precisely). The impact of this reduction was indeed confirmed by the migration and invasion assays. P-MAPA was able to reduce the migration and invasion capacity, and the delayed wound closure in IL-12-treated cells may be likely due to its decreased metabolic activity. Given that lower doses of P-MAPA and IL-12 are recommended to be well-tolerated, OC cell apoptosis could be prevented by the low-level toxicity of chemicals; conversely, these concentrations are safely used to activate immune responses and modulate cell metabolism. When associated with PTX, P-MAPA was able to increase cell death and apoptosis/necrosis ratio without potentiating the PTX effects on cell cycle. In accordance with a previous study in which approximately 50% of SKOV-3 cells died after 48 h exposure to 5 μM of PTX [21], we observed that P-MAPA not only was effective to increase cell death in the presence of PTX but also to maintain cell toxicity even after considerably lower levels of PTX. This increase in cell death might be a result of apoptosis induction, since the apoptosis/necrosis ratio was significantly higher in animals treated with the combination of P-MAPA and PTX. Because apoptosis lead to the release of the damage-associated molecular pattern (DAMP), this higher ratio may facilitate immunogenic cell death (ICD) [22].

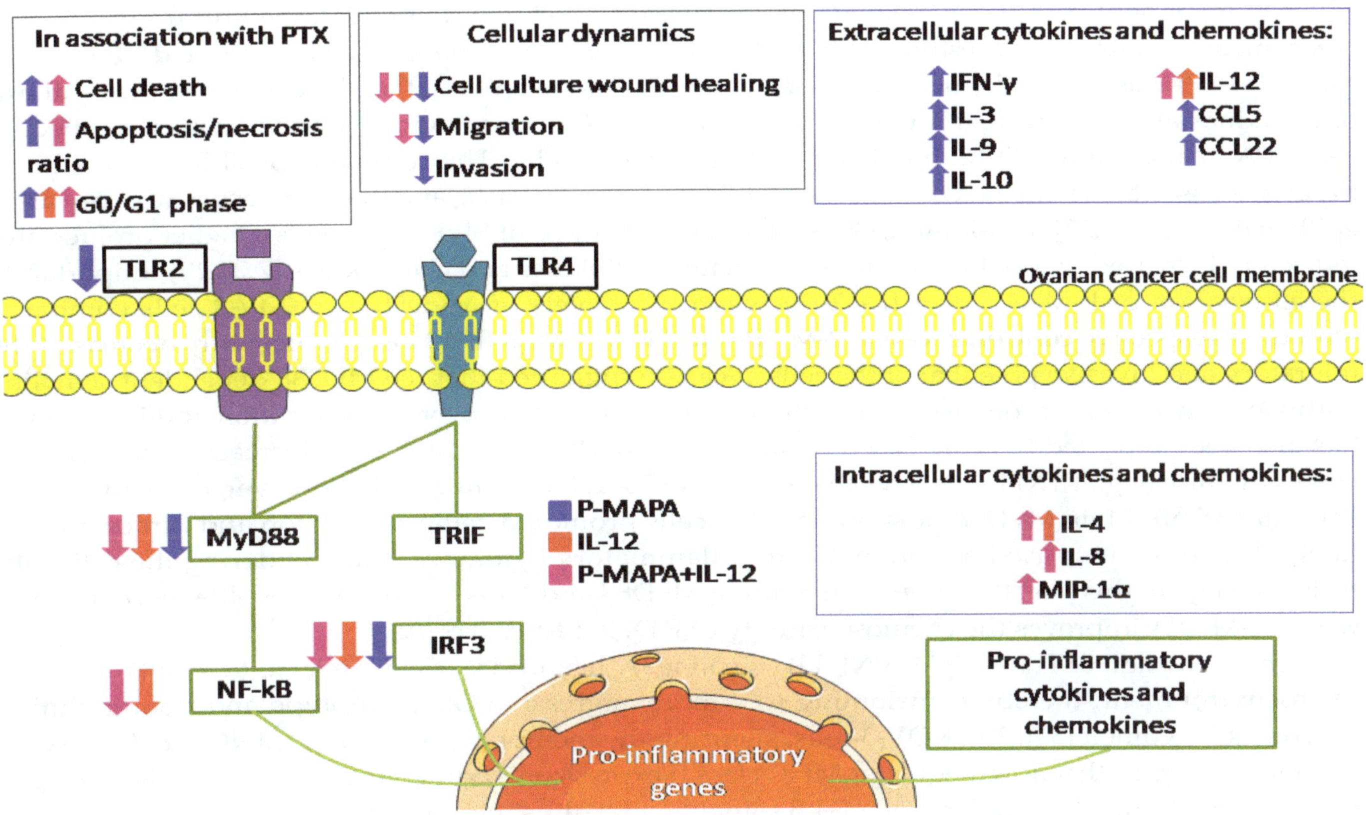

Figure 7. Schematic view of the effects of P-MAPA and IL-12 on human SKOV-3 cells. The effect of each treatment is shown by its representative color. Up and down arrows indicate whether the treatment increased or decreased, respectively, such as cellular function or molecule at these levels. The treatments reduced the downstream molecules (MyD88, NF-kB, and IRF3, with the exception of P-MAPA in reducing NF-kB) of both canonical and non-canonical toll-like receptor (TLR) signaling pathways, and only P-MAPA significantly downregulated the TLR2 levels. The intracellular cytokine/chemokine levels were increased after treatment with IL-12 (IL-4) or P-MAPA+IL-12 (IL-4, IL-8 and MIP-1α); P-MAPA was more effective in increasing the secretion of the following cytokines/chemokines: IFN-γ, IL-3, IL-9, IL-10, RANTES/CCL5, MDC/CCL22). As expected, IL-12 was used to treat SKOV-3 cells and appeared increased after IL-12 and P-MAPA+IL-12 treatments. Although IL-12 only reduced the SKOV-3 cells' wound closure, P-MAPA efficiently regulated the cellular dynamics by reducing the wound closure, cell migration and invasion. The combination of P-MAPA with IL-12 decreased the period of wound closure and cell migration rate. MyD88, myeloid differentiation primary response 88; NF-kB, nuclear factor kappa B; TRIF, TIR-domain-containing adapter-inducing interferon-β; IRF-3, interferon regulatory factor 3; TLR2, toll-like receptor 2; TLR4, toll-like receptor 4; P-MAPA, protein aggregate magnesium-ammonium phospholinoleate-palmitoleate anhydride; IL, interleukin; MIP-1α, macrophage inflammatory protein 1α; IFN-γ, interferon gamma; RANTES, regulated on activation, normal T cell expressed and secreted; MDC, macrophage-derived chemokine; CCL, C-C motif chemokine ligand.

The pro-inflammatory actions of TLR signaling in cancer cells and immune cells may severely affect tumor progression [23], and, particularly, the immunosuppressive OC microenvironment needs to be continuously immunostimulated [23,24]. Although TLR4 was unchanged by the treatments, P-MAPA induces a reduction in the TLR2 levels together with downstream molecules in SKOV-3 cells. Additionally, we found TLR2 nuclear expression in SKOV-3 cells treated with P-MAPA. Although we are not the first to observe nuclear staining of TLR2 and TLR4 [25], the effect of the switch of cytoplasmic to nuclear expression in SKOV-3 cells remains unclear. Based on our results, this nuclear expression seems not to have any negative effect favoring cancer development. Although the TLR2-induced MyD88-dependent pathway is related to an increase in IL-12 secretion [26], the immunoregulatory mechanisms whereby IL-12 restores TLR2 to levels close to control remain to be elucidated. In immune cells, P-MAPA has reportedly been described as a TLR4 agonist [9–11], thereby enhancing the synthesis of cytokines and activating a Th1-polarized response. Our data evidenced the protective effect of P-MAPA in attenuating TLR2-mediated signaling in OC cells. The activation of TLR, especially via MyD88, is associated with increased tumor growth, chemoresistance, and the early recurrence of ovarian epithelial tumors [7,27]. In addition, OC expressing high levels of MyD88 presents a higher proliferative index and increased production of pro-inflammatory cytokines and chemokines [7,28,29]. Importantly, the association of P-MAPA and IL-12 decreased the levels of MyD88 in SKOV-3 cells compared with their respective control; because P-MAPA and P-MAPA + IL-12 also significantly decreased the migratory and invasive potential of the cells, it can be suggested that the MyD88-dependent signaling pathway may be one of the mechanisms by which SKOV-3 cells promote migration and invasion. It has also been reported that increased expression of MyD88 is related to a decreased sensitivity to chemotherapy (e.g., PTX) in the MyD88-negative OC A2780 cell line [30]; moreover, the activation of MyD88 and NF-kB in MyD88-positive SKOV-3 cells promoted cell proliferation and tumor growth, likely due to the increased secretion of pro-inflammatory cytokines, thus rendering the cells PTX resistant [13]. In this line, the downregulation of MyD88 and NF-kB may be a possible mechanism by which P-MAPA improves the chemosensitivity of PTX in SKOV-3 cells.

The activation of TLR4/MyD88/NF-kB signaling by ligands is strongly related to an inflammatory microenvironment, thereby contributing to a more aggressive OC phenotype and poorer clinical outcomes in women [31]. In SKOV-3 cells, silencing the membrane-associated RING-CH (MARCH), an ubiquitin ligase that downregulates MHC class II expression, resulted in reduced cell migration and invasion in addition to inhibition of NF-kB signaling [32], thus reinforcing that NF-kB may play a role in the regulation of numerous cellular dynamics. Taken together, the combination of P-MAPA and IL-12 was efficient to induce the downregulation of both MyD88 and NF-kB, which can be of great value to enhance the overall survival of patients while attenuating OC progression and metastasis.

TRIF activation is responsible for triggering the TLR non-canonical pathway, thus activating several transcriptional factors, such as NF-kB, IRF3 and AP-1, and resulting in cytokines and type I IFN production [33,34]. Although few studies have explored the role of TRIF/IRF3 in OC cells, they seem to be critical for therapy [35]. Recently, Chuffa et al. [23] reported the downregulation of TRIF and IRF3 in OC-induced rats, whereby the immunomodulatory agent dramatically reduced the volume and mass of ovarian tumors. Importantly, P-MAPA and IL-12, either alone or in association, significantly downregulated IRF3 levels, evidencing the potential of immunotherapies to act by both canonical and non-canonical TLR pathways.

Immunostimulatory and immunosuppressive molecules can contribute to either inhibiting or enhancing anti-tumor immune activity of such a response by immunotherapy. We screened a number of molecules displaying important effects in OC, but most of them displayed no changes in SKOV-3 cells after P-MAPA and IL-12 treatments. Treatment of SKOV-3 with rhIL-12 showed its availability in both IL-12 and P-MAPA+IL-12 groups, thus proving that the agent was present in the supernatants; whether IL-12 therapy was still capable of stimulating more IL-12 production by the cells is uncertain. IL-3 levels are stimulated by P-MAPA therapy, and this increase might be protective for patients during OC chemotherapy; administration of rhIL-3 to patients with platelet count $< 75{,}000/mm^3$ is effective to fight thrombocytopenia and neutropenia after chemotherapy [36]. Moreover, IL-3 is able to intensify the dose of carboplatin for primary advanced OC [37]. P-MAPA also enhanced IL-9 secretion by SKOV-3 cells, and this effect seems to have a dual impact on the immune system. IL-9 was initially recognized as a T-cell growth factor with oncogenic potential. However, Th9 cell-secreted IL-9 has been revisited for the immunity of some tumors [38]. IL-9 activates innate immune cells like mast cells, contributing to tumor growth prevention [38], and in addition to Th9 cell-derived IL-3, induction of adaptive anti-cancer responses that favor DCs survival has been reported in various cancers [39].

Regulatory T (Treg) cells can infiltrate into solid OC or ascitic fluid, contributing to an immunosuppressive microenvironment by secreting IL-10 and TGFB-1 while reducing the IFN-γ levels [40]. Because these cytokines participate either in stimulating or inhibiting the activities of other immune cells, P-MAPA seems to work as a double-edge sword regarding the SKOV-3 cells. Although mechanistically unclear, P-MAPA contributes partially to reducing the immunosuppression, likely due to the increased levels of IFN-γ rather than IL-10. In fact, high IFN-γ secretion meets our proposal by enhancing OC-cell immunogenicity through the recruitment of CD8+T and natural killer (NK) cells, in addition to increasing the anti-tumor activity of macrophages; we recently found that P-MAPA reduces Treg cells and stimulates CD8+T effector cells in OC-bearing animals (unpublished data). Recently, the expression of programmed death-ligand 1 (PD-L1) on tumor cells represents an important pathway by which malignant cells evade the immune system. In SKOV-3 cells, PD-L1 was variably found in the surface and cytoplasm [41], and its expression was correlated with high levels of TNF-α, IL-10, and IL-6 released from tumor-associated macrophages (TAMs). Because P-MAPA and IL-12 attenuated the downstream mediators of the TLR signaling, the altered expression of some cytokines may be independent of TLR-mediated inflammatory response.

A complex network represented by chemokines and its receptors, growth factors, inflammatory products, and other molecules (e.g., NF-kB), is responsible for tumor progression or rejection. Chemokines signal not only for tumor cells but may control tumor development through activation of specific receptors expressed in a variety of cells, thereby regulating the traffic of infiltrating macrophages, lymphocytes, DCs, and neutrophils [42]. The secretion of CCL5, which binds to the CCR4 receptor, is strongly associated with the presence of tumor-infiltrating CD8+T cells; the upregulation of its receptor in activated vaccine-primed T cells improved tumor homing in OC [43]. In SKOV-3 cells, the levels of CCL22/MDC and CCL5/RANTES were higher after P-MAPA therapy. Although these chemokines appear to be associated with a poor prognosis when released by immune cells, the functional meaning of their production by OC cells as to their significance in the OC microenvironment remains to be investigated. CCL22 is secreted by DCs and macrophages and acts on target cells by interacting with the CCR4 receptor located in the cell surface [44]. CCL22 is correlated to the chemoattraction of Treg cells in advanced stages of OC, and its expression was increased in response to IFN-γ signaling [45]. This finding partially corroborates our results in which both CCL22 and IFN-γ were higher in SKOV-3 cells after P-MAPA therapy; in contrast, P-MAPA does not promote elevation in the number of Treg cells (data not shown). A previous study by Giuntoli et al. [46] showed that ascites specimens originating from patients with malignant OC were accomplished by elevated levels of IL-6, IL-8, IL-10, IL-15, IP-10, MCP-1, MIP-1β, and VEGF, in contrast to significantly reduced levels of IL-2, IL-5, IL-7, IL-17, and CCL5/RANTES. Although controversial, IL-8 production by human OC cells plays a role in controlling tumor growth [47], and MIP-1α is involved in the recruitment of Th1 and cytotoxic effector T cells [48]. We found a higher secretion IL-8 and MIP-1α after combinatory treatment of P-MAPA and IL-12. Partially supporting our results, IL-8 levels have already been reported to be augmented in OC, even after the downregulation of NF-kB [49]; however, the alternative mechanism involved with this production remains unclear. Additionally, we observed increased levels of RANTES after P-MAPA treatment. RANTES is responsible for recruiting T cells, macrophages, eosinophils, and basophils into the inflammatory sites. In addition to IL-2 and IFN-γ, RANTES is thought to induce the activation and proliferation of NK cells while enhancing the anti-tumor response in animal models [46]. In addition to the overexpression of VEGF and MCP-1, a reduction in RANTES levels is associated with activating pathways for tumor growth. Normally, OCs produce large amounts of RANTES, and this production is correlated with the infiltration of TAMs, CD8+T cells, and tumor progression [50,51]; these chemokines are further related to the acquisition of polarized immune responses (Th1 versus Th2). Although some negative effects are associated with the efficacy of chemotherapy related to RANTES, therapy with P-MAPA may be helpful against tumor expansion.

4. Materials and Methods

4.1. Cell Line and Cell Culture

The human OC cell line SKOV-3 was purchased from the American Type Culture Collection (ATCC, Rockville, MD, USA). The SKOV-3 cells were routinely incubated in RPMI 1640 (Life Technologies, Grand Island, NY, USA) supplemented with 10% Fetal Bovine Serum (FBS) and 1% anti-anti solution (100 mg/mL penicillin G, and 100 μg/mL streptomycin (Merck, Darmstadt, Germany). The culture medium was changed every 2 to 3 days. All cells were maintained at 37 °C in a humidified atmosphere of 5% CO_2.

4.2. Treatments with P-MAPA and IL-12

To evaluate the in vitro effect of the treatments, different doses of P-MAPA (25 μg/mL, 50 μg/mL, and 100 μg/mL) were tested in accordance with Favaro et al. [9]. Initially, 5 mg P-MAPA was diluted in 1 mL of saline solution to achieve the desired stock solution of 5 mg/mL, which were then diluted in the cell culture medium to obtain the testing doses. For the treatment with recombinant (rh)IL-12, concentrations of 0.5 ng/mL, 1 ng/mL, and 2 ng/mL were diluted in the culture medium based on the previous report by Su et al. [52]. For the combination of P-MAPA and IL-12, the most effective dose and incubation period were determined after performing an MTT assay. The saline solution was used as a solvent vehicle control and prepared in the same volume and dilution for both treatments. All experiments were performed at 0, 24, 48, and 72 h time exposure and assayed in three technical and biological replicates.

4.3. Cell Cytotoxicity (MTT Assay)

The SKOV-3 cells were seeded in a 96-well plate at a density of 1×10^3 cells/well. The cellular activity and/or toxicity were evaluated in different concentrations of P-MAPA and IL-12 and periods (0, 24, and 48 h) to define the best treatment protocol. For this experiment, the choice of dose and period of treatment was the combination of high cellular viability with low toxicity and efficient signaling regulation. Thereafter, different doses of PTX were associated with P-MAPA and IL-12 to verify the sensitivity effects. An MTT solution (5 mg/mL) was added to the wells for 4 h, and the crystals were diluted with DMSO under agitation. The concentration was determined by an Epoch microplate reader (BioTek Instruments, Highland Park, PO, USA) at 540 nm, being the reference curve fixed at 650 nm. The percentage of crystal formation was calculated by fixing the control group crystal formation as 100%.

4.4. *Apoptosis Rate by Annexin V-FITC/PI Staining*

During the apoptosis process, cells normally externalize the phospholipid phosphatidylserine (PS), which binds with high affinity to Annexin V in the presence of calcium. Herein, we used the Annexin V assay with the BD Pharmingen™ Annexin V-FITC Apoptosis Detection Kit (ApoAlert Annexin V, Clontech, CA, USA). The SKOV-3 cells (1×10^5 cells) were placed in a 6-well plate and left for 6 h to attach. The cells were then treated with 25 μg/mL of P-MAPA, 1 ng/mL of rhIL-12 or their association for 48 h. In addition, P-MAPA and IL-12 were added to the lowest dose of PTX (0.625 μM) to confirm chemosensitivity. After the treatment period, cells were trypsinized and centrifuged (Centrifuge 5804 R, Eppendorf, Hamburg, Germany)) for 10 min at 1200 rpm for culture medium removal. The cell pellet was washed twice with phosphate-buffered saline (PBS) and centrifuged at 10,000 rpm for 30 s, followed by resuspension with 100 μL Annexin V binding buffer and incubation with Annexin V and propidium iodide (PI) for 15 min in the dark at room temperature. After the incubation, the prepared cells were then analyzed by flow cytometry in a FACSCantoTMII with FACSDiva (BD Biosciences, Clontech, CA, USA) software. The flow cytometric results were analyzed by the FlowJo software (vX.10.6 version, Tree Stars Inc., Ashland, OR, USA).

4.5. *Cell Cycle Determination by PI Staining*

The cell cycle stages (G0/G1, S, and G2/M) were performed by flow cytometry analysis through the DNA content measurement of nuclei stained with PI dye. After all the treatments, the SKOV-3 cells (1×10^5) were trypsinized, washed with PBS, and centrifuged for 5 min at 1500 rpm. After the cells were fixed in 70% cold ethanol at 4 °C for 1 h, they were incubated with PI staining solution of 50 μg/mL PI and 10 mg/mL RNase A for 1 h at room temperature in a dark room. Flow cytometry was performed in a FACSCantoTMII with FACSDiva (BD Biosciences, Clontech, CA, USA) software to analyze DNA content. The relative ratios of cells in the G0/G1, S, and G2/M phases were calculated using FlowJo software (vX.10.6 version, Tree Stars Inc.).

4.6. *Wound-Healing Assay*

The wound-healing method was performed to verify the effects of P-MAPA and rhIL-12 alone or in combination on cell migration capacity. Briefly, 3×10^5 SKOV-3 cells were placed in 6-well plates with a serum-free culture medium for cell starvation. When the cells reached high confluence, a wound was created through the confluent cell monolayer using an angled tip at 45°, and the SKOV-3 cells were then immediately treated with the pre-determined doses of P-MAPA, rhIL-12, or both, diluted in 2 mL of complete RPMI 1640 medium. Images were obtained at 0 h, 6 h, 12 h, 24 h, 36 h, and 48 h until the wound closure. Migration area (%) was measured using Image-J software. All experiments were analyzed in biological and technical triplicate.

4.7. *Cell Migration Using Transwell Insert*

To evaluate the migratory potential of the cells, 1×10^4 SKOV-3 cells were seeded in triplicates into the upper chambers of 24-well ThinCert™ cell culture inserts (GBO, Americana, SP, Brazil) with PVDF filters (8.0 μm pore size) containing the corresponding treatment diluted in serum free RPMI 1640 medium. In the lower chamber, RPMI supplemented with 10% FBS was added as a chemotactic factor. After the plates were incubated at 37 °C and 5% CO_2 for 24 h, the cells in the upper chamber were gently removed with a cotton swab. The cells that had migrated to the lower surface of the insert through the 8.0 μm pore were fixed in methanol for 8 min and stained with hematoxylin for 45 s. The migrated cells were photographed with 20× objectives under an inverted microscope (ZeissAxiovert®, Germany).

Four non-overlapped images were randomly analyzed for each well and the migrated cells were counted using Image J software.

4.8. Invasion Assay

The invasion assay was performed using a 24-well ThinCert™ cell culture insert (GBO, Americana, SP, Brazil) with PVDF filters (8.0 µm pore size). Briefly, 24-well plates were previously coated with Geltrex® (ThermoFisher, Waltham, MA, USA), which mimics the biological basement membrane matrix, and 1×10^4 cells were placed in the upper chamber with a serum-free culture medium containing the treatments. After 24 h, the invasive potential was determined by the amount of cells capable of crossing the barrier when chemotactically attracted by the RPMI 1640 medium supplemented with 10% FBS in the lower chamber. The protocol of cell fixing and staining was the same described for cell migration. Finally, four non-overlapped images were randomly analyzed per well and the invasive cells were counted using Image J software.

4.9. Immunofluorescence Assay

After the SKOV-3 cells were seeded in coverslips and treated with P-MAPA, rhIL-12, or their association for 48 h, they were fixed in methanol for 8 min at room temperature and then washed in sterile ice-cold PBS. To avoid nonspecific bindings, a blocking solution containing 3% (*v*/*v*) bovine serum albumin (BSA) was added for 1 h. Then, cells were incubated overnight with rabbit polyclonal anti-TLR2 and anti-TLR4 antibodies diluted 1:200 (Abcam, Cambridge, MA) for 4 h, followed by post incubation with secondary polyclonal anti-IgG conjugated to FITC (1:200 dilution in 1% BSA, Santa Cruz Biotechnology, Inc., CA) for 1 h. After the reactions, 4,6-diamidino-2-phenylindole (DAPI; Sigma, St Louis, MO) was used for nuclei staining. Positive staining was analyzed using a confocal fluorescence microscope Zeiss Axiophot II (Carl Zeiss, Oberköchen, Germany) at different magnification (excitation filter 590 nm, emission filter 650 nm) and for DAPI staining (excitation filter 365 nm, emission filter 485 nm). The relative fluorescence in FITC images was calculated using Image J software.

4.10. Western Blot Analysis

After the treatments, five replicates of each experiment were used. After being washed with cold PBS, 1×10^6 SKOV-3 cells were added to radioimmunoprecipitation assay buffer (RIPA) lysis buffer containing protease inhibitors and rapidly frozen for 24 h. Under constant agitation for 30 min at 4 °C, the cells were resuspended and transferred to 1.5 mL tubes and centrifuged for 20 min at 12,000 rpm. Protein quantification was performed using a Bradford assay, and the same amount of protein (40 µg) was solubilized in 1.5×Laemmli buffer and then used for 4–20% SDS-PAGE (Bio-Rad Laboratories, Hercules, CA, USA). After electrophoresis was carried out on tris-glycine running buffer system (120 V for 2 h), the proteins were electro-transferred (350 mA) to nitrocellulose membranes, and then blocked with 3% BSA in tris-buffered saline plus tween 20 (TBS-T) solution for 1 h. Afterward, the proteins were incubated with respective primary antibodies (1:500; Abcam, Cambridge, UK) at 4 °C overnight: anti-TLR2, anti-TLR4, anti-MyD88, anti-NF-kB p65, anti-TRIF, anti-IRF3. Subsequently, the membranes were washed three times and then incubated for 90 min with specific secondary antibodies (Sigma-Aldrich, St. Louis, MO, USA) diluted 1:20,000 in 1% BSA. After sequential washes, positive reactions were performed using ECL kit (Thermo Fisher Scientific, MA). All of the blots were calculated using individual samples obtained from three replicates/group and were represented as the mean optical density (band intensity/housekeeping protein). β-actin was used as the endogenous control.

4.11. *Cytokine and Chemokine Assay*

Levels of different cytokines and chemokines were determined in both supernatants and cell homogenates using a MilliPlex® Map Kit (EMD Millipore, Darmstadt, Germany) with a standard 20-plex detection kit according to the manufacturer's protocols. The human cytokine/chemokine Panel I kit (cat. no. HCYTOMAG-60K) included the following analytes: interferon-gamma (IFN-γ), interleukin (IL)-1β, IL-2, IL-3, IL-4, IL-6, IL-7, IL-8, IL-9, IL- 10, IL-12, IL-13, IL-15, IL-17, IP-10, macrophage-derived chemokine (MDC/CCL22), monocyte chemotactic protein-1 (MCP-1), macrophage inflammatory protein-1 (MIP)-1α, MIP-1β, and regulated upon activation normal T cell expressed and secreted (RANTES/CCL5). The concentrations were ranged between 0 and the lowest detectable level in each assay before log transformation. The analyses combined fluorescent cytometry and ELISA technology, so that each magnetic bead was added to a specific anti-cytokine to achieve a specific binding. For this experiment, the levels of analytes varied from 0.4 to 3500 pg/mL and the intra-assay CV was < 10%, inter-assay CV < 15%. No cross-reactivity was observed among cytokines and other molecules. The fluorescence intensity was measured using the MAGPIX system (Luminex Corporation, Austin, TX, USA).

4.12. *Statistical Analysis*

All data were evaluated using the analysis of variance (ANOVA) and presented as the mean ± standard deviation (SD). Significant results were then compared by Tukey or Newman-Keuls *post hoc* tests, and statistical significance was set at $p < 0.05$ for all analyses. Data were analyzed and constructed using GraphPad Prism 5.0 scientific graphing software (GraphPad Software, San Diego, CA, USA).

5. Conclusions

In summary, we demonstrated that P-MAPA in association with IL-12, both considered potent immunomodulatory agents, exhibited anti-cancer activities on human SKOV-3 cells. Although P-MAPA combined with IL-12 promotes a reduction in cell viability and cell migration, P-MAPA alone reduces the invasion capacity and enhances apoptosis in the presence of PTX. Similarly to either P-MAPA or IL-12 alone, the combinatory therapy induced the downregulation of TLR-downstream molecules involved with inflammation, which may result in protection against chemoresistance; these effects seem to be associated with TLR2 suppression rather than TLR4 signaling. P-MAPA alone stimulated the secretion of pro- and anti-inflammatory mediators, and its association with IL-12 increased the production of IL-4, -8, and MIP-1α by the SKOV-3 cells; this may promote changes in the immune responsiveness of the OC microenvironment. In addition to the effect on OC-infiltrated immune cells, these immunotherapies might provide a sustained opportunity for a novel combined strategy against malignant OC cells.

Author Contributions: L.A.L., L.G.d.A.C., F.K.D.: conceived the hypothesis of the study, collected and analyzed the data, and drafted the manuscript. W.J.F., F.E.M., M.M., G.G.R., R.K., M.S.C., R.F.D., I.d.S.N.: participated in its design, intellectual conception of the study, and in the acquisition of data. All authors have read and agreed to the published version of the manuscript.

Acknowledgments: We are grateful to HélioKushima and Valeria Sandrim from Department of Pharmacology, IBB/UNESP, Botucatu, SP, Brazil, for excellent technical assistance and support.

Abbreviations

BSA	Bovine serum albumin
CEEA	Ethical Committee of the Institute of Bioscience/UNESP
CEMIB	Multidisciplinary Center for Biological Investigation
DAB	Diaminobenzidine
DAPI	6-diamidino-2-phenylindole
DCs	Dendritic cells
FITC	Fluorescein Isothiocyanate
HRP-conjugated	Horseradish peroxidase-conjugated
H	Hematoxylin
IFN	Interferon
IFN-γ	Interferon gamma
IL-6	Interleukin 6
IL-8	Interleukin 8
IRF3	Interferon regulatory factor 3
MyD88	Myeloid differentiation factor 88
NF-kB p65	Nuclear factor kappa B subunit p65
NK	natural killer cells
OC	ovarian cancer
PBS	phosphate-buffered saline
P-MAPA	Protein aggregate magnesium-ammonium phospholinoleate-palmitoleate anhydride
PTX	paclitaxel
RIPA	Radioimmunoprecipitation assay buffer
SDS-PAGE	Sodium dodecyl sulphate-polyacrylamide gel electrophoresis
TBS-T	Tris-Buffered Saline plus Tween 20
CD4 + T	CD4-positive T cells
CD8 + T	CD8-positive T cells
Th1	T helper 1
TLR (s)	Toll-like receptor (s)
TLR2	Toll-like receptor 2
TLR4	Toll-like receptor 4
TRIF	TIR domain-containing adaptor inducing interferon-beta

References

1. Siegel, R.L.; Miller, K.D.; Jemal, A. Cancer statistics, 2018. *CA Cancer J. Clin.* **2018**, *68*, 7–30. [CrossRef] [PubMed]
2. Fallows, S.; Price, J.; Atkinson, R.J.; Johnston, P.G.; Hickey, I.; Russell, S.E. P53 mutation does not affect prognosis in ovarian epithelial malignancies. *J. Pathol.* **2001**, *194*, 68–75. [CrossRef] [PubMed]
3. Cannistra, S.A. Cancer of the ovary. *N. Engl. J. Med.* **2004**, *351*, 2519–2565. [CrossRef] [PubMed]
4. Chuffa, L.G.; Fioruci-Fontanelli, B.A.; Mendes, L.O.; Fávaro, W.J.; Pinheiro, P.F.; Martinez, M.; Martinez, F.E. Characterization of chemically induced ovarian carcinomas in an ethanol-preferring rat model: Influence of long-term melatonin treatment. *PLoS ONE* **2013** *8*, e81676. [CrossRef] [PubMed]

5. Chuffa, L.G.; Lupi-Júnior, L.A.; Costa, A.B.; Amorim, J.P.; Seiva, F.R. The role of sex hormones and steroid receptors on female reproductive cancers. *Steroids* **2017**, *118*, 93–108. [CrossRef]
6. Ebell, M.H.; Culp, M.B.; Radke, T.J. A systematic review of symptoms for the diagnosis of ovarian cancer. *Am. J. Prev. Med.* **2016**, *50*, 384–394. [CrossRef]
7. Kelly, M.G.; Alvero, A.B.; Chen, R.; Silasi, D.A.; Abrahams, V.M.; Chan, S.; Visintin, I.; Rutherford, T.; Mor, G. TLR-4 signaling promotes tumor growth and paclitaxel chemoresistance in ovarian cancer. *Cancer Res.* **2006**, *66*, 3859–3868. [CrossRef]
8. Bronte, G.; Cicero, G.; Sortino, G.; Pernice, G.; Catarella, M.T.; D'Alia, P.; Cusenza, S.; Lo Dico, S.; Bronte, E.; Sprini, D.; et al. Immunotherapy for recurrent ovarian cancer: A further piece of the puzzle or a striking strategy? *Expert Opin. Biol. Ther.* **2014**, *14*, 103–114. [CrossRef]
9. Fávaro, W.J.; Nunes, O.S.; Seiva, F.R.; Nunes, I.S.; Woolhiser, L.K.; Durán, N.; Lenaerts, A.J. Effects of P-MAPA immunomodulator on Toll-like receptors and p53: Potential therapeutic strategies for infectious diseases and cancer. *Infect. Agent. Cancer* **2012**, *7*, 1–15.
10. Garcia, P.V.; Seiva, F.R.; Carniato, A.P.; de Mello Júnior, W.; Duran, N.; Macedo, A.M.; de Oliveira, A.G.; Romih, R.; de Oliveira, A.G.; Romih, R.; et al. Increased toll-like receptors and p53 levels regulate apoptosis and angiogenesis in non-muscle invasive bladder cancer: Mechanism of action of P-MAPA biological response modifier. *BMC Cancer* **2016**, *16*, 422. [CrossRef]
11. de Almeida Chuffa, L.G.; de Moura Ferreira, G.; Lupi, L.A.; da Silva Nunes, I.; Fávaro, W.J. P-MAPA immunotherapy potentiates the effect of cisplatin on serous ovarian carcinoma through targeting TLR4 signaling. *J. Ovarian Res.* **2018**, *11*, 8. [CrossRef]
12. Chen, R.; Alvero, A.B.; Silasi, D.A.; Steffensen, K.D.; Mor, G. Cancers take their Toll–the function and regulation of Toll-like receptors in cancer cells. *Oncogene* **2008**, *27*, 225–233. [CrossRef]
13. Szajnik, M.; Szczepanski, M.J.; Czystowska, M.; Elishaev, E.; Mandapathil, M.; Nowak-Markwitz, E.; Spaczynski, M.; Whiteside, T.L. TLR4 signaling induced by lipopolysaccharide or paclitaxel regulates tumor survival and chemoresistance in ovarian cancer. *Oncogene* **2009**, *28*, 4353–4363. [CrossRef] [PubMed]
14. Wang, A.C.; Su, Q.B.; Wu, F.X.; Zhang, X.L.; Liu, P.S. Role of TLR4 for paclitaxel chemotherapy in human epithelial ovarian cancer cells. *Eur. J. Clin. Investig.* **2009**, *39*, 157–164. [CrossRef] [PubMed]
15. Trinchieri, G. Interleukin-12 and the regulation of innate resistance and adaptive immunity. *Nat. Rev. Immunol.* **2003**, *3*, 133–146. [CrossRef] [PubMed]
16. Cohen, C.A.; Shea, A.A.; Heffron, C.L.; Schmelz, E.M.; Roberts, P.C. Interleukin-12 Immunomodulation Delays the Onset of Lethal Peritoneal Disease of Ovarian Cancer. *J. Interferon Cytokine Res.* **2016**, *36*, 62–73. [CrossRef] [PubMed]
17. Colombo, M.P.; Trinchieri, G. Interleukin-12 in anti-tumor immunity and immunotherapy. *Cytokine Growth Factor Rev.* **2002**, *13*, 155–168. [CrossRef]
18. Hurteau, J.A.; Blessing, J.A.; DeCesare, S.L.; Creasman, W.T. Evaluation of recombinanthuman interleukin-12 in patients with recurrent or refractory ovarian cancer: Agynecologic oncology group study. *Gynecol. Oncol.* **2001**, *82*, 7–10. [CrossRef]
19. Lenzi, R.; Edwards, R.; June, C.; Seiden, M.V.; Garcia, M.E.; Rosenblum, M.; Freedman, R.S. Phase II study of intraperitoneal recombinant interleukin-12 (rhIL-12) in patients with peritoneal carcinomatosis (residual disease <1 cm) associated with ovarian cancer or primary peritoneal carcinoma. *J. Transl. Med.* **2007**, *5*, 66.
20. Präbst, K.; Engelhardt, H.; Ringgeler, S.; Hübner, H. Cell Viability Assays: Methods and Protocols. *Methods Mol. Biol.* **2017**, *1601*, 117.
21. Ahn, H.J.; Kim, Y.S.; Kim, J.U.; Han, S.M.; Shin, J.W.; Yang, H.O. Mechanism of taxol-inducedapoptosis in human SKOV3 ovarian carcinoma cells. *J. Cell Biochem.* **2004**, *91*, 1043–1052. [CrossRef]
22. Wang, Y.J.; Fletcher, R.; Yu, J.; Zhang, L. Immunogenic effects of chemotherapy-induced tumor cell death. *Genes Dis.* **2018**, *5*, 194–203. [CrossRef]
23. Chuffa, L.G.; Fioruci-Fontanelli, B.A.; Mendes, L.O.; Ferreira Seiva, F.R.; Martinez, M.; Fávaro, W.J.; Domeniconi, R.F.; Pinheiro, P.F.; Delazari Dos Santos, L.; Martinez, F.E. Melatonin attenuates the TLR4-mediated inflammatory response through MyD88- and TRIF-dependent signaling pathways in an in vivo model of ovarian cancer. *BMC Cancer* **2015**, *15*, 34. [CrossRef]
24. Lavoue, V.; Thedrez, A.; Leveque, J.; Foucher, F.; Henno, S.; Jauffret, V.; Belaud-Rotureau, M.A.; Catros, V.; Cabillic, F. Immunity of human epithelial ovarian carcinoma: The paradigm of immunesuppression in cancer. *J. Transl. Med.* **2013** *11*, 1–12. [CrossRef]

25. Jouhi, L.; Koljonen, V.; Böhling, T.; Haglund, C.; Hagström, J. The expression of toll-like receptors 2, 4, 5, 7 and 9 in Merkel cell carcinoma. *Anticancer Res.* **2015**, *35*, 1843–1849.
26. Zhu, G.; Gui, Z. Effect of silkworm peptide on inducting M1 type polarization andTh1 activation via TLR2-induced MyD88-dependent pathway. *Food Sci. Nutr.* **2019**, *7*, 1251–1260. [CrossRef] [PubMed]
27. d'Adhemar, C.J.; Spillane, C.D.; Gallagher, M.F.; Bates, M.; Costello, K.M.; Barry-O'Crowley, J.; Haley, K.; Kernan, N.; Murphy, C.; Smyth, P.C.; et al. The MyD88+ phenotype is an adverse prognostic factor in epithelial ovarian cancer. *PLoS ONE* **2014**, *9*, e100816. [CrossRef]
28. Kim, K.H.; Jo, M.S.; Suh, D.S.; Yoon, M.S.; Shin, D.H.; Lee, J.H.; Choi, K.U. Expression and significance of the TLR4/MyD88 signaling pathway in ovarian epithelial cancers. *World J. Surg. Oncol.* **2012**, *10*, 193. [CrossRef] [PubMed]
29. Gaikwad, S.M.; Thakur, B.; Sakpal, A.; Singh, R.K.; Ray, P. Differential activation of NF-κB signaling is associated with platinum and taxane resistance in MyD88deficient epithelial ovarian cancer cells. *Int. J. Biochem. Cell Biol.* **2015**, *61*, 90–102. [CrossRef] [PubMed]
30. Zhan, Y.; Xiang, F.; Wu, R.; Xu, J.; Ni, Z.; Jiang, J.; Kang, X. MiRNA-149 modulates chemosensitivity of ovarian cancer A2780 cells to paclitaxel by targeting MyD88. *J. Ovarian Res.* **2015**, *8*, 48. [CrossRef] [PubMed]
31. Li, Z.; Block, M.S.; Vierkant, R.A.; Fogarty, Z.C.; Winham, S.J.; Visscher, D.W.; Kalli, K.R.; Wang, C.; Goode, E.L. The inflammatory microenvironment in epithelial ovarian cancer: A role for TLR4 and MyD88 and related proteins. *Tumour Biol.* **2016**, *37*, 13279–13286. [CrossRef] [PubMed]
32. Meng, Y.; Hu, J.; Chen, Y.; Yu, T.; Hu, L. Silencing MARCH1 suppresses proliferation, migration and invasion of ovarian cancer SKOV3 cells via downregulation of NF-κB and Wnt/β-catenin pathways. *Oncol. Rep.* **2016**, *36*, 2463–2470. [CrossRef] [PubMed]
33. Yamamoto, M.; Sato, S.; Hemmi, H.; Hoshino, K.; Kaisho, T.; Sanjo, H.; Takeuchi, O.; Sugiyama, M.; Okabe, M.; Takeda, K.; et al. Role of adaptor TRIF in the MyD88-independent toll-like receptor signaling pathway. *Science* **2003**, *301*, 640–643. [CrossRef] [PubMed]
34. Ullah, M.O.; Sweet, M.J.; Mansell, A.; Kellie, S.; Kobe, B. TRIF-dependent TLR signaling, its functions in host defense and inflammation, and its potential as a therapeutic target. *J. Leukoc. Biol.* **2016**, *100*, 27–45. [CrossRef] [PubMed]
35. Muccioli, M.; Sprague, L.; Nandigam, H.; Pate, M.; Benencia, F. Toll-like receptors as novel therapeutic targets for ovarian cancer. *ISRN Oncol.* **2012**, *2012*, 642141. [CrossRef] [PubMed]
36. Yamamoto, K.; Yajima, A.; Terashima, Y.; Nozawa, S.; Taketani, Y.; Yakushiji, M.; Noda, K. Phase II clinical study on the effects of recombinant human interleukin-3 onthrombocytopenia after chemotherapy for advanced ovarian cancer. SDZ ILE 964[IL-3] Study Group. *J. Immunother.* **1999**, *22*, 539–545. [CrossRef]
37. Veldhuis, G.J.; Willemse, P.H.; van Gameren, M.M.; Aalders, J.G.; Mulder, N.H.; Mull, B.; Biesma, B.; deVries, E.G. Recombinant human interleukin-3 to dose-intensify carboplatin and cyclophosphamide chemotherapy in epithelial ovarian cancer: A phase I trial. *J. Clin. Oncol.* **1995**, *13*, 733–740. [CrossRef]
38. Rivera-Vargas, T.; Humblin, E.; Végran, F.; Ghiringhelli, F.; Apetoh, L. Th9 cells inanti-tumor immunity. *Semin. Immunopathol.* **2017**, *39*, 39–46. [CrossRef]
39. Park, J.; Li, H.; Zhang, M.; Lu, Y.; Hong, B.; Zheng, Y.; He, J.; Yang, J.; Qian, J.; Yi, Q. Murine Th9 cells promote the survival of myeloid dendritic cells in cancerimmunotherapy. *Cancer Immunol. Immunother.* **2014**, *63*, 835–845. [CrossRef]
40. Singh, M.; Loftus, T.; Webb, E.; Benencia, F. Minireview: Regulatory T Cells and Ovarian Cancer. *Immunol. Investig.* **2016**, *45*, 712–720. [CrossRef]
41. Qu, Q.X.; Xie, F.; Huang, Q.; Zhang, X.G. Membranous and cytoplasmic expression ofPD-L1 in ovarian cancer cells. *Cell. Physiol. Biochem.* **2017**, *43*, 1893–1906. [CrossRef] [PubMed]
42. Barbieri, F.; Bajetto, A.; Florio, T. Role of chemokine network in the development and progression of ovarian cancer: A potential novel pharmacological target. *J. Oncol.* **2010**, *2010*, 426956. [CrossRef] [PubMed]
43. Zsiros, E.; Duttagupta, P.; Dangaj, D.; Li, H.; Frank, R.; Garrabrant, T.; Hagemann, I.S.; Levine, B.L.; June, C.H.; Zhang, L.; et al. The ovarian cancer chemokine landscape isconducive to homing of vaccine-primed and CD3/CD28-costimulated T cells prepared for adoptive therapy. *Clin. Cancer Res.* **2015**, *21*, 2840–2850. [CrossRef]
44. Vulcano, M.; Albanesi, C.; Stoppacciaro, A.; Bagnati, R.; D'Amico, G.; Struyf, S.; Transidico, P.; Bonecchi, R.; Del Prete, A.; Allavena, P.; et al. Dendritic cells as a major source of macrophage-derived chemokine/CCL22 in vitro and in vivo. *Eur. J. Immunol.* **2001**, *31*, 812–822. [CrossRef]

45. Fialová, A.; Partlová, S.; Sojka, L.; Hromádková, H.; Brtnický, T.; Fučíková, J.; Kocián, P.; Rob, L.; Bartůňková, J.; Spíšek, R. Dynamics of T-cell infiltration during thecourse of ovarian cancer: The gradual shift from a Th17 effector cell response toa predominant infiltration by regulatory T-cells. *Int. J. Cancer* **2013**, *132*, 1070–1079.
46. Giuntoli, R.L., 2nd; Webb, T.J.; Zoso, A.; Rogers, O.; Diaz-Montes, T.P.; Bristow, R.E.; Oelke, M. Ovarian cancer-associated ascites demonstrates altered immune environment: Implications for antitumor immunity. *Anticancer Res.* **2009**, *29*, 2875–2884.
47. Lee, L.F.; Hellendall, R.P.; Wang, Y.; Haskill, J.S.; Mukaida, N.; Matsushima, K.; Ting, J.P. IL-8 reduced tumorigenicity of human ovarian cancer in vivo due to neutrophil infiltration. *J. Immunol.* **2000**, *164*, 2769–2775. [CrossRef]
48. Colvin, E.K. Tumor-associated macrophages contribute to tumor progression in ovarian cancer. *Front. Oncol.* **2014**, *4*, 137. [CrossRef]
49. Tino, A.B.; Chitcholtan, K.; Sykes, P.H.; Garrill, A. Resveratrol and acetyl-resveratrol modulate activity of VEGF and IL-8 in ovarian cancer cell aggregates via attenuation of the NF-κB protein. *J. Ovarian Res.* **2016**, *9*, 84. [CrossRef]
50. Milliken, D.; Scotton, C.; Raju, S.; Balkwill, F.; Wilson, J. Analysis of chemokinesand chemokine receptor expression in ovarian cancer ascites. *Clin. Cancer Res.* **2002**, *8*, 1108–1114.
51. Soria, G.; Ben-Baruch, A. The inflammatory chemokines CCL2 and CCL5 in breastcancer. *Cancer Lett.* **2008**, *267*, 271–285. [CrossRef] [PubMed]
52. Su, W.; Ito, T.; Oyama, T.; Kitagawa, T.; Yamori, T.; Fujiwara, H.; Matsuda, H. The direct effect of IL-12 on tumor cells: IL-12 acts directly on tumor cells to activate NF-kB and enhance IFN-g-mediated STAT1 phosphorylation. *Biochem. Biophys. Res. Commun.* **2001**, *280*, 503–5121. [CrossRef] [PubMed]

6

Biophysical Characterization and Anticancer Activities of Photosensitive Phytoanthraquinones Represented by Hypericin and its Model Compounds

Valéria Verebová [1], Jiří Beneš [2] and Jana Staničová [1,2,*]

[1] Department of Chemistry, Biochemistry and Biophysics, University of Veterinary Medicine & Pharmacy, Komenského 73, 041 81 Košice, Slovakia; valeria.verebova@uvlf.sk

[2] Institute of Biophysics and Informatics, First Faculty of Medicine, Charles University, Kateřinská 1, 121 08 Prague, Czech Republic; jiri.benes@lf1.cuni.cz

* Correspondence: jana.stanicova@uvlf.sk;

Academic Editors: José Antonio Lupiáñez, Amalia Pérez-Jiménez and Eva E. Rufino-Palomares

Abstract: Photosensitive compounds found in herbs have been reported in recent years as having a variety of interesting medicinal and biological activities. In this review, we focus on photosensitizers such as hypericin and its model compounds emodin, quinizarin, and danthron, which have antiviral, antifungal, antineoplastic, and antitumor effects. They can be utilized as potential agents in photodynamic therapy, especially in photodynamic therapy (PDT) for cancer. We aimed to give a comprehensive summary of the physical and chemical properties of these interesting molecules, emphasizing their mechanism of action in relation to their different interactions with biomacromolecules, specifically with DNA.

Keywords: natural photosensitive compounds; anticancer activity; hypericin; emodin; quinizarin; danthron; interaction; DNA

---

1. Photodynamic Therapy

Photodynamic therapy (PDT) is part of photochemotherapy and requires the presence of a photosensitive substance (drug, PS), oxygen, and a powerful light source in the area of absorption of the PS used. The main requirements for activating the properties of a PS are its selective accumulation in tumor tissue, high intensity of absorption in the visible and near-infrared region of the spectrum, low level of dark toxicity, and absence of side-effects [1,2]. Selective accumulation and retention of PS in tumor tissues rather than in the surrounding healthy tissue lead to selective destruction of the tumor in PDT, while the surrounding healthy tissue remains intact. Such selectivity is one of the biggest advantages of this method, which may be substituted in some cases for chemotherapy, radiotherapy, or surgery in the treatment of cancer. Due to drug excretion [3] and redistribution, the effective therapeutic dose entering tumor cells is only a fraction of the administered PS. Administration of increased amounts of therapeutics is not possible because they have cytotoxic effects, which could cause significant toxicity in healthy cells. It is very important therefore to find alternative approaches, which increase the efficacy of the drug dose in the tumor and decrease the dose in healthy tissue [4]. Higher selectivity of PSs for tumor cells can be achieved by combining them with transport agents, which preferentially interact with tumor cells, ensure the selective accumulation of the drug within the diseased tissue, and deliver the desired therapeutic drug concentration to a targeted site in the patient's body. Transport systems commonly used for photosensitizers are polymers, liposomes, oil emulsions, certain metals, some proteins, and carbon-based nanoparticles [5–10]. Stable and biocompatible transport systems with a long half-life in the blood are ideal. Selective drug delivery to tumor tissue, transport of nanoparticles containing a PS, and a tumor cell with a receptor is the objectives for achieving high selectivity and low drug concentration [11]. Several research groups have confirmed the hypothesis that one possible approach to achieving these goals is to prepare low-density lipoprotein (LDL)-based particles [12–17].

1.1. PDT in Cancer Therapy

PDT has been a promising, non-invasive method for the treatment of certain types of cancer for more than 25 years [18–23]; in addition, PDT has also been studied in various non-oncological applications; leishmaniasis [24], psoriasis [25,26], age-related macular degeneration [27,28], hyperplasia [27], restenosis [25], and in cardiology [29], urology [30], immunology [31], ophthalmology [28,32], dental medicine [33,34], and dermatology [35,36]. The combination of light and PS also shows promising results in the treatment of bacterial, fungal, parasitic, and viral infections [37–40].

The basic process in tumor PDT is shown in the diagram in Figure 1. The photosensitizer is usually administered intravenously (systematically) or topically, and the administration of PS has also been studied orally, mostly in patients with extensive damage (not always caused by cancer) [1,41].

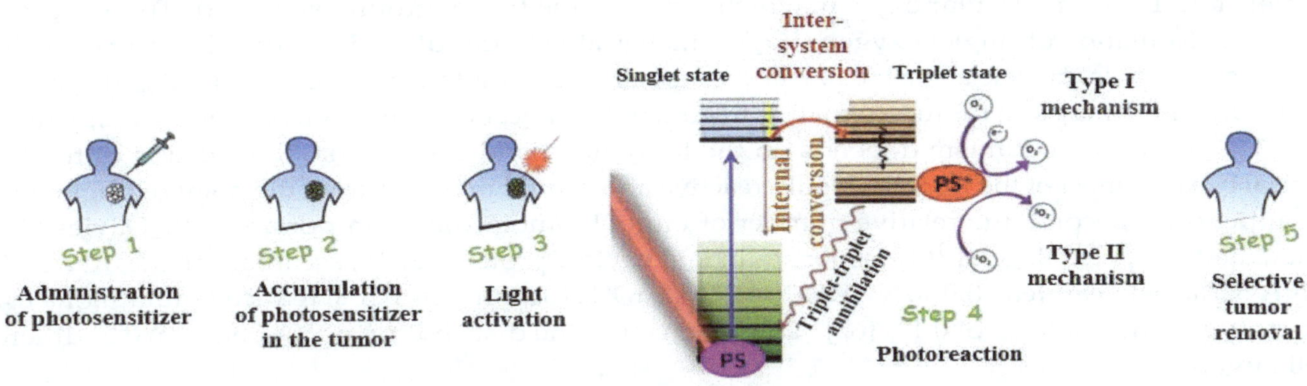

Figure 1. Scheme of photodynamic therapy (PDT; edited by [42,43]).

PS accumulates in the tumor tissue, which is subsequently irradiated with a light source of suitable wavelength, leading, in the presence of oxygen, to the formation of reactive oxygen species (ROS) and destruction of tissue and whole cells [1,41], while deactivation of important enzymes occurs and changes in the properties of biomacromolecules [44]. After activation of the photoactive substance by light and its interaction with molecular oxygen, singlet oxygen is formed. The singlet oxygen released in this photochemical reaction is highly toxic and can directly cause the death of tumor cells, through apoptosis, necrosis, or autophagy mechanism [45]. The release of singlet oxygen evokes oxidative stress, increases cytotoxicity, and DNA damage in cancer cells, modifies cellular metabolism, alters cancer cell death signaling pathways [46]. It also damages the blood vessels in tumor cells, resulting in indirect cell death through hypoxia (deficiency of oxygen) or aging (cell starvation). Diffuse distance of singlet oxygen obtained from photobleaching experiments has been appointed as 10–20 nm [47]. More recent time-resolved phosphorescence measurements show higher diffuse distance corresponding to 100 nm [48]. An explanation of this discrepancy was given by Hatz et al. [48] considering a fact that singlet oxygen behaves as a selective rather than reactive intermediate upon encountering other molecules in the cell.

Tissue damage depends on the depth of light penetration used to activate the PS. Membranes are damaged by cell death, triggering a number of inflammatory and immune processes, which cascade and cause the death of other tumor cells [49]. However, it was found out that singlet oxygen might cause membrane destruction directly. The cell membrane can be the main target of the singlet oxygen reaction for the bacterial membrane [50] and eukaryotic plasma membrane [51].

After surface irradiation PDT, the deeper connective tissues are only slightly damaged, so the patient's body can begin to restore the structure and flexibility of the damaged cells, and subsequently the tissues [52,53].

1.2. Physicochemical Mechanism of PDT

The photodynamic effect can be induced by two mechanisms called Type I and Type II (Figure 1—Step 4). After photon absorption, the PS molecule goes from the ground state (S_0) to the singlet excited state (S_1). From this excited state, the PS can be returned to the ground state by energy emission through non-radiative and/or radiant processes (fluorescence). In its excited state, the PS can also spontaneously move from the singlet state S_1 to the excited triplet state (T_1) by means of the intersystem conversion process. In this state, the transition to the ground state through a phosphorescence process can occur [54].

The type I mechanism involves electron transfer reactions between the PS molecule in the excited states of S_1 and T_1 and the substrate. This process results in the formation of ionic radicals, which tend to react immediately with oxygen to form a mixture of highly reactive oxygen radicals, such as superoxide radical ($\cdot O_2$), hydrogen peroxide (H_2O_2), and hydroxyl radical ($\cdot OH$), which oxidize a wide range of biomacromolecules [2,55].

The type II mechanism is characterized by energy transfer reactions between PS in the excited triplet state T_1 and molecular oxygen, which is also in the triplet ground state (T_0). These reactions cause the formation of singlet oxygen ($^1O_2$), which is able to rapidly oxidize cellular structures such as proteins, lipids, nucleic acids [56,57], and organelles leading to tumor cell death [58,59]. This also means that PDT may be a useful alternative treatment for cancer cells resistant to chemotherapy [60,61].

The reaction mechanism depends on the following conditions. First, the location of the PS is crucial because most of the ROS are highly reactive and cannot move far from the point of origin before disappearing. Second, the relative number of target biomolecules is important [43]. Davies (2003) calculated the percentage of $^1O_2$ responses in leukocytes: protein 68.5%, ascorbate 16.5%, RNA 6.9%, DNA 5.5%, beta-carotene 0.9%, NADH/NADPH 0.69%, tocopherols 0.5%, reduced glutathione 0.4%, lipids 0.2%, and cholesterol 0.1% [62]. This means that the distribution of $^1O_2$ may vary in different cell targets.

Both mechanisms can occur simultaneously. Their proportional representation is significantly influenced by the PS, the substrate, the oxygen concentration, and the binding of PS to the substrate. In addition, the type II mechanism appears to be more efficient as it has a higher rate constant than electron transfer reactions (type I mechanism). As a result, energy transfer to other compounds that can compete with oxygen is less important, so type II is more often dominant [58,63].

1.3. PDT Applications

PDT currently occupies an increasingly important place in clinical medicine. Its most promising application is the treatment of small and superficial tumors, e.g., some types of skin, neck, stomach [64], lung [65–67], bronchial [68] or oral cancer [69], esophagus [70,71], bladder [71,72], brain [73], prostate and pleura [74] tumors, breast [75] but also skin disease [76], atherosclerosis, and viral diseases therapy [77], including AIDS [78].

The future of PDT lies in efforts to find or synthesize new photosensitizers with properties allowing their greater selectivity for tumor tissues, and to find new approaches for the specific localization of already-known PS in tumor cells. This should contribute to the wider and more effective application of PDT in clinical practice. Targeted PDT has several advantages they are important in participation in the treatment of oncological diseases. Some of them are listed below: high selectivity, negligible side effects, low level of complications during and after treatment, high quality of life for patients, diagnostics and therapy in one step, and lower financial costs [79]. It can be a convenient complementary therapeutic method to classical surgery, chemotherapy, radiotherapy, and independent limited diagnosis.

2. Plant-Derived Photosensitive Substances

Photoactive compounds occurring in medicinal plants with potential utilization in PDT have been found to be less toxic than synthetic agents. The reduction of side effects using natural PSs in cancer treatment is another advantage of this therapeutic approach. However, their clinical applications have been limited by several imperfections such as accumulation in tissues, a lack of chemical purity, or low penetration [80]. Muniyandi et al. [81] have published a comprehensive review article about the role of photoactive phytocompounds in PDT. Phototoxic effects, potential applications in the PDT of cancer of the main natural PSs groups (furanocoumarins, thiophenes, alkaloids, curcumins, polyacetylenes, and anthraquinones) have been described [81]. Our paper focuses on the four anthraquinones, of which hypericin is the most promising PS in the PDT of cancer. With regard to the hydrophobicity of studied anthraquinones, which is important for their penetration through membranes, the following types of PSs have been distinguished.

Types of Photosensitive Substances by Hydrophobicity

PDT either uses chemotherapeutics commonly applied in chemotherapy, which must also be photosensitive, or new PSs are proposed. All photosensitizers (except uroporphyrin and photophrin), which have been proposed as drugs for use in PDT, interact more or less with serum proteins after intravenous administration. From the point of view of PDT, however, the interaction of the drugs with DNA is also quite important, as it is necessary to disrupt and stop the division of tumor cells, and this can be achieved only through their interaction with DNA [62,82]. In some cases, this interaction is not very significant (as these drugs have a greater affinity for proteins), so it is necessary to find a transporter that will help deliver the drug to the cell nucleus, thereby mediating the drug–DNA interaction [83,84]. Success in the treatment of cancer requires sufficiently hydrophobic drugs to cross the lipid membrane. For this reason, the hydrophobicity of drugs plays an important role in their distribution, metabolism, and excretion from the patient´s body. Due to these facts, we distinguish four groups of drugs with the ability to localize and accumulate in the tumor. Moreover, there are no rigid boundaries between these groups of drugs, and there is some overlapping between them, in some cases a continuous transition.

1. Hydrophobic PSs—compounds requiring the presence of transporters, such as liposomes or Cremophor EL, or Tween 80. They have the ability to localize in the inner lipid part of lipoproteins, mainly in LDL and high-density lipoproteins (HDLs), but also in very-low-density lipoproteins (VLDLs). This group includes phthalocyanines (ZnPC, C1A1PC), naphthalocyanines (isoBOSINC), tin-etiopurpurine (SnET2) [84], and hypericin [85].
2. Amphiphilic PSs—asymmetric compounds, which can be incorporated into the outer phospholipid and apoprotein layer of lipoprotein particles, e.g., disulfonates ($TPPS_{2a}$, $C1A1PCS_{2a}$), lutetium teraphyrin (LuTex), and monoaspartyl chlorine (MACE), which forms a barrier between albumin and HDL [84]. Emodin can be included in this group [86].
3. Hydrophilic PSs—drugs that predominantly bind to albumins and globulins, e.g., tetra-sulfone derivates of tetraphenylporfin ($TPPS_3$ and $TPPS_4$) and chloroaluminum phthalocyanine ($C1A1PCS_3$ and $C1A1PCS_4$) [84].
4. Intercalators—drugs that are used mainly in chemotherapy, which intercalate into DNA and are also photoactive, e.g., doxorubicin [87], daunorubicin [88], adriamycin [89], quinizarin [90], and danthron [91].

In this work, we focused in more detail on a very prospective PS in PDT of cancer hypericin. During a study of hypericin molecule incorporation into biomacromolecules (we focused on DNA) model compounds are using for simplification of the problem. Anthraquinones emodin, quinizarin, and danthron represent a significantly smaller part of the larger hypericin molecule with the same chemical groups. This fact facilitates the creation of a proper model for interaction between hypericin and biomacromolecules. Moreover, chosen hypericin derivatives themselves originate from medicinal plants, as the PS can be utilized in PDT and their anticancer effects are known. With respect to the above-mentioned sorting of PSs into groups, they can be representatives of highly hydrophobic (hypericin), mildly hydrophobic (emodin), and intercalating molecules (quinizarin and danthron).

Scientists and physicians are currently working on how to increase the effectiveness of cancer treatment. One option that has been shown to be very effective is a combination of therapies (PDT and chemotherapy), which involve the direct or mediated interaction of anticancer drugs with DNA and other bioactive macromolecules (serum albumins, lipoproteins) [92–94]. Hypericin, emodin, quinizarin, and danthron are examples of anticancer drugs which are chemotherapeutics synthesized by medicinal plants and PSs, and which can be used, in PDT. The discovery of new natural drugs is very important because they have many benefits for the patients. Drugs derived from medicinal plants are less toxic to the body, their use poses less risk of adverse side effects, does not depends on them, they are suitable for all age groups of patients, and can be easily combined with conventional drugs, i.e., do not show contraindications.

3. Hypericin

Hypericin, a naturally occurring pigment, is found in certain plant species of the genus *Hypericum*. The most important representative is Saint John´s Wort (*Hypericum perforatum*) from the family *Hypericaceae*, a plant with golden-yellow flowers that grows to a height of 30–90 cm [95]. Hypericin has also been reported as occurring in some species of Australian insects [96]. Hypericin, 7,14 dione-1,3,4,6,8,12-hexahydroxy 10,11 dimethyl-phenanthrol [1,10,9,8-opgra] perylene (Figure 2) is an aromatic polycyclic dione, which exhibits a wide range of biological activities.

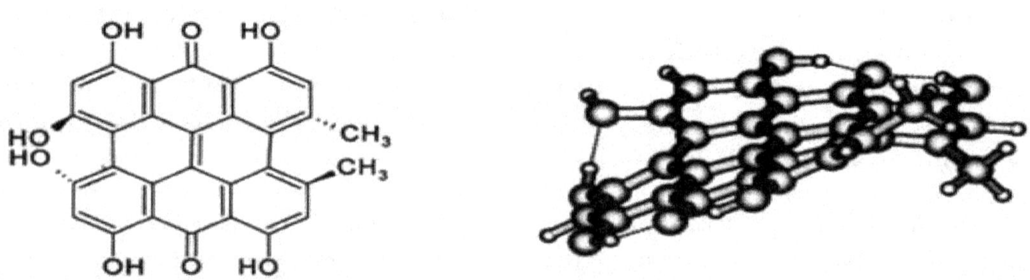

(a) (b)

Figure 2. Two-dimensional (**a**) and three-dimensional (**b**) structure of hypericin [97].

It has long been used to treat depression caused by a disorder of the brain neurotransmitters responsible for human moods [98,99]. Hypericin has antiviral [100,101] and antitumor activity [102–105] and is used to heal wounds, neuralgic sites, and hypertrophic scar [106–108]. Hypericin has been demonstrated to be very effective on bacteria [109–114]. Studies of hypericin´s antiviral activity confirm that it is known to effectively deactivate enveloped viruses, but it is ineffective against non-enveloped viruses. The antiviral activity of hypericin has been demonstrated against several types of viruses: herpes simplex virus, murine cytomegalovirus, sindbis virus [115,116], hepatitis B [117], anemia, some types of leukemic viruses [118], and HIV [119–121], so it has also been used in the clinical treatment of AIDS patients [122]. Hypericin activity depends to a large extent on the presence of light and oxygen. These two factors determine the extent of its antiviral activity and both antiviral and antitumor activities increase significantly after visible light irradiation [123].

Hypericin, together with two other hydroxyquinones, hypocrellin A and calphostin, is characterized by negligible dark toxicity, significant photocytotoxicity to tumor cells, intense absorption at higher wavelengths (>550 nm), higher selectivity for tumor tissues, and faster leaching than hematoporphyrins [124]. Hypericin is soluble in most solvents. In organic solvents (DMSO, ethanol) its solution is red; in basic media, it is green; and in aqueous solutions, it forms purple dispersed particles [125]. The absorption spectrum of hypericin in neutral organic solvents has two main transitions in the visible region, $S_0 \rightarrow S_1$ (500–600 nm) and $S_0 \rightarrow S_2$ (425–485 nm), and two intense absorption bands. Hypericin forms non-fluorescent aggregates in aqueous solutions. The absorption and fluorescence spectra of hypericin in hexane, chloroform, and toluene are similar to those in water, so it can be assumed that hypericin molecules also form aggregates in these solvents. An indicator of the formation of aggregates in solution is the absence of fluorescence [126]. Several physical and chemical properties of hypericin are shown in Table 1.

Table 1. Physical and chemical properties of selected photosensitizers (hypericin, emodin, quinizarin, and danthron).

Photosensitizer		**Hypericin**	**Emodin**	**Quinizarin**	**Danthron**
Hydrophobicity		high	amphiphilic with mild hydrophobicity	low	Low
AlogP		5.040	2.568	2.324	2.324
Absorption maximum in DMSO λ_{max} (nm)		560 600	440	475	430
Fluorescence maximum $\lambda_{exc.}$ (nm)		603 560	520 440	540 475	575 430
Dissociated form (nm)	PS^0	560	440	475	430
	PS^{1-}	600 [127]	480	560	475
	PS^{2-}	650 [127]	525	595	500
	PS^{4-}	630 [127]			
	PS^{6-}	640 [127]			
Dissociated constant	pKa_1	2 [127]	7.2	11.3	10.5
	pKa_2	7.8 [127]	10.6	12.7	12.9
	pKa_3	11.5 [127]			
	pKa_4	13 [127]			

The photophysics of hypericin is very complicated, and some effort to interpret its photophysical and photochemical properties is necessary to elucidate its pharmacological and biological activities. Phenols are known to be good electron donors, while quinones act as electron acceptors. Hypericin contains both phenolic and quinone moieties. This structural characteristic places it in the group of amphi-electron compounds. The results of experiments suggest that hypericin has the potential to be a good oxidizing and reducing agent [128]. At present, the mechanisms leading to the selective accumulation of hypericin in tumor tissue compared to normal tissue are not known, nor the mechanism of its antiviral and antitumor action has been clearly determined. Thomas et al. proposed a mechanism of hypericin activity that depends on the presence of molecular oxygen, consisting of transferring energy from the excited triplet state of hypericin to the ground state of molecular oxygen, thereby generating oxygen in the singlet state, which is a highly-reactive molecule [129]. Singlet oxygen production has been theoretically confirmed [118] and experimentally demonstrated in organic solvents and lipid media [130–132]. Other studies suggest that although oxygen may play an important role in some cases, it is not always necessary for the antiviral activity of hypericin [133]. According to the work of the J.W. Petrich group, the origin of the photoinduced antiviral activity of hypericin may lie in its ability to produce a local pH drop in cells after irradiation [134]. The close relationship between the mechanism of hypericin antitumor activity and photoactivated local acidification in cells has been confirmed in experiments on tumor cell membrane experiments [102].

Hypericin is currently considered as a potential antitumor drug in PDT. It belongs in the group of highly hydrophobic PSs (AlogP = 5.04) [135]. Its cytotoxic and antitumor activity has been demonstrated, and its inhibitory effects on epidermal growth factor-R and a wide range of protein kinases (protein tyrosine kinase, MAP-kinase, and protein kinase C) [136]. The significant photosensitivity properties of hypericin together with its selective uptake in tumor tissues, especially in bladder cancer cells and its minimal cytotoxicity in the dark, are major positive indications for the clinical use of hypericin in the photodynamic cancer treatment [137]. Hypericin is a photosensitizer found in the endoplasmic reticulum, which, when activated by light, mediates the rapid emptying of calcium Ca^{2+} from the endoplasmic reticulum, which is linked to programmed cell death [138]. Although hypericin has been shown to be a potent inducer of cell death in PDT, some in vivo studies suggest that cells treated with PDT may activate rescue-signaling pathways, which may ultimately lead to tumor survival and recurrence [18,139].

Hypericin is a very good fluorescent probe for super-resolution microscopy [140]. Knowledge of the distribution of this molecule in the individual components of a living system is essential in detecting the modes of action of hypericin in biological organisms. The accumulation of hypericin in cells is determined by the diffuse and soluble properties of the molecule. It is known that after the initial accumulation in the cell membranes (20 min), an increased concentration of hypericin in the cell nucleus is observed with increasing time [141]. This indicates the possible interaction of hypericin with nucleic acids, the most essential component of the cell nucleus. Ultraviolet resonance Raman spectroscopy with 257 nm excitation was used to study nucleic acid-hypericin complexes. The excitation used amplifies the vibrational modes of nucleic acid bases. Resonance Raman spectra for complexes of polynucleotides with hypericin showed that hypericin preferentially interacts with purines at the N7 position, and this interaction is stronger in guanine than in adenine [142]. In addition, the spectra of the complex of hypericin with polyrG and calf thymus DNA, which were studied by means of surface-enhanced Raman spectroscopy, are dominated by bands corresponding to hypericin vibrations. Based on the spectra obtained, the importance of the guanine base in the interaction of hypericin with nucleic acid was confirmed. The spectrum of the polyrG complex contains changes similar to those in the spectrum of the DNA complex. Based on these results, it can be assumed that DNA induces changes in the stretching vibrations of the hypericin skeleton associated with the vibrations of the hydroxyl groups, suggesting that the hydroxyl groups of hypericin participate in the interaction with nucleic acid [143].

The mechanism of hypericin distribution in tissues, cells, and cellular organelles is also thought to be a relatively complex process, which is affected by hypericin concentration, incubation time, and properties of biological units. The bio distribution of hypericin in human organisms also depends on the mode of transport in the bloodstream. Hypericin binds to serum proteins, where lipoprotein particles appear to be a more efficient transporter than albumin. The interaction of hypericin with albumin is specific [144], while its interaction with lipoproteins is non-specific [145]. After binding with macromolecules (lipid structures, serum proteins, and sugars), hypericin forms biologically active monomers with an emission band around 600 nm, thus overcoming problems with its solubility in physiological solutions, which is very important in terms of its activity [97,137].

4. Emodin

Emodin, (1,3,8-trihydroxy-6-methylanthraquinone, Figure 3) is an anthraquinone derivate, a naturally-occurring pigment isolated from the underground part of the traditional Chinese medicinal plant *Rheum palmatum*, which is used mainly for its antitumor, immunosuppressive, antiinflammatory [146], antibacterial, diuretic, laxative [147], antiulcerogenic (antiulcer) [148], and vasorelaxant effects [149]. It is also found in other plant species, such as *Cassia*, *Aloe*, and *Rhamnus* [150–154]. In practice, it is available in the form of an orange crystalline substance. It is insoluble in aqueous media, and it forms aggregates (mostly in the acidic pH range). Emodin shows poor solubility in chloroform, ether, and benzene, but is highly soluble in DMSO and ethanol.

The antiviral properties of emodin have also been confirmed, mainly on enveloped viruses. This property of emodin is related to its high affinity for the phospholipid membrane, in which it inhibits hydrophobic interactions between individual hydrocarbon chains [155]. Emodin has been proposed as a major precursor of the microbial metabolic pathway in the isolation of hypericin [156,157]. It is a redox catalyst and plays an important role in many processes, such as electron transport, photosynthesis, or cellular respiration [158]. Its effect on cell death has been widely studied both in the dark and after light activation [155,159]. The stimulatory effects and the prokinetic effect of emodin on gastrointestinal smooth muscle have been described in several studies [147,160]. In recent years, its effect on the contractility of smooth muscle cells has been studied [161,162].

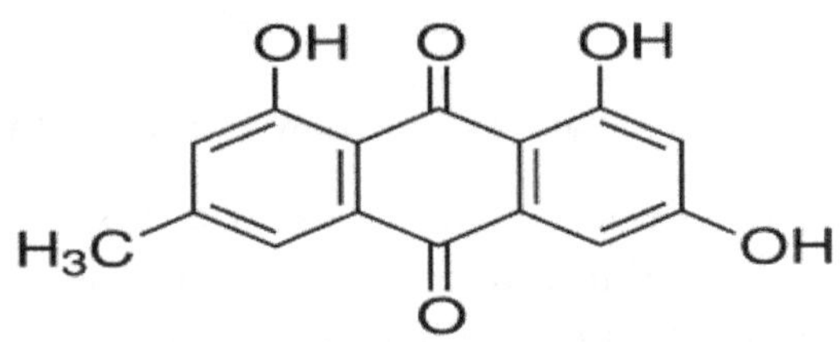

Figure 3. Structural formula of emodin.

In addition to the pharmacological properties mentioned above, emodin also has toxicological effects. Under aerobic conditions, it is photolabile in visible light and phototoxic in vitro and it can cause testicular toxicity in mice leading to hypospermatogenesis [163,164]. It inhibits protein kinase casein kinase II (CK2). Genetic disorder of the catalytic subunits of CK2 protein kinase leads to changes in sperm shape in mice during spermatogenesis and is also responsible for male infertility [165,166]. Several authors have studied the interaction of emodin with DNA [167–169]; for example, it causes the formation of DNA double-strand breaks by stabilizing topoisomerase II-DNA cleavage complexes and inhibiting ATP hydrolysis by topoisomerase II [170]. Emodin has a high binding affinity for serum proteins and is known to bind non-covalently to DNA in intact cells in the presence of serum proteins [159]. The interaction of emodin with proteins has been studied using several techniques surface-enhanced Raman spectroscopy, NMR, fluorescence spectroscopy, circular dichroism, and the stopped-flow method [171–174]. The formation of emodin–protein complexes is very important with regard to understanding the mode of drug delivery and transport in tumor cells [174]. Emodin belongs in the drug of amphiphilic PSs with mild hydrophobic properties (Alog P = 2.568) [135]. It has an anticancer effect on some types of human liver and lung tumors. However, the molecular mechanisms of emodin-mediated tumor regression have not been precisely defined [150]. Emodin has specific antineuroectodermal tumor activity in vitro and in vivo [175]. It suppresses tyrosine kinase activity on HER-2 breast cancer cells, inhibits the transformation of the phenotype of these cells, and can affect androgen receptors directly by inhibiting cell growth in prostate cancer cells [146]. The antitumor activity of emodin on the human chronic myeloid leukemia cell line K562 has also been demonstrated in vitro and in vivo [176]. Emodin is toxic for glioma cells by inhibiting their proliferation and inducing apoptosis of C6 cells [177]. It is known to increase the sensitivity of tumor cells to chemotherapeutics, but the mechanism of the emodin-mediated chemotherapeutic effect on cancer cells has been the subject of intense study for many years [150,178]. Important physical properties of emodin are listed in Table 1.

5. Quinizarin

Quinizarin (1,4-dihydroxyanthraquinone, Figure 4) is a polycyclic aromatic hydrocarbon containing two opposite carboxyl groups (C=O) at positions 9,10. It takes the form of a yellow crystalline substance and occurs in nature in plants (*Aloe*, Cascara Sagrada, Senna, and rhubarb), fungi, some lichens, and insects [179]. Quinizarin is soluble in basic solutions, acetone, chloroform, and DMSO. It is almost insoluble in aqueous solutions, but its solubility increases with increasing temperature. It is used as a pesticide as a fungicide and as an additive in lubricants [180]. In addition, it is used as a colorant in the food, textile, dyeing, and photographic industries [181]. Quinizarin inhibits HIV proteinase [182] and acts as a mutagenic agent on some mammalian bacteria [183]. Immunological analysis studies have shown that it stimulates the P450 enzyme in rat epithelial and liver cells [184].

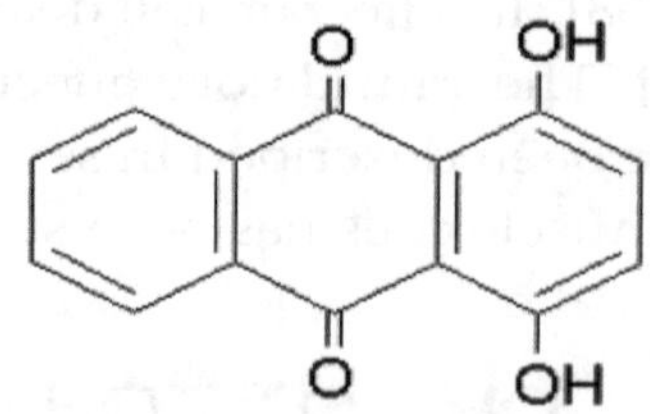

Figure 4. Structural formula of quinizarin.

The structure of quinizarin has been studied using several spectroscopic methods, such as fluorescence measurements [185], resonance Raman and infrared spectroscopy [186], and X-ray structural analysis [187]. It has planar C_{2v} molecular symmetry and crystallizes in a monoclonal system. Quinizarin is a highly fluorescent substance. The fact that it is almost insoluble in water significantly complicates the application of Raman spectroscopy in its study. However, infrared FT Raman and surface-enhanced Raman spectroscopy can also be used to characterize it in aqueous media [188].

Quinizarin is the simplest model molecule of a chromophore typical of some biologically and pharmaceutically significant compounds, including the antitumor anthracycline antibiotics doxorubicin, daunorubicin, and adriamycin, which are used in antineoplastic therapy. The quinizarin-like quinoid moiety is probably responsible for the cytotoxicity and cardiotoxicity of anthracycline drugs [180]. It is thought to be able to intercalate into DNA [189,190]. We can classify it among the photosensitive intercalators with low hydrophobicity (AlogP = 2.324), which could be applied in PDT [135]. The physical properties of quinizarin are shown in Table 1.

6. Danthron

Danthron (1,8-dihydroxyanthraquinone or chrysazine, Figure 5) is a hydroxyanthraquinone that occurs wild in nature found in many plants but also in some insect species (e.g., *Pyrrhalta luteola* larvae). It is very often isolated from dry leaves and stems of the plant *Xyris semifuscata* growing in Madagascar [191]. It is commercially available in the form of an orange, red, or red-yellow crystalline powder. Like quinizarin, it is soluble in basic solutions, chloroform, and DMSO. It is practically insoluble in water. Danthron and quinizarin are derivatives of emodin and hypericin. Danthron is part of the anticancer drug aclacinomycin. It is thought to intercalate into DNA and therefore can be used as an example of a low hydrophobicity intercalator (AlogP = 2.324) in PDT. However, it can also be a carcinogen, causing the development of adenoma or adenocarcinoma of the colon and increased incidence of liver cancer cells [191,192]. Danthron is one of the hydroxyanthraquinone derivatives causing topoisomerase II inhibition [193], which is involved in various cellular processes, including chromosome segregation [194], and it is essential for maintaining genome stability [195].

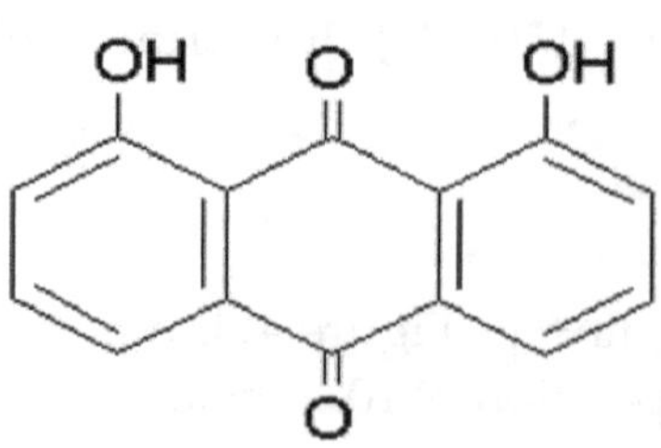

Figure 5. Structural formula of danthron.

Danthron is used as a laxative [159,196]. It is currently applied as an antioxidant, a fungicide to control powdery mildew, and has an irreplaceable role in the research into anticancer agents. Together with emodin, it is the basic structure of aglycones, which are naturally occurring laxative glycosides [191]. Danthron shows mutagenic activity [197] and indicates mutations in cells of the lymphatic system [192].

Its structure has been studied using fluorescence, resonance Raman and infrared spectroscopy. The danthron crystal is tetragonal and its planar molecule has an asymmetric structure with two different intramolecular O . . . . .O distances. The optical properties of danthron can be discussed in terms of C_{2v} pseudosymmetry [188]. Danthron and quinizarin form two intramolecular hydrogen bonds, which cause small changes in the structure of anthraquinone molecules. The presence of two hydrogen bonds in quinizarin allows for double proton transfer, which can take place in two steps or a one-step process. Conversely, the geometry of the danthron molecule allows only single proton transmission. The structure of danthron and quinizarin has been intensively studied and experimentally determined. For quinizarin, X-ray structural analysis identified the values of the distance O . . . . .O and O . . . . .H bounds, which are 2.57 and 1.77–1.79 Å respectively. This technique helped to define the O . . . . .O distance for danthron and setting its value at 2.49 Å, but it did not provide any information about proton binding [198]. Table 1 shows characteristic physical properties.

7. Hypericin and Its Derivatives Interaction with DNA

In recent years the interaction of hypericin, emodin, quinizarin, and danthron with biomacromolecules has been studied, especially with DNA, LDL, and human serum albumin (HSA) has been investigated [199–202]. The results of our studies in this area supplement the scientific knowledge on this subject. The measurements indicate that PSs incorporate into DNA, LDL, and HSA, but interact most easily with LDL particles. Distribution of molecules has been studied at two different conditions: (i) DNA–ligand complexes were exposed to the presence of free LDL particles or HSA molecules, respectively and (ii) LDL- or HSA-ligand, respectively, complexes were in the presence of free DNA molecules. From measurements at the first conditions, it is clear that while the fluorescence intensity for the DNA-hypericin complex increases with the addition of LDL to the solution, a less pronounced effect can be observed for the other PSs, DNA–emodin, DNA–quinizarin, and DNA–danthron. Similarly, HSA molecules added to the solution slightly increase the fluorescence intensity in the DNA–hypericin complex. In a competitive environment, they redistribute and rebind from DNA macromolecule to LDL (hypericin) or HSA (emodin, quinizarin, and danthron). In contrast, the fluorescence intensity did not change for the DNA–emodin complex, and a slight decrease in fluorescence has been observed in the DNA–quinizarin and DNA–dantron complexes. The presence of free DNA leads to a decrease in the fluorescence intensity of the LDL–emodin, LDL–quinizarin, and LDL–danthron/HSA–quinizarin and HSA–danthron complexes. For LDL–hypericin and HSA–hypericin complexes, an increase in fluorescence with the addition of DNA was recorded. The fluorescence intensity of the HSA–emodin complex remains unchanged [135]. It is noteworthy that the quenching of fluorescence in the presence of DNA has been observed for intercalating molecules [190]. These results allowed us to state that the molecules of the studied PSs can be extracted from DNA by HSA molecules rather than LDL particles, with the exception of hypericin, where there is a more significant binding from DNA in the presence of LDL particles. Experiments in fluorescence analysis of native and denatured DNA were designed to determine if and how the interaction of hypericin, emodin, quinizarin, and danthron with native and denatured DNA differed. Significant changes were detected for quinizarin and danthron, where fluorescence increased significantly in the presence of denatured DNA. It can be assumed that DNA denaturation increased the distances between the individual quinizarin and danthron molecules (there is a decrease in fluorescence quenching) and helped to better visualize the molecules inside the DNA. This applies in particular to molecules that intercalate into the DNA structure, i.e., quinizarin and danthron. For hypericin and emodin, it has been noted only a slight change in the intensity of fluorescence in the presence of denatured DNA, respectively from which it can again predict a different interaction mode of these PSs with DNA [135].

As a representative of highly hydrophobic PSs, hypericin binds to DNA by means of a large groove [203,204]. A binding constant, whose value was also determined, is 4.0×10^4 L/mol [204]. Emodin, with mild hydrophobic properties, interacts with DNA by binding into a small groove. This interaction is characterized by binding constant 8.1×10^4 L/mol. These ligands are incorporated into the DNA groove with hydrophobic or hydrogen bounds [204]. An intercalating mode of interaction with DNA has been confirmed for quinizarin and danthron, which is very clearly supported by atomic force microscopy measurements. Quinizarin and dathron cause DNA to unwind due to intercalation, increasing the contour length of linear DNA by 10%. By the action of natural photosensitizers studied by us, more rigid molecules of linear DNA have been detected. It is known that this is not only the type of reaction they are involved in. Quinizarin and danthron can also bind to the surface of DNA molecules by means of electrostatic forces. The size of the binding constant of this interaction type for both PSs is 1.1×10^4 L/mol [190].

Cell experiments have been performed with the aim of better understanding the mechanisms of the interaction of hypericin, emodin, quinizarin, and danthron with DNA. Success in the treatment of cancer requires sufficient hydrophobic drugs to cross the lipid membrane. The hydrophobicity of drugs therefore plays an important role in their distribution, metabolism, and excretion from the patient´s body. The main barrier preventing the interaction of nuclear DNA with anticancer drugs is the nuclear envelope. On the other hand, the detoxification process is accompanied by a decrease in drug concentration during the active outflow of these drugs. P-glycoprotein, a member of the transport protein family, is involved in this process [205]. The function of these proteins is to remove toxins from cells [206], so it is possible to regulate drug resistance by manipulating P-glycoprotein activity [207,208]. Another approach to preventing cancer cell resistance to drugs could be based on photochemical activation at a well-defined site/organelle [209]. With this in mind, the intracellular interaction of the drugs discussed here with DNA directly in the nucleus was studied using selective photoactivation and regulation of P-glycoprotein function. Selective photoactivation facilitates entry of emodin, quinizarin, and danthron molecules into the nucleus of tumor cells by means of passive diffusion (this phenomenon has not been observed in the case of hypericin). Inhibition of P-glycoprotein may increase the intracellular concentration of the molecules studied and aid their interaction with DNA. Inhibition of P-glycoprotein stimulates the passive transport of these molecules to the nucleus of tumor cells. In addition, emodin is known to significantly promote the entry of other drugs into the nucleus of tumor cells, with the exception of strongly hydrophobic ones (hypericin-like), which are characterized by a high binding affinity for P-glycoprotein [135].

The treatment of tumor cells with natural photosensitive drugs significantly depends on the degree of hydrophobicity, lipophilicity, and DNA intercalation properties of the drugs used.

8. Conclusions

Cancer is a group of diseases characterized by abnormal and uncontrolled cell growth, which can affect a particular tissue or organ in a very aggressive manner and are able to spread to other parts of the body, they can metastasize. Cancer can be treated by classical therapeutic procedures (surgery, chemotherapy, and radiotherapy) and modern, very promising therapeutic methods. These include PDT. These studies show that the most effective way to treat cancer is to combine PDT with traditional therapies, respectively in some cases, PDT can even replace conventional treatment. It is very likely that PDT will be used in the future as the therapeutic approach in the treatment of specific cancers and non-cancerous diseases. This method minimizes the side effects of traditional therapeutic methods, is less invasive, more effective, and affordable. The condition for the successful treatment of cancer with PDT is the disruption of DNA macromolecule, which stops the division of tumor cells. Therefore, it is necessary to find suitable drugs that interact with DNA directly, respectively mediated by transporters that transport them to the nucleus of the tumor cell. A great advantage of newly discovered drugs is that they are natural, easier to prepare, and do not burden the patient´s body as much as synthetically produced drugs. The success of cancer treatment is highly dependent on the application of hydrophobic drugs, which can more easily cross the lipid membrane of tumor cells. Therefore, the interaction of drugs with different hydrophobicity with DNA macromolecule is the subject of many studies.

Author Contributions: Conceptualization, J.S. and V.V.; methodology, J.B.; software, J.B.; validation, J.S., V.V. and J.B.; formal analysis, V.V.; investigation, V.V.; resources, V.V.; data curation, J.S.; writing—original draft preparation, V.V.; writing—review and editing, J.S.; visualization, J.B.; supervision, J.S.; project administration, J.S.; funding acquisition, J.S. All authors have read and agreed to the published version of the manuscript.

References

1. Castano, A.P.; Demidova, T.N.; Hamblin, M.R. Mechanisms in photodynamic therapy: Part one—Photosensitizers, photochemistry and cellular localization. *Photodiagn. Photodyn. Ther.* **2004**, *1*, 279–293. [CrossRef]
2. Deda, D.K.; Araki, K. Nanotechnology, light and chemical action: An effective combination to kill cancer cells. *J. Braz. Chem. Soc.* **2015**, *26*, 2448–2470. [CrossRef]
3. Allen, T.M.; Hansen, C.B.; Demenzes, D.E.L. Pharmacokinetics of long circulating liposomes. *Adv. Drug Deliv. Rev.* **1995**, *16*, 267–284. [CrossRef]
4. Loomis, K.; McNeeley, K.; Bellamkonda, R.V. Nanoparticles with targeting triggered release and imaging functionality for cancer application. *Soft Matter* **2011**, *7*, 839–856. [CrossRef]
5. Reddi, E. Role of delivery vehicles for photosensitizers in the photodynamic therapy of tumors. *J. Photochem. Photobiol. B* **1997**, *37*, 189–195. [CrossRef]
6. Huntošová, V.; Buzová, D.; Petrovajová, D.; Kasak, P.; Nad'ová, Z.; Jancura, D.; Sureau, F.; Miškovský, P. Development of a new LDL-based transport system for hydrophobic/amphiphilic drug delivery to cancer cells. *Int. J. Pharm.* **2012**, *436*, 463–471. [CrossRef]
7. Hally, C.; Delcanale, P.; Nonell, S.; Viappiani, C.; Abbruzzetti, S. Photosensitizing proteins for antibacterial photodynamic inactivation. *Transl. Biophotonics* **2020**, e201900031. [CrossRef]
8. Ghorbani, J.; Rahban, D.; Aghamiri, S.; Teymouri, A.; Bahador, A. Photosensitizers in antibacterial photodynamic therapy: An overview. *Laser Ther.* **2018**, *27*, 293–302. [CrossRef] [PubMed]
9. Buriankova, L.; Buzova, D.; Chorvat, D.; Sureau, F.; Brault, D.; Miskovsky, P.; Jancura, D. Kinetics of hypericin association with low-density lipoproteins. *Photochem. Photobiol.* **2011**, *87*, 56–63. [CrossRef]
10. Lenkavska, L.; Blascakova, L.; Jurasekova, Z.; Macajova, M.; Bilcik, B.; Cavarga, I.; Miskovsky, P.; Huntosova, V. Benefits of hypericin transport and delivery by low- and high-density lipoproteins to cancer cells: From in vitro to ex ovo. *Photodiagn. Photodyn. Ther.* **2019**, *25*, 214–224. [CrossRef]
11. Konan, Y.N.; Gurny, R.; Allemann, E. State of the art in the delivery of photosensitizers for photodynamic therapy. *J. Photochem. Photobiol. B Biol.* **2002**, *66*, 89–106. [CrossRef]
12. Firestone, R.A. Low-density lipoprotein as a vehicle for targeting antitumor compounds to cancer cells. *Bioconjugate Chem.* **1994**, *5*, 105–113. [CrossRef] [PubMed]
13. Versluis, A.J.; van Geel, P.J.; Oppellar, H.; van Berkel, T.J.; Bijsterbosch, M.K. Receptor-mediated uptake of low-density lipoprotein by B16 melanoma cells in vitro and in vivo in mice. *Br. J. Cancer* **1996**, *4*, 525–532. [CrossRef] [PubMed]
14. Rensen, P.C.; de Vrueh, R.L.; Kuiper, J.; Bijsterbosch, M.K.; Biessen, E.A.; van Berkel, T.J. Recombinant lipoproteins: Lipoprotein-like lipid particles for drug targeting. *Adv. Drug Deliv. Rev.* **2001**, *47*, 251–276. [CrossRef]
15. Kader, A.; Pater., A. Loading anticancer drugs into HDL as well as LDL has little affect on properties of complexes and enhances cytotoxicity to human carcinoma cells. *J. Control. Release* **2002**, *80*, 29–44. [CrossRef]
16. Zheng, G.; Chen, J.; Li, H.; Glickson, J.D. Rerouting lipoprotein nanoparticles to selected alternate receptors for the targeted delivery of cancer diagnostic and therapeutic agents. *Proc. Natl. Acad. Sci. USA* **2005**, *102*, 17757–17762. [CrossRef]
17. Song, L.; Li, H.; Sunar, U.; Chen, J.; Corbin, I.; Yodh, A.G.; Zheng, G. Naphthalocyanine-reconstituted LDL nanoparticles for in vivo cancer imaging and treatment. *Int. J. Nanomed.* **2007**, *2*, 767–774.
18. Dougherty, T.J.; Gomer, C.J.; Henderson, B.W.; Jori, G.; Kessel, D.; Korbelik, M.; Moan, J.; Peng, Q. Photodynamic therapy. *J. Natl. Cancer Inst.* **1998**, *90*, 889–905. [CrossRef]
19. Wilson, B.C.; Patterson, M.S. The physics, biophysics and technology of photodynamic therapy. *Phys. Med. Biol.* **2008**, *53*, R61–R109. [CrossRef]
20. Yano, S.; Hirohara, S.; Obata, M.; Hagiya, Y.; Ogura, S.; Ikeda, A.; Kataoka, H.; Tanaka, M.; Joh, T. Current states and future views in photodynamic therapy. *J. Photochem. Photobiol. C Photochem. Rev.* **2011**, *12*, 46–67. [CrossRef]

21. Lim, C.K.; Heo, J.; Shin, S.; Jeong, K.; Seo, Y.H.; Jang, W.D.; Park, C.R.; Park, S.Y.; Kim, S.; Kwon, I.C. Nanophotosensitizers toward advanced photodynamic therapy of cancer. *Cancer Lett.* **2013**, *334*, 176–187. [CrossRef] [PubMed]
22. Bechet, D.; Mordon, S.R.; Guillemin, F.; Barberi-Heyob, M.A. Photodynamic therapy of malignant brain tumours: A complementary approach to conventional therapies. *Cancer Treat. Rev.* **2014**, *40*, 229–241. [CrossRef] [PubMed]
23. Benov, L. Photodynamic therapy: Current status and future direction. *Med. Princ. Pract.* **2015**, *24*, 14–28. [CrossRef] [PubMed]
24. Miguel-Gomez, L.; Vano-Galvan, S.; Perez-Garcia, B.; Carrillo-Gijon, R.; Jaen-Olasolo, P. Treatment of folliculitis decalvans with photodynamic therapy: Results in 10 patients. *J. Am. Acad. Dermatol.* **2015**, *72*, 1085–1087. [CrossRef]
25. Sharman, W.M.; Allen, C.M.; van Lier, J.E. Photodynamic therapeutics: Basic principles and clinical applications. *Drug Discov. Today* **1999**, *4*, 507–517. [CrossRef]
26. Jin, Y.; Zhang, X.; Kang, H.; Du, L.; Li, M. Nanostructures of an amphiphilic zinc phthalocyanine polymer conjugate for photodynamic therapy of psoriasis. *Colloids Surf. B* **2015**, *128*, 405–409. [CrossRef]
27. Sharman, W.M.; van Lier, J.E.; Allen, C.M. Targeted photodynamic theory via receptor mediated delivery systems. *Adv. Drug Deliv. Rev.* **2004**, *56*, 53–76. [CrossRef]
28. Cruess, A.F.; Zlateva, G.; Pleil, A.M.; Wirostko, B. Photodynamic therapy with verteporfin in age-related macular degeneration: A systematic review of efficacy, safety, treatment modifications and pharmacoeconomic properties. *Acta Ophthalmol.* **2009**, *87*, 118–132. [CrossRef]
29. Rockson, S.G.; Lorenz, D.P.; Cheong, W.F.; Woodburn, K.W. Photoangioplasty: An emerging clinical cardiovascular role for photodynamic therapy. *Circulation* **2000**, *102*, 591–596. [CrossRef]
30. Bozzini, G.; Colin, P.; Betrouni, N.; Nevoux, P.; Ouzzane, A.; Puech, P.; Willers, A.; Mordon, S. Photodynamic therapy in urology: What can we do now and where are we heading. *Photodiagn. Photodyn. Ther.* **2012**, *9*, 261–273. [CrossRef]
31. Panzarini, E.; Inguscio, V.; Dini, L. Immunogenic cell death: Can it be exploited in photodynamic therapy for cancer. *Biomed. Res. Int.* **2013**, *2013*, 482160. [CrossRef] [PubMed]
32. Lang, G.E.; Mennel, S.; Spital, G.; Wachtlin, J.; Jurklies, B.; Heimann, H.; Damato, B.; Meyer, C.H. Different indications of photodynamic therapy in ophthalmology. *Klin. Monbl. Augenheilkd.* **2009**, *226*, 725–739. [CrossRef] [PubMed]
33. Trindade, A.C.; De Figueiredo, J.A.P.; Steier, L.; Weber, J.B.B. Photodynamic therapy in endodontics: A literature review. *Photomed. Laser Surg.* **2015**, *33*, 175–182. [CrossRef] [PubMed]
34. Vohra, F.; Al-Kheraif, A.A.; Qadri, T.; Hassan, M.I.A.; Ahmedef, A.; Warnakulasuriya, S.; Javed, F. Efficacy of photodynamic therapy in the management of oral premalignant lesions. A systematic review. *Photodiagn. Photodyn. Ther.* **2015**, *12*, 150–159. [CrossRef]
35. Karrer, S.; Kohl, E.; Feise, K.; Hiepe-Wegener, D.; Lischner, S.; Philipp-Dormston, W.; Podda, M.; Prager, W.; Walker, T.; Szeimies, R.M. Photodynamic therapy for skin rejuvenation: Review and summary of the literature-results of a consensus conference of an expert group for aesthetic photodynamic therapy. *J. Dtsch. Dermatol. Ges.* **2013**, *11*, 137–148. [CrossRef]
36. Fuhrmann, G.; Serio, A.; Mazo, M.; Nair, R.; Stevens, M.M. Active loading into extracellular vesicles significantly improves the cellular uptake and photodynamic effect of porphyrins. *J. Control. Release* **2015**, *205*, 35–44. [CrossRef]
37. Baptista, M.S.; Wainwright, M. Photodynamic antimicrobial chemotherapy (PACT) for the treatment of malaria, leishmaniasis and trypanosomiasis. *Braz. J. Med. Res.* **2011**, *44*, 1–10. [CrossRef]
38. Goslinski, T.; Piskorz, J. Fluorinated porphyrinoids and their biomedical applications. *J. Photochem. Photobiol. C Photochem. Rev.* **2011**, *12*, 304–321. [CrossRef]
39. Hanakova, A.; Bogdanova, K.; Tomankova, K.; Pizova, K.; Malohlava, J.; Binder, S.; Bajgar, R.; Langova, K.; Kolar, M.; Mosinger, J.; et al. The application of antimicrobial photodynamic therapy on *S. aureus* and *E. coli* using porphyrin photosensitizers bound to cyclodextrin. *Microbiol. Res.* **2014**, *169*, 163–170. [CrossRef]
40. Baltazar, L.M.; Ray, A.; Santos, D.A.; Cisalpino, P.S.; Friedman, A.J.; Nosanchuk, J.D. Antimicrobial photodynamic therapy: An effective alternative approach to control fungal injections. *Front. Microbiol.* **2015**, *6*, 202. [CrossRef]
41. Bonnett, R. Progress with heterocyclic photosensitizers for the photodynamic therapy (PDT) of tomours. *J. Heterocyclic Chem.* **2002**, *39*, 455. [CrossRef]

42. Photolitec, LLC. Tumor Specific Imaging Therapy. *Photodynamic Therapy.* Available online: http://photolitec.org/Tech_PDT.html (accessed on 10 August 2020).
43. Vatansever, F.; de Melo, W.C.M.A.; Avci, P.; Vecchio, D.; Sadasivam, M.; Gupta, A.; Chandran, R.; Karimi, M.; Parizotto, N.A.; Yin, R.; et al. Antimicrobial strategies centered around reactive oxygen species—bactericidal antibiotics, photodynamic therapy, and beyond. *Microbiol. Rev.* **2013**, *37*, 955–989. [CrossRef] [PubMed]
44. Henderson, B.W.; Dougherty, T.J. How does photodynamic therapy work. *Photochem. Photobiol.* **1992**, *55*, 145–157. [CrossRef]
45. Agostinis, P.; Berg, K.; Cengel, K.A.; Foster, T.H.; Girotti, A.W.; Gollnick, S.O.; Hahn, S.M.; Hamblin, M.R.; Juzeniene, A.; Kessel, D.; et al. Photodynamic therapy of cancer: An update. *CA Cancer J. Clin.* **2011**, *61*, 250–281. [CrossRef] [PubMed]
46. Senapathy, G.J.; George, B.P.; Abrahamse, H. Exloring the role of phytochemicals as potent natural photosensitizers in photodynamic therapy. *Anticancer Agents Med. Chem.* **2020**, *20*, 1831–1844. [CrossRef] [PubMed]
47. Moan, J.; Berg, K. The photodegradation of porphyrins in cells can be used to estimate the lifetime of singlet oxygen. *Photochem. Photobiol.* **1991**, *53*, 549–553. [CrossRef]
48. Hatz, S.; Poulsen, L.; Ogilby, P.R. Time-resolved singlet oxygen phosphorescence measurements from photosensitized experiments in single cells: Effects of oxygen diffusion and oxygen concentration. *Photochem. Photobiol.* **2008**, *84*, 1284–1290. [CrossRef]
49. Nyst, H.J.; Tan, I.B.; Stewart, F.A.; Balm, A.J.M. Is photodynamic therapy a good alternative to surgery and radiotherapy in the treatment of head and neck cancer. *Photodiagn. Photodyn. Ther.* **2009**, *6*, 3–11. [CrossRef]
50. Schafer, M. High sensitivity of Deinococcus radiodurans to photodynamically-produced singlet oxygen. *Int. J. Radiat. Biol.* **1998**, *74*, 249–253. [CrossRef]
51. Kochevar, I.E.; Lambert, C.R.; Lynch, M.C.; Tedesco, A.C. Comparison of photosensitized plasma membrane damage caused by singlet oxygen and free radicals. *Biochim. Biophys. Acta* **1996**, *1280*, 223–230. [CrossRef]
52. Barr, H.; Tralau, C.J.; Boulos, P.B.; MacRobert, A.J.; Tilly, R.; Bown, S.G. The contrasting mechanisms of colonic collagen damage between photodynamic therapy and thermal injury. *Photochem. Photobiol.* **1987**, *46*, 795–800. [CrossRef] [PubMed]
53. Hopper, C. Photodynamic therapy. A clinical reality in the treatment of cancer. *Lancet. Oncol.* **2000**, *1*, 212–219. [CrossRef]
54. Allison, R.R.; Bagnato, V.S.; Sibata, C.H. Future of oncologic photodynamic therapy. *Future Oncol.* **2010**, *6*, 929–940. [CrossRef] [PubMed]
55. Foote, C. Mechanisms of photo-oxygenation. In *Porphyrin Localization and Treatment of Tumors*, 1st ed.; Doiron, D.R., Gomer, C.J., Eds.; Alan R. Liss: New York, NY, USA, 1984; pp. 3–18.
56. Boegheim, J.P.; Scholte, H.; Dubbehman, T.M.; Beems, E.; Raap, A.K.; van Steveninck, J. Photodynamic effects of hematoporphyrin-derivative on enzyme activities of murine L929 fibroblasts. *J. Photochem. Photobiol. B* **1987**, *1*, 61–73. [CrossRef]
57. Gibson, S.L.; Hilf, R. Interdependence of fluence, drug, dose and oxygen on hematoporphyrin derivate induced photosensitization of tumor mitochondria. *Photochem. Photobiol.* **1985**, *42*, 367–373. [CrossRef]
58. Dolmans, D.E.; Fukumura, D.; Jain, R.K. Photodynamic therapy for cancer. *Nat. Rev. Cancer* **2003**, *3*, 380–387. [CrossRef]
59. Ochsner, M. Photophysical and photobiological processes in the photodynamic therapy of tumors. *J. Photochem. Photobiol. B* **1997**, *39*, 1–18. [CrossRef]
60. Canti, G.; Lattuada, D.; Morelli, S.; Nicolin, A.; Cubeddu, R.; Taroni, P.; Valentini, G. Efficacy of photodynamic therapy against doxorubicin-resistant murine tumors. *Cancer Lett.* **1995**, *93*, 255–259. [CrossRef]
61. Lofgren, L.A.; Hallgren, S.; Nilsson, E.; Westerborn, A.; Nilsson, C.; Reizenstein, J. photodynamic therapy for recurrent nasopharyngeal cancer. *Arch. Otolaryngol. Head Neck Surg.* **1995**, *121*, 997–1002. [CrossRef]
62. Davies, M.J. Singlet oxygen-mediated damage to proteins and its consequences. *Biochem. Biophys. Res. Commun.* **2003**, *305*, 761–770. [CrossRef]
63. Bicalho, L.S.; Longo, J.P.F.; Pereira, L.O.; Santos, M.F.M.A.; Azevedo, R.B. Photodynamic therapy, a new approach in the treatment of oral cancer. *Rev. Univ. Ind. Santander. Salud.* **2010**, *42*, 167–174.
64. Yoo, J.O.; Lim, Y.C.; Kim, Y.M.; Ha, K.S. Differential cytotoxic responses to low-and high-dose photodynamic therapy in human gastric and bladder cancer cells. *J. Cell Biochem.* **2011**, *112*, 3061–3071. [CrossRef]
65. Moghissi, K.; Dixon, K.; Parson, R.J. A controlled trial of Nd-YAG laser vs photodynamic therapy for odvanced malignant bronchial obstruction. *Laser Med. Sci.* **1993**, *8*, 269–273. [CrossRef]

66. Kato, H.; Okunaka, T.; Shimatani, H. Photodynamic therapy for early state bronchogenic carcinoma. *J. Clin. Laser Med. Surg.* **1996**, *14*, 235–238. [CrossRef] [PubMed]
67. Manoto, S.L.; Abrahamse, H. Effect of a newly synthesized Zn sulfophthalocyanine derivative on cell morphology, viability, proliferation, and cytotoxicity in a human lung cancer cell line (A549). *Lasers Med. Sci.* **2011**, *26*, 523–530. [CrossRef]
68. Jheon, S.; Lee, J.M.; Kim, J.K.; Kim, K.H.; Seo, S.J. Photodynamic therapy for tracheobronchial cancer. *Photodiagn. Photodyn. Ther.* **2011**, *6*, 177. [CrossRef]
69. Grant, W.E.; MacRobert, A.J.; Bown, S.G.; Hopper, C.; Speight, P.M. Photodynamic therapy of oral cancer: Photosensitization with systemic aminolaevulinic acid. *Lancet* **1993**, *342*, 147–148. [CrossRef]
70. Barr, H.; Shepherd, N.A.; Dix, A.; Roberts, D.J.H.; Tan, W.C.; Krasner, N. Eradication of high-grade dysplasia in columnar-lined (Barrett´s) oesophagus by photodynamic therapy with endogenously generated protoporphyrin IX. *Lancet* **1996**, *348*, 584–585. [CrossRef]
71. Miller, J.D.; Baron, E.D.; Scull, H.; Hsia, A.; Berlin, J.C.; McCormick, T.; Colussi, V.; Kenney, M.E.; Cooper, K.D.; Oleinick, N.L. Photodynamic therapy with the phtalocyanin photosensitizer Pc 4: The case experience with preclinical mechanistic and early clinical-tranlational studies. *Toxicol. Appl. Pharmacol.* **2007**, *224*, 290–299. [CrossRef]
72. Nseyo, U.O.; DeHaven, J.; Dougherty, T.J.; Potter, W.R.; Merrill, D.L.; Lundahl, S.L.; Lamm, D.L. Photodynamic therapy (PDT) in the treatment of patients with resistant superficial bladder cancer: A long-term experience. *J. Clin. Laser Med. Surg.* **1998**, *16*, 61–68. [CrossRef]
73. Leon, S.P.; Folkerth, R.D.; Black, P. Microvessel density is a prognostic indicator for patients with astroglial brain tumors. *Cancer* **1996**, *77*, 362–372. [CrossRef]
74. Zhu, T.C.; Finlay, J.C. The role of photodynamic therapy (PDT) physics. *Med. Phys.* **2008**, *35*, 3127–3136. [CrossRef] [PubMed]
75. George, B.P.A.; Abrahamse, H. A review on novel breast cancer therapies: Photodynamic therapy and plant derived agent induced cell death mechanisms. *Anticancer Agents Med. Chem.* **2016**, *16*, 793–801. [CrossRef] [PubMed]
76. Kostović, K.; Pastar, Z.; Ceović, R.; Mokos, Z.B.; Buzina, D.S.; Stanimirović, A. Photodynamic therapy in dermatology: Current treatments and implications. *Coll. Antropol.* **2012**, *36*, 1477–1481. [PubMed]
77. Kessel, D. Photosensitization of viral particles. *J. Lab. Clin. Med.* **1990**, *116*, 428. [PubMed]
78. Tardivo, J.P.; Del Giglio, A.; Paschoal, L.H.; Baptista, M.S. New photodynamic therapy protocol to treat AIDS-related Kaposi´s sarcoma. *Photomed. Laser Surg.* **2006**, *24*, 528–531. [CrossRef] [PubMed]
79. Mĺkvy, P. Position and possibilities of photodynamic therapy in oncology. *Oncology* **2007**, *5*, 299–301.
80. Castano, A.P.; Demidova, T.N.; Hamblin, M.R. Mechanisms in photodynamic therapy: Part three—Photosensitizer pharmacokinetics, biodistribution, tumor localization and modes of tumor destruction. *Photodiagn. Photodyn. Ther.* **2005**, *2*, 91–106. [CrossRef]
81. Muniyandi, K.; George, B.; Parimelazhagan, T.; Abrahamse, H. Role of photoactive phytocompounds in photodynamic therapy of cancer. *Molecules* **2020**, *25*, 4102. [CrossRef]
82. Doherty, R.E.; Sazanovich, I.V.; McKenzie, L.K.; Stasheuski, A.S.; Coyle, R.; Baggaley, E.; Bottomley, S.; Weinstein, J.A.; Bryant, H.E. Photodynamic killing of cancer cells by a platinum(II) complex with cyclometallating ligand. *Sci. Rep.* **2016**, *6*, 22668. [CrossRef]
83. Pouton, C.W.; Wagstaff, K.M.; Roth, D.M.; Moseley, G.W.; Jans, D.A. Targeted delivery to the nucleus. *Adv. Drug Deliv. Rev.* **2007**, *59*, 698–717. [CrossRef] [PubMed]
84. Sobolev, A.S. Novel modular transporters delivering anticancer drugs and foreign DNA to the nuclei of target cancer cells. *J. Buon.* **2009**, *14* (Suppl. 1), S33–S42.
85. de Melo, W.C.M.A.; Lee, A.N.; Perussi, J.R.; Hamblin, M.R. Electroporation enhances antimicrobial photodynamic therapy mediated by the hydrophobic photosensitizer, hypericin. *Photodiagn. Photodyn. Ther.* **2013**, *10*, 647–650. [CrossRef] [PubMed]
86. Alves, D.S.; Pérez-Fons, L.; Estepa, A.; Micol, V. Membrane-related effects underlying the biological activity of the anthraquinones emodin and barbaloin. *Biochem. Pharmacol.* **2004**, *68*, 549–561. [CrossRef]
87. Du, K.; Xia, Q.; Heng, H.; Feng, F. Temozolomide-doxorubicin conjugate as a double intercalating agent and delivery by apoferritin for glioblastoma chemotherapy. *ACS Mater. Interfaces* **2020**, *12*, 34599–34609. [CrossRef] [PubMed]

88. Mandelli, F.; Vignetti, M.; Suciu, S.; Stasi, R.; Petti, M.C.; Meloni, G.; Muus, P.; Marmont, F.; Marie, J.P.; Labar, B.; et al. Daunorubicin versus mitoxantrone versus idarubicin as induction and consolidation chemotherapy for adults with acute myeloid leukemia: The EORTC and GIMEMA groups study AML-10. *J. Clin. Oncol.* **2009**, *27*, 5397–5403. [CrossRef] [PubMed]
89. Wójcik, K.; Zarebski, M.; Cossarizza, A.; Dobrucki, J.W. Daunomycin, an antitumor DNA intercalator, influences histone-DNA interactions. *Cancer Biol. Ther.* **2013**, *14*, 823–832. [CrossRef] [PubMed]
90. Hu, X.; Cao, Y.; Yin, X.; Zhu, L.; Chen, Y.; Wang, W.; Hu, J. Design and synthesis of various quinizarin derivatives as potential anticancer agents in acute T lymphoblastic leukemia. *Bioorganic Med. Chem.* **2019**, *27*, 1362–1369. [CrossRef] [PubMed]
91. Chen, H.; Zhao, C.; He, R.; Zhou, M.; Liu, Y.; Guo, X.; Wang, M.; Zhu, F.; Qin, R.; Li, X. Danthron suppresses autophagy and sensitizers pancreatic cancer cells to doxorubicin. *Toxicol. In Vitro* **2019**, *54*, 345–353. [CrossRef]
92. Wang, Y.; Yang, M.; Qian, J.; Xu, W.; Wang, J.; Hou, G.; Ji, L.; Suo, A. Sequentially self-assembled polysaccharide-based nanocomplexes for combined chemotherapy and photodynamic therapy of breast cancer. *Carbohydr. Polym.* **2019**, *203*, 203–213. [CrossRef]
93. Lee, H.; Han, J.; Shin, H.; Han, H.; Na, K.; Kim, H. Combination of chemotherapy and photodynamic therapy for cancer treatment with sonoporation effects. *J. Control. Release* **2018**, *283*, 190–199. [CrossRef] [PubMed]
94. He, C.; Liu, D.; Lin, W. self-assembled core-shell nanoparticles for combined chemotherapy and photodynamic therapy of resistant head and neck cancers. *ACS Nano* **2015**, *9*, 991–1003. [CrossRef] [PubMed]
95. Gleason, H.A.; Cronquist, A. *Manual of Vascular Plants of Northeastern United States and Adjacent Canada*, 2nd ed.; New York Botanical Garden: Bronx, New York, NY, USA, 1991; p. 910.
96. Rahman, A. Bioactive natural products (Part C). In *Studies in Natural Products Chemistry*, 1st ed.; Rahman, A., Ed.; Elsevier: Amsterdam, The Netherlands, 2000; Volume 22, p. 647.
97. Miškovský, P. Hypericin—A new antiviral and antitumor photosensitizer: Mechanism of action and interaction with biological macromolecules. *Curr. Drug Targets* **2002**, *3*, 55–84. [CrossRef] [PubMed]
98. Thornett, A. Use of hypericin as antidepressant. Valid measure of antidepressant efficacy in primary care is needed. *Brit. Med. J.* **2000**, *320*, 1141.
99. Butterweck, V.; Winterhoff, H.; Herkenham, M. St John´s wort, hypericin, and imipramine: A comparative analysis of mRNA levels in brain areas involved in HPA axis control following short-term and long-term administration in normal and stressed rats. *Mol. Psychiatry* **2001**, *6*, 547–564. [CrossRef]
100. Eberman, R.; Alth, G.; Kreitner, M.; Kubin, A. Natural products derived from plants as potential drugs for the photodynamic destruction of tumor cells. *J. Photochem. Photobiol. B* **1996**, *36*, 95–97. [CrossRef]
101. Pengelly, A. *The Constituents of Medical Plants: An Introduction to the Chemistry and Therapeutics of Herbal Medicine*, 2nd ed.; CABI Publishing: Cambridge, UK, 2004; pp. 20–50.
102. Miroššay, A.; Mirossay, L.; Tóthová, J.; Miškovský, P.; Onderková, H.; Mojžiš, J. Potentiation of hypericin and hypocrellin-induced phototoxicity by omeprazole. *Phytomedicine* **1999**, *6*, 311–317. [CrossRef]
103. Cavarga, I.; Brezani, P.; Fedorocko, P.; Miskovsky, P.; Bobrov, N.; Longauer, F.; Rybarova, S.; Mirossay, L.; Stubna, J. Photoinduced antitumor effect of hypericin can be enhanced by fractionated dosing. *Photomedicine* **2005**, *12*, 680–683. [CrossRef]
104. Plenagl, N.; Duse, L.; Seitz, B.S.; Goergen, N.; Pinnapireddy, S.R.; Jedelska, J.; Brűβler, J.; Bakowsky, U. Photodynamic therapy—hypericin tetraether liposome conjugates and their antitumor and antiangiogenic activity. *J. Drug Deliv.* **2019**, *26*, 23–33. [CrossRef]
105. Bianchini, P.; Cozzolino, M.; Oneto, M.; Pesce, L.; Pennacchietti, F.; Tognolini, M.; Giorgio, C.; Nonell, S.; Cavanna, L.; Delcanale, P.; et al. Hypericin-apomyoglobin an enhanced photosensitizer complex for the treatment of tumor cells. *Biomacromolecules* **2019**, *20*, 2024–2033. [CrossRef]
106. Fiebich, B.L.; Lieb, A.H. Inhibition of substance P induced cytokine synthesis by St John's Wort extracts. *Pharmacopsychiatry* **2001**, *34*, 526–528. [CrossRef] [PubMed]
107. Samadi, S.; Khadivzadeh, T.; Emami, A.; Moosavi, N.S.; Tafaghodi, M.; Behnam, H.R. The effect of Hypericum perforatum on the wound healing and scar of cesarean. *J. Altern. Complement. Med.* **2010**, *16*, 113–117. [CrossRef]
108. Hajhashemi, M.; Ghanbari, Z.; Movahedi, M.; Rafieian, M.; Keivani, A.; Haghollahi, F. The effect of Achillea millefolium and Hypericum perforatum ointments on episiotomy wound healing in primiparous women. *J. Matern. Fetal Neonatal Med.* **2018**, *31*, 63–69. [CrossRef] [PubMed]

109. García, I.; Ballesta, S.; Gilaberte, Y.; Rezusta, A.; Pascual, Á. Antimicrobial photodynamic activity of hypericin against methicillin-susceptible and resistant Staphylococcus aureus biofilms. *Future Microbiol.* **2015**, *10*, 347–356. [CrossRef] [PubMed]
110. Engelhardt, V.; Krammer, B.; Plaetzer, K. Antibacterial photodynamic therapy using water-soluble formulations of hypericin or mTHPC is effective in inactivation of Staphylococcus aureus. *Photochem. Photobiol. Sci.* **2010**, *9*, 365–369. [CrossRef] [PubMed]
111. Yow, C.; Tang, H.M.; Chu, E.S.; Huang, Z. Hypericin-mediated photodynamic antimicrobial effect on clinically isolated pathogens. *Photochem. Photobiol.* **2012**, *88*, 626–632. [CrossRef]
112. Rodríguez-Amigo, B.; Delcanale, P.; Rotger, G.; Juárez-Jiménez, J.; Abbruzzetti, S.; Summer, A.; Agut, M.; Luque, F.J.; Nonell, S.; Viappiani, C. The complex of hypericin with β-lactoglobulin has antimicrobial activity with perspective applications in dairy industry. *J. Dairy Sci.* **2015**, *98*, 89–94. [CrossRef]
113. Delcanale, P.; Rodríguez-Amigo, B.; Juárez-Jiménez, J.; Luque, F.J.; Abbruzzetti, S.; Agut, M.; Nonell, S.; Viappiani, C. Tuning the local solvent composition at a drug carrier surface: Effect of dimethyl sulfoxide/water mixture on the photofunctional properties of hyperici-β-lactoglobulin. *Mat. Chem. B* **2017**, *5*, 1633–1641. [CrossRef]
114. Pezzuoli, D.; Cozzolino, M.; Montali, C.; Brancaleon, L.; Bianchini, P.; Zantedeschi, M.; Bonardi, S.; Viappiani, C.; Abbruzzetti, S. Serum albumins are efficient delivery systems for the photosensitizer hypericin in photosensitization-based treatments against Staphylococcus aureus. *Food Control.* **2018**, *94*, 254–262. [CrossRef]
115. Lopez-Bazzocchi, I.; Hudson, J.B.; Towers, G.H. Antiviral activity of photoactive plant pigment hypericin. *Photochem. Photobiol.* **1991**, *54*, 95–98. [CrossRef]
116. Hudson, J.B.; Lopez-Bazzocchi, I.; Towers, G.H. Antiviral activities of hypericin. *Antivir. Res.* **1991**, *15*, 101–112. [CrossRef]
117. Moraleda, G.; Wu, T.T.; Jilbert, A.R.; Aldrich, C.E.; Condreay, L.D.; Larsen, S.H.; Tang, J.C.; Colacino, J.M.; Mason, W.S. Inhibition of duck hepatitis B virus replication by hypericin. *Antivir. Res.* **1993**, *20*, 235–247. [CrossRef]
118. Guedes, R.C.; Eriksson, L.A. Effects of halogen substitution on the photochemical properties of hypericin. *J. Photochem. Photobiol. A Chem.* **2006**, *178*, 41–49. [CrossRef]
119. Meruelo, D.; Lavie, G.; Lavie, D. Therapeutic agents with dramatic antiretroviral activity and little toxicity at effective doses: Aromatic polycyclic diones hypericin and pseudohypericin. *Proc. Natl. Acad. Sci. USA* **1988**, *85*, 5230–5234. [CrossRef]
120. Hudson, J.B.; Imperial, V.; Haugland, R.P.; Diwu, Z. Antiviral activities of photoactive perylenequinones. *Photochem. Photobiol.* **1997**, *65*, 352–354. [CrossRef]
121. Xu, Y.; Lu, C. Raman spectroscopy study on structure of human immunodeficiency virus (HIV) and hypericin-induced photosensitive damage of HIV. *Sci. China Ser. C* **2005**, *48*, 117–132.
122. Gulick, R.M.; McAuliffe, V.; Holden-Wiltse, J.; Crumpacker, C.; Liebes, L.; Stein, D.S.; Meehan, P.; Hussey, S.; Forcht, J.; Valentine, F.T. Phase I studies of hypericin, the active compound in St. John's Wort, as an antiretroviral agent in HIV-infected adults: AIDS clinical trials group protocols 150 and 258. *Ann. Intern. Med.* **1999**, *130*, 510–514. [CrossRef]
123. Kerb, R.; Reum, T.; Brockmöller, J.; Bauer, S.; Roots, I. No clinically relevant photosensitization after single-dose and steady state in treatment with hypericum extract in man. *Eur. J. Clin. Pharmacol.* **1995**, *49*, A156.
124. Diwu, Z. Novel therapeutic and diagnostic applications of hypocrellins and hypericins. *Photochem. Photobiol.* **1995**, *61*, 529–539. [CrossRef]
125. Wynn, J.L.; Cotton, T.M. Spectroscopic properties of hypericin in solution and at surfaces. *J. Phys. Chem.* **1995**, *99*, 4317–4323. [CrossRef]
126. Yamazaki, T.; Ohta, N.; Yamazaki, I.; Song, P.S. Excited-state properties of hypericin: Electronic spectra and fluorescence decay kinetics. *J. Phys. Chem.* **1993**, *97*, 7870–7875. [CrossRef]
127. Keša, P.; Antalík, M. Determination of pKa constants of hypericin in aqueous solution of the anti-allergic hydrotropic drug Cromolyn disodium salt. *Chem. Phys. Lett.* **2017**, *676*, 112–117. [CrossRef]
128. Redepenning, J.; Tao, N. Measurement of formal potentials for hypericin in dimethylsulfoxide. *Photochem. Photobiol.* **1993**, *58*, 532–535. [CrossRef] [PubMed]
129. Thomas, C.; Pardini, R.S. Oxygen dependence of hypericin-induced phototoxicity to EMT6 mouse mammary carcinoma cells. *Photochem. Photobiol.* **1992**, *55*, 831–837. [CrossRef]
130. Ehrenberg, B.; Anderson, J.L.; Foote, C.S. Kinetics and yield of singlet oxygen photosensitized by hypericin inorganic and biological media. *Photochem. Photobiol.* **1998**, *68*, 135–140. [CrossRef]

131. Roslaniec, M.; Weitman, H.; Freeman, D.; Mazur, Y.; Ehrenberg, B. Liposome binding constant and singlet oxygen quantum yields of hypericin, tetrahydroxyhelianthrone and their derivatives: Studies in organic solutions and in liposomes. *J. Photochem. Photobiol. B Biol.* **2000**, *57*, 149–158. [CrossRef]
132. Gbur, P.; Dedič, R.; Jancura, D.; Miškovský, P.; Hala, J. Time-resolved luminescence and singlet oxygen formation under illumination of hypericin in acetone. *J. Lumin.* **2008**, *128*, 765–767. [CrossRef]
133. Fehr, M.J.; Carpenter, S.L.; Petrich, J.W. The role of oxygen in the photoinduced antiviral activity of hypericin. *Bioorg. Med. Chem. Lett.* **1994**, *4*, 1339–1344. [CrossRef]
134. Carpenter, S.; Fehr, J.M.; Kraus, G.A.; Petrich, J.W. Chemiluminescent activation of the antiviral activity of hypericin: A molecular flashlight. *Proc. Natl. Acad. Sci. USA* **1994**, *91*, 12273–12277. [CrossRef] [PubMed]
135. Verebová, V.; Belej, D.; Joniová, J.; Jurašeková, Z.; Miškovský, P.; Kožár, T.; Horváth, D.; Staničová, J.; Huntošová, V. Deeper insights into the drug defense of glioma cells against hydrophobic molecules. *Int. J. Pharm.* **2016**, *503*, 56–67. [CrossRef]
136. de Witte, P.; Agostinis, P.; Van Lint, J.; Merlevede, W.; Vandenheede, J.R. Inhibition of epidermal growth factor receptor tyrosine kinase activity by hypericin. *Biochem. Pharmacol.* **1993**, *46*, 1929–1936. [CrossRef]
137. Agostinis, P.; Vantieghem, A.; Merlevede, W.; de Witte, P. Hypericin in cancer treatment: More light on the way. *Int. J. Biochem. Cell Biol.* **2002**, *34*, 221–241. [CrossRef]
138. Buytaert, E.; Callewaert, G.; Hendrickx, N.; Scorrano, L.; Hartmann, D.; Missiaen, L.; Vandenheede, J.R.; Heirman, I.; Grooten, J.; Agostinis, P. Role of endoplasmic reticulum depletion and multidomain proapoptic BAX and BAK proteins in shaping cell death after hypericin-mediated photodynamic therapy. *Faseb. J.* **2006**, *20*, 756–758. [CrossRef]
139. Ferrario, A.; von Tiehl, K.; Wong, S.; Luna, M.; Gomer, C.J. Cyclooxygenase-2 inhibitor treatment enhances photodynamic therapy-mediated tumor response. *Cancer Res.* **2002**, *62*, 3956–3961.
140. Delcanale, P.; Pennacchietti, F.; Maestrini, G.; Rodríguez-Amigo, B.; Bianchini, P.; Diaspro, A.; Iagatti, A.; Patrizi, B.; Foggi, P.; Agut, M.; et al. Subdiffraction localization of a nanostructured photosensitizer in bacterial cells. *Sci. Rep.* **2015**, *5*, 15564. [CrossRef] [PubMed]
141. Miškovský, P.; Sureau, F.; Chinsky, L.; Turpin, P.Y. Subcellular distribution of hypericin in human cancer cells. *Photochem. Photobiol.* **1995**, *62*, 546–549. [CrossRef]
142. Miškovský, P.; Chinsky, L.; Wheeler, G.V.; Turpin, P.Y. Hypericin site specific interactions within polynucleotides used as DNA model compounds. *J. Biomol. Struct. Dyn.* **1995**, *13*, 547–552. [CrossRef]
143. Sánchez-Cortés, S.; Miškovský, P.; Jancura, D.; Bertoluzza, A. Specific interactions of antiretroviraly active drug hypericin with DNA as studied by surface-enhanced resonance Raman spectroscopy. *J. Phys. Chem.* **1996**, *100*, 1938–1944. [CrossRef]
144. Das, K.; Smirnov, A.V.; Wen, J.; Miškovský, P.; Petrich, J.W. Photophysics of hypericin and hypocrellin A in complex with subcellular components: Interactions with human serum albumin. *Photochem. Photobiol.* **1999**, *69*, 633–645. [CrossRef]
145. Senthil, V.; Jones, L.R.; Senthil, K.; Grossweiner, L.J. Hypericin photosensitization in aqueous model system. *Photochem. Photobiol.* **1994**, *59*, 40–47. [CrossRef]
146. Mijatovic, S.; Maksimovic-Ivanic, D.; Radovic, J.; Milijkovic, D.; Kaludjerovic, G.N.; Sabo, T.J.; Trajkovic, V. Aloe emodin decreases the ERK-dependent anticancer activity of cisplatin. *Cell Mol. Life Sci.* **2005**, *62*, 1275–1282. [CrossRef] [PubMed]
147. Ma, T.; Qi, Q.H.; Yang, W.X.; Xu, J.; Dong, Z.L. Contractile effects and antracellular Ca^{2+} signaling induced by emodin in circular smooth muscle cells of rat colon. *World J. Gastroenterol.* **2003**, *9*, 1804–1807. [CrossRef] [PubMed]
148. Janeczko, M.; Masčyk, M.; Kubiński, K.; Golczyk, H. Emodin, a natural inhibitor of protein kinase CK2, suppresses growth, hyphal development, and biofilm formation of Candida Albicans. *Yeast* **2017**, *34*, 253–265. [CrossRef]
149. Huang, H.C.; Lee, C.R.; Lee Chao, P.D.; Chen, C.C.; Chu, S.H. Vasorelaxant effects of emodin, an antraquinone from a Chinese herb. *Eur. J. Pharmacol.* **1991**, *205*, 289–294.
150. Su, Y.T.; Chang, H.L.; Shyue, S.K.; Hsu, S.L. Emodin induces apoptosis in human lung adenocarcinoma cells through a reactive oxygen species-dependent mitochondrial signaling pathway. *Biochem. Pharmacol.* **2005**, *70*, 229–241. [CrossRef] [PubMed]
151. Chukwujelwu, J.C.; Coombes, P.H.; Mulholland, D.A.; van Staden, J. Emodin, an antibacterial anthraquinone from the roots of Cassia occidentalis. *S. Afr. J. Bot.* **2006**, *72*, 295–297. [CrossRef]

152. Srinivas, G.; Babykutty, S.; Sathiadevan, P.P.; Srinivas, P. Molecular mechanism of emodin action: Transition from laxative ingredient to an antitumor agent. *Med. Res. Rev.* **2007**, *27*, 591–608. [CrossRef] [PubMed]
153. Fernand, V.E.; Dinh, D.T.; Washington, S.J.; Fakayode, S.O.; Loss, J.N.; van Ravenswaay, R.O.; Warner, I.M. Determination of pharmacologically active compounds in root extracts of Cassia Alata L. by use of high performance liquid chromatography. *Talanta* **2008**, *74*, 896–902. [CrossRef]
154. Hennebelle, T.; Weniger, B.; Joseph, H.; Sahpaz, S.; Bailleul, F. Senna alata. *Fitoterapia* **2009**, *80*, 385–393. [CrossRef]
155. Andersen, D.O.; Weber, N.D.; Wood, S.G.; Hughes, B.G.; Murray, B.K.; North, J.A. In vitro virucidal activity of selected anthraquinones and anthraquinone derivatives. *Antiviral Res.* **1991**, *16*, 185–196. [CrossRef]
156. Kusari, S.; Lamshöft, M.; Zühlke, S.; Spiteller, M. An endophytic fungus from hypericum perforatum that produces hypericin. *J. Nat. Prod.* **2008**, *71*, 159–162. [CrossRef] [PubMed]
157. Karioti, A.; Bilia, A.R. Hypericins as potential leads for new therapeutics. *Int. J. Mol. Sci.* **2010**, *11*, 562–594. [CrossRef] [PubMed]
158. Bogdanska, A.; Chmurzyński, L.; Ossowski, T.; Liwo, A.; Jeziorek, D. Protolytic equilibria of dihydroxyanthraquinones in non-aqueous solutions. *Anal. Chim. Acta* **1999**, *402*, 339–343. [CrossRef]
159. Mueller, S.O.; Lutz, W.K.; Stopper, H. Factors affecting the genotoxic potency ranking of natural anthraquinones in mammalian cell culture systems. *Mutat. Res.* **1998**, *414*, 125–129. [CrossRef]
160. Li, J.; Yang, W.; Hu, W.; Wang, J.; Jin, Z.; Wang, X.; Xu, W. Effects of emodin on the activity of K channel in guinea pig taenia coli smooth muscle cells. *Acta Pharm. Sin.* **1998**, *33*, 321–325.
161. Ma, T.; Qi, Q.H.; Xu, J.; Dong, Z.L.; Yang, W.X. Signal pathways involved in emodin-induced contraction of smooth muscle cells from rat colon. *World J. Gastroenterol.* **2004**, *10*, 1476–1479. [CrossRef] [PubMed]
162. Chen, D.; Xiong, Y.; Wang, L.; Lv, B.; Lin, Y. Characteristics of emodin on modulating the contractility of jejunal smooth muscle. *Can. J. Physiol. Pharmacol.* **2012**, *90*, 455–462. [CrossRef]
163. Vargas, F.; Fraile, G.; Velásquez, M.; Correia, H.; Fonseca, G.; Marin, M.; Marcano, E.; Sánchez, Y. Studies on the photostability and phototoxicity of aloe-emodin, emodin and rhein. *Pharmazie* **2002**, *57*, 399–404.
164. Oshida, K.; Hirakata, M.; Maeda, A.; Miyoshi, T.; Miyamoto, Y. Toxicological effect of emodin in mouse testicular gene expression profile. *J. Appl. Toxicol.* **2011**, *31*, 790–800. [CrossRef]
165. Xu, X.; Toselli, A.; Russell, L.D.; Seldin, D.C. Globozospermia in mice lacking the casein kinase II α'catalytic subunit. *Nat. Genet.* **1999**, *23*, 118–121. [CrossRef] [PubMed]
166. Escalier, D.; Silvius, D.; Xu, X. Spermatogenesis of mice lacking CK2alpha'failure of germ cell survival and characteristic modifications of the spermatid nucleus. *Mol. Reprod. Dev.* **2003**, *66*, 190–201. [CrossRef] [PubMed]
167. Wang, L.; Lin, L.; Ye, B. Electrochemical studies of the interaction of the anticancer herbal drug emodin with DNA. *J. Pharm. Biomed. Anal.* **2006**, *42*, 625–629. [CrossRef] [PubMed]
168. Bi, S.; Zhang, H.; Qiao, C.; Sun, Y.; Liu, C. Studies of interaction of emodin and DNA in the presence of ethidium bromide by spectroscopic method. *Spectrochim. Acta A Mol. Biomol. Spectrosc.* **2008**, *69*, 123–129. [CrossRef] [PubMed]
169. Saito, S.T.; Silva, G.; Pungartnik, C.; Brendel, M. Study of DNA-emodin interaction by FTIR and UV-Vis spectroscopy. *J. Photochem. Photobiol. B: Biol.* **2012**, *111*, 59–63. [CrossRef]
170. Li, Y.; Luan, Y.; Qi, X.; Li, M.; Gong, L.; Xue, X.; Wu, X.; Wu, Y.; Chen, M.; Xing, G.; et al. Emodin triggers DNA double-strand breaks by stabilizing topoisomerase II-DNA cleavage complexes and by inhibiting ATP hydrolysis of topoisomerase II. *Toxicol. Sci.* **2010**, *118*, 435–443. [CrossRef]
171. Fabriciova, G.; Sanchez-Cortes, S.; Garcia-Ramos, J.V.; Miskovsky, P. Surface-enhanced Raman spectroscopy study of the interaction of the antitumoral drug emodin with serum albumin. *Biopolymers* **2004**, *74*, 125–130. [CrossRef]
172. Bi, S.Y.; Song, D.O.; Kan, Y.H.; Xu, D.; Tian, Y.; Zhou, X.; Zhang, H.Q. Spectroscopic characterization of effective components anthraquinones in Chinese medicinal herbs binding with serum albumins. *Spectrochim. Acta A Biomol. Spectrosc.* **2005**, *62*, 203–212. [CrossRef]
173. Koistinen, K.M.; Soininen, P.; Venalainen, T.A.; Hayrinen, J.; Laatikainen, R.; Perakyla, M.; Tervahauta, A.I.; Karenlampi, S.O. Birch PR-10c interacts with several biologically important ligands. *Phytochemistry* **2005**, *66*, 2524–2533. [CrossRef]
174. Sevilla, P.; Rivas, J.M.; García-Blanco, F.; García-Ramos, J.V.; Sánchez-Cortés, S. Identification of the antitumoral drug emodin binding sites in bovine serum albumin by spectroscopic methods. *BBA-Proteins Proteom.* **2007**, *1774*, 1359–1369. [CrossRef]

175. Pecere, T.; Gazzola, M.V.; Mucignat, C.; Parolin, C.; Dalla, V.F.; Cavaggioni, A.; Basso, G.; Diaspro, A.; Salvato, B.; Carli, M.; et al. Aloe-emodin is a new type of anticancer agent with selective activity against neuroectodermal tumors. *Cancer Res.* **2000**, *60*, 2800–2804.
176. Chun-Guan, W.; Jun-Qing, Y.; Bei-Zhong, L.; Dan-Ting, J.; Chong, W.; Liang, Z.; Dan, Z.; Yan, W. Anti-tumor activity of emodin against human chronic myelocytic leukemia K562 cell lines in vitro and in vivo. *Eur. J. Pharmacol.* **2010**, *627*, 33–41. [CrossRef] [PubMed]
177. Kuo, T.C.; Yang, J.S.; Lin, M.W.; Hsu, S.C.; Lin, J.J.; Lin, H.J.; Hsia, T.C.; Liao, L.; Yang, M.D.; Fan, M.J.; et al. Emodin has cytotoxic and pretoctive effect in rat c6 glioma cells: Roles of Mdr1a and nuclear factor κB in cell survival. *J. Pharmacol. Exp. Ther.* **2009**, *330*, 736–744. [CrossRef] [PubMed]
178. Ko, J.C.; Su, Y.J.; Lin, S.T.; Jhan, J.Y.; Ciou, S.C.; Cheng, C.M.; Lin, Y.W. Suppression of ERCC1 and Rad51 expression through ER1/2 inactivation is essential in emodin-mediated cytotoxicity in human non-small cell lung cancer cells. *Biochem. Pharmacol.* **2010**, *79*, 655–664. [CrossRef] [PubMed]
179. Chemicalland21. Quinizarin. Available online: http://www.chemicalland21.com/specialtychem/finechem/QUINIZARIN.htm (accessed on 7 September 2020).
180. Quinti, L.; Allen, N.S.; Edge, M.; Murphy, B.P.; Perotti, A. A study of the strongly fluorescent species formed by the interaction of the dye 1,4-dihydroxyanthraquinone (quinizarin) with A(III). *J. Photochem. Photobiol. A Chem.* **2003**, *155*, 79–91. [CrossRef]
181. Yohida, M. Chemistry and hair dyes application of dihydroxy derivates of anthraquinone and naphtoquinone. *Prog. Org. Coat.* **1997**, *31*, 63–72. [CrossRef]
182. Brinkworth, R.I.; Fairle, D.P. Hydroxyquinones are competitive nonpeptide inhibitors of HIV-1 proteinase. *Biochim. Biophys. Acta* **1995**, *1253*, 5–8. [CrossRef]
183. Brown, J.P. A review of the genetic effects of naturally occurring flavonoids, anthraquinones and related compounds. *Mutat. Res.* **1980**, *75*, 243–277. [CrossRef]
184. Longo, V.; Amato, G.; Salvetti, A.; Gervasi, P.G. Heterogenous effect of anthraquinones on drug-metabolizing enzymes in the liver and small intestine of rat. *Chem. Biol. Interact.* **2000**, *126*, 63–77. [CrossRef]
185. Carter, T.P.; Gillispie, G.D.; Connoll, M.A. Intramolecular hydrogen bonding in substituted anthraquinones by laser-induced fluorescence. 1. 1,4-dihydroxyanthraquinone (quinizarin). *J. Phys. Chem.* **1982**, *86*, 192–196. [CrossRef]
186. Smulevich, G.; Angeloni, L.; Giovannardi, S.; Marzocchi, M.P. Resonance Raman and polarized light infrared spectra of 1,4-dihydroxyanthraquinone, vibrational studies of the ground and excited electronic states. *Chem. Phys.* **1982**, *65*, 313–322. [CrossRef]
187. Nigam, G.; Deppisch, B. Redetermination of the structure of 1,4-dihydroxyanthraquinone ($C_{14}H_8O_4$). *Z. Kristallogr.* **1980**, *151*, 185–191. [CrossRef]
188. Fabriciová, G.; Garcia-Ramos, J.V.; Miškovský, P.; Sanchez-Cortes, S. Absorption and acidic behavior of anthraquinone drugs quinizarin and danthron on Ag nanoparticles studied by Raman spectroscopy. *Vib. Spectrosc.* **2004**, *34*, 273–281. [CrossRef]
189. Bondy, G.S.; Armstrong, C.L.; Dawson, B.A.; Héroux-Metcalf, C.; Neville, G.A.; Rogers, C.G. Toxicity of structurally related anthraquinones and anthrones to mammalian-cell in vitro. *Toxicol. In Vitro* **1994**, *8*, 329–335. [CrossRef]
190. Verebová, V.; Adamčík, J.; Danko, P.; Podhradský, D.; Miškovský, P.; Staničová, J. Anthraquinones quinizarine and danthron unwind negatively supercoiled DNA and lengthen linear DNA. *Biochem. Biophys. Res. Commun.* **2014**, *444*, 50–55. [CrossRef] [PubMed]
191. IARC. Dantron (chrysazin; 1,8-dihydroxyanthraquinone). In *Pharmaceutical Drugs*; International Agency for Research on Cancer: Lyon, France, 1990; pp. 265–275.
192. Mueller, S.O.; Stopper, H.; Dekant, W. biotransformation of the anthraquinones emodin and chrysophanol by cytochrome P450 enzymes. Bioactivation to genotoxic metabolites. *Drug Metab. Dispos.* **1998**, *26*, 540–546.
193. Müller, S.O.; Eckert, I.; Lutz, W.K.; Stopper, H. Genotoxicity of the laxative drug components emodin, aloe-emodin and danthron in mammalian cells: Topoisomerase II mediated. *Mutat. Res. Genet. Toxicol.* **1996**, *371*, 165–173. [CrossRef]
194. Downes, C.S.; Mullinger, A.M.; Johnson, R.T. Inhibitors of DNA topoisomerase II prevent chromatid separation in mammalians cells but do not prevent exit from mitosis. *Proc. Natl. Acad. Sci. USA* **1991**, *88*, 8895–8899. [CrossRef]

195. Wang, J.R.; Caron, P.R.; Kim, R.A. The role of DNA topoisomerases in recombination and genomic stability: A double-edged sword. *Cell* **1990**, *62*, 403–406. [CrossRef]
196. Neimeikaité-Čéniené, A.; Sergediené, E.; Nivinskas, H.; Čénas, N. Cytotoxicity of natural hydroxyanthraquinones: Role of oxidative stress. *Z. Naturforsch. C* **2002**, *57*, 822–827. [CrossRef]
197. Lieberman, D.F.; Fink, R.C.; Schaefer, F.L.; Mulcahy, R.J.; Stark, A. Mutagenicity of anthraquinone and hydroxylated anthraquinones in the Ames/Salmonella microsome system. *Appl. Environ. Microbiol.* **1982**, *43*, 1354–1359. [CrossRef]
198. Ferreiro, M.L.; Rodriguez-Otero, J. Ab inition study of the intramolecular proton transfer in dihydroxyanthraquinones. *J. Mol. Struct.* **2001**, *542*, 63–77. [CrossRef]
199. Ansari, S.S.; Khan, R.H.; Naqvi, S. Probing the intermolecular interactions into serum albumin and anthraquinone systems: A spectroscopic and docking approach. *J. Biomol. Struct. Dyn.* **2018**, *36*, 3362–3375. [CrossRef] [PubMed]
200. Jutkova, A.; Chorvat, D.; Miskovsky, P.; Jancura, D.; Datta, S. Encapsulation of anticancer drug curcumin and co-loading with photosensitizer hypericin into lipoproteins investigated by fluorescence resonance energy transfer. *Int. J. Pharm.* **2019**, *564*, 369–378. [CrossRef] [PubMed]
201. Kozsup, M.; Dömötör, O.; Nagy, S.; Farkas, E.; Enyedy, E.A.; Buglyó, P. Synthesis, characterization and albumin binding capabilities of quinizarin containing ternary cobalt(III) complexes. *J. Inorg. Biochem.* **2020**, *204*, 110963. [CrossRef]
202. Crlikova, H.; Kostrhunova, H.; Pracharova, J.; Kozsup, M.; Nagy, S.; Buglyó, P.; Brabec, V.; Kasparkova, J. Antiproliferative, DNA binding, and cleavage properties of dinuclear Co(III) complexes containing the bioactive quinizarin ligand. *J. Biol. Inorg. Chem.* **2020**, *25*, 339–350. [CrossRef]
203. Kočišová, E.; Chinsky, L.; Miškovský, P. Sequence specific interaction of the photoactive drug hypericin depends on the structural arrangement and the stability of the structure containing its specific 5′AG3′target: A resonance Raman spectroscopy study. *J. Biomol. Struct. Dyn.* **1999**, *17*, 51–59. [CrossRef]
204. Staničová, J.; Verebová, V.; Strejčková, A. Potential anticancer agent hypericin and its model compound emodin: Interaction with DNA. *Čes. Slov. Farm.* **2016**, *65*, 28–31.
205. Gottesman, M.M.; Fojo, T.; Bates, S.E. Multidrug resistance in cancer: Role of ATP-dependent transporters. *Nat. Rev. Cancer* **2002**, *2*, 48–58. [CrossRef]
206. Aller, S.G.; Yu, J.; Ward, A.; Weng, Y.; Chittaboina, S.; Zhou, R.P.; Harrell, P.M.; Trinh, Y.T.; Zhang, Q.H.; Urbatsch, I.L.; et al. Structure of P-glycoprotein reveals a molecular basis for poly-specific drug binding. *Science* **2009**, *323*, 1718–1722. [CrossRef]
207. Regina, A.; Demeule, M.; Laplante, A.; Jodoin, J.; Dagenais, C.; Berthelet, F.; Moghrabi, A.; Beliveau, R. Multidrug resistance in brain tumors: Roles of the blood-brain barrier. *Cancer Metastasis Rev.* **2001**, *20*, 13–25. [CrossRef]
208. Szaflarski, W.; Sujka-Kordowska, P.; Januchowski, R.; Wojtowicz, K.; Andrzejewska, M.; Nowicki, M.; Zabel, M. Nuclear localization of P-glycoprotein is responsible for protection of the nucleus from doxorubicin in the resistant LoVo cell line. *Biomed. Pharmacother.* **2013**, *67*, 497–502. [CrossRef] [PubMed]
209. Weyergang, A.; Berstad, M.E.; Bull-Hansen, B.; Olsen, C.E.; Selbo, P.K.; Berg, K. Photochemical activation of drug for the treatment of therapy-resistant cancers. *Photochem. Photobiol. Sci.* **2015**, *14*, 1465–1475. [CrossRef] [PubMed]

7

New Zampanolide Mimics: Design, Synthesis and Antiproliferative Evaluation

Guanglin Chen [1], Ziran Jiang [1], Qiang Zhang [2], Guangdi Wang [2] and Qiao-Hong Chen [1,*]

1 Department of Chemistry, California State University, Fresno, CA 93740, USA; chen.bmc@gmail.com (G.C.); ziranjiang@mail.fresnostate.edu (Z.J.)
2 Department of Chemistry and RCMI Cancer Research Center, Xavier University of Louisiana, New Orleans, LA 70125, USA; qzhang1@xula.edu (Q.Z.); gwang@xula.edu (G.W.)
* Correspondence: qchen@csufresno.edu;

Abstract: Zampanolide is a promising microtubule-stabilizing agent (MSA) with a unique chemical structure. It is superior to the current clinically used MSAs due to the covalent nature of its binding to β-tubulin and high cytotoxic potency toward multidrug-resistant cancer cells. However, its further development as a viable drug candidate is hindered by its limited availability. More importantly, conversion of its chemically fragile side chain into a stabilized bioisostere is envisioned to enable zampanolide to possess more drug-like properties. As part of our ongoing project aiming to develop its mimics with a stable side chain using straightforward synthetic approaches, 2-fluorobenzyl alcohol was designed as a bioisosteric surrogate for the side chain based on its binding conformation as confirmed by the X-ray structure of tubulin complexed with zampanolide. Two new zampanolide mimics with the newly designed side chain have been successfully synthesized through a 25-step chemical transformation for each. Yamaguchi esterification and intramolecular Horner–Wadsworth–Emmons condensation were used as key reactions to construct the lactone core. The chiral centers at C17 and C18 were introduced by the Sharpless asymmetric dihydroxylation. Our WST-1 cell proliferation assay data in both docetaxel-resistant and docetaxel-naive prostate cancer cell lines revealed that compound **6** is the optimal mimic and the newly designed side chain can serve as a bioisostere for the chemically fragile *N*-acetyl hemiaminal side chain in zampanolide.

Keywords: natural product; anticancer agent; synthesis; zampanolide

1. Introduction

Prostate cancer is still one of the big health concerns, as evidenced by its high incidence and mortality rate in American men. In 2019, 174,650 new prostate cancer cases that account for nearly 20% of all cancer cases and 31,620 prostate cancer deaths are projected to occur in the United States [1]. Prostate cancer is driven by the androgen receptor (AR)-regulated gene expression that is initiated by the binding of androgen to the AR [2]. Androgen deprivation therapy (ADT) has thus been the main treatment for prostate cancer over 70 years. However, the median duration of ADT response is merely 18–24 months due to inevitable progression to castration-resistant prostate cancer (CRPC) [3]. Consequently, approximately 30,000 prostate cancer deaths in the United State each year are caused by CRPC as well as resistance to the current treatments. The critical driving force for the continued progression of lethal CRPC is the reactivation of AR transcriptional activity [4,5]. The current first-line and second-line chemotherapeutics for CRPC are two microtubule-stabilizing cytotoxic agents (MSA), docetaxel and cabazitaxel [6–8]. Promotion of mitotic arrest is the initially well-established mechanism underlying the action of MSAs as anticancer agents [9]. The MSAs were recently revealed to impair AR transcriptional activity by suppressing nuclear importation of AR as downstream of microtubule stabilization [10]. This alternative mechanism is independent of MSA-induced mitotic arrest and can explain in part the efficacy of MSA in AR-driven CRPC.

The marine macrolide (−)-zampanolide (**1**, Figure 1) [11] has been demonstrated as a unique and promising MSA, which distinguishes it from the current clinically used MSAs due to (1) the covalent nature of its binding to the taxane pocket in β-tubulin as confirmed by a high-resolution X-ray structure of zampanolide in complex with α,β-tubulin, and (2) the very high cytotoxic potency as evidenced by low nanomolar IC_{50} values in suppressing multidrug-resistant cancer cell proliferation [12].

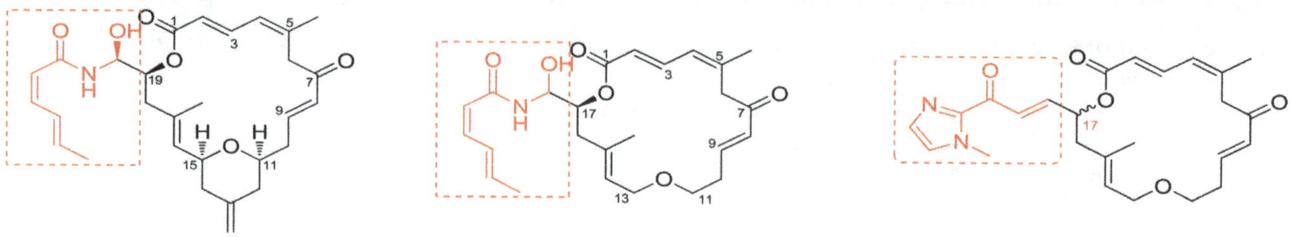

(-)-zampanolide (**1**) desTHP-(-)-zampanolide (**2**) desTHPzampanolide mimic **3**, 17S desTHPzampanolide mimic **4**, 17R

Figure 1. Zampanolide, desTHP-(−)-zampanolide, desTHPzampanolide mimics **3** and **4**.

Although (−)-zampanolide has shown great potential in becoming a more effective chemotherapeutic for CRPC, no in vivo assessment of its antitumor efficacy, pharmacokinetics, and toxicity in animal models has so far been reported yet mainly because of its limited supply. Unfortunately, the supply issue of (−)-zampanolide cannot be addressed either by isolation from marine sponge sources or by current reported total syntheses. The best yield for isolation of (−)-zampanolide from marine sponge sources is merely 0.001% [12,13], and the highest yield for its syntheses is only 0.9% [14–18]. More importantly, the chemically fragile *N*-acyl hemiaminal side chain of zampanolide can compromise its pharmacokinetic profiles as well as the feasibility as a viable drug candidate. The easy cleavage of the *N*-acyl hemiaminal side chain has been confirmed by a thermolysis reaction carried out by Professor Smith and his coworkers [16], and the instability of zampanolide in $CDCl_3$ has been reported by Higa and coworkers when they first identified its structure [13]. The *N*-acyl hemiaminal side chain of zampanolide is, however, very vital to retain its excellent cytotoxic potency, and the derivative without the side chain has 10- to 1000-fold less potency in certain cell models [12,19,20]. Our previous study has confirmed that a suitably designed side chain (e.g., the side chain in desTHPzampanoide mimics **3** and **4**) can function as a bioisostere for the chemically unstable *N*-acyl hemiaminal side chain in desTHPzampanolide (**2**) [21]. However, the bioisosteric side chains that we reported previously do not contain a hydroxyl substituent, corresponding to the C20 alcohol of zampanolide that is hydrogen-bonded to the carbonyl oxygen of Thr276 in β-tubulin. As part of our ongoing project to develop simplified and stabilized zampanolide mimics, this paper presents the design, total synthesis, and antiproliferative evaluation of zampanolide mimics in which the *N*-acyl hemiaminal side chain is substituted by more stable 2-fluorobenzyl alcohol appendages.

2. Results and Discussion

2.1. Design of New Zampanolide Mimics

The first group of side chains in the zampanolide mimics (e.g., **3**–**4**) previously published by us [21] do not contain a hydroxyl group in order to render a more simplified synthesis. However, the binding conformation confirmed by the high-resolution crystal structure of zampanolide tubulin complex [22] indicates the hydroxyl group at the C20 position in zampanolide is hydrogen-bonded to the carbonyl oxygen of Thr276 in β-tubulin. With this point in mind, a new side chain (S-2) was designed as a bioisosteric substitution for the N-acyl hemiaminal side chain, an unstable moiety in zampanolide but important for its potent cytotoxic properties. The stabilized side chain (S-2) was designed to replace the chemically fragile N-acylhemiaminal moiety (blue circle in Figure 2) with a benzyl alcohol. The 20OH group is retained in the target side chain so that it can be hydrogen-bonded to the main-chain carbonyl oxygen of Thr^{276} in β-tubulin. The 1′O atom of zampanolide's side chain is replaced with fluorine atom in the designed side chain so that it can be hydrogen-bonded to the NH group of Thr^{276} in β-tubulin. The E,Z-hexadienoyl amide in zampanolide side chain is replaced with a planar conjugate phenyl ring to preserve the hydrophobic contacts between the proposed side chain and residues of β-tubulin. The Almann's desTHP-dactylolide and its enantiomer [23] were further adopted as the core structure of the new zampanolide mimics (**5** and **6**) in the current study because of the acceptable in vitro potency of desTHP-(−)-zampanolide (**2**) and the practical synthesis of the core. Consequently, we set **5** and **6** as our new target mimics of zampanolide in this study.

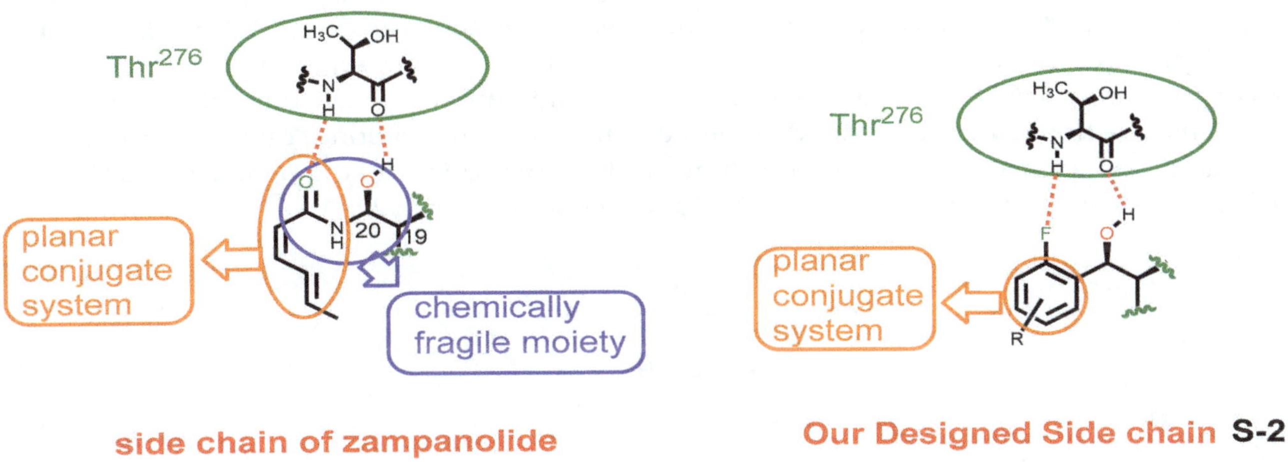

Figure 2. Design of a new stabilized side chain for zampanolide mimics.

2.2. Synthesis

Our retrosynthetic analysis of the zampanolide mimics **5** and **6**, using Yamaguchi esterification and intramolecular Horner–Wadsworth–Emmons condensation as key reactions, is illustrated in Scheme 1. The Yamaguchi esterification was employed to connect Fragment C1–C8 (carboxylic acid **9**) with Fragment C9–C18 (alcohol **7** or **8**) via the ester bond between C1 and C17. The intramolecular Horner–Wadsworth–Emmons condensation was used to close the macrolactone ring at C8–C9. These two key reactions were successfully applied to our syntheses of desTHPdactylolide and the mimics of desTHPzampanolides [21,23]. The known Fragment C1–C8 (**9**) was readily synthesized via 10 steps from commercially available 2-butyn-1-ol according to the reported procedure [24].

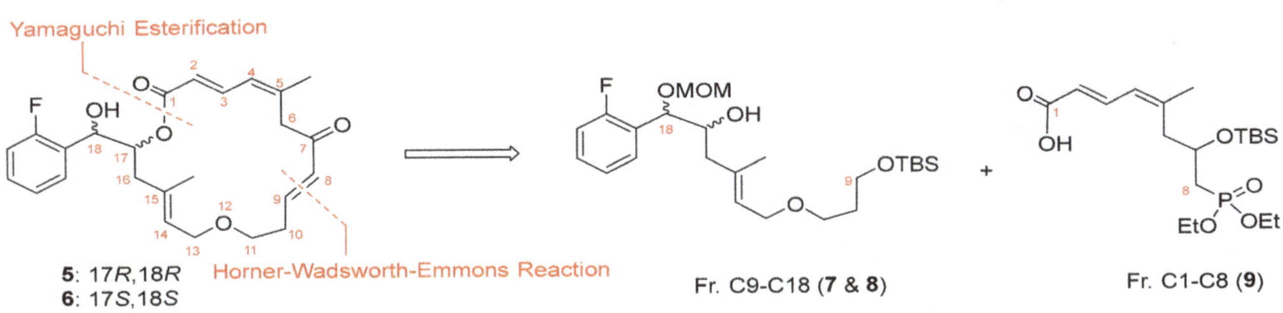

Scheme 1. Retrosynthetic analysis of zampanolide mimics **5** and **6**.

The preparation of Fragment C9–C18 (**7** and **8**) with the desired side chain is shown in Scheme 2. The chiral centers at C17 and C18 in the Fragment C9–C18 (**7** and **8**) were introduced by the Sharpless asymmetric dihydroxylation using the commercially available AD-mix formulations (AD-mix-α and AD-mix-β, respectively) with the ligand and the osmium salt as the critical trace component (0.6%

by wt) and ferricyanide and carbonate as the bulk ingredient (99.4% by wt.) [25]. Compound (*E*)-ethyl 3-(2-fluorophenyl)acrylate was synthesized by the Wittig reaction of the commercially available 2-fluorobenzaldehyde (**10**) with ethyl 2-(triphenyl- phosphoranylidene)acetate (**11**) according to the procedure described in the literature [26]. (*E*)-3-(2-Fluorophenyl)prop-2-en-1-ol (**13**) was synthesized by reducing (*E*)-ethyl 3-(2-fluorophenyl)acrylate (**12**) with diisobutylaluminium hydride (DIBAL) based on the procedure reported in the literature [27]. The Sharpless asymmetric dihydroxylation of the allylic alcohol (**13**) with AD-mix-*α* or AD-mix-*β* was performed following the standard experimental procedure reported in the literature and sulfonamide was used to accelerate the hydrolysis of osmate ester [25]. Epoxy alcohols (**18** with *R,R* configuration, **19** with *S,S* configuration) have been synthesized by sequential selective mesylation of primary alcohol (**14** or **15**) and intermolecular Williamson ether synthesis [28]. The hydroxy group in epoxy alcohols (**18** with *R,R* configuration, **19** with *S,S* configuration) was then protected as the corresponding methoxymethyl (MOM) ethers (**20** with *R,R* configuration, **21** with *S,S* configuration). Iodo ether **22** was prepared using the optimized protocol previously developed in our laboratory [23]. Its lithiation with *tert*-butyllithium followed by nucleophilic reaction with epoxy MOM ether (**20** with *R,R* configuration, **21** with *S,S* configuration) in toluene at −90 °C mediated by boron trifluoride etherate furnished Fragment C9–C18 (**7** with *R,R* configuration, **8** with *S,S* configuration) in 22–23% overall yield from **22**.

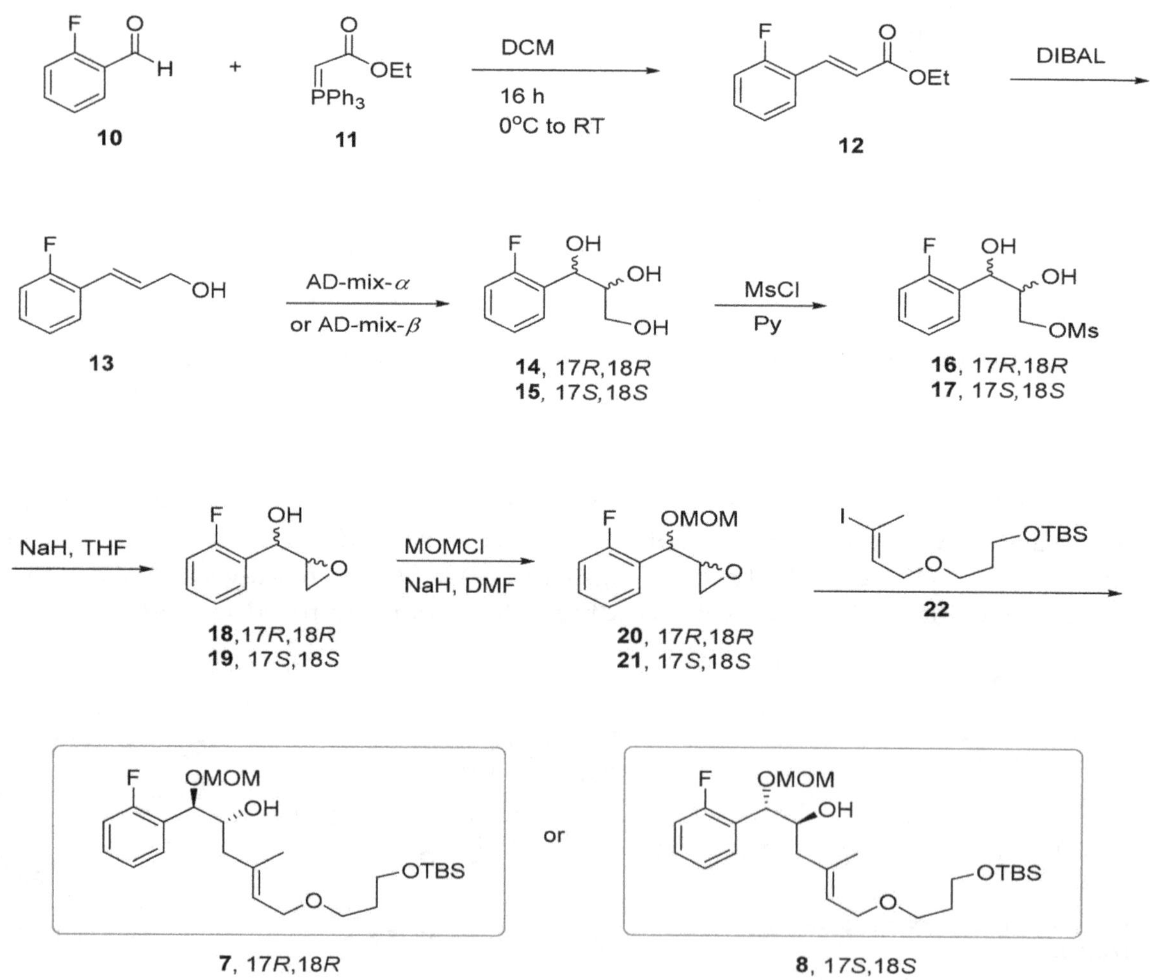

Scheme 2. Synthesis of Fragment C9–C18 (**7** and **8**).

As illustrated in Scheme 3, the union of Fragment C1–C8 (alcohol **9**) and Fragment C9–C18 (carboxylic acid, **7** with *R,R* configuration, **8** with *S,S* configuration) has been accomplished by the Yamaguchi esterification to yield bis-TBS ethers (**23** with *R,R* configuration, **24** with *S,S* configuration). Removal of the protecting TBS groups at C7 and C9 with HF-pyridine complex followed by double oxidation of the corresponding diol (**25** with *R,R* configuration and **26** with *S,S* configuration) with Dess–Martin periodinane afforded the keto aldehydes (**27** with *R,R* configuration, **28** with *S,S* configuration). Without further chromatographic purification, the crude keto aldehydes were directly subjected to the synthesis of zampanolide mimics (**29** with *R,R* configuration, **30** with *S,S* configuration) through the intramolecular HWE condensation catalyzed by $Ba(OH)_2$. Since extractive work-up resulted in significant hydrolysis of the ester [21], the reaction was quenched by filtration of the reaction mixture through a pad of silica gel and the crude product was subjected to preparative TLC purification. The MOM group in **29** was initially planned to be removed using methanolic HCl, but the methanol participated in a Michael addition to the enone, which resulted in the byproduct **31** (Scheme 4). The removal of the MOM with HCl was, therefore, carried out using THF rather than methanol as solvent, leading to the desired zampanolide mimics (**5** with *R,R* configuration at C17 and C18, **6** with *S,S* configuration at C17 and C18).

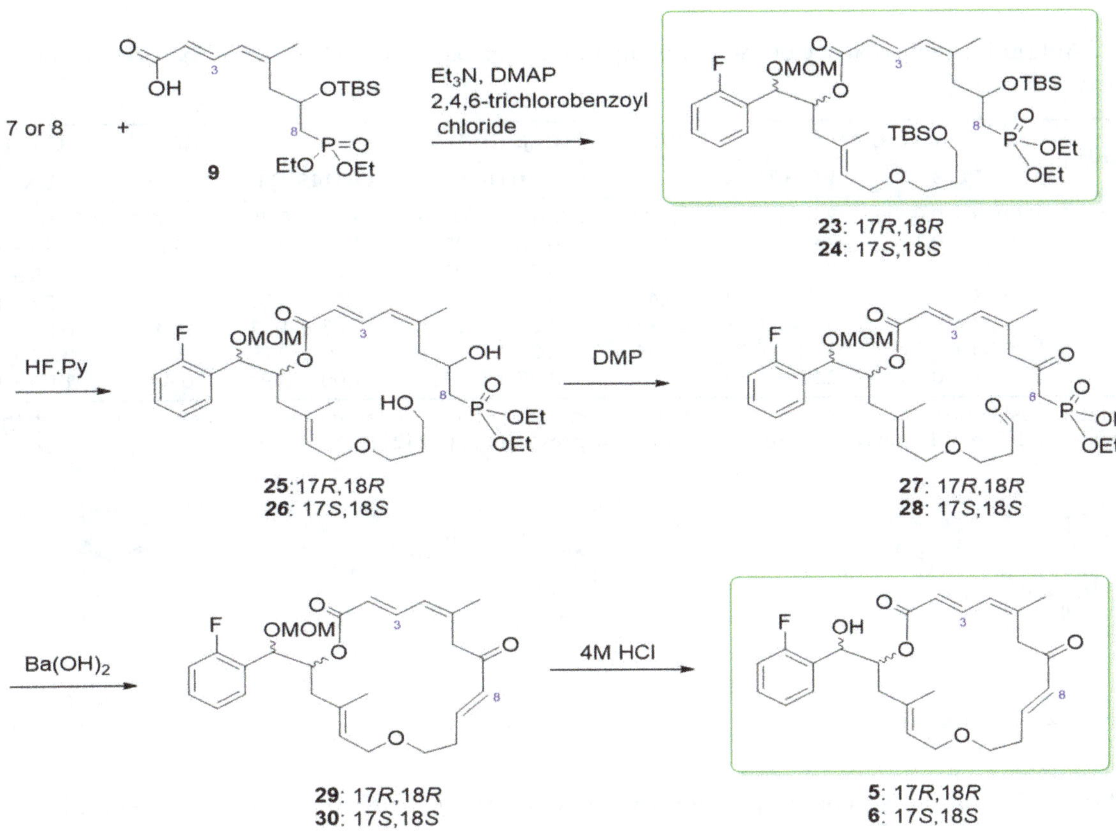

Scheme 3. Synthesis of zampanolide mimics 5 and 6.

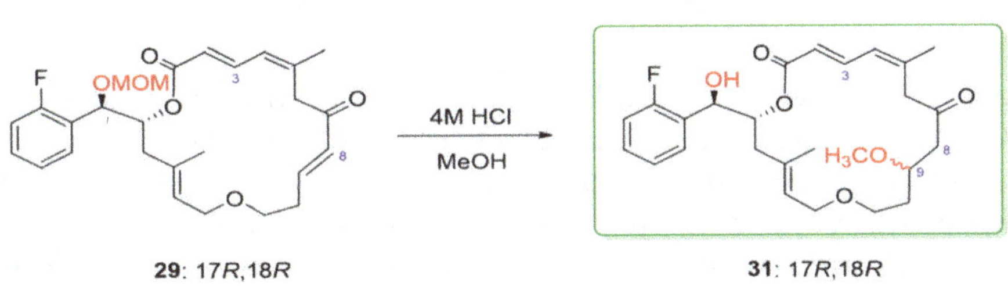

Scheme 4. Deprotection of MOM ether 29 with methanolic HCl.

2.3. *Antiproliferative Activity toward Prostate Cancer Cell Lines*

The in vitro antiproliferative activity of two pairs of enantiomeric macrolides, **5** and **6**, **29** and **30**, has been assessed against a panel of prostate cancer cell lines, including three docetaxel-sensitive prostate cancer cell models (PC-3 DU145, and LNCaP) and two docetaxel-resistant prostate cancer cell lines (PC-3/DTX and DU145/DTX). WST-1 cell proliferation assay was used for the in vitro evaluation according to the procedure described in the Experimental Section. Docetaxel was used as a positive control while DMSO as a negative control. The half-maximal inhibitory concentrations (IC_{50} values) were measured by WST-1 cell proliferation assay after 3 days of exposure, calculated from the dose–response curves, and presented as the mean ± standard deviation of the mean in Table 1. The IC_{50} values for these four new zampanolide mimics are in the range of 1.00–9.36 μM. Mimic **6** has a set of smallest IC_{50} values (1.00–3.91 μM) among the four test macrolides. As summarized in Figure 3, the IC_{50} values of new mimic **6** are very close to those for mimic **3** (0.86–2.97 μM) and mimic **32** (1.92–3.16 μM). The mimic **3** has been evidenced to have similar potency as desTHPzampanolide **2** with the *N*-acetyl hemiaminal side chain of zampanolide against prostate cancer cells [21]. The side chain in mimic **6** was thus identified as a new bioisostere for the chemically unstable *N*-acetyl hemiaminal side chain of zampanolide. The relative resistance for Mimic **6** of PC-3/DTX over PC-3 and DU145/DTX over DU145 is 0.59 and 0.44, respectively.

Table 1. Antiproliferative potency of zampanolide mimics against docetaxel-sensitive and docetaxel-resistant prostate cancer cells.

Compounds	IC_{50}: (μM) [a]		R/S [a]	IC_{50}: (μM) [a]		R/S [a]	IC_{50}: (μM)
	PC-3	PC-3/DTX		DU145	DU145/DTX		LNCaP
Docetaxel	0.0019 ± 0.0006	2.34 ± 0.25	1232	0.0012 ± 0.0003	8.58 ± 0.39	7150	0.0002 ± 0.00005
3 [b]	0.88 ± 0.19	2.97 ± 0.09	1.3	0.86 ± 0.25	2.78 ± 0.16	3.2	0.76 ± 0.29
4 [b]	0.35 ± 0.05	0.30 ± 0.05	0.9	0.29 ± 0.03	0.46 ± 0.10	1.6	0.35 ± 0.02
29	9.36 ± 0.15	3.97 ± 0.24	0.42	3.98 ± 0.57	4.42 ± 0.55	1.1	5.29 ± 0.49
5	8.72 ± 2.21	3.63 ± 0.11	0.42	3.87 ± 0.23	5.03 ± 1.11	1.3	6.51 ± 0.60
30	5.80 ± 0.21	3.71 ± 0.72	0.64	2.28 ± 0.51	4.30 ± 0.79	1.9	3.15 ± 0.19
6	3.91 ± 0.73	2.31 ± 0.32	0.59	2.27 ± 0.39	1.00 ± 0.91	0.44	1.92 ± 0.29

[a] The relative resistance of the two cell lines obtained by dividing the IC_{50} value of the resistance cell line by that of the parental cell line. [b] These data were reported in our previous paper [21].

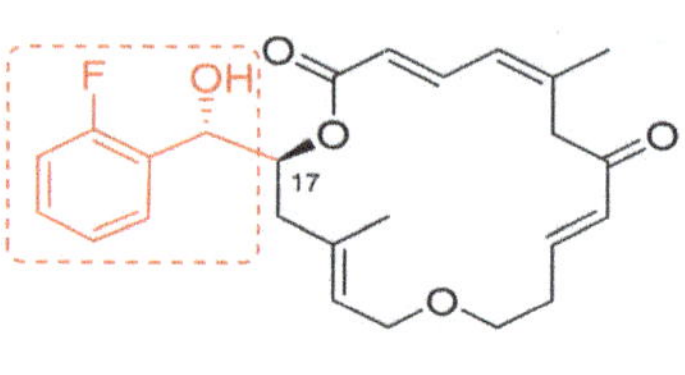

6
IC_{50} Values in the five cell lines:
1.00 - 3.91 μM

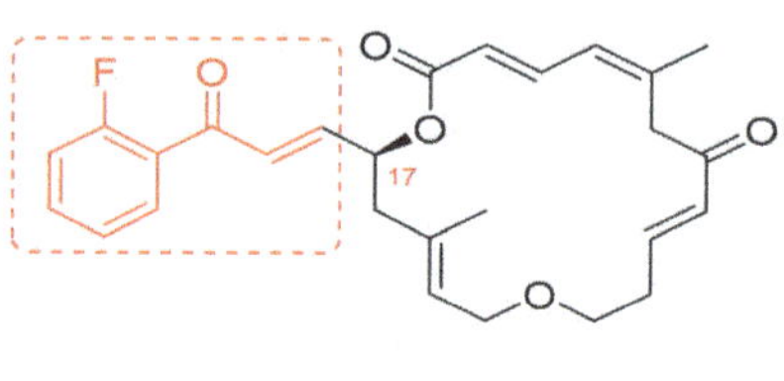

32
IC_{50} Values in the five cell lines:
1.92 - 3.16 μM

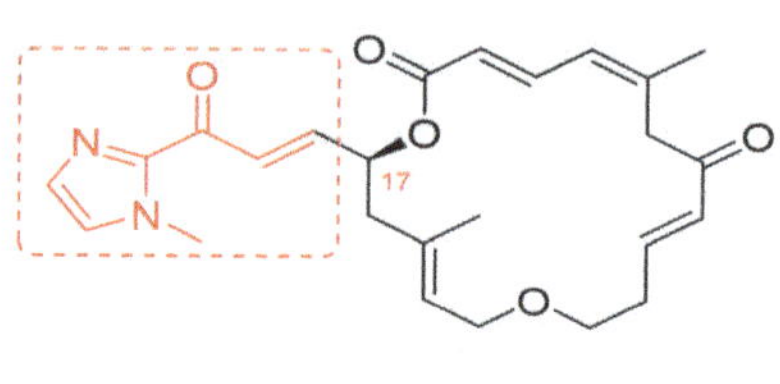

3
IC_{50} Values in the five cell lines:
0.86 - 2.97 μM

Figure 3. Comparison of antiproliferative potency among different zampanolide mimics.

3. Materials and Methods

3.1. General Procedures

Optical rotations were measured on a RUDOLPH Research Analytical Autopol III Automatic Polarimeter (RUDOLPH Research Analytical, Hackettstown, NJ, USA). IR spectra were recorded on a Nicolet Nexus 470 FTIR spectrophotometer (Thermo Fisher Scientific, Waltham, MA, USA). High-Resolution MS were obtained on an Orbitrap mass spectrometer (Thermo Fisher Scientific, Waltham, MA, USA) with electrospray ionization (ESI). NMR spectra (see Supplementary Materials) were obtained on a Bruker Fourier 300 spectrometer (Billerica, MA, USA) in $CDCl_3$. The chemical shifts are given in ppm referenced to the respective solvent peak, and coupling constants are reported in Hz. Anhydrous THF and dichloromethane were purified by PureSolv MD 7 Solvent Purification System from Innovative Technologies (MB-SPS-800) (Herndon, VA, USA). All other reagents and solvents were purchased from commercial sources (Fisher Scientific, Portland, OR, USA) and were used without further purification. Silica gel column chromatography was performed using silica gel (32–63 μM). Preparative thin-layer chromatography (PTLC) separations were carried out on thin-layer chromatography plates loaded with silica gel 60 GF254 (EMD Millipore Corporation, Berlington, MA, USA). Starting materials **22** and **9** were synthesized using the procedure previously described by us [23]. (*E*)-ethyl 3-(2-fluorophenyl)acrylate (**12**) was prepared from commercially available 2-fluorobenzaldehyde (**10**, CAS 446-52-6) according to the reported procedure [26]. (*E*)-3-(2-Fluorophenyl)prop-2-en-1-ol (**13**) was synthesized by reducing (*E*)-ethyl 3-(2-fluorophenyl)acrylate (**12**) with DIBAL based on the procedure reported in the literature [27]. Its structure was confirmed by ^{1}H NMR and high resolution mass spectrometry (HRMS) data (calculated for $C_9H_{10}FO$ (M + H): 153.0716; Found: 153.0710).

3.2. *Synthesis of (1R,2R)-1-(2-Fluorophenyl)propane-1,2,3-triol [(17R,18R) triol* **14**]

AD-mix-α (5.9 g) was dissolved in a mixture of *tert*-butyl alcohol (21 mL) and water (21 mL). The solution was stirred vigorously at room temperature until two clear phases were observed. At this point, the lower aqueous phase emerged as bright yellow. Methanesulfonamide (399 mg, 4.2 mmol, 1 equiv) was added and the reaction mixture was cooled down to 0 °C. A solution of 13 (640 mg, 4.2 mmol, 1 equiv) in 1 mL of *tert*-butyl alcohol was then added. The resulting mixture was stirred vigorously at 0 °C overnight and the reaction progress was monitored with TLC. The reaction was quenched by adding solid sodium sulfate (6.3 g) at 0 °C. The mixture was warmed to room temperature and stirred for 30–60 min. The *tert*-butyl alcohol was removed under vacuum, and saturated sodium bicarbonate (30 mL) and water (300 mL) were added to the residue. The mixture was stirred for additional 30 min and then extracted with ethyl acetate (150 mL × 3). The combined extracts were rinsed with brine, dried over anhydrous sodium sulfate, and concentrated. The crude product was purified through column chromatography eluting with ethyl acetate. The product after purification, with quantitative yield, still contained a trace amount of methanesulfonamide, which is good enough to be used for the next-step reaction. ^{1}H NMR (300 MHz, $CDCl_3$) δ. 7.38 (t, J = 7.2 Hz, 1H, aromatic H), 7.21 (dd, J = 13.5, 5.7 Hz, 1H, aromatic H), 7.06 (t, J = 7.5 Hz, 1H, aromatic H), 6.95 (t, J = 8.4 Hz, 1H, aromatic H), 4.88 (d, J = 6.3 Hz, 1H, H-18), 4.23 (br.s, 3H, 3 × OH), 3.77 (q, J = 5.1 Hz, 1H, H-17), 3.45 (d, J = 4.8 Hz, 2H, H_2 16). ^{13}C NMR (75 MHz, $CDCl_3$) δ 159.9 (d, J_{CF} = 243.8 Hz), 129.6, 128.5, 127.9 (d, J_{CF} = 12.8 Hz), 124.6, 115.4 (d, J_{CF} = 21.8 Hz), 75.3, 68.8, 63.5. IR (film) ν_{max}: 3384, 2988, 1617, 1490, 1455, 1320, 1222, 1054 cm^{-1}. HRMS (ESI): *m/z* calculated for $C_9H_{12}FO_3$ $[M + H]^+$: 187.0770. Found: 187.0766.

3.3. *Synthesis of (2R,3R)-3-(2-Fluorophenyl)-2,3-dihydroxypropyl methanesulfonate [(17R,18R) mesylate* **16**]

To a solution of triol **14** (1.37 g, 7.39 mmol) in pyridine (15 mL, 0.5 M), methane sulfonyl chloride (0.57 mL, 7.39 mmol) was added dropwise at 0 °C under argon. The reaction mixture was stirred at room temperature for 20 h and the reaction progress was monitored by TLC (Hexane/EtOAc, 1:1, *v/v*). The reaction was quenched by diluting with ethyl acetate (800 mL), and the resulting solution was rinsed with brine (50 mL × 3) and dried over anhydrous sodium sulfate. After removing the organic solvent, the residue was subjected to column chromatography, using 40% ethyl acetate in hexane as eluent, to give the desired product. Colorless oil; 81% yield. ^{1}H NMR (300 MHz, $CDCl_3$) δ 7.47 (dt, J = 7.5, 1.8 Hz, 1H, aromatic H), 7.34–7.27 (m, 1H, aromatic H), 7.17 (dt, J = 7.5, 0.9 Hz, 1H, aromatic H), 7.04 (ddd, J = 10.5, 8.1, 0.9 Hz, 1H, aromatic H), 5.00 (d, J = 5.7 Hz, 1H, H-18), 4.27–4.16 (m, 2H, H_2-16), 4.06–4.01 (m, 1H, H-17), 3.18 (br.s, 2H, 2 × OH), 3.03 (s, 3H, SO_2CH_3). ^{13}C NMR (75 MHz, $CDCl_3$) δ 159.9 (d, J_{CF} = 244.3 Hz), 130.1 (d, J_{CF} = 8.3 Hz), 128.4 (d, J_{CF} = 3.8 Hz), 127.0 (d, J_{CF} = 12.8 Hz), 124.8 (d, J_{CF} = 3.8 Hz), 115.7 (d, J_{CF} = 21.8 Hz), 72.9, 70.4, 67.9 (d, J_{CF} = 2.3 Hz), 37.6. IR (film) ν_{max}: 3502, 3029, 2940, 1617, 1587, 1490, 1456, 1346, 1171 cm^{-1}. HRMS (ESI): *m/z* calculated for $C_{10}H_{14}FO_5S$ $[M + H]^+$: 265.0546. Found: 265.0547.

3.4. *Synthesis of (R)-(2-Fluorophenyl)((R)-oxiran-2-yl)methanol [(17R,18R) epoxide* **18**]

To a suspension of sodium hydride (275 mg, 60%, 6.87 mmol, 1.5 equiv) in anhydrous THF (36 mL), a solution of **16** (1.21 g, 4.58 mmol, 1 equiv) in anhydrous THF was added at about −30 °C under argon. The reaction mixture was stirred at 0 °C overnight and the reaction progress was monitored with TLC (hexane:EtOAc, 3:1). The mixture was filtered through a silica gel pad eluting with ethyl acetate. After concentration to remove the solvent, the residue was subjected to PTLC purification eluting with toluene:EtOAc (3:1, *v/v*) to furnish the desired epoxide. Colorless oil; 57% yield. ^{1}H NMR (300 MHz, $CDCl_3$) δ 7.57 (dd, J = 7.8, 1.8 Hz, 1H, aromatic H), 7.35–7.28 (m, 1H, aromatic H), 7.20 (dt, J = 7.5, 1.2 Hz, 1H, aromatic H), 7.06 (ddd, J = 10.5, 8.1, 1.2 Hz, 1H, aromatic H), 4.84 (t, J = 6.6 Hz, 1H, H-18), 3.26–3.22 (m, 1H, H-17), 2.92–2.85 (overlapped, 2H, H_2-16), 2.47 (d, J = 5.7 Hz, 1H, OH). ^{13}C NMR (75 MHz, $CDCl_3$) δ 159.9 (d, J_{CF} = 244.5 Hz), 129.6 (d, J_{CF} = 8.3 Hz), 127.9 (d, J_{CF} = 4.5 Hz), 127.3 (d, J_{CF} = 13.5 Hz), 124.5 (d, J_{CF} = 3.8 Hz), 115.4 (d, J_{CF} = 21.8 Hz), 68.7 (d, J_{CF} = 2.3 Hz), 55.6, 45.5 (d, J = 2.3 Hz). IR (film) ν_{max}: 3420, 3067, 3002, 2928, 1617, 1586 1488, 1456, 1224 cm^{-1}. HRMS (ESI): *m/z* calculated for $C_9H_{10}FO_2$ [M + H]$^+$: 169.0665. Found: 169.0657.

3.5. *Synthesis of (R)-2-((R)-(2-Fluorophenyl)(methoxymethoxy)methyl)oxirane [(17R,18R)MOM ether* **20**]

To a solution of alcohol **18** (716 mg, 4.3 mmol) in DMF (4.2 mL), sodium hydride (204 mg, 60%, 5.1 mmol) was added at 4 °C, and the mixture was stirred at 4 °C for 30 min. Methoxymethyl chloride (0.39 mL, 5.1 mmol) followed by tetrabutylammonium iodide (157 mg, 0.43 mmol) was added to the reaction mixture. The reaction was proceeded with stirring at room temperature for 20 h. The reaction mixture was diluted with ethyl acetate (300 mL) and diethyl ether (300 mL) and then rinsed with brine (50 mL × 3). The organic layer was dried over anhydrous sodium sulfate and concentrated to give a crude mass, which was purified by column chromatography eluting with hexane/ethyl acetate (3:1, *v/v*) to furnish the MOM ether **20** as a pale-yellow oil in 67% yield. ^{1}H NMR (300 MHz, $CDCl_3$) δ 7.51 (dt, J = 7.2, 1.8 Hz, 1H, aromatic H), 7.33–7.25 (m, 1H, aromatic H), 7.17 (dt, J = 7.5, 1.2 Hz, 1H, aromatic H), 7.04 (ddd, J = 9.9, 8.1, 1.2 Hz, 1H, aromatic H), 4.75 (d, J = 6.9 Hz, 1H, OCH_2OCH_3), 4.67 (d, J = 6.9 Hz, 1H, OCH_2OCH_3), 4.62 (d, J = 6.6 Hz, 1H, H-18), 3.36 (s, 3H, OCH_3), 3.26–3.22 (m, 1H, H-17), 2.73–2.72 (overlapped, 2H, H_2-16). ^{13}C NMR (75 MHz, $CDCl_3$) δ 160.3 (d, J = 244.5 Hz), 129.8 (d, J = 8.3 Hz), 128.6 (d, J = 4.5 Hz), 125.2 (d, J = 14.3 Hz), 124.4 (d, J = 3.0 Hz), 115.5 (d, J = 21.8 Hz), 94.6, 73.0, 55.6, 54.4, 44.2 (d, J = 2.3 Hz). IR (film) ν_{max}: 2891, 1615, 1587, 1488, 1455, 1022 cm^{-1}. HRMS (ESI): *m/z* calculated for $C_{11}H_{14}FO_3$ [M + H]$^+$: 213.0927. Found: 213.0921.

3.6. *Synthesis of (5R,6R,E)-5-(2-Fluorophenyl)-8,16,16,17,17-pentamethyl-2,4,11,15-tetraoxa-16-silaoctadec-8-en-6-ol [(17R,18R) Fragment C9–C18 (***7***)]*

To a solution of vinyliodide **22** (164 mg, 0.44 mmol; co-evaporated twice with pentane) in toluene (3 mL) at −78 °C, *tert*-butyllithium (0.46 mL, 1.9 M, 0.89 mmol) was added, and the mixture was stirred at −78 °C for 45 min prior to being cooled down to −90 °C. Epoxide **20** (188 mg, 0.89 mmol; co-evaporated twice with pentane) in toluene (1.5 mL) was added dropwise to make sure that interior temperature lower than −78 °C. The reaction solution was re-cooled to −90 °C before BF_3•OEt_2 (0.11 mL, 0.89 mmoL) was added dropwise. The resulting solution was then stirred at −78 °C overnight prior to being quenched with ethyl acetate (15 mL) and saturated aqueous sodium bicarbonate (35 mL) was added. The organic layer was separated and the aqueous layer was extracted with ethyl acetate (60 mL × 3). The combined organic layers were dried over anhydrous sodium sulfate and concentrated *in Vacuum* to remove ethyl acetate. The crude mass was subjected to PTLC purification over silica gel using hexane/ethyl acetate (4:1, *v/v*) as eluent to yield secondary alcohol **7** as a pale-yellow oil in 23% yield. ^{1}H NMR (300 MHz, $CDCl_3$) δ. 7.41 (dt, J = 7.2, 1.5 Hz, 1H, aromatic H), 7.32–7.24 (m, 1H, aromatic H), 7.15 (dt, J = 7.5, 0.9 Hz, 1H, aromatic H), 7.53 (ddd, J = 9.9, 8.1, 0.9 Hz, 1H, aromatic H), 5.41 (t, J = 6.6 Hz, 1H, H-14), 4.81 (d, J = 6.3 Hz, 1H, H-17), 4.62 (d, J = 6.9 Hz, 1H, OCH_2OCH_3), 4.58 (d, J = 6.6 Hz, 1H, OCH_2OCH_3), 3.94 (d, J = 6.6 Hz, 2H, H_2-13), 3.67 (t, J = 6.3 Hz, 2H, H_2-11), 3.46 (t, J = 6.3 Hz, 2H, H_2-9), 3.36 (s, 3H), OCH_3), 1.75 (quin, J = 6.3 Hz, 2H, H_2-10), 1.64 (s, 3H, 15-CH_3), 0.87 (s, 9H, TBS), 0.03 (s, 6H, TBS). ^{13}C NMR (75 MHz, $CDCl_3$) δ 160.9 (d, J_{CF} = 244.8 Hz), 136.4, 129.8, 129.1, 128.7, 126.1 (d, J_{CF} = 13.5 Hz), 124.5 (d, J_{CF} = 3.8 Hz), 115.6 (d, J_{CF} = 21.8 Hz), 95.3, 75.6, 72.5 (d, J_{CF} = 12.1 Hz), 67.3, 67.0, 60.2, 56.2, 43.0, 33.2, 26.1, 26.07, 18.5, 16.6, 16.5. IR (film) ν_{max}: 3420, 2929,

1715, 1647, 1615, 1488, 1029 cm^{-1}. HRMS (ESI): *m/z* calculated for $C_{24}H_{42}FO_5Si$ [M + H]$^+$: 457.2786. Found: 457.2780.

3.7. Synthesis of (2E,4Z)-(5R,6R,E)-5-(2-Fluorophenyl)-8,16,16,17,17-pentamethyl-2,4,11,15-tetraoxa-16-silaoctadec-8-en-6-yl 7-((tert-butyldimethylsilyl)oxy)-8-(diethoxyphosphoryl)-5- methylocta-2,4-dienoate [(17R,18R) ester **23***]*

To a solution of Fragment C1–C8 (**9**, 37 mg, 0.09 mmol; co-evaporated with pentane twice) in toluene (0.5 mL) at room temperature, trimethylamine (28 μL, 0.20 mmol) and 2,4,6-trichlorobenzoyl chloride (18 μL, 0.12 mmol) was sequentially added, and the reaction mixture was stirred at room temperature for 1.5 h. A solution of alcohol **7** (35 mg, 0.08 mmol) and DMAP (9.3 mg, 0.08 mmol) in toluene (0.5 mL) was then added to the reaction mixture. The reaction was allowed to proceed with stirring at room temperature for 19 h prior to being quenched with water (5 mL) and saturated aqueous sodium bicarbonate (5 mL). The mixture was extracted with ethyl acetate (5 mL × 3), the combined organic extracts were dried over anhydrous sodium sulfate and concentrated *in vacuum*. PTLC purification of the crude product over silica gel eluting with hexane/ethyl acetate (60:40, *v/v*) yielded the ester **23** as a mixture of diastereoisomers in a 1:1 ratio as a colorless oil in 77% yield. ^{1}H NMR (300 MHz, $CDCl_3$) δ 7.50 (dd, *J* = 15.0, 11.7 Hz, H-3), 7.42 (t, *J* = 7.5 Hz, 1H, aromatic H), 7.25–7.20 (m, 1H, aromatic H), 7.10 (t, *J* = 7.5 Hz, 1H, aromatic H), 7.00 (t, *J* = 8.4 Hz, 1H, aromatic H), 6.03 (d, *J* = 11.4 Hz, H-4), 5.75 (d, *J* = 15.3 Hz, 1H, H-2), 5.43–5.37 (m, 1H, H-17), 5.33 (t, *J* = 6.6 Hz, 1H, H-14), 5.08 (d, *J* = 5.4 Hz, 1H, H-18), 4.58 (d, *J* = 6.6 Hz, 1H, -OCH_2OCH_3), 4.51 (d, *J* = 6.6 Hz, 1H, OCH_2OCH_3), 4.18–4.04 (overlapped, 5H, 2 x OCH_2CH_3, H-7), 3.93–3.79 (m, 2H, H_2-13), 3.64 (t, *J* = 6.3 Hz, 2H, H_2-11), 3.40 (t, *J* = 6.3 Hz, 2H, H_2-9), 3.32 (s, 3H, -OCH_2OCH_3), 2.58–2.48 (m, 2H, H_2-16), 2.33–2.24 (m, 2H, H_2-8), 2.00–1.92 (m, 2H, H_2-6), 1.87 (s, 3H, 5-CH_3), 1.72 (quin, *J* = 6.3 Hz, 2H, H_2-10), 1.64 (1.63) (s, 3H, 15-CH_3), 1.31 (t, *J* = 7.2 Hz, 6H, 2 × OCH_2CH_3), 0.86 (s, 9H, TBS), 0.81 (0.80) (s, 9H, TBS), 0.04 (0.03) (s, 3H, TBS), 0.01 (s, 6H, TBS), −0.04(−0.05) (s, 3H, TBS). ^{13}C NMR (75 MHz, $CDCl_3$) δ 166.8 (166.7), 160.8 (d, *J* = 244.5 Hz), 146.4 (d, *J* = 9.8 Hz), 141.6, 135.2 (d, *J* = 3.8 Hz), 129.7, 129.0, 126.8, 125.7 (d, *J* = 13.5 Hz), 125.1, 124.3, 119.3, 115.6 (115.3), 95.0, 72.9, 72.3, 67.3, 66.8, 61.7(61.6), 60.5, 60.1, 56.1, 41.8 (41.2), 36.1, 34.3, 33.1, 27.0, 26.11, 26.05, 25.90, 25.87, 25.2, 25.0, 18.5, 18.0, 16.6 (16.5), −4.6, −5.2. IR (film) ν_{max}: 2929, 2856, 1716, 1489, 1251, 1020 cm^{-1}. HRMS (ESI): *m/z* calculated for $C_{43}H_{77}FO_{10}PSi_2$ [M + H]$^+$: 859.4777. Found: 859.4756.

3.8. Synthesis of (2E,4Z)-(1R,2R,E)-1-(2-Fluorophenyl)-6-(3-hydroxypropoxy)-1-(methoxymethoxy) -4-methylhex-4-en-2-yl 8-(diethoxyphosphoryl)-7-hydroxy-5-methylocta-2,4-dienoate [(17R,18R) diol **25***]*

To a solution of di-TBS ether **23** (90 mg, 0.105 mmol) in THF (4.2 mL) at 0 °C in a plastic bottle, hydrogen fluoride-pyridine complex (70%, 1.0 mL) was added dropwise. The solution was stirred at 0 °C for 5 min and then at room temperature for 16 h. Saturated sodium bicarbonate (30 mL) was added to quench the reaction and the suspension was extracted with ethyl acetate (30 mL × 3). The combined organic extracts were dried over anhydrous sodium sulfate and the dried extract was concentrated under vacuum. The crude product was purified by PTLC, eluting with dichloromethane/methanol (93:7. *v/v*), and the pure diol was washed out from the PTLC silica gel with acetone as a pale-yellow oil in 92% yield. ^{1}H NMR (300 MHz, $CDCl_3$) δ 7.50 (7.49) (dd, *J* = 15.3, 11.7 Hz, 1H, H-3), 7.43 (t, *J* = 9.0 Hz, 1H, aromatic H), 7.30–7.23 (m, 1H, aromatic H), 7.13 (7.12) (t, *J* = 7.5 Hz, 1H, aromatic H), 7.031 (7.028) (dd, *J* = 10.2, 9.0 Hz, 1H, aromatic H), 6.11 (d, *J* = 11.4 Hz, 1H, H-4), 5.80 (d, *J* = 15.3 Hz, 1H, H-2), 5.47–5.40 (m, 1H, H-17), 5.32 (t, *J* = 5.7 Hz, 1H, H-14), 5.09 (d, *J* = 5.7 Hz, 1H, H-18), 4.58 (d, *J* = 6.9 Hz, 1H, -OCH_2OCH_3), 4.51 (d, *J* = 6.9 Hz, 1H, OCH_2OCH_3), 4.18–4.06 (overlapped, 5H, 2 × OCH_2CH_3, H-7), 3.90 (t, *J* = 5.7 Hz, 2H, H_2-13), 3.69 (3.68) (t, *J* = 5.7 Hz, 2H, H_2-11), 3.48 (3.47) (t, *J* = 5.7 Hz, 2H, H_2-9), 3.33 (3.32) (s, 3H, -OCH_2OCH_3), 3.03 (s, 2H, 2 × OH), 2.66–2.53 (m, 1H, H-16), 2.46–2.19 (m, 3H, H_2-8 & H-16), 1.92 (S, 3H, 5-CH_3), 1.96–1.88 (m, 2H, H_2-6), 1.75 (quin, *J* = 5.7 Hz, 2H, H_2-10), 1.65 (s, 3H, 15-CH_3), 1.33 (t, *J* = 7.2 Hz, 6H, 2 × OCH_2CH_3). ^{13}C NMR (75 MHz, $CDCl_3$) δ 167.0 (166.8), 160.9 (d, *J* = 247.5 Hz), 146.0, 140.8 (d, *J* = 17.3 Hz), 135.7 (d, *J* = 9.0 Hz), 129.8, 129.0,

126.8, 125.6 (d, J = 12.8 Hz), 124.8 (d, J = 11.3 Hz), 124.4, 119.7 (d, J = 11.3 Hz), 115.7 (115.4), 94.9, 73.0, 72.4, 68.8, 67.4, 65.3, 62.2, 61.8, 56.1, 41.1, 34.6 (34.5), 32.7, 32.3, 25.3, 25.0, 16.6 (16.5). IR (film) ν_{max}: 3366, 2929, 1711, 1633, 1488, 1222, 1019 cm^{-1}. HRMS (ESI): *m/z* calculated for $C_{31}H_{49}FO_{10}P$ $[M + H]^+$: 631.3048. Found: 631.3041.

3.9. Synthesis of (R,3E,9E,11Z,15E)-6-((R)-(2-Fluorophenyl)(methoxymethoxy)methyl)-4,12-dimethyl-1,7-dioxacyclooctadeca-3,9,11,15-tetraene-8,14-dione [(17R,18R) macrolactone **29***]*

To a solution of diol **25** (65 mg, 0.10 mmol) in dichloromethane (6.2 mL) at room temperature, Dess–Martin periodinane (DMP, 131 mg, 0.30 mmol) was added. The reaction mixture was stirred for 30 min before a second portion of DMP (131 mg, 0.30 mmol) was added. The reaction was allowed to proceed with stirring at room temperature for an additional 1 h. The reaction mixture was poured into a stirred mixture of saturated sodium bicarbonate (30 mL) and saturated sodium thiosulfate (30 mL), and the resulting suspension was stirred for 30 min before being extracted with dichloromethane (30 mL × 3). The combined organic extracts were dried over anhydrous sodium sulfate and the dried extract was concentrated under vacuum. The crude product was used for the next reaction without further purification. To a solution of the crude ketoaldehyde (0.10 mmol) obtained above in THF (103 mL) at 0 °C was added water (2.2 mL) followed by activated barium hydroxide (15 mg, 0.08 mmol). The reaction mixture was stirred at 0 °C for 30 min and at room temperature for 2.5 h, then was filtered through a pad of sodium sulfate and a pad of silica gel that was rinsed with ethyl acetate. After evaporation of the solvent, the crude product was subjected to PTLC purification, using hexane/ethyl acetate (73:37) as eluent, to yield the pure macrolactone **29**. Colorless oil, 46% yield for two steps. $[\alpha]$: −15.6 (c = 0.23, MeOH). ^1H NMR (300 MHz, $CDCl_3$) δ 7.60 (dd, J = 15.0, 11.4 Hz, 1H, H-3), 7.46 (dt, J = 7.5, 1.8 Hz, 1H, aromatic H), 7.33–7.25 (m, 1H, aromatic H), 7.16 (dt, J = 7.5, 1.2 Hz, 1H, aromatic H), 7.05 (ddd, J = 9.9, 8.4, 1.2 Hz, 1H, aromatic H), 6.82 (dt, J = 16.2, 6.6 Hz, 1H, H-9), 6.12 (d, J = 11.4 Hz, 1H, H-4), 6.01 (d, J = 16.2 Hz, 1H, H-8), 5.91 (d, J = 15.0 Hz, 1H, H-2), 5.51 (ddd, J = 11.4, 6.3, 1.2 Hz, 1H, H-17), 5.27 (dd, J = 7.8, 4.8 Hz, 1H, H-14), 5.12 (d, J = 6.3 Hz, 1H, H-18), 4.60 (d, J = 6.9 Hz, 1H, *O-CH_2*OCH_3), 4.53 (d, J = 6.9 Hz, 1H, O*CH_2*OCH_3), 3.99 (dd, J = 12.0, 8.1 Hz, 1H, H-16), 3.88–3.81 (m, 2H, H_2-13), 3.47–3.28 (m, 2H, H_2-11), 3.34 (s, 3H, OCH_2O*CH_3*), 3.14 (d, J = 12.6 Hz, 1H, H-16), 2.43–2.36 (m, 2H, H_2-10), 2.33 (d, J = 12.0 Hz, 1H, H-6), 2.05 (d, J = 12.1 Hz, 1H, H-6), 1.83 (s, 3H, 5-CH_3), 1.63 (S, 3H, 15-CH_3). ^{13}C NMR (75 MHz, $CDCl_3$) δ 197.2, 166.6, 160.9 (d, J = 244.5 Hz), 146.8, 142.5, 139.7, 138.9, 134.3, 130.3, 128.9 125.9 (d, J = 7.5 Hz), 125.6 (d, J = 13.5 Hz), 125.2 (d, J = 5.6 Hz), 124.5, 120.9 (d, J = 5.3 Hz), 115.6 (d, J = 21.8 Hz), 94.9, 72.9, 72.6, 67.9, 67.8, 56.0, 46.0, 41.4, 33.1, 24.09, 16.7. IR (film) ν_{max}: 2931, 1713, 1633, 1489, 1358, 1226, 1030 cm^{-1}. HRMS (ESI): *m/z* calculated for $C_{27}H_{34}FO_6$ $[M + H]^+$: 473.2339. Found: 473.2333.

3.10. Synthesis of (R,3E,9E,11Z,15E)-6-((R)-(2-Fluorophenyl)(hydroxy)methyl)-4,12-dimethyl-1,7-dioxacyclooctadeca-3,9,11,15-tetraene-8,14-dione [(17R,18R) macrolactone **5***]*

To a solution of **29** (30 mg, 0.064 mmol) in a mixture of tetrahydrofuran/water (0.92 mL, 1:1, *v/v*), concentrated hydrochloric acid (130 µL) was added. The two more portions of concentrated hydrochloric acid (130 µL × 2) were added sequentially after each one-hour stirring at room temperature. The reaction mixture was stirred at room temperature overnight before the reaction was quenched by adding saturated ammonium chloride (60 mL). The subsequent mixture was extracted with ethyl acetate (40 mL × 3). The combined extracts were dried over anhydrous sodium sulfate and the solvents were evaporated *in vacuum*. The crude product was purified over preparative thin layer chromatography eluting with toluene/ethyl acetate (3:1, *v/v*) to furnish the desired product (11 mg). Colorless syrup, 41% yield. ^1H NMR (300 MHz, $CDCl_3$) δ 7.62 (dd, J = 15.0, 11.7 Hz, 1H, H-3), 7.49 (dt, J = 7.5, 1.8 Hz, 1H, aromatic H), 7.31–7.27 (m, 1H, aromatic H), 7.17 (dt, J = 7.5, 1.2 Hz, 1H), 7.05 (ddd, J = 10.2, 8.1, 0.9 Hz, 1H), 6.83 (dt, J = 15.9, 6.9 Hz, 1H, H-9), 6.12 (d, J = 11.4 Hz, 1H, H-4), 6.02 (d, J = 16.2 Hz, 1H, H-8), 5.91 (d, J = 15.0 Hz, 1H, H-2), 5.48–5.38 (m, 1H, H-17), 5.27 (t, J = 6.0 Hz, 1H, H-14), 5.10 (d, J = 6.3 Hz, 1H, H-18), 3.99 (dd, J = 12.0, 8.1 Hz, 1H, H-16), 3.86 (br.s, 1H, H-13), 3.82 (br.s, 1H, H-13),

3.51–3.36 (m, 2H, H_2-11), 3.18 (d, J = 12.9 Hz, 1H, H-16), 2.44–2.34 (m, 3H, H_2-10, H-6), 2.06 (d, J = 14.4 Hz, 1H, H-6), 1.83 (s, 3H, 5-CH_3), 1.62 (s, 3H, 15-CH_3). ^{13}C NMR (75 MHz, $CDCl_3$) δ 197.2, 167.0, 160.1 (d, J_{CF} = 244.5 Hz), 146.9, 143.0, 140.1 (d, J_{CF} = 12.8 Hz), 134.2, 130.2, 129.9, 128.8, 127.6 (d, J_{CF} = 12.8 Hz), 126.0, 125.2, 124.6, 120.7, 115.6 (d, J_{CF} = 21.8 Hz), 79.4, 74.4, 70.3, 68.0, 45.9, 41.4, 33.0, 24.1, 16.7. [α]: −15.2 (c = 0.16, MeOH). IR (film) ν_{max}: 3428, 2924, 2854, 1706, 1633, 1558, 1488, 1360, 1221, 1036 cm^{-1}. HRMS (ESI): m/z calculated for $C_{25}H_{30}FO_5$ $[M + H]^+$: 429.2077. Found: 429.2074.

3.11. *Synthesis of (1S,2S)-1-(2-Fluorophenyl)propane-1,2,3-triol [(17S,18S) triol* **15***]*

Triol **15** was prepared in 68% yield from 13 catalyzed by AD-mix-β using a similar procedure used to synthesize its antipode **14**. ^{1}H NMR (300 MHz, $CDCl_3$) δ 7.39 (t, J = 7.5 Hz, 1H, aromatic H), 7.22 (dd, J = 13.8, 7.2 Hz, 1H, aromatic H), 7.07 (t, J = 7.5 Hz, 1H, aromatic H), 6.96 (t, J = 9.3 Hz, 1H, aromatic H), 4.90 (d, J = 6.3 Hz, 1H, H-18), 4.21 (br.s, 3H, 3 × OH), 3.78 (dd, J = 10.2, 4.8 Hz, 1H, H-17), 3.48 (d, J = 4.8 Hz, 2H, H_2-16). ^{13}C NMR (75 MHz, $CDCl_3$) δ 160.0 (d, J_{CF} = 244.5 Hz), 129.6, 128.5 (d, J_{CF} = 16.5 Hz), 127.8 (d, J_{CF} = 12.8 Hz), 124.6, 115.5 (d, J_{CF} = 21.8 Hz), 75.4, 68.8, 63.4. IR (film) ν_{max}: 3375, 2930, 1781, 1489, 1456, 1319 cm^{-1}. HRMS (ESI): m/z calculated for $C_9H_{12}FO_3$ $[M + H]^+$: 187.0770. Found: 187.0765.

3.12. *Synthesis of (2S,3S)-3-(2-Fluorophenyl)-2,3-dihydroxypropyl methanesulfonate [(17S,18S) mesylate* **17***]*

Mesylate **17** was prepared from triol **15** as a colorless oil in 72% yield, employing a procedure similar to that used for the mesylation of triol **14**. ^{1}H NMR (300 MHz, $CDCl_3$) δ 7.48 (dt, J = 7.5, 1.8 Hz, 1H, Aromatic H), 7.32–7.29 (m, 1H, aromatic H), 7.18 (dt, J = 8.4, 0.9 Hz, 1H, aromatic H), 7.05 (ddd, J = 9.3, 8.1, 0.9 Hz, 1H, aromatic H), 5.01 (d, J = 5.7 Hz, 1H, H-18), 4.28–4.15 (m, 2H, H_2-16), 4.08–4.03 (m, 1H, H-17), 3.04 (s, 3H, SO_2CH_3). ^{13}C NMR (75 MHz, $CDCl_3$) δ 159.9 (d, J_{CF} = 244.5 Hz, 1H), 130.1, 128.4, 127.0 (d, J_{CF} = 12.8 Hz, 1H), 124.8, 115.7 (d, J_{CF} = 21.8 Hz, 1H), 72.9, 70.3, 67.9, 37.6. IR (film) ν_{max}: 3482, 3029, 2939, 1616, 1587, 1489, 1456, 1332, 1168 cm^{-1}. HRMS (ESI): m/z calculated for $C_{10}H_{14}FO_5S$ $[M + H]^+$: 265.0546. Found: 265.0542.

3.13. *Synthesis of (S)-(2-Fluorophenyl)((S)-oxiran-2-yl)methanol [(17S,18S) epoxide* **19***]*

Epoxide **19** (52%, pale yellow oil) was obtained from mesylate **17** according to the internal Williamson ether synthesis procedure employed for the conversion of mesylate **16** to epoxide **18**. ^{1}H NMR (300 MHz, $CDCl_3$) δ 7.57 (dt, J = 7.5, 1.8 Hz, 1H, aromatic H), 7.35–7.25 (m, 1H, aromatic H), 7.20 (dt, J = 7.5, 1.2 Hz, 1H, aromatic H), 7.06 (ddd, J = 10.5, 8.1, 1.2 Hz, 1H, aromatic H), 4.83 (d, J = 5.1 Hz, 1H, H-18), 3.26–3.21 (m, 1H, H-17), 2.92–2.84 (m, 2H, H_2-16). ^{13}C NMR (75 MHz, $CDCl_3$) δ 160.0 (d, J_{CF} = 244.5 Hz), 129.8, 127.6 (d, J_{CF} = 9.0 Hz), 127.4 (d, J_{CF} = 13.5 Hz), 124.7, 115.6 (d, J_{CF} = 21.0 Hz), 68.6, 55.4, 45.6. IR (film) ν_{max}: 3482, 3029, 2939, 1617, 1587, 1489, 1456, 1331, 1168 cm^{-1}. HRMS (ESI): m/z calculated for $C_9H_{10}FO_2$ $[M + H]^+$: 169.0665. Found: 169.0659.

3.14. *Synthesis of (S)-2-((S)-(2-Fluorophenyl)(methoxymethoxy)methyl)oxirane [(17S,18S) MOM ether* **21***]*

MOM ether **21** was prepared from epoxide **19** as a pale-yellow oil in 73% yield employing a procedure similar to that used for conversion of **18**. ^{1}H NMR (300 MHz, $CDCl_3$) δ 7.44 (dt, J = 7.5, 1.8 Hz, 1H, aromatic H), 7.32–7.27 (m, 1H, aromatic H), 7.17 (dt, J = 7.5, 0.9 Hz, 1H, aromatic H), 7.05 (ddd, J = 10.2, 8.4, 1.2 Hz, 1H, aromatic H), 4.76 (d, J = 6.6 Hz, 1H, -OCH_2OCH_3), 4.68 (d, J = 6.9 Hz, 1H, H-18), 4.63 (d, J = 6.6 Hz, 1H, -OCH_2OCH_3), 3.37 (s, 3H, -OCH_2OCH_3), 3.27 – 3.23 (m, 1H, H-17), 2.75–2.73 (m, 2H, H_2-16). ^{13}C NMR (75 MHz, $CDCl_3$) δ 160 (d, J_{CF} = 245.3 Hz), 129.9 (d, J_{CF} = 8.3 Hz), 128.7 (d, J_{CF} = 3.8 Hz), 125.3 (d, J_{CF} = 14.3 Hz), 124.5 (d, J_{CF} = 3.8 Hz), 115.7 (d, J_{CF} = 21.8 Hz), 94.8, 73.1, 55.8, 54.6, 44.4. IR (film) ν_{max}: 2891, 2825, 1616, 1587, 1488, 1455, 1149, 1022 cm^{-1}. HRMS (ESI): m/z calculated for $C_{11}H_{14}FO_3$ $[M + H]^+$: 213.0927. Found: 213.0920.

*3.15. Synthesis of (5S,6S,E)-5-(2-Fluorophenyl)-8,16,16,17,17-pentamethyl-2,4,11,15-tetraoxa-16-silaoctadec-8-en-6-ol [(17S, 18S) Fragment C9–C18 (**8**)]*

(17*S*,18*S*) Fragment C9–C18 (**8**) was synthesized as a colorless oil in 22% yield from MOM ether **21** in a similar way to the synthesis of its antipode (17*R*,18*R*) Fragment C9–C18 (7). ^{1}H NMR (300 MHz, $CDCl_3$) δ 7.41 (dt, J = 7.5, 1.8 Hz, 1H, aromatic H), 7.32–7.24 (m, 1H, aromatic H), 7.15 (dt, J = 7.5, 1.2 Hz, 1H, aromatic H), 7.03 (ddd, J = 10.2, 8.4, 1.2 Hz, 1H, aromatic H), 5.41 (t, J = 6.6 Hz, 1H, H-14), 4.81 (d, J = 6.6 Hz, 1H, H-18), 4.63 (d, J = 6.6 Hz, 1H, OCH_2OCH_3), 4.58 (d, J = 6.6 Hz, 1H, OCH_2OCH_3), 3.95 (d, J = 6.6 Hz, 2H, H_2-13), 3.82 (dt, J = 10.2, 5.7 Hz, 1H, H-17), 3.67 (t, J = 6.0 Hz, 2H, H_2-11), 3.46 (t, J = 6.6 Hz, 2H, H_2-9), 3.36 (s, 3H, OCH_3), 2.23 (dd, J = 12.6, 9.6 Hz, 1H, H-16), 2.05 (dd, J = 12.6, 2.7 Hz, 1H, H-16), 1.76 (quin, J = 6.3 Hz, 2H, H_2-10), 1.64 (s, 3H, 15-CH_3), 0.87 (s, 9H, TBS), 0.03 (s, 6H, TBS). ^{13}C NMR (75 MHz, $CDCl_3$) δ 160.9 (d, J_{CF} = 244.7 Hz), 136.4, 129.2, 128.9, 128.6, 126.1 (d, J_{CF} = 12.8 Hz), 124.5, 115.5, 95.3, 75.6, 72.7, 67.3, 67.0, 60.2, 56.2, 43.0, 33.2, 26.0, 18.5, 16.6, 16.5. IR (film) ν_{max}: 3461, 2928, 2855, 1616, 1586, 1252, 1090, 1031 cm^{-1}. HRMS (ESI): *m/z* calculated for $C_{24}H_{42}FO_5Si$ [M + H]$^+$: 457.2786. Found: 457.2782.

*3.16. Synthesis of (2E,4Z)-(5S,6S,E)-5-(2-Fluorophenyl)-8,16,16,17,17-pentamethyl-2,4,11,15-tetraoxa-16-silaoctadec-8-en-6-yl 7-((tert-butyldimethylsilyl)oxy)-8-(diethoxyphosphoryl)-5-methylocta-2,4-dienoate [(17S,18S) ester **24**]*

(17*S*,18*S*) Ester **24** was obtained as a pale-yellow oil in 91% yield from (17*S*,18*S*) Fragment C9–C18 (**8**) and Fragment C1–C8 (**9**), according to the esterification procedure employed for the preparation of ester **23**. ^{1}H NMR (300 MHz, $CDCl_3$) δ 7.50 (dd, J = 14.4, 12.0 Hz, 1H, H-3), 7.42 (t, J = 7.2 Hz, 1H, aromatic H), 7.34–7.21 (m, 1H, aromatic H), 7.10 (t, J = 7.5 Hz, 1H, aromatic H), 7.01 (t, J = 9.3 Hz, 1H, aromatic H), 6.03 (d, J = 11.7 Hz, 1H, H-4), 5.76 (d, J = 15.0 Hz, 1H, H-2), 5.45–5.37 (m, 1H, H-17), 5.33 (t, J = 6.0 Hz, 1H, H-14), 5.08 (d, J = 5.1 Hz, 1H, H-18), 4.58 (d, J = 6.9 Hz, 1H, OCH_2OCH_3), 4.51 (d, J = 6.6 Hz, 1H, OCH_2OCH_3), 4.23–4.04 (m, 5H, 2 × OCH_2CH_3, H-7), 3.93–3.80 (m, 2H, H_2-13), 3.65 (t, J = 6.6 Hz, 2H, H_2-11), 3.41 (t, J = 6.3 Hz, H_2-9), 3.32 (s, 3H, OCH_2OCH_3), 2.58–2.54 (m, 2H, H_2-16), 2.33–2.28 (m, 2H, H_2-8), 2.03–1.93 (m, 2H, H_2-6), 1.87 (s, 3H, 5-CH_3), 1.77–1.70 (m, 2H. H_2-10), 1.64 (s, 3H, 15-CH_3), 1.31 (t, J = 6.9 Hz, 6H, 2 × OCH_2CH_3), 0.90 (0.88) (s, 3H, TBS), 0.86 (s, 6H, TBS), 0.81 (0.80) (s, 9H, TBS), 0.08 (0.04) (s, 6H, TBS), 0.02 (-0.04) (s, 6H, TBS). ^{13}C NMR (75 MHz, $CDCl_3$) δ 166.7, 160.8 (d, J_{CF} = 245.3 Hz), 146.5 (146.4), 146.3 (146.2), 135.7 (135.2), 129.8, 129.0, 126.8, 125.8 (125.6),125.1 (124.7), 124.3 119.2, 115.5 (d, J_{CF} = 27.5 Hz), 95.0, 72.9, 72.3, 68.9, 66.8, 61.8, 61.7, 60.1, 56.1, 41.7 (41.2), 36.0 (34.2), 33.1, 32.3, 29.8, 27.0, 26.0, 25.9, 25.8, 24.9, 18.5, 18.1, 18.0, 16.6, 16.5. IR (film) ν_{max}: 2928, 2856, 1714, 1636, 1250, 1020 cm^{-1}. HRMS (ESI): *m/z* calculated for $C_{43}H_{77}FO_{10}PSi_2$ [M + H]$^+$: 859.4777. Found: 859.4774.

*3.17. Synthesis of (2E,4Z)-(1S,2S,E)-1-(2-Fluorophenyl)-6-(3-hydroxypropoxy)-1-(methoxymethoxy)-4-methylhex-4-en-2-yl 8-(diethoxyphosphoryl)-7-hydroxy-5-methylocta-2,4-dienoate [(17S,18S) diol **26**]*

(17*S*,18*S*) Diol **26** was obtained as a colorless syrup in 65% yield according to the TBS deprotection procedure used for the conversion of (17*R*,18*R*) ester **23** to (17*R*,18*R*) diol **25**. ^{1}H NMR (300 MHz, CD_3COCD_3) δ 7.63–7.55 (m, 1H, H-3), 7.52 (t, J = 7.8 Hz, 1H, aromatic H), 7.41–7.33 (m, 1H, aromatic H), 7.23 (t, J = 7.2 Hz, 1H, aromatic H), 7.14 (t, J = 9.0 Hz, 1H, aromatic H), 6.16 (d, J = 11.4 Hz, 1H, H-4), 5.80 (d, J = 15.0 Hz, 1H, H-2), 5.46 (quin, J = 5.1 Hz, 1H, H-17), 5.31 (t, J = 6.6 Hz, 1H, H-14), 5.10 (d, J = 5.7 Hz, 1H, H-18), 4.61 (d, J = 6.6 Hz, 1H, -OCH_2OCH_3), 4.51 (d, J = 6.6 Hz, 1H, -OCH_2OCH_3), 4.22–4.04 (overlapped, 5H, 2 × –OCH_2CH_3, H-7), 3.88 (d, J = 6.0 Hz, 2H, H_2-13), 3.57 (t, J = 4.8 Hz, 2H, H_2-11), 3.40 (t, J = 6.3 Hz, 2H, H_2-9), 3.30 (s, 3H, -OCH_2OCH_3), 2.92 (br.s, 2H, 2 × OH), 2.60–2.57(overlapped, 2H, H_2-16), 2.29 (d, J = 9.3 Hz, 2H, H_2-8), 2.07–2.04 (m, 2H, H_2-6), 1.95 (s, 3H, 5-CH_3), 1.68 (quin, J = 6.0 Hz, H_2-10), 1.65 (s, 3H, 15-CH_3), 1.29 (t, J = 7.2 Hz, 6H, 2 × –OCH_2CH_3). ^{13}C NMR (75 MHz, $CDCl_3$) δ 166.0, 160.7 (d, J_{CF} = 243.8 Hz), 147.0 (d, J_{CF} = 9.8 Hz), 140.8, 134.2, 129.8, 129.3, 125.8 (d, J_{CF} = 9.8 Hz), 125.6, 125.4 (d, J_{CF} = 4.5 Hz), 124.3, 119.1, 115.3 (115.0), 94.7, 72.3, 66.8, 66.7, 65.5, 61.4(61.3), 61.2 (61.1), 59.1, 55.1, 41.2, 40.7, 34.6, 33.02(32.98), 32.0, 24.4, 15.91(15.86), 15.7(15.6). IR (film) ν_{max}: 3381,

2927, 1709, 1633, 1488, 1019 cm^{-1}. HRMS (ESI): *m/z* calculated for $C_{31}H_{49}FO_{10}P$ $[M + H]^+$: 631.3048. Found: 631.3045.

3.18. Synthesis of (2E,4Z)-(1S,2S,E)-1-(2-Fluorophenyl)-1-(methoxymethoxy)-4-methyl-6-(3-oxopropoxy) hex-4-en-2-yl 8-(diethoxyphosphoryl)-5-methyl-7-oxoocta-2,4-dienoate [ketoaldehyde (17S,18S) **28***]*

The crude product was obtained from (17*S*,18*S*) diol **26** employing the oxidation procedure used for the synthesis of its antipode **27**. After being confirmed by its ^{1}H NMR data, the crude product was directly used for the next step reaction without further purification. ^{1}H NMR (300 MHz, $CDCl_3$) δ 9.72 (t, J = 1.8 Hz, 1H, CHO), 7.41 (dt, J = 7.5, 1.8 Hz, 1H, aromatic H), 7.31 (dd, J = 15.0, 11.7 Hz, 1H, H-3), 7.29–7.22 (m, 1H), 7.11 (dt, J = 7.5, 0.9 Hz, 1H), 7.51 (ddd, J = 10.2, 8.1, 0.9 Hz, 1H), 6.17 (d, J = 11.1 Hz, 1H, H-4), 5.83 (d, J = 15.0 Hz, 1H, H-2), 5.45–5.38 (m, 1H), 5.31 (t, J = 5.7 Hz, 1H, H-14), 5.07 (d, J = 5.4 Hz, 1H), 4.57 (d, J = 6.9 Hz, 1H, OCH_2OCH_3), 4.50 (d, J = 6.9 Hz, 1 H, OCH_2OCH_3), 4.20–4.11 (m, 5H, 2 × OCH_2CH_3, H-7), 3.90 (t, J = 7.2 Hz, 2H, H_2-13), 3.65 (t, J = 6.0 Hz, 2H, H_2-11), 3.31 (s, 3H, OCH_3), 3.10 (d, J = 22.8 Hz, 2H, H_2-8), 2.39–2.19 (m, 2H, H_2-10), 1.87 (s, 3H, 5-CH_3), 1.63 (s, 3H, 15-CH_3).

3.19. Synthesis of (S,3E,9E,11Z,15E)-6-((S)-(2-Fluorophenyl)(methoxymethoxy)methyl)-4,12-dimethyl-1,7-dioxacyclooctadeca-3,9,11,15-tetraene-8,14-dione [(17S,18S) macrolide **30***]*

(17*S*,18*S*) Macrolide **30** was synthesized according to the HWE ring closing procedure employed for the conversion of **27** to **29**. Colorless syrup, 68% yield for two steps. [α]: +8.1 (c = 0.22, MeOH). ^{1}H NMR (300 MHz, $CDCl_3$) δ 7.59 (dd, J = 15.0, 11.4 Hz, 1H, H-3), 7.46 (dt, J = 7.5, 1.8 Hz, 1H, aromatic H), 7.36–7.25 (m, 1H, aromatic H), 7.15 (dt, J = 7.5, 1.2 Hz, 1H, aromatic H), 7.04 (ddd, J = 9.9, 8.1, 1.2 Hz, 1H, aromatic H), 6.81 (dt, J = 15.9, 6.9 Hz, 1H, H-9), 6.11 (d, J = 11.4 Hz, 1H, H-4), 6.00 (d, J = 16.2 Hz, 1H, H-8), 5.90 (d, J = 15.0 Hz, 1H, H-2), 5.50 (dd, J = 11.4, 6.3 Hz, 1H, H-17), 5.26 (dd, J = 7.5, 4.5 Hz, 1H, H-14), 5.11 (d, J = 6.3 Hz, 1H, H-18), 4.59 (d, J = 6.9 Hz, 1H,–OCH_2OCH_3), 4.52 (d, J = 6.6 Hz, 1H, –OCH_2OCH_3), 3.98 (dd, J = 12.0, 8.1 Hz, 1H, H-16), 3.88 – 3.81 (overlapped, 2H, H_2-13), 3.46 – 3.31 (overlapped, 2H, H_2-11), 3.33 (s, 3H, OCH_3), 3.14 (d, J = 12.6 Hz, 1H, H-16), 2.42–2.35 (m, 2H, H_2-10), 2.33 (d, J = 11.7 Hz, 1H, H-6), 2.04 (d, J = 11.7 Hz, 1H, H-6), 1.82 (s, 3H, 5-CH_3), 1.63 (s, 3H, 15-CH_3). ^{13}C NMR (75 MHz, $CDCl_3$) δ 197.1, 166.6, 160.9 (d, J_{CF} = 244.5 Hz), 146.8, 142.5, 139.8, 134.3, 130.2, 129.9, 129.0, 125.9 (d, J_{CF} = 7.5 Hz), 125.5 (d, J = 13.5 Hz), 125.2 (d, J_{CF} = 4.5 Hz), 124.5, 120.9 (d, J_{CF} = 3.8 Hz), 115.6 (d, J_{CF} = 21.0 Hz), 94.9, 72.9, 72.6, 67.9, 67.8, 56.0, 45.9, 41.4, 33.1, 24.1, 16.7. IR (film) ν_{max}: 2925, 2854, 1714, 1669, 1634, 1489, 1359, 1280 cm^{-1}. HRMS (ESI): *m/z* calculated for $C_{27}H_{34}FO_6$ $[M + H]^+$: 473.2339. Found: 473.2332.

3.20. Synthesis of (S,3E,9E,11Z,15E)-6-((S)-(2-Fluorophenyl)(hydroxy)methyl)-4,12-dimethyl-1,7-dioxacyclooctadeca-3,9,11,15-tetraene-8,14-dione [(17S,18S) zampanolide mimic **6***]*

(17*S*,18*S*) Zampanolide mimic **6** was obtained according to the MOM deprotection procedure used for the conversion of (17*R*,18*R*) macrolide **29** to (17S,18S) zampanolide mimic **5**. Colorless syrup, 45% yield. [α]: +15.6 (c = 0.15, MeOH). ^{1}H NMR (300 MHz, CD_3COCD_3) δ 7.61 (dd, J = 15.0, 11.1 Hz, 1H, H-3), 7.34 (dd, J = 14.4, 7.2 Hz, 1H, aromatic H), 7.21 (t, J = 7.5 Hz, 1H, aromatic H), 7.10 (dd, J = 10.5, 8.1 Hz, 1H, aromatic H), 6.83 (dt, J = 16.2, 6.3 Hz, 1H, H-9), 6.20 (d, J = 11.1 Hz, 1H, H-4), 6.06 (d, J = 15.9 Hz, H-8), 5.88 (d, J = 12.6 Hz, 1H, H-2), 5.44 (dd, J = 11.1, 5.4 Hz, 1H, H-17), 5.27 (t, J = 5.4 Hz, 1H, H-14), 5.17 (t, J = 5.4 Hz, 1H, H-18), 4.81 (d, J = 5.4 Hz, 1H, OH), 4.07–3.97 (m, 1H, H-16), 3.90 (d, J = 12.9 Hz, 1H, H-13), 3.83 (dd, J = 12.3, 4.5 Hz, 1H, H-13), 3.48– 3.32 (m, 2H, H_2-11), 3.17 (d, J = 12.6 Hz, 1H, H-16), 2.42–2.33 (overlapped, 3H, H_2-10, H-6), 2.19 (d, J = 13.8 Hz, 1H, H-6), 1.81 (s, 3H, 5-CH_3), 1.64 (s, 3H, 15-CH_3). ^{13}C NMR (75 MHz, CD_3COCD_3) δ 196.5, 166.5, 160.5 (d, J_{CF} = 242.3 Hz), 146.6, 142.7, 139.8, 134.7, 130.6, 129.7, 129.5, 126.3, 126.2, 125.7, 124.8, 121.7, 115.6, 73.8, 69.0, 68.9, 68.2, 45.8, 41.6, 33.2, 23.8, 16.3. IR (film) ν_{max}: 3447, 2916, 2855, 1710, 1669, 1633, 1489, 1456, 1359, 1281, 1148 cm^{-1}. HRMS (ESI): *m/z* calculated for $C_{25}H_{30}FO_5$ $[M + H]^+$: 429.2077. Found: 429.2073.

3.21. Cell Culture

All cell lines were initially purchased from American Type Culture Collection (ATCC). The PC-3, PC-3/DTX, and LNCaP prostate cancer cell lines were routinely cultured in RPMI-1640 medium supplemented with 10% FBS and 1% penicillin/streptomycin. Cultures were maintained in a high humidity environment supplemented with 5% carbon dioxide at a temperature of 37 °C. The DU145 and DU145/DTX prostate cancer cells were routinely cultured in Eagle's Minimum Essential Medium (EMEM) supplemented with 10% FBS and 1% penicillin/streptomycin.

The procedure illustrated in the literature [29,30] was adapted to establish docetaxel-resistant prostate cancer cell lines. Specifically, docetaxel-resistant DU145 and PC-3 cell lines (DU145/DTX and PC-3/DTX) were developed over a period of one year by stepwise increased concentrations of docetaxel. Cells were repeatedly conserved in an appropriate concentration of docetaxel, starting with IC_{50} value of the respective parent cell lines. Docetaxel-containing media will be replaced every 2–3 days. The concentration of docetaxel was increased when cells exhibited resistance to treatments.

3.22. WST-1 Cell Proliferation Assay

PC-3, PC-3/DTX, DU145, DU145/DTX, or LNCaP cells were placed in 96-well plates at a density of 3200 cells each well in 200 μL of culture medium. The cells were then treated with synthesized mimics, or positive reference separately at different doses for 3 days, while equal treatment volumes of DMSO were used as vehicle control. After the cells were cultured in a CO_2 incubator at 37 °C for three days, the premixed WST-1 cell proliferation reagent (10 μL, Clontech) was added to each well. The cells were incubated for additional 3 h at 37 °C before mixing gently for one minute on an orbital shaker to ensure homogeneous distribution of color. A microplate-reader (Synergy HT, BioTek) was used to measure the absorbance of each well at a wavelength of 430 nm. The half-maximal inhibitory concentration (IC_{50} value) is the concentration of each compound that inhibits cell proliferation by 50% under the experimental conditions. Each of IC_{50} value is represented as the average from triplicate determinations that were reproducible and statistically significant. The IC_{50} values were calculated based on dose–response curves from at least five dosages for each compound.

3.23. Statistical Analysis

All data are represented as the mean ± standard deviation (S.D.) for the number of experiments indicated. Other differences between treated and control groups were analyzed using the Student's t-test. A p-value < 0.05 was considered statistically significant.

4. Conclusions

In summary, two new zampanolide mimics have been designed and each of them has been achieved through a 25-step chemical transformation starting from commercially available 2-butyn-1-ol. Yamaguchi esterification and intramolecular Horner–Wadsworth–Emmons condensation were employed as crucial reactions to build up the C-17 and C-1 ester moiety and to close the lactone ring. The chiral centers at C17 and C18 in the Fragment C9–C18 (**7** and **8**) were introduced by the Sharpless asymmetric dihydroxylation using the commercially available AD-mix formulations. Our WST-1 cell proliferation assay data in both docetaxel-resistant and docetaxel-sensitive prostate cancer cell lines revealed that compound **6** is the optimal mimic and the newly designed side chain can act as a bioisostere for the chemically fragile *N*-acetyl hemiminal side chain in zampanolide.

Author Contributions: Conceptualization and design, Q.C.; experimentation and data analysis, G.C., Z.J., Q.Z., G.W., and Q.-H.C.; funding acquisition, Q.-H.C. and G.W.; all authors finally reviewed and approved the manuscript. All authors have read and agreed to the published version of the manuscript.

Acknowledgments: We thank the Department of Chemistry and College of Science and Mathematics at CSU-Fresno for all administrative support.

References

1. Siegel, R.L.; Miller, K.D.; Jamal, A. Cancer Statistics, 2019. *CA Cancer J. Clin.* **2019**, *69*, 7–34. [CrossRef] [PubMed]
2. Tan, M.H.; Li, J.; Xu, H.E.; Melcher, K.; Yong, E.-L. Androgen receptor: Structure, role in prostate cancer, and drug discovery. *Acta Pharmacol. Sin.* **2015**, *36*, 3–23. [CrossRef] [PubMed]
3. Elshan, N.G.R.D.; Rettig, M.B.; Jung, M.E. Molecules targeting the androgen receptor (AR) signaling axis beyond the AR-ligand binding domain. *Med. Res. Rev.* **2019**, *39*, 910–960. [CrossRef] [PubMed]
4. Ojo, D.; Lin, X.; Wong, N.; Gu, Y.; Tang, D. Prostate cancer stem-like cells contribute to the development of castration-resistant prostate cancer. *Cancers* **2015**, *7*, 2290–2308. [CrossRef] [PubMed]
5. Schweizer, M.T.; Yu, E.Y. Persistent androgen receptor addiction in castration-resistant prostate cancer. *J. Hematol. Oncol.* **2015**, *8*, 128. [CrossRef] [PubMed]
6. De Bono, J.S.; Oudard, S.; Ozguroglu, M.; Hansen, S.; Machiels, J.-P.; Kocak, I.; Gravis, G.; Bodrogi, I.; Mackenzie, M.; Shen, L.; et al. Prednisone plus cabazitaxel or mitoxantrone for metastatic castration-resistant prostate cancer progressing after docetaxel treatment: A randomized open-label trial. *Lancet* **2010**, *376*, 1147–1154. [CrossRef]
7. Tannock, I.F.; de Wit, R.; Berry, W.R.; Horti, J.; Pluzanska, A.; Chi, K.N.; Oudard, S.; Theodore, C.; James, N.D.; Turesson, I.; et al. Docetaxel plus prednisone or mitoxantrone plus prednisone for advanced prostate cancer. *Engl. J. Med.* **2004**, *351*, 1502–1512. [CrossRef]
8. Petrylak, D.P.; Tangen, C.M.; Hussain, M.H.A.; Lara, P.N.; Jones, J.A.; Taplin, M.E.; Burch, P.A.; Berry, D.; Moinpour, C.; Kohli, M.; et al. Docetaxel and estramustine compared with mitoxantrone and prednisone for advanced refractory prostate cancer. *N. Engl. J. Med.* **2004**, *351*, 1513–1520. [CrossRef]
9. Jordan, M.A.; Wilson, L. Microtubules as a target for anticancer drugs. *Nat. Rev. Cancer* **2004**, *4*, 253–265. [CrossRef]
10. Thadani-Mulero, M.; Nanus, D.M.; Giannakakou, P. Androgen receptor on the move: Boarding the microtubule expressway to the nucleus. *Cancer Res.* **2012**, *72*, 4611–4615. [CrossRef]
11. Chen, Q.-H.; Kingston, D.G.I. Zampanolide and dactylolide: Cytotoxic tubulin-assembly agents and promising anticancer leads. *Nat. Prod. Rep.* **2014**, *31*, 1202–1226. [CrossRef] [PubMed]
12. Field, J.J.; Singh, A.J.; Kanakkanthara, A.; Halafihi, T.I.; Northcote, P.T.; Miller, J.H. Microtubule stabilizing activity of zampanolide, a potent macrolide isolated from the Tongan marine sponge Cacospongia mycofijensis. *J. Med. Chem.* **2009**, *52*, 7328–7332. [CrossRef] [PubMed]
13. Tanaka, J.; Higa, T. Zampanolide, a new cytotoxic macrolide from a marine sponge. *Tetrahedron Lett.* **1996**, *37*, 5535–5538. [CrossRef]
14. Hoye, T.R.; Hu, M. Macrolactonization via Ti(IV)-mediated epoxy-acid coupling: A total synthesis of (−)-dactylolide [and zampanolide]. *J. Am. Chem. Soc.* **2003**, *125*, 9576–9577. [CrossRef]
15. Ghosh, A.K.; Cheng, X. Enantioselective total synthesis of (−)-zampanolide, a potent microtubule-stabilizing agent. *Org. Lett.* **2011**, *13*, 4108–4111. [CrossRef]
16. Smith, A.B.; Safonov, I.G.; Corbett, R.M. Total synthesis of (+)-zampanolide and (+)-dactylolide. *J. Am. Chem. Soc.* **2002**, *124*, 11102–11113. [CrossRef]
17. Uenishi, J.; Iwamoto, T.; Tanaka, J. Total synthesis of (−)-zampanolide and questionable existence of (−)-dactylolide as the elusive biosynthetic precursor of (−)-zampanolide in an Okinwan sponge. *Org. Lett.* **2009**, *11*, 3262–3265. [CrossRef]
18. Zurwerra, D.; Glaus, F.; Betschart, L.; Schuster, J.; Gertsch, J.; Ganci, W.; Altmann, K.-H. Total synthesis of (−)-zampanolide and structure-activity relationship studies on (−)-dactylolide derivatives. *Chem. Eur. J.* **2012**, *18*, 16868–16883. [CrossRef]
19. Field, J.J.; Pera, B.; Calvo, E.; Canales, A.; Zurwerra, D.; Trigili, C.; Rodriguez-Salarichs, J.; Matesanz, R.; Kanakkanthara, A.; Wakefield, S.J.; et al. Zampanolide, a potent new microtubule-stabilizing agent, covalently reacts with the taxane luminal site in tubulin α, β-heterodimers and microtubules. *Chem. Biol.* **2012**, *19*, 686–698. [CrossRef]
20. Ding, F.; Jennings, M.P. Total synthesis of (−)-dactylolide and formal synthesis of (−)-zampanolide via target oriented β-C-glycoside formation. *J. Org. Chem.* **2008**, *73*, 5965–5976. [CrossRef]

21. Chen, G.; Patanapongpibu, M.; Jiang, Z.; Zhang, Q.; Zheng, S.; Wang, G.; White, J.D.; Chen, Q.-H. Synthesis and antiproliferative evaluation of new zampanolide mimics. *Org. Biomole. Chem.* **2019**, *10*, 3830–3844. [CrossRef] [PubMed]
22. Prota, A.E.; Bargsten, K.; Zurwerra, D.; Field, J.J.; Diaz, J.F.; Altmann, K.-H.; Steinmetz, M.O. Molecular mechanism of action of microtubule-stabilizing anticancer agents. *Science* **2013**, *339*, 587–590. [CrossRef] [PubMed]
23. Chen, G.; Wang, R.; Vue, B.; Patanapongpibul, M.; Zhang, Q.; Zheng, S.; Wang, G.; White, J.D.; Chen, Q.-H. Optimized synthesis and antiproliferative activity of desTHPdactylolides. *Bioorg. Med. Chem.* **2018**, *26*, 3514–3520. [CrossRef] [PubMed]
24. Zurwerra, D.; Gertsch, J.; Altmann, K.-H. Synthesis of (−)-dactylolide and 13-desmethylene-(−)-dactylolide and their effects on tubulin. *Org. Lett.* **2010**, *12*, 2302–2305. [CrossRef] [PubMed]
25. Sharpless, K.B.; Amberg, W.; Bennani, Y.L.; Crispino, G.A.; Hartung, J.; Jeong, K.-S.; Kwong, H.-L.; Morikawa, K.; Wang, Z.M.; Xu, D.; et al. The osmium-catalyzed asymmetric dihydroxylation: A new ligand class and a process improvement. *J. Org. Chem.* **1992**, *57*, 2768–2771. [CrossRef]
26. Lad, N.P.; Kulkarni, S.; Sharma, R.; Mascarenhas, M.; Kulkarni, M.R.; Pandit, S.S. Piperlongumine derived cyclic sulfonamides (sultams): Synthesis and in vitro exploration for therapeutic potential against HeLa cancer cell lines. *Eur. J. Med. Chem.* **2017**, *126*, 870–878. [CrossRef] [PubMed]
27. Huang, J.; Wang, W.; He, H.-Y.; Jian, L.; Fu, H.-Y.; Zheng, X.-L.; Li, R.-X. An approach to the synthesis of 1-propenylnaphthols and 3-arylnaphtho[2,1-*b*]furans. *J. Org. Chem.* **2017**, *82*, 2523–2534. [CrossRef]
28. Banwell, M.G.; Chand, S.; Savage, G.P. An enantioselective total synthesis of the stilbenolignan (−)-aiphanol and the determination of its absolute stereochemistry. *Tetrahedron Asymmetry* **2005**, *16*, 1645–1654. [CrossRef]
29. O'Neill, A.J.; Prencipe, M.; Dowline, C.; Fan, Y.; Mulrane, L.; Gallagher, W.M.; O'Connor, D.; Devery, A.; Corcoran, C.; Rani, S.; et al. Characterisation and manipulation of docetaxel resistant prostate cancer cell lines. *Mol. Cancer* **2011**, *10*, 126. [CrossRef]
30. Shiota, M.; Kashiwagi, E.; Yokomizo, A.; Takeuchi, A.; Dejima, T.; Song, Y.; Tatsugami, K.; Inokuchi, J.; Uchiumi, T.; Naito, S. Interaction between docetaxel resistance and castration resistance in prostate cancer: Implications of twistI, YB-I, and androgen receptor. *Prostate* **2013**, *73*, 1336–1344. [CrossRef]

8

Synthesis, Antiproliferative and Antioxidant Evaluation of 2-Pentylquinazolin-4(3*H*)-one(thione) Derivatives with DFT Study

Amira A. El-Sayed [1], Mahmoud F. Ismail [1], Abd El-Galil E. Amr [2,3,*] and Ahmed M. Naglah [2,4]

1 Department of Chemistry, Faculty of Science, Ain Shams University, 11566 Abbassia, Cairo 11566, Egypt; amira_aa47@hotmail.com (A.A.E.-S.); fawzy2010@sci.asu.edu.eg (M.F.I.)

2 Pharmaceutical Chemistry Department, Drug Exploration & Development Chair (DEDC), College of Pharmacy, King Saud University, Riyadh 11451, Saudi Arabia; amnaglah@gmail.com

3 Applied Organic Chemistry Department, National Research Center, Cairo, Dokki 12622, Egypt

4 Peptide Chemistry Department, Chemical Industries Research Division, National Research Centre, Dokki, Cairo 12622, Egypt

* Correspondence: aamr@ksu.edu.sa;

Academic Editor: Qiao-Hong Chen

Abstract: The current study was chiefly designed to examine the antiproliferative and antioxidant activities of some novel quinazolinone(thione) derivatives **6–14**. The present work focused on two main points; firstly, comparing between quinazolinone and quinazolinthione derivatives. Whereas, antiproliferative (against two cell lines namely, HepG2 and MCF-7) and antioxidant (by two methods; ABTS and DPPH) activities of the investigated compounds, the best quinazolinthione derivatives were **6** and **14**, which exhibited excellent potencies comparable to quinazolinone derivatives **5** and **9**, respectively. Secondly, we compared the activity of four series of Schiff bases which included the quinazolinone moiety (**11a–d**). In addition, the antiproliferative and antioxidant activities of the compounds with various aryl aldehyde hydrazone derivatives (**11a–d**) analogs were studied. The compounds exhibited potency that increased with increasing electron donating group in *p*-position (OH > OMe > Cl) due to extended conjugated systems. Noteworthy, most of antiproliferative and antioxidant activities results for the tested compounds are consistent with the DFT calculations.

Keywords: quinazolin-4(3*H*)-one; quinazolin-4(3*H*)-thione; Schiff base; antiproliferative activity; antioxidant activity; DFT study

1. Introduction

Cancer is the second leading cause of death globally, and the contribution of cancer disease to the overall mortality rate is increasing. Economically, the total annual cost of cancer in 2010 was estimated at approximately US$ 1.16 trillion [1]. So that, more rational design, synthesis, and evaluation of new compounds as anticancer, with higher efficiency is considered as urgent mission in the medicinal chemistry field.

Quinazoline and quinazolinone derivatives are considered as tremendous targets for the medicinal chemists, due to the fact that they are the scaffold of different potent anticancer drugs, such as Gefitinib (trade name Iressa®), Erlotinib (trade name Tarceva®) [2–4], Methaqualone [5], Afloqualone (as anticonvulsant activity) [6,7], Chloroqualone (as antitussive), and Diproqualone (as sedative-hypnotic agents) [8] (Figure 1).

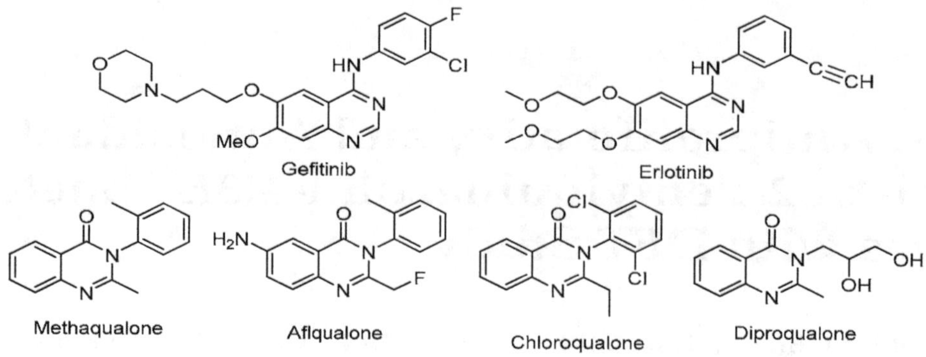

Figure 1. Some structures of synthetic drugs scaffold quinazoline and quinazolinone derivatives.

In the last decades and until now, various compounds including quinazolinone moiety conspicuously exhibited broad spectrum in numerous pharmacological activities such as anticancer [9–14], anticonvulsants [15], antiproliferative [16], anti-inflammatory [17], antihypertensive [18], antifungal [19], antibacterial, antioxidant [20], antimicrobial [21], anti-allergic [22], antimalarial [23], antileishmanial [24], and treatment of Alzheimer's disease (AD) [25].

Generally, the natural products are considered as one of the most interesting sources of biologically active compounds. Among them, naturally occurring quinazolin-4(3*H*)-one derivatives, which can be isolated from various plants and microorganisms such as Luotonin A (sources; *Peganum nigellastrum*) [26], 2-(heptan-3-yl)quinazolinone (sources; *Bacillus cereus*) [27], Dictyoquinazol A (sources; *Dictyophora indusiata*) [28], and Echinozolinone (sources; *Echinops echinatus*) [29] (Figure 2).

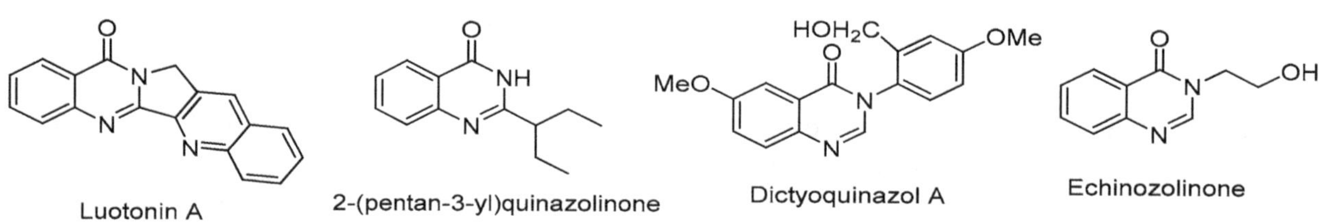

Figure 2. Some structures of naturally occurring quinazolin-4(3*H*)-one derivatives.

Quinazolinones have been synthesized by different methodologies [28,30–37], in the present study, the conventional methodology to construct novel qunizolinone compounds has been adopted, followed by the study of the antiproliferative activity, antioxidant activity, and DFT calculations for the synthesized compounds.

2. Results and Discussion

2.1. Chemistry

In this interesting work, curing of anthranilic acid **1** with hexanoyl chloride **2** in dry pyridine afforded the corresponding *N*-hexanoyl derivative **3** [38], which was cyclized by heating in distilled acetic anhydride to give 2-pentyl-4*H*-benzo[*d*][1,3]oxazin-4-one **4** [39,40] (Scheme 1).

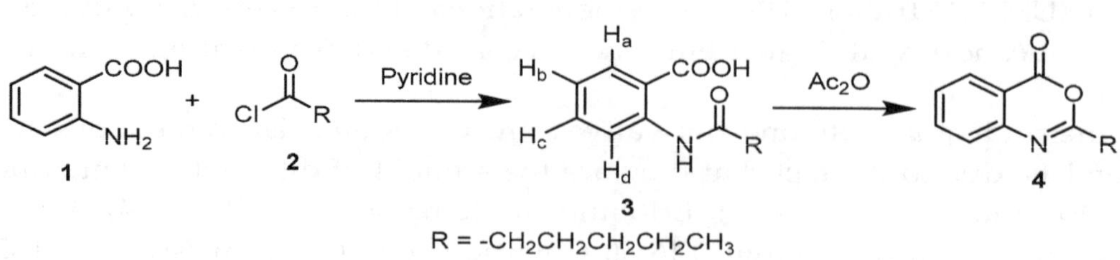

Scheme 1. The strategy for synthesis of compound **4**.

Benzoxazinone derivative **4** was utilized in situ as a precursor to construct new quinazolinone derivatives. For instance, reaction of benzoxazinone derivative **4** with formamide afforded 2-pentylquinazolin-4(3*H*)-one **5** [41] (Scheme 2). The ^{1}H NMR spectrum of **5** exhibited a singlet peak at 12.13 ppm exchangeable with D_2O corresponding to NH proton, two doublet and two triplet peaks in the aromatic region at 8.05–7.42 ppm corresponding to four aromatic protons, and four characteristic peaks upfield at 2.56–0.84 ppm for *n*-pentyl protons.

Afterwards, sulfuration of 2-pentylquinazolin-4(3*H*)-one **5** by utilizing of phosphorus pentasulfide in dry toluene afforded 2-pentylquinazoline-4(3*H*)-thione **6** (Scheme 2). The formation of compound **6** was unambiguously elaborated by the presence of intense band at 1236 cm^{-1} corresponding to $\upsilon_{C=S}$ and the absence of the stretching band of $\upsilon_{C=O}$ in the IR spectrum. On the other hand, the incorporation of β-D-glucose pentaacetate with quinazolinone derivative **5** at the nitrogen atom of the later awarded *N*-(β-D-glucopyranosyl-2,3,4,6-tetraacetate)-2-pentyl quinazolin-4(3*H*)-one **7** (Scheme 2), via attacking of the lone pair of nitrogen atom of quinazolinone derivative **5** at the anomeric carbon (C_1) of β-D-glucose pentaacetate, followed by ring opening and then ring closure with expulsion of acetate as a leaving group.

The chemical structure of compound **7** was explained by the IR spectrum, whereas it showed a band at 1746 cm^{-1} compatible with $\upsilon_{C=O}$ of the acetate groups and lacked the absorption band for the NH group. Moreover, this structure was also interpreted by the ^{1}H-NMR spectrum which revealed seven signals at 5.92–3.51 ppm and four singlet signals at 1.97–1.91 ppm all of them corresponding to the protons of β-D-glucopyranosyl-2,3,4,6-tetraacetate moiety.

Curing of the benzoxazinone derivative **4** with ethanolamine under reflux for 3 h afforded 3-(2-hydroxyethyl)-2-pentylquinazolin-4(3*H*)-one **8** as the sole product. The IR spectrum of compound **8** showed a broad band at 3395 cm^{-1} corresponding to OH functionality. Furthermore, the ^{1}H-NMR spectrum appreciably emerged a triplet peak at 4.95 ppm exchangeable with D_2O corresponding to OH proton, triplet, and quartet peaks at 4.11 and 3.65 ppm, respectively, compatible with ethyl protons of 2-hydroxyethyl moiety. As well, the ^{13}C-NMR spectrum exhibited two peaks at 58.8 and 46.1 ppm corresponding to the two carbons of 2-hydroxyethyl moiety.

3-Amino-2-pentylquinazolin-4(3*H*)-one **9** was commenced by refluxing of compound **4** with hydrazine monohydrate in absolute ethanol for 4 h (Scheme 2). The formation of compound **9** was confirmed by spectroscopic and elemental data. In particular, the ^{1}H-NMR spectrum of compound **9** manifested a singlet signal commutable in D_2O at 5.70 ppm corresponding to NH_2 protons.

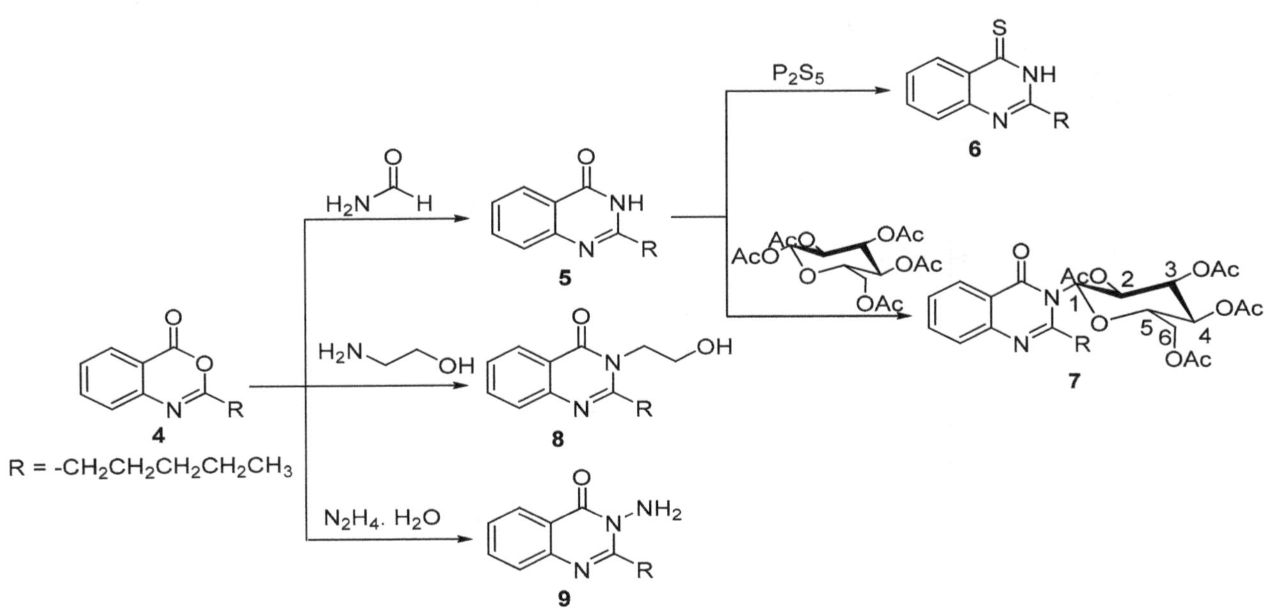

Scheme 2. Synthetic route to compounds **5–9**.

Reaction of 3-amino-2-pentylquinazolin-4(3*H*)-one **9** with various aldehydes **10a–d** gave Schiff bases **11a–d** as the sole product in each case (Scheme 3). The ^{1}H-NMR spectra of compounds **11a–d** exhibited the appearance of a singlet signal in the region between 8.81–8.69 ppm compatible with methine proton of N=CH group.

The thiazolidin-4-one moiety **12** was constructed by the reaction of Schiff base **11a** with methyl thioglycolate in absolute ethanol including a small amount of piperidine as a catalyst for 3 h (Scheme 3). The prospective structure **12** is in keeping with its spectral and elemental analyses.

Additionally, the nucleophilicity of the amino group of compound **9** was also estimated by fusion of it with 4,5,6,7-tetrachloroisobenzofuran-1,3-dione in oil bath for an hour and that afforded phthalimido derivative **13** in an excellent yield (Scheme 3). The foreseeable structure of compound **13** was elucidated by their spectral data and elemental analysis. Obviously, its IR spectrum showed stretching absorption bands at 1788, and 1746 cm^{-1} corresponding to the carbonyl groups of phthalimido moiety and at 1707 cm^{-1} corresponding to carbonyl group of the quinazolinone moiety. The ^{1}H-NMR spectrum exhibited four peaks for four aromatic protons and another four peaks for n-pentyl protons. Furthermore, its ^{13}C-NMR spectrum emerged variant peaks, all of them fit with the proposed structure.

Eventually, the thione derivative **14** was obtained via sulfuration of compound **9** by utilizing phosphorus pentasulfide as the above pervious method (Scheme 3). The structure of **14** was unequivocally explained via the existence of a peak in the ^{13}C NMR spectrum at 182.1 ppm compatible with the carbon of the thione functional group.

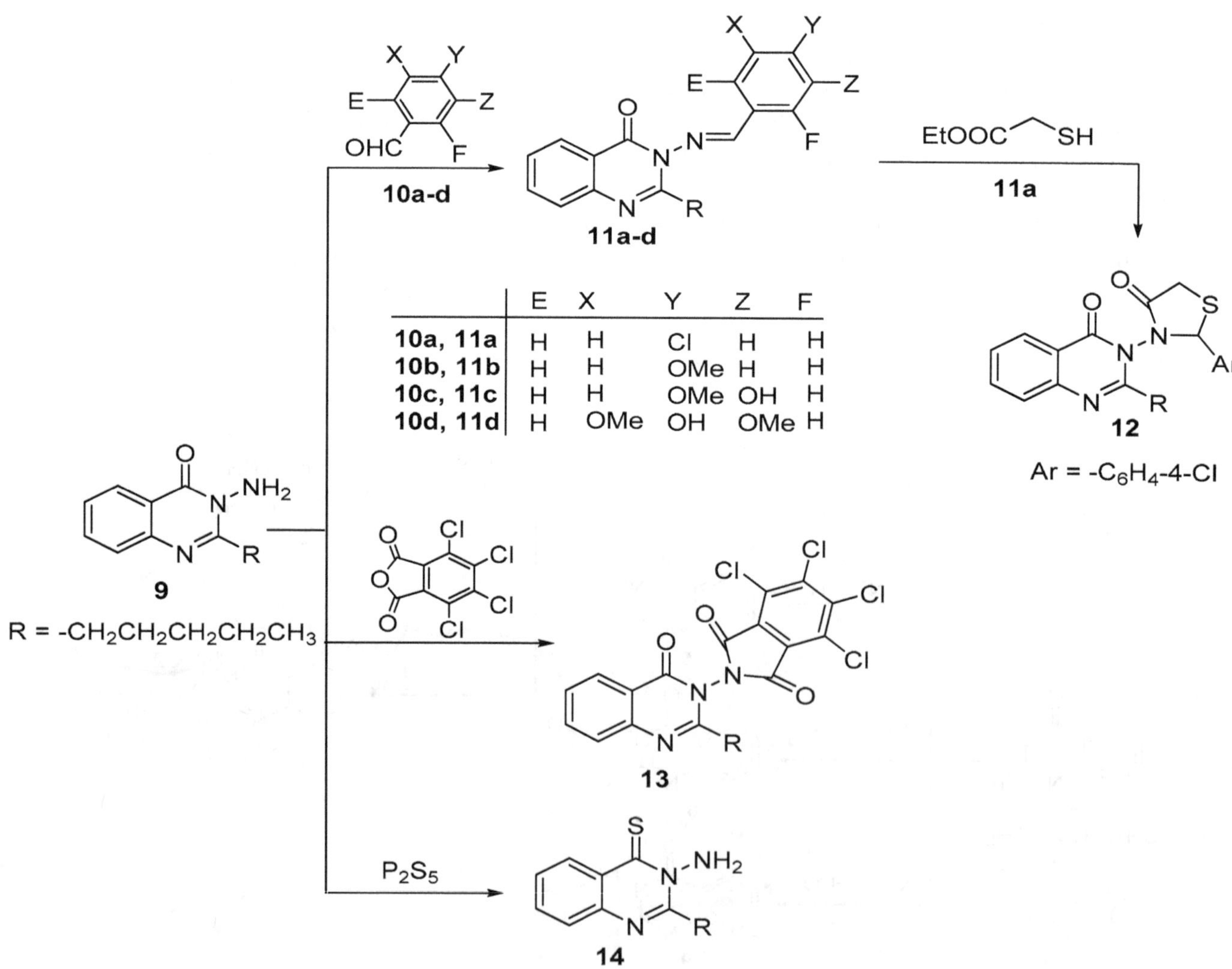

	E	X	Y	Z	F
10a, 11a	H	H	Cl	H	H
10b, 11b	H	H	OMe	H	H
10c, 11c	H	H	OMe	OH	H
10d, 11d	H	OMe	OH	OMe	H

Scheme 3. Synthetic route to compounds **11–14**.

2.2. *Biological Evaluation*

2.2.1. Antiproliferative Screening

Twelve compounds possessing quinazolinone(thione) moieties **5–14** along with compound **3** were screened against two cell lines, namely hepatocellular carcinoma (HepG2) and mammary gland (MCF-7) in vitro by utilizing MTT assay [42,43]. The latter assay is a colorimetric test based on the change of the yellow MTT (3-(4,5-dimethylthiazolyl-2)-2,5-diphenyltetrazolium bromide) to a purple formazan derivative by mitochondrial succinate dehydrogenase in viable cells and the Doxorubicin (DOX) was used as a standard reference.

The results listed in Table 1 and illustrated in Figure 3, demonstrate that compounds **6** and **11d** have a very strong efficacy against HePG2 cell line with IC_{50} values at 5.20 ± 0.5 and 7.63 ± 0.6 μM, respectively. Meanwhile, compounds **6, 11d,** and **14** have a very strong efficacy against the MCF-7 cell line with IC_{50} values at 6.88 ± 0.4, 8.60 ± 0.7, and 10.78 ± 0.9 μM, respectively. Compounds **11b, 11c** have a strong efficacy against both cell lines with IC_{50} values in the range (12.54 ± 1.1–19.68 ± 1.6 μM). For the HePG2 cell line, compounds **5, 9, 11a,** and **14** have a moderate efficacy with IC_{50} values in the range (23.75 ± 1.9–41.92 ± 2.8 μM). Where, for the MCF-7 cell line, compounds **3, 5, 9,** and **11a** have a moderate efficacy with IC_{50} in the range (21.98 ± 1.8–47.53 ± 2.9 μM). Ultimately, the remaining compounds in both cases have weak efficacies with IC_{50} values > 50 μM.

Table 1. Cytotoxic efficacy of thirteen compounds against hepatocellular carcinoma (HePG2) and mammary gland (MCF-7) cell lines.

Compounds	**In Vitro Cytotoxicity IC_{50} (μM)**	
	HePG2	**MCF-7**
DOX	4.50 ± 0.3	4.17 ± 0.2
3	52.01 ± 3.3	47.53 ± 2.9
5	23.75 ± 1.9	21.98 ± 1.8
6	5.20 ± 0.5	6.88 ± 0.4
7	66.84 ± 4.0	54.23 ± 3.2
8	85.55 ± 4.5	70.86 ± 4.1
9	33.27 ± 2.5	28.69 ± 2.2
11a	41.92 ± 2.8	33.39 ± 2.5
11b	17.27 ± 1.4	19.68 ± 1.6
11c	12.54 ± 1.1	14.10 ± 1.3
11d	7.63 ± 0.6	8.60 ± 0.7
12	76.14 ± 4.3	59.15 ± 3.8
13	60.34 ± 3.8	56.28 ± 3.5
14	27.39 ± 2.3	10.78 ± 0.9

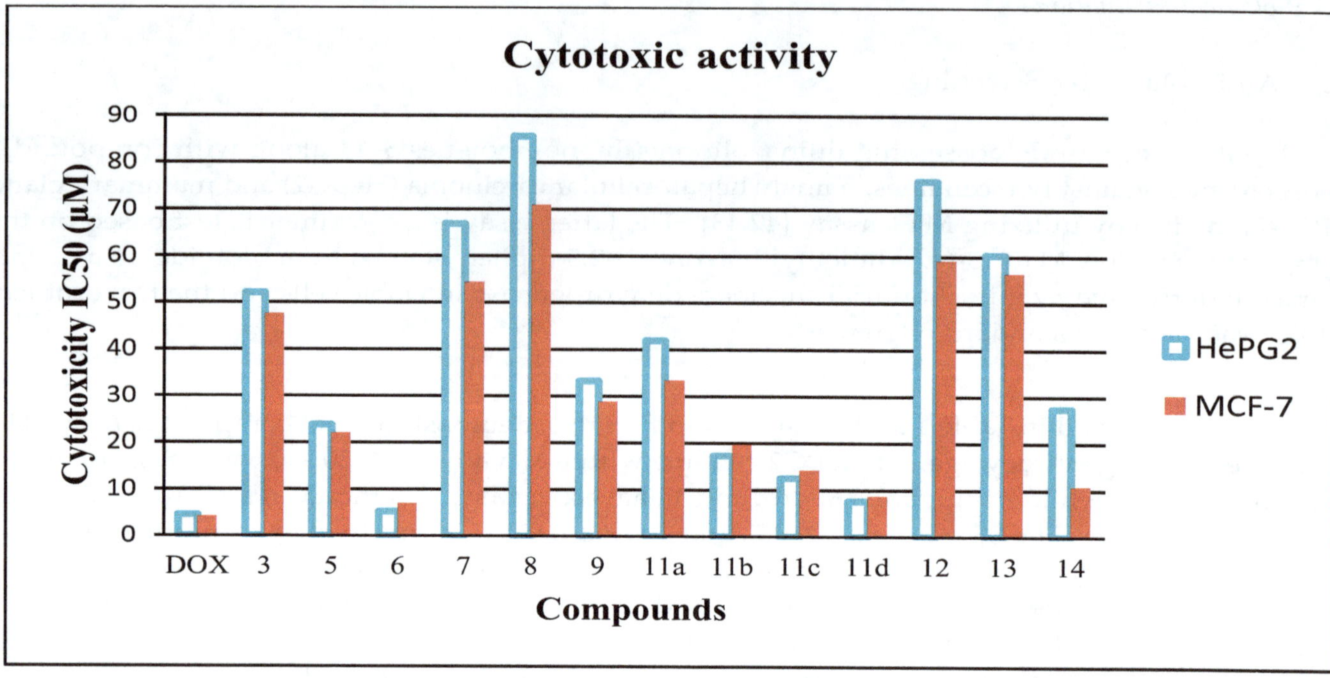

Figure 3. Cytotoxic efficacy of thirteen compounds against HePG2 and MCF-7 cell lines.

Through our screening of the antiproliferative efficacy of the synthesized compounds, it was determined that the average of relative viability of cells (%) with different concentrations such as 100, 50, 25, 12.5, 6.25, 3.125, and 1.56 µM against two cell lines (HePG2 and MCF-7) as shown in Figures 4 and 5.

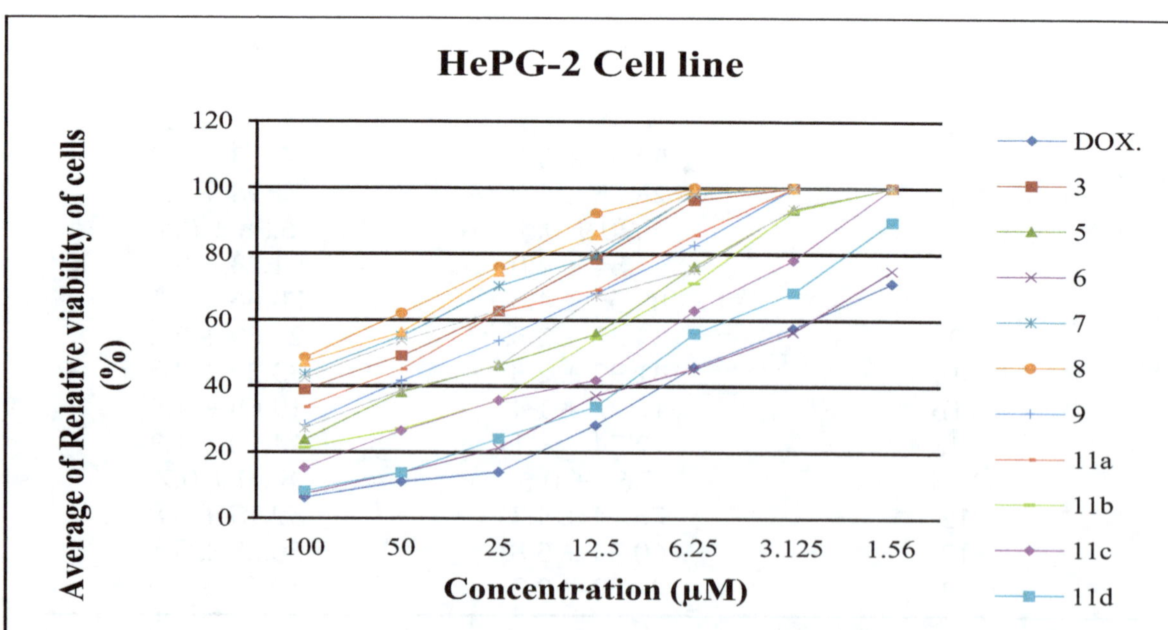

Figure 4. Average of relative viability of HePG-2 cell line (%) with different concentrations.

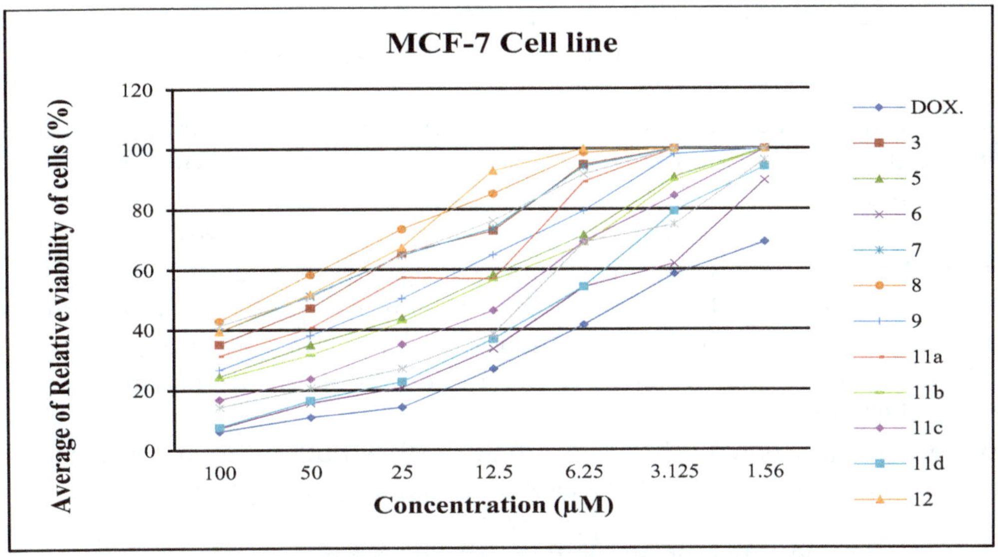

Figure 5. Average of relative viability of MCF-7 cell line (%) with different concentrations.

Structure Activity Relationship (SAR)

By comparing the antiproliferative efficacy of the thirteen synthesized compounds in this study to their chemical structures, it was concluded that the following structure activity relationship's (SAR's) is hypothesized:

1. Conversion of quinazolin-4(3*H*)-one derivative **5** to quinazolin-4(3*H*)-thione derivative **6** enhanced the antiproliferative activity against both cell lines from moderate activity to very strong activity.
2. Similarly, conversion of 3-amino-2-pentylquinazolin-4(3*H*)-one **9** to 3-amino-2-pentylquinazoline-4(3*H*)-thione **14** enhanced the antiproliferative activity against both cell lines.
3. Reaction of **9** with various aryl aldehydes afforded hydrazone derivatives **(11a–d)** analoges with variable potencies according to the following sequence: 3,5-$(OMe)_2$-4-OH-C_6H_2 **11d** > 3-OH-4-(OMe)-C_6H_3 **11c > ** 4-(OMe)-C_6H_4 **11b >** 4-Cl-C_6H_4 **11a**, whereas, the OH group in *p*-position is more electron donating group than the OMe group and Cl atom (i.e., the delocalization of n-π electrons decreased in the above sequence).
4. Construction of the thiazolidinone ring in compound **12** decreased the antiproliferative activity comparable with the hydrazone derivative **11a**, due to decreasing of the delocalization of n-π electrons after replacement of the C=N group (electron attracting group) by the thiazolidinone ring.

2.2.2. Antioxidant Activity Screening

One of the aims of this work is the screening of all synthesized compounds for antioxidant activity using two different methods, namely ABTS [2,2′-azino-bis(3-ethyl benzothiazoline-6-sulfonic acid)] and DPPH assays. DPPH (2,2-diphenyl-1-picryl-hydrazyl-hydrate) free radical assay based on electron-transfer that produces a violet solution in ethanol. This free radical is stable at ambient temperature and reduced in the presence of an antioxidant molecule, leading to colorless ethanol solution. After investigation of these results as listed in Table 2 and Figure 6, it was realized that, compounds **6** and **11d** have promising activity through using ABTS assay. Meanwhile, in the case of using DPPH assay, compounds **6, 11d** and **14** have also very high activity. Ascorbic acid was used as a reference through the antioxidant activity screening.

The results depicted in Table 2 and Figure 6 demonstrated that, DPPH assay findings are very approximately related to those of ABTS assay with only one exception, compound **14** has an excellent antioxidant activity against DPPH (IC_{50} = 26.87 ± 0.23 μM) than that of the ABTS method (IC_{50} = 71.42 ± 0.52 μM). Noteworthy, all the screened compounds in the case of the DPPH method exhibited IC_{50}

smaller than the corresponding ones of the same compounds in the case of the ABTS method, and it proposed that these compounds are more promising scavengers of the DPPH radical than those of the ABTS radical.

By comparing the antioxidant efficacy of the thirteen synthesized compounds in this study to their chemical structures, it was concluded that the following structure antioxidant activity relationship's (SAR's) is hypothesized:

1. The presence of C=S enhanced antioxidant activity than the presence of C=O, as shown in compounds **6** and **14** comparable with compounds **5** and **9**, respectively.

2. The hydrazone derivatives **(11a–d)** analogs have variable potencies according to the following sequence: 3,5-$(OMe)_2$-4-OH-C_6H_2 **11d** > 3-OH-4-(OMe)-C_6H_3 **11c** > 4-(OMe)-C_6H_4 **11b** > 4-Cl-C_6H_4 **11a**, whereas, OH group in *p*-position is a more electron donating group (has more conjugated system) than OMe group and Cl atom.

3. In compound **12**, replacement of C=N group by the thiazolidinone ring decreased the antioxidant activity comparable with **11a**, because of the lack of the conjugated system.

Table 2. Antioxidant activities of all synthesized compounds by using 2,2'-azino-bis(3-ethyl benzothiazoline-6-sulfonic acid (ABTS) and 2,2-diphenyl-1-picryl-hydrazyl-hydrate (DPPH) methods.

Compounds	ABTS IC_{50} (μM)	DPPH IC_{50} (μM)
Ascorbic acid	31.26 ± 0.20	16.83 ± 0.15
3	93.24 ± 0.70	52.14 ± 0.65
5	65.13 ± 0.46	41.16 ± 0.42
6	35.48 ± 0.23	19.25 ± 0.18
7	114.63 ± 0.73	59.43 ± 0.68
8	160.92 ± 0.94	92.36 ± 0.76
9	77.38 ± 0.56	46.23 ± 0.48
11a	89.10 ± 0.64	50.12 ± 0.54
11b	58.03 ± 0.41	38.47 ± 0.37
11c	52.87 ± 0.36	32.69 ± 0.29
11d	46.25 ± 0.28	22.91 ± 0.21
12	154.51 ± 0.85	73.03 ± 0.72
13	131.95 ± 0.77	65.58 ± 0.66
14	71.42 ± 0.52	26.87 ± 0.23

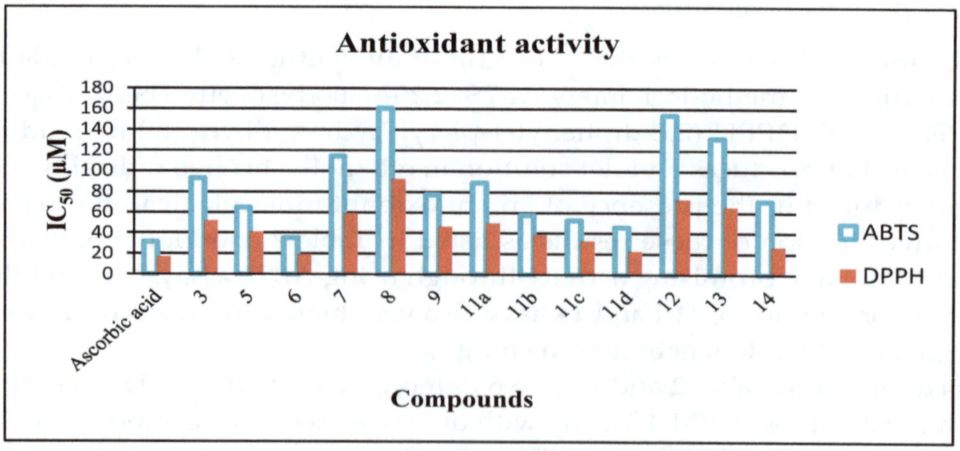

Figure 6. Antioxidant activities of all synthesized compounds by using ABTS and DPPH methods.

Previous reports of structurally similar compounds (in quinazoline ring) but with different substituents have demonstrated different results in antiproliferative and antioxidant activities from our results [9,33,44].

2.3. Density Functional Theory

According to the frontier molecular orbital (FMO) theory, the highest occupied molecular orbital (HOMO) acts as an electron-donor and the lowest unoccupied molecular orbital (LUMO) acts as an electron-acceptor [45]. Meanwhile, both play remarkable roles in the electronic studies by using quantum chemical calculations and they are also of significant importance in modern biochemistry and molecular biology [46]. A molecule is considered as a softer and has an excellent chemical reactivity when it has a smaller energy gap. Meanwhile, a molecule is considered to have a higher chemical hardness and assumed to have good stability when it has a larger energy gap [47–51].

The quantum chemical calculations were implemented by the density functional theory (DFT) method by using the Gaussian(R) 09 program at the B3LYP level in conjunction with 6-31G(d,p) basis set and computed parameters are summarized in Table 3.

By computing and using the energy gap ($\Delta E = E_{LUMO} - E_{HOMO}$) and dipole moment values beside another quantum chemical parameters such as ionization energy ($I = -E_{HOMO}$), electron affinity ($A = -E_{LUMO}$) [52], chemical hardness ($\eta = (I - A)/2$), chemical softness ($S = 1/\eta$) [53], and binding energy, we can rationally explicate the relation between the chemical structure and the antiproliferative activity (SAR's). Whereas, the energy gap of compound **6** ($\Delta E = 3.98$ eV) is smaller than that corresponding of compound **5** ($\Delta E = 4.85$ eV) and also compound **6** has a higher chemical softness value ($S = 0.50$ eV^{-1}) than that corresponding of compound **5** ($S = 0.41$ eV^{-1}). These results are matching with the results of the antiproliferative screening whereas, compound **6** has a higher potency comparable with compound **5** for both cell lines (HepG2 and MCF-7) as shown in Table 1 and Figure 3. Similarly, compound **14** has a smaller energy gap and a higher chemical softness than that corresponding to compound **9** as listed in Table 2. In addition, in vitro compound **14** showed a remarkable higher efficacy comparable with compound **9** as shown in Table 1 and Figure 3. Notably, the dipole moment values of compounds **6** ($\mu = 3.4641$ D) and **14** ($\mu = 1.852$ D) are higher than that of compounds **5** ($\mu = 3.2867$ D) and **9** ($\mu = 1.764$ D), respectively.

On the other hand, compounds **11a–d** possess antiproliferative activity in the following order **11d** > **11c** > **11b** > **11a**, meanwhile, the energy gaps of these compounds increase in the following order **11a** ($\Delta E = 2.99$ eV) < **11d** ($\Delta E = 3.05$ eV) < **11c** ($\Delta E = 3.10$ eV) < **11b** ($\Delta E = 3.13$ eV). The lower of the antiproliferative activity of compound **11a** may be explained by values of the dipole moment whereas; the dipole moment of compound **11a** is smaller than that of compounds **11b–d** as shown in Table 3.

Table 3. Quantum chemical parameters of the selected compounds with Density Functional Theory (DFT) at B3LYP/6-31G (d,p) basis set.

Comp. No.	5	6	9	14	11a	11b	11c	11d
E HOMO (eV)	−5.9432	−5.6352	−5.9405	−4.7724	−5.7277	−5.6363	−5.6717	−5.6602
E LUMO (eV)	−1.0917	−1.6515	−1.1298	−1.6836	−2.7301	−2.4983	−2.5709	−2.6009
(ΔE) Energy gap (eV)	4.8515	3.9837	4.8107	3.0888	2.9976	3.1380	3.1008	3.0593
(I) Ionization energy (eV)	5.9432	5.6352	5.9405	4.7724	5.7277	5.6363	5.6717	5.6602
(A) Electron affinity (eV)	1.0917	1.6515	1.1298	1.6836	2.7301	2.4983	2.5709	2.6009
(η) Chemical hardness (eV)	2.4258	1.9919	2.4054	1.5444	1.49881	1.56901	1.5504	1.52969
(S) Chemical softness (eV^{-1})	0.4122	0.5020	0.4157	0.6475	0.6672	0.6374	0.6450	0.6537
(E_T) Binding energy (a.u)	−689.79	−1012.73	−745.11	−1068.05	−1473.81	−1128.73	−1203.94	−1318.44
(μ) Dipole moment (D)	3.2867	3.4641	1.764	1.852	3.2722	4.4472	4.1944	6.232

The distributions of the HOMO and LUMO orbitals of the selected compounds are computed at the same level of the DFT theory and are provided in Figures 7 and 8. The results manifested that possible reactive sites exist as shown below:

1. The HOMO of compounds **5** and **9** are nearly similar and the distribution of orbitals are mainly situated on the quinazolinone moiety, also, the LUMO of these compounds are situated on the same moiety.

2. The HOMO of compounds **6** and **14** are nearly similar and the distribution of orbitals are mainly situated on C=S, while, the LUMO of these compounds are mainly situated on the quinazolinthione moiety.

3. The HOMO of compounds **11a–d** are nearly similar and the distribution of orbitals are mainly situated on the quniazolinone moiety, meanwhile, the LUMO of these compounds are mainly situated on the aryl aldehyde hydrazone system.

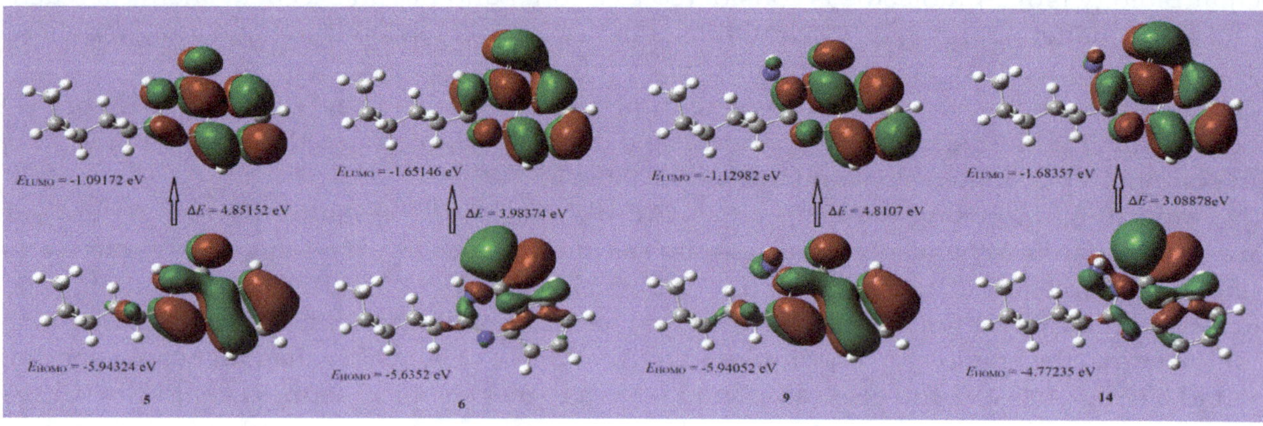

Figure 7. Schematic representation of HOMO and LUMO coefficient distribution of compounds **5, 6, 9,** and **14.**

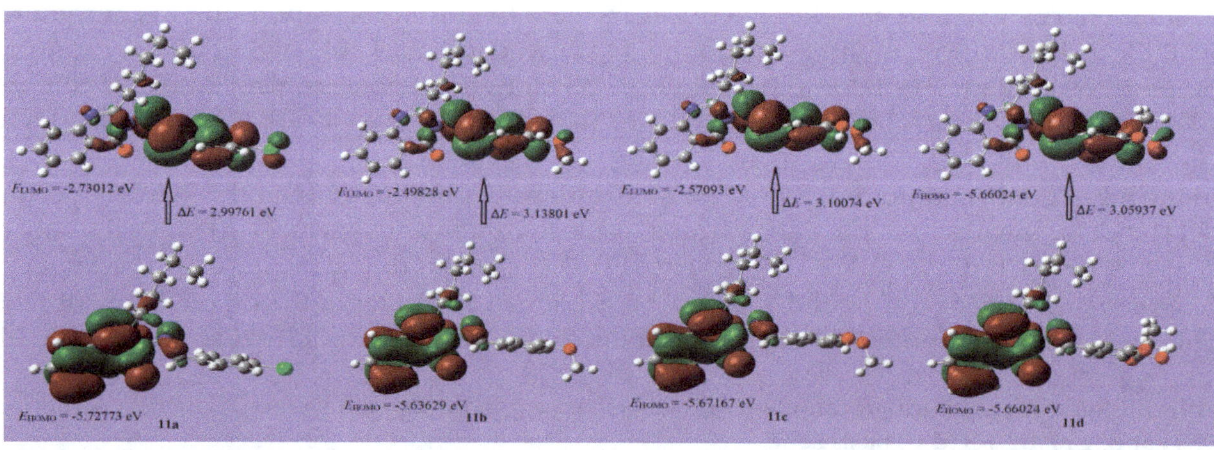

Figure 8. Schematic representation of highest occupied molecular orbital (HOMO) and loest unoccupied molecular orbital (LUMO) coefficient distribution of compounds **11a–d**.

3. Materials and Methods

3.1. Chemistry

The melting point is uncorrected and was measured on a Stuart SMP 30 advanced digital electric melting point apparatus (Cole-Parmer, Staffordshire, UK). All reactions were monitored by TLC (Kieselgel 60 F_{254}, Merck, Munchen, Germany) and spots were visualized using UV (254 nm), In the region (400–4000 cm^{-1}), the IR spectrum was measured in the KBr phase by using the Nicolet iS10 FT-IR spectrometer (Shimadzu Corporation, Kyoto, Japan). The ^{1}H-NMR (at 400 MHz) and ^{13}C-NMR (at 100 MHz) spectra were performed at chemical warfare labs, Egypt, with a Varian Gemini spectrometer (Metrohim, California, United States) in DMSO-d_6 as a solvent by using tetramethylsilane (TMS) as a reference. Perkin-Elmer 2400 CHN elemental analyzer (Waltham, MA, USA) was used to record CHN elemental analysis at the Faculty of Science, Cairo University, Egypt. The mass spectrum was measured on Shimadzu GC-MS QP1000EX apparatus (Shimadzu Corporation, Kyoto, Japan) at the central analytical lab, Ain Shams University, Cairo, Egypt.

3.1.1. 2-Hexanamidobenzoic Acid **3**

Hexanoyl chloride **2** (1.39 mL, 0.01 mol) was added dropwise to anthranilic acid **1** (1.37 g, 0.01 mol) dissolved in dry pyridine (20 mL) at ambient temperature with stirring. The stirring was continued for an hour, and then the resulting emulsion was acidified with cold 10% HCl solution. The white solid which separated was collected by filtration and then recrystallized from benzene to give **3** [38] as white crystals; m.p.: 92–95 °C (Lit. m.p.: 93–95 °C) [38], yield: 92%. IR (KBr, cm^{-1}): 3426–2463 (br) (OH), 3206 (NH), 2959, 2934, 2861 ($CH_{aliph.}$), 1691, 1637 (C=O). ^{1}H-NMR (400 MHz, DMSO-d_6) δ (ppm): 13.51 (br.s, 1H, OH, exchangeable with D_2O), 11.09 (s, 1H, NH, exchangeable with D_2O), 8.48 (d, 1H, Ar-H, H_a, J = 8.8 Hz), 7.95 (d, 1H, Ar-H, H_d, J = 8.0 Hz), 7.55 (t, 1H, Ar-H, H_c, J = 7.8 Hz, J = 8.0 Hz), 7.11 (t, 1H, Ar-H, H_b, J = 7.4 Hz, J = 7.8 Hz), 2.35 (t, 2H, $COCH_2$, J = 7.2 Hz, J = 7.6 Hz), 1.60 (quintet, 2H, $COCH_2\underline{CH_2}$, J = 7.2 Hz, J = 7.6 Hz), 1.31–1.26 (m, 4H, $CH_3\underline{CH_2CH_2}$), 0.85 (t, 3H, CH_3, J = 6.8 Hz, J = 7.2 Hz), MS m/z (%): 235 ($M^{\cdot+}$; 29.4). Anal. Calcd. for $C_{13}H_{17}NO_3$ (235.28): C, 66.36; H, 7.28; N, 5.95. Found: C, 66.36; H, 7.28; N, 5.95.

3.1.2. 2-Pentyl-4*H*-benzo[*d*][1,3]oxazin-4-one **4**

A suspension of 2-hexanamidobenzoic acid **3** (2.35 g, 0.01 mol) in freshly distilled acetic anhydride (10 mL) was heated in water bath for an hour followed by a concentration of the mixture in vacuo and used in situ [39,40].

3.1.3. 2-Pentylquinazolin-4(3*H*)-one **5**

A solution of benzoxazinone **4** (2.17 g, 0.01 mol) in formamide (15 mL) was refluxed for 7 h. After cooling, the reaction mixture was poured onto ice cold water, the obtained solid was filtered off, dried, and recrystallized from petroleum ether 60–80 °C to give **5** [41] as white crystals; m.p.: 142–144 °C (Lit. m.p.: 153–154 °C) [41], yield: 92%. IR (KBr, cm^{-1}): 3171 (NH), 2958, 2928, 2860 ($CH_{aliph.}$), 1680 (C=O), 1614 (C=N or C=C). ^{1}H-NMR (400 MHz, DMSO-d_6) δ (ppm): 12.13 (s, 1H, NH, exchangeable with D_2O), 8.05 (d, 1H, Ar-H, H_a, J = 8.0 Hz), 7.74 (t, 1H, Ar-H, H_c, J = 7.6 Hz, J = 7.8 Hz), 7.56 (d, 1H, Ar-H, H_d, J = 8 Hz), 7.42 (t, 1H, Ar-H, H_b, J = 7.6 Hz), 2.56 (t, 2H, N=CCH_2, J = 7.6 Hz, J = 8.0 Hz), 1.70 (quintet, 2H, N=$CCH_2\underline{CH_2}$, J = 7.6 Hz, J = 7.2 Hz), 1.30–1.26 (m, 4H, $CH_3\underline{CH_2CH_2}$), 0.84 (t, 3H, CH_3, J = 6.8 Hz, J = 7.2 Hz). ^{13}C-NMR (100 MHz, DMSO-d_6) δ (ppm): 162.2, 157.9, 149.4, 134.7, 127.2, 126.3, 126.1, 121.2, 34.9, 31.1, 26.9, 22.2, 14.2. MS m/z (%): 216 ($M^{\cdot+}$; 26.3). Anal. Calcd. for $C_{13}H_{16}N_2O$ (216.28): C, 72.19; H, 7.46; N, 12.95. Found: C, 72.26; H, 7.49; N, 12.86.

3.1.4. 2-Pentylquinazoline-4(3*H*)-thione **6**

To a solution of quinazolinone **5** (2.16 g, 0.01 mol) in dry toluene (30 mL), P_2S_5 (2.22 g, 0.01 mol) was added. The reaction mixture was refluxed for 1 h, and then filtered off. The obtained filtrate was evaporated under reduced pressure, the formed solid was collected by filtration, dried, and recrystallized from ethanol to give **6** as light brown crystals; m.p.: 101–103 °C, yield: 76%. IR (KBr, cm^{-1}): 3184, 3141 (NH), 2967, 2935, 2852 ($CH_{aliph.}$), 1618 (C=N), 1604 (C=C), 1236 (C=S). ^{1}H-NMR (400 MHz, DMSO-d_6) δ (ppm): 13.69 (s, 1H, NH, exchangeable with D_2O), 8.52 (d, 1H, Ar-H, H_d, J = 8.4 Hz), 7.83 (t, 1H, Ar-H, H_c, J = 7.6 Hz), 7.63 (d, 1H, Ar-H, H_a, J = 8.4 Hz), 7.52 (t, 1H, Ar-H, H_b, J = 7.4 Hz, J = 7.8 Hz), 2.70 (t, 2H, N=CCH_2, J = 7.6 Hz, J = 8.0 Hz), 1.72 (quintet, 2H, N=$CCH_2\underline{CH_2}$, J = 7.6 Hz, J = 7.2 Hz), 1.31–1.26 (m, 4H, $CH_3\underline{CH_2CH_2}$), 0.85 (t, 3H, CH_3, J = 6.8 Hz). MS m/z (%): 232 ($M^{\cdot+}$; 16.7). Anal. Calcd. for $C_{13}H_{16}N_2S$ (232.35): C, 67.20; H, 6.94; N, 12.06; S, 13.80. Found: C, 67.31; H, 7.03; N, 12.01; S, 13.85.

3.1.5. *N*-(β-D-Glucopyranosyl-2,3,4,6-tetraacetate)-2-pentylquinazolin-4(3H)-one **7**

Quinazolinone **5** (2.16 g, 0.01 mol) was refluxed with β-D-glucose pentaacetate (3.90 g, 0.01 mol) in absolute ethanol (50 mL) for 3 h. the solid obtained after slow evaporation of the resulting solution was collected and recrystallized from ethanol to give **7** as white crystals; m.p.: 135–137 °C, yield: 62%. IR (KBr, cm^{-1}): 2955, 2924, 2854 ($CH_{aliph.}$), 1746 ($C{=}O_{ester}$), 1678 ($C{=}O_{quinazolinone}$), 1613 (C=N). ^{1}H-NMR (400 MHz, DMSO-d_6) δ (ppm): 8.05 (d, 1H, Ar-H, H_a, J = 8.0 Hz), 7.74 (t, 1H, Ar-H, H_c, J = 8.4 Hz, J = 6.8 Hz), 7.56 (d, 1H, Ar-H, H_d, J = 8.4 Hz), 7.43 (t, 1H, Ar-H, H_b, J = 8.0 Hz, J = 7.2 Hz), 5.92 (d, 1H, C_1-H, J = 8.4 Hz), 5.39 (t, 1H, C_2-H, J = 9.6 Hz), 4.93 (t, 1H, C_3-H, J = 9.6 Hz), 4.90 (t, 1H, C_4-H, J = 8.4 Hz, J = 10.0 Hz), 4.14, 412 (d,d, 1H, C_6-H, J = 10.4 Hz, J = 5.6 Hz), 3.97 (d, 1H, C_6-H, J = 10.4 Hz), 3.51 (m, 1H, C_5-H), 2.56 (t, 2H, N=CCH_2, J = 8.0 Hz, J = 7.6 Hz), 1.978 (s, 3H, CH_3), 1.973 (s, 3H, CH_3), 1.961 (s, 3H, CH_3), 1.917 (s, 3H, CH_3), 1.69 (quintet, 2H, N=C$CH_2\underline{CH_2}$, J = 7.6 Hz, J = 6.8 Hz), 1.31−1.26 (m, 4H, $CH_3\underline{CH_2CH_2}$), 0.84 (t, 3H, CH_3, J = 6.8 Hz, J = 7.2 Hz). MS *m/z* (%): 546 (M^+; 32.4). Anal. Calcd. for $C_{27}H_{34}N_2O_{10}$ (546.57): C, 59.33; H, 6.27; N, 5.13. Found: C, 59.18; H, 6.21; N, 5.08.

3.1.6. 3-(2-Hydroxyethyl)-2-pentylquinazolin-4(3*H*)-one **8**

A solution of benzoxazinone **4** (2.17 g, 0.01 mol) in ethanolamine (15 mL) was heated under reflux for 3 h. The reaction mixture was poured onto ice cold water, the obtained solid was filtered off, dried, and then recrystallized from ethanol to give **8** as white crystals; m.p.: 84–85 °C, yield: 47%. IR (KBr, cm^{-1}): 3395 (OH), 2953, 2931, 2872 ($CH_{aliph.}$), 1648 (C=O), 1611 (C=N). ^{1}H-NMR (400 MHz, DMSO-d_6) δ (ppm): 8.07 (d, 1H, Ar-H, H_a, J = 8.0 Hz), 7.75 (t, 1H, Ar-H, H_c, J = 7.8 Hz, J = 7.6 Hz), 7.57 (d, 1H, Ar-H, H_d, J = 8.0 Hz), 7.44 (t, 1H, Ar-H, H_b, J = 7.6 Hz, J = 7.2 Hz), 4.95 (t, 1H, OH, exchangeable with D_2O, J = 5.6 Hz), 4.11 (t, 2H, $\underline{CH_2}CH_2OH$, J = 5.6 Hz, J = 6.0 Hz), 3.65 (q, 2H, $\underline{CH_2}OH$, J = 6.0 Hz, J = 5.6 Hz), 2.93 (t, 2H, N=C$\underline{CH_2}$, J = 7.6 Hz, J = 8.0 Hz), 1.75 (quintet, 2H, N=C$CH_2\underline{CH_2}$, J = 7.6 Hz, J = 7.6 Hz), 1.40−1.32 (m, 4H, $CH_3\underline{CH_2CH_2}$), 0.88 (t, 3H, CH_3, J = 7.2 Hz). ^{13}C-NMR (100 MHz, DMSO-d_6) δ (ppm): 161.7, 158.4, 147.4, 134.6, 127.1, 126.5, 126.4, 120.4, 58.8, 46.1, 34.6, 31.3, 26.3, 22.4, 14.3. MS *m/z* (%): 260 (M^+; 41.2). Anal. Calcd. for $C_{15}H_{20}N_2O_2$ (260.34): C, 69.20; H, 7.74; N, 10.76. Found: C, 69.17; H, 7.68; N, 10.81.

3.1.7. 3-Amino-2-pentylquinazolin-4(3*H*)-one **9**

A mixture of benzoxazinone **4** (2.17 g, 0.01 mol) and hydrazine hydrate (1.5 mL) in absolute ethanol (20 mL) was refluxed for 3 h. The mixture was poured onto ice cold water, the formed solid was filtered off, and recrystallized from ethanol to give **9** as buff crystals; m.p.: 58–60 °C, yield: 43%. IR (KBr, cm^{-1}): 3306, 3263 (NH_2), 2954, 2931, 2910, 2856 ($CH_{aliph.}$), 1673 (C=O), 1630 (C=N). ^{1}H NMR (400 MHz, DMSO-d_6) δ (ppm): 8.08 (d, 1H, Ar-H, H_a, J = 7.8 Hz), 7.75 (t, 1H, Ar-H, H_c, J = 7.4 Hz, J = 7.8 Hz), 7.59 (d, 1H, Ar-H, H_d, J = 7.6 Hz), 7.45 (t, 1H, Ar-H, H_b, J = 7.2 Hz, J = 7.6 Hz), 5.70 (s, 2H, NH_2, exchangeable with D_2O), 2.90 (t, 2H, N=CCH_2, J = 7.2 Hz, J = 8.0 Hz), 1.74 (quintet, 2H, N=C$\underline{CH_2}CH_2$, J = 7.6 Hz, J = 7.2 Hz), 1.37−1.30 (m, 4H, $CH_3\underline{CH_2CH_2}$), 0.87 (t, 3H, CH_3, J = 6.4 Hz, J =7.2 Hz). ^{13}C-NMR (400 MHz, DMSO-d_6) δ (ppm): 160.9, 158.8, 147.0, 134.3, 127.2, 126.39, 126.31, 120.2, 34.0, 31.4, 26.0, 22.3, 14.3. MS *m/z* (%): 231 (M^+; 41.1). Anal. Calcd. for $C_{13}H_{17}N_3O$ (231.30): C, 67.51; H, 7.41; N, 18.17. Found: C, 67.39; H, 7.34; N, 18.24.

3.1.8. General Procedure for Synthesis of **11a–d**

A mixture of compound **9** (2.31 g, 0.01 mol) and the appropriate aldehydes **10a–d** (0.01 mol) in absolute ethanol (30 mL) was refluxed for 4–6 h. The reaction mixture was evaporated under reduced pressure; the obtained residue was collected and recrystallized from the proper solvent to give the corresponding benzylidene derivatives **11a–d**, respectively.

3-((4-Chlorobenzylidene)amino)-2-pentylquinazolin-4(3*H*)-one **11a**

Yellow crystals; m.p.: 176–178 °C (ethanol), yield: 72%. IR (KBr, cm^{-1}): 2943, 2866 ($CH_{aliph.}$), 1667 (C=O), 1624 (C=N). ^{1}H-NMR (400 MHz, DMSO-d_6) δ (ppm): 8.69 (s, 1H, N=CH), 7.95 (d, 1H, Ar-H, H_a, J = 7.8 Hz), 7.88 (d, 2H, Ar-H, $H_E + H_F$, J = 8.8 Hz), 7.66 (t, 1H, Ar-H, H_c, J = 8.4 Hz), 7.57 (d, 3H, Ar-H, $H_d + H_X + H_Z$), 7.46 (t, 1H, Ar-H, H_b, J = 8.4 Hz), 2.34 (t, 2H, N=CCH_2, J = 7.6 Hz), 1.60 (quintet, 2H, N=CCH_2CH_2, J = 7.2 Hz), 1.31–1.26 (m, 4H, $CH_3CH_2CH_2$), 0.85 (t, 3H, CH_3, J = 6.8 Hz). MS *m/z* (%): 353 (M^+; 4.0). Anal. Calcd. for $C_{20}H_{20}ClN_3O$ (353.85): C, 67.89; H, 5.70; Cl, 10.02; N, 11.88. Found: C, 67.78; H, 5.62; Cl, 9.89; N, 11.79.

3-((4-Methoxybenzylidene)amino)-2-pentylquinazolin-4(3*H*)-one **11b**

White crystals; m.p.: 83–84 °C (petroleum ether 60–80 °C), yield: 64%. IR (KBr, cm^{-1}): 2946, 2912, 2882, 2843 ($CH_{aliph.}$), 1669 (C=O), 1606 (C=N or C=C). ^{1}H-NMR (400 MHz, DMSO-d_6) δ (ppm): 8.81 (s, 1H, N=CH), 8.12 (d, 1H, Ar-H, H_a, J = 7.8 Hz), 7.89 (d, 2H, Ar-H, $H_E + H_F$, J = 8.8 Hz), 7.80 (t, 1H, Ar-H, H_c, J = 8.2, Hz, J = 7.4 Hz), 7.65 (d, 1H, Ar-H, H_d, J = 8.0 Hz), 7.50 (t, 1H, Ar-H, H_b, J = 7.6, Hz, J = 7.4 Hz), 7.12 (d, 2H, Ar-H, $H_X + H_Z$, J = 8.8 Hz), 3.85 (s, 3H, OCH_3), 2.80 (t, 2H, N=CCH_2, J = 7.6 Hz, J = 8.0 Hz), 1.71 (quintet, 2H, N=CCH_2CH_2, J = 7.6 Hz, J = 7.2 Hz), 1.33–1.26 (m, 4H, $CH_3CH_2CH_2$), 0.81 (t, 3H, CH_3, J = 7.2 Hz). MS *m/z* 7(%): 349 (M^+; 11.). Anal. Calcd. for $C_{21}H_{23}N_3O_2$ (349.43): C, 72.18; H, 6.63; N, 12.03. Found: C, 72.29; H, 6.69; N, 11.88.

3-((3-Hydroxy-4-methoxybenzylidene)amino)-2-pentylquinazolin-4(3*H*)-one **11c**

White crystals; m.p.: 150–152 °C (ethanol), yield: 57%. IR (KBr, cm^{-1}): 3277 (OH), 2956, 2927, 2892, 2863, 2845 ($CH_{aliph.}$), 1678 (C=O), 1603 (C=N or C=C). ^{1}H-NMR (400 MHz, DMSO-d_6) δ (ppm): 9.49 (s, 1H, OH, exchangeable with D_2O), 8.70 (s, 1H, N=CH), 8.12 (d, 1H, Ar-H, H_a, J = 8.0 Hz), 7.79 (t, 1H, Ar-H, H_c, J = 8.0 Hz, J =8.4 Hz), 7.65 (d, 1H, Ar-H, H_d, J = 7.6 Hz), 7.49 (t, 1H, Ar-H, H_b, J = 8.0 Hz, J = 7.2 Hz), 7.42 (d, 1H, H_F, J_m = 2 Hz), 7.30, 7.28 (d,d, 1H, Ar-H, H_E, J_o = 8.4 Hz, J_m = 2 Hz), 7.07 (d, 1H, Ar-H, H_X, J = 8.4 Hz), 3.85 (s, 3H, OCH_3), 2.78 (t, 2H, N=CCH_2, J = 7.6 Hz), 1.71 (quintet, 2H, N=CCH_2CH_2, J = 7.6 Hz, J = 7.2 Hz), 1.31–1.28 (m, 4H, $CH_3CH_2CH_2$), 0.81 (t, 3H, CH_3, J = 6.8 Hz, J = 7.2 Hz). MS *m/z* (%): 365 (M^+; 23.4). Anal. Calcd. for $C_{21}H_{23}N_3O_3$ (365.43): C, 69.02; H, 6.34; N, 11.50. Found: C, 68.88; H, 6.28; N, 11.62.

3-((4-Hydroxy-3,5-dimethoxybenzylidene)amino)-2-pentylquinazolin-4(3*H*)-one **11d**

White crystals; m.p.: 148–150 °C (benzene), yield: 61%. IR (KBr, cm^{-1}): 3408 (OH), 2952, 2911, 2844 ($CH_{aliph.}$), 1668 (C=O), 1591 (C=N or C=C). ^{1}H-NMR (400 MHz, DMSO-d_6) δ (ppm): 9.36 (br.s, 1H, OH, exchangeable with D_2O), 8.72 (s, 1H, N=CH), 8.12 (d, 1H, Ar-H, H_a, J = 8.2 Hz), 7.79 (t, 1H, Ar-H, H_c, J = 8.0 Hz, J = 7.4 Hz), 7.65 (d, 1H, Ar-H, H_d, J = 7.6 Hz), 7.50 (t, 1H, Ar-H, H_b, J = 8.0 Hz, J = 7.2 Hz), 7.23 (s, 2H, $H_E + H_F$), 3.82 (s, 6H, 2OCH_3), 2.81 (t, 2H, N=CCH_2, J = 7.6 Hz, J = 8.0 Hz), 1.72 (quintet, 2H, N=CCH_2CH_2, J = 7.6 Hz, J = 7.2 Hz), 1.36–1.26 (m, 4H, $CH_3CH_2CH_2$), 0.81 (t, 3H, CH_3, J = 6.8 Hz, J =7.2 Hz). ^{13}C-NMR (100 MHz, DMSO-d_6) δ (ppm): 169.8, 158.0, 156.5, 148.6 (2), 146.7, 140.8, 134.6, 127.4, 127.0, 126.7, 122.8, 121.3, 106.8 (2), 56.5 (2), 34.5, 31.3, 26.0, 22.2, 14.2. MS *m/z* (%): 395 (M^+; 62.1), Anal. Calcd. for $C_{22}H_{25}N_3O_4$ (395.46): C, 66.82; H, 6.37; N, 10.63. Found: C, 66.95; H, 6.41; N, 10.58.

3.1.9. 2-(4-Chlorophenyl)-3-(4-oxo-2-pentylquinazolin-3(4*H*)-yl)thiazolidin-4-one **12**

A mixture of compound **11a** (3.53 g, 0.01 mol) and methyl thioglycolate (0.89 mL, 0.01 mol) in absolute ethanol (30 mL) containing piperidine (0.5 mL) was refluxed for 3 h. The obtained solid after evaporation of the solvent was collected and recrystallized from petroleum ether 60–80 °C to give **12** as pale yellow crystals; m.p.: 78–80 °C, yield: 47%. IR (KBr, cm^{-1}): 2951, 2925, 2868 ($CH_{aliph.}$), 1736 ($C=O_{thiazolidinone}$), 1671 ($C=O_{quinazolinone}$), 1608 (C=N or C=C). ^{1}H-NMR (100 MHz, DMSO-d_6) δ (ppm): 8.13 (d, 1H, Ar-H, H_a, J = 8.2 Hz), 7.96 (d, 2H, Ar-H, $H_E + H_F$, J = 8.0 Hz), 7.80 (t, 1H, Ar-H,

H_c, J = 7.6 Hz), 7.65 (d, 1H, Ar-H, H_d, J = 8.0 Hz), 7.64 (d, 2H, Ar-H, $H_X + H_Z$, J = 8.4 Hz), 7.51 (t, 1H, Ar-H, H_b, J = 7.6 Hz, J = 7.8 Hz), 5.70 (s, 1H, SCH), 3.75, 3.67 (d,d, 2H, $CH_{2(thiazolidinone)}$, J = 23.6 Hz, J = 23.2 Hz), 2.81 (t, 2H, N=CCH_2, J = 8.0 Hz, J = 7.6 Hz), 1.71 (quintet, 2H, N=$CCH_2\underline{CH_2}$, J = 7.6 Hz, J = 8.0 Hz), 1.35–1.17 (m, 4H, $CH_3\underline{CH_2CH_2}$), 0.80 (t, 3H, CH_3, J = 7.2 Hz). MS *m/z* (%): 427 (M^+; 11.8). Anal. Calcd. for $C_{22}H_{22}ClN_3O_2S$ (427.95): C, 61.75; H, 5.18; Cl, 8.28; N, 9.82; S, 7.49. Found: C, 61.66; H, 5.12; Cl, 8.31; N, 9.75; S, 7.55.

3.1.10. 4,5,6,7-Tetrachloro-2-(4-oxo-2-pentylquinazolin-3(4*H*)-yl)isoindoline-1,3-dione **13**

Compound **9** (2.31 g, 0.01 mol) was fused with 4,5,6,7-tetrachloroisobenzofuran-1,3-dione (2.85 g, 0.01 mol) in oil bath for an hour. The resulting solid was recrystallized from ethanol to give **13** as orange crystals; m.p.: 178–180 °C, yield: 86%. IR (KBr, cm^{-1}): 2943, 2856 ($CH_{aliph.}$), 1788, 1746 ($C{=}O_{imide}$), 1705 ($C{=}O_{quinazolinone}$), 1606 (C=N or C=C). ^{1}H-NMR (400 MHz, DMSO-d_6) δ (ppm): 8.08 (d, 1H, Ar-H, H_a, J = 8 Hz), 7.94 (t, 1H, Ar-H, H_c, J = 8.0 Hz, J = 7.2 Hz), 7.76 (d, 1H, Ar-H, H_d, J = 8.0 Hz), 7.60 (t, 1H, Ar-H, H_b, J = 7.6 Hz), 2.73 (t, 2H, N=CCH_2, J = 6.8 Hz, J = 8.0 Hz), 1.70–1.60 (m, 2H, N=$CCH_2\underline{CH_2}$), 1.29–1.27 (m, 4H, $CH_3\underline{CH_2CH_2}$), 0.81 (t, 3H, CH_3, J = 6.8 Hz, J =7.2 Hz). ^{13}C-NMR (100 MHz, DMSO-d_6) δ (ppm): 161.5, 161.3, 157.9, 157.7, 147.4, 146.7, 140.0, 138.8, 136.6 (2), 128.2 (2), 128.0, 127.1, 126.8, 119.8, 32.6, 30.9, 26.0, 22.2, 14.2. MS *m/z* (%): 231 (M^+; 41.1). Anal. Calcd. for $C_{21}H_{15}C_{14}N_3O_3$ (499.17): C, 50.53; H, 3.03; Cl, 28.41; N, 8.42. Found: C, 50.61; H, 3.09; Cl, 28.37; N, 8.53.

3.1.11. 3-Amino-2-pentylquinazoline-4(3*H*)-thione **14**

A mixture of compound **9** (2.31 g, 0.01 mol) and P_2S_5 (2.22 g, 0.01 mol) in dry toluene (15 mL) was heated under reflux for 4 h. The mixture was filtered off, the filtrate was evaporated under reduced pressure, the obtained solid was collected, dried, and recrystallized from ethanol to give **14** as yellow crystals; m.p.: 57–59 °C, yield: 53%. IR (KBr, cm^{-1}): 3240, 3200 (NH_2), 2925, 2855 ($CH_{aliph.}$), 1591 (C=N or C=C), 1238 (C=S). ^{1}H-NMR (400 MHz, DMSO-d_6) δ (ppm): 8.51 (d, 1H, Ar-H, H_a, J = 8.2 Hz), 7.82 (t, 1H, Ar-H, H_c, J = 7.6 Hz, J = 7.8 Hz), 7.69 (d, 1H, Ar-H, H_d, J = 7.6 Hz), 7.57 (t, 1H, Ar-H, H_b, J = 7.6 Hz), 7.04 (s, 2H, NH_2, exchangeable with D_2O), 3.06 (t, 2H, N=CCH_2, J = 7.2 Hz, J = 8.0 Hz), 1.81 (quintet, 2H, N=$CCH_2\underline{CH_2}$, J = 7.6 Hz, J = 7.2 Hz), 1.42–1.32 (m, 4H, $CH_3\underline{CH_2CH_2}$), 0.88 (t, 3H, CH_3, J = 6.8 Hz, J =7.2 Hz). ^{13}C NMR (100 MHz, DMSO-d_6) δ (ppm): 182.1, 155.5, 142.0, 134.5, 130.6, 128.1 (2), 127.4, 34.4, 31.3, 25.5, 22.4, 14.3. MS *m/z* (%): 247 (M^+; 74.3). Anal. Calcd. for $C_{13}H_{17}N_3S$ (247.36): C, 63.12; H, 6.93; N, 16.99; S, 12.96. Found: C, 63.19; H, 6.96; N, 17.11; S, 12.82.

3.2. Cytotoxicity and Antiproliferative Evaluation

MTT Assay

The implement of MTT methodology for the antiproliferative screening of quinazolinone derivatives **5–14** along with compound **3** against two cell lines, namely, hepatocellular carcinoma (HepG2) and mammary gland (MCF-7) were obtained from ATCC through the Holding company for biological products and vaccines (VACSERA), Cairo, Egypt. The reference anticancer drug used was Doxorubicin. The MTT assay was carried out at the pharmacology department, Faculty of pharmacy, Mansoura University, Egypt according to the reported literatures [42,43,54]. The cells were cultured in a RPMI-1640 medium with 10% fetal bovine serum, followed by the addition of antibiotics (100 units/mL penicillin and 100 μg/mL streptomycin) at 37 °C in a 5% CO_2 incubator. The cells were seeded in a 96-well plate at a density of (1.0×10^4 cells/well) at 37 °C for 48 h under 5% CO_2. Treatment of cells with different concentrations of compounds such as 100, 50, 25, 12.5, 6.25, 3.125, and 1.56 μM was carried out and placed in the incubator for 24 h. Then, 20 μL of MTT solution at 5 mg/mL was added and incubated for 4 h. DMSO (100 μL) was added into each well to dissolve the purple formazan formed. At 570 nm absorbance the colorimetric assay was measured and recorded by using a plate reader (BioTek EL ×800 Microplate Reader, BioTek Instruments, Inc, Winooski, VT, USA).

Calculation of the relative cell viability (%) = (A of treated samples /A of untreated sample) × 100.

3.3. *Antioxidant Assay*

3.3.1. Antioxidant Activity Screening Assay

ABTS Method

By the bleaching of ABTS derived radical cations, the detections of antioxidant activities were estimated. The radical cation was prepared by the reaction of ABTS [2,2′-azino-bis(3-ethyl benzothiazoline-6-sulfonic acid)] (60 μL) with MnO_2 (3 mL, 25 mg/mL) in a phosphate buffer solution (10 μM, pH 7, 5 mL). The solution was shaken for 3 min, centrifuged, filtered, and recorded at λ_{max} 734 nm the absorbance $A_{(control)}$ of the resulting ABTS radical solution (green-blue). Upon the addition of the tested sample solution (20 μl) with different concentrations of compounds such as 200, 100, 50, 25, and 12.5 μM in spectroscopic grade MeOH/buffer (1:1 *v*/*v*) to the ABTS solution, the absorbance $A_{(test)}$ was measured. The decreasing in the absorbance is expressed as % inhibition which was calculated according to the following equation [55]:

$$\% \text{ Inhibition} = [A_{(control)} - A_{(test)}/A_{(control)}] \times 100 \quad (1)$$

where; the reference and standard antioxidant compound in this test is the ascorbic acid solution (20 μL, 2 mM) and the blank sample was performed by the solvent without ABTS.

DPPH Method

According to the methodology described by Brand-Williams et al. [56], the measurement of the DPPH radical scavenging activity was implemented. The samples with different concentrations of compounds such as 200, 100, 50, 25, and 12.5 μM were allowed to react with the stable DPPH radical in ethanol solution. Whereas, the reaction mixture consisted of sample (0.5 mL), absolute ethanol (3 mL), and DPPH radical solution (0.3 mL) 0.5 mM in ethanol. DPPH is reduced when it reacts with an antioxidant compound, which can donate hydrogen. The changes in color (from deep violet to light yellow) were recorded [absorbance (*Abs*)] at λ_{max} 517 nm after 100 min of reaction using a UV-Vis spectrophotometer (Schimadzu Co., Tokyo, Japan). The blank solution was prepared by mixing ethanol (3.3 mL) and the sample (0.5 mL). Meanwhile, the mixture of ethanol (3.5 mL) and DPPH radical solution (0.3 mL) serve as a positive control.

The scavenging activity percentage (*AA* %) was determined according to Mensor et al. [57]:

$$AA\ \% = 100 - [(Abs_{(sample)} - Abs_{(blankl)}/Abs_{(control)}) \times 100] \quad (2)$$

3.4. *Computational Procedures*

All theoretical calculations and results of the studied compounds were implemented by utilizing Gaussian(R) 09 D.01 [58] (Semichem Inc., Shawnee Mission, KS, USA) by applying the DFT operation with the hybrid functional B3LYP level [59,60] in conjunction with the 6−31G(d,p) basis set. The visualization of these results was achieved using GaussView 6.0.16 software (Semichem Inc., Shawnee Mission, KS, USA).

4. Conclusions

In conclusion, this work focused on the study of the antiproliferative and antioxidant activities in vitro in addition to the theoretical calculation of the DFT theory of some novel quinazolinone(thione) derivatives **6–14**. Two main points were the principal targets; firstly, by comparing the activities of quinazolinone and quinazolinthione derivatives. Secondly, comparing the activities of four series of Schiff bases, that have quinazolinone moiety. The results of this study imply that the quinazolinthione derivatives **6** and **14** have promising potent antiproliferative activity comparable with quinazolinone derivatives **5** and **9**, respectively. According to the DFT study, compounds **6** and **14** have a smaller energy gap and a higher chemical softness than that of compounds **5** and **9**, respectively. Additionally, screening of various aryl aldehyde hydrazone derivatives **(11a–d)** analogs exhibited that the potency increased with increasing the electron donating group in *p*-position due to increasing of the conjugated system, and that was supported by the DFT study.

On the other hand, compounds **6** and **11d** showed promising antioxidant activity using ABTS assay. While in the DPPH assay, compounds **6, 11d,** and **14** have showed potent activities comparable to the ascorbic acid which was used as a reference drug. Noteworthy, the results of both antiproliferative and antioxidant activities for each compound individually are nearly the same.

Author Contributions: The listed authors contributed to this work as described in the following: A.A.E.-S., M.F.I., and A.E.-G.E.A. designed the research idea, implemented the synthesis and characterization of novel compounds, and contributed to the data interpretation. A.E.-G.E.A. and A.M.N. contributed to discuss the results, writing the original draft manuscript, and revisions. All authors read and approved the final manuscript.

References

1. Stewart, B.W.; Wild, C.P. (Eds.) *World Cancer Report*; International Agency for Research on Cancer: Lyon, France, 2014.
2. Spanò, V.; Montalbano, A.; Carbone, A.; Parrino, B.; Diana, P.; Cirrincione, G.; Castagliuolo, I.; Brun, P.; Issinger, O.G.; Tisi, S.; et al. Synthesis of a new class of pyrrolo[3,4-h]quinazolines with antimitotic activity. *Eur. J. Med. Chem.* **2014**, *74*, 340–357. [CrossRef] [PubMed]
3. Sordella, R.; Bell, D.W.; Haber, D.A.; Settleman, J. Gefitinib-sensitizing EGFR mutations in lung cancer activate anti-apoptotic pathways. *Science* **2004**, *305*, 1163–1167. [CrossRef] [PubMed]
4. Raymond, E.; Faivre, S.; Armand, J.P. Epidermal growth factor receptor tyrosine kinase as a target for anticancer therapy. *Drugs* **2000**, *60*, 15–23. [CrossRef] [PubMed]
5. Ko, H.C.; Wang, Y.H.; Liou, K.T.; Chen, C.M.; Chen, C.H.; Wang, W.Y.; Chang, S.; Hou, Y.C.; Chen, K.T.; Chen, C.F.; et al. Antiinflammatory effects and mechanisms of the ethanol extract of Evodia rutaecarpa and its bioactive components on neutrophils and microglial cells. *Eur. J. Pharmacol.* **2007**, *555*, 211–217. [CrossRef] [PubMed]
6. Keller, T.L.; Zocco, D.; Sundrud, M.S.; Hendrick, M.; Edenius, M.; Yum, J.; Kim, Y.J.; Lee, H.K.; Cortese, J.F.; Wirth, D.F.; et al. Halofuginone and other febrifugine derivatives inhibit prolyl-tRNA synthetase. *Nat. Chem. Biol.* **2012**, *8*, 311–317. [CrossRef]
7. El-Azab, A.S.; Eltahir, K.E. Synthesis and anticonvulsant evaluation of some new 2,3,8-trisubstituted-4(3*H*)-quinazoline derivatives. *Bioorg. Med. Chem. Lett.* **2012**, *22*, 327–333. [CrossRef]
8. Shcherbakova, I.; Balandrin, M.F.; Fox, J.; Ghatak, A.; Heaton, W.L.; Conklin, R.L. 3*H*-Quinazolin-4-ones as a new calcilytic template for the potential treatment of osteoporosis. *Bioorg. Med. Chem. Lett.* **2005**, *15*, 1557–1560. [CrossRef]
9. Reddy, A.G.; Babu, V.H.; Rao, Y.J.P. A review on quinazolines as anticancer agents. *J. Chem. Pharm.Sci.* **2017**, *10*, 1492–1504.
10. Mohamed, M.A.; Ayyad, R.R.; Shawer, T.Z.; Abdel-Aziz, A.A.-M.; El-Azab, A.S. Synthesis and antitumor evaluation of trimethoxyanilides based on 4(3*H*)-quinazolinone scaffolds. *Eur. J. Med. Chem.* **2016**, *112*, 106–113. [CrossRef]
11. Chinigo, G.M.; Paige, M.; Grindrod, S.; Hamel, E.; Dakshanamurthy, S.; Chruszcz, M.; Minor, W.; Brown, M.L. Asymmetric synthesis of 2,3-dihydro-2-arylquinazolin-4-ones: methodology and application to a potent fluorescent tubulin inhibitor with anticancer activity. *J. Med. Chem.* **2008**, *51*, 4620–4631. [CrossRef]
12. Kubo, K.; Shimizu, T.; Ohyama, S.; Murooka, H.; Iwai, A.; Nakamura, K.; Hasegawa, K.; Kobayashi, Y.; Takahashi, N.; Takahashi, K.; et al. Novel potent orally active selective VEGFR-2 tyrosine kinase inhibitors: synthesis, structure-activity relationships, and antitumor activities of *N*-phenyl-*N'*-{4-(4-quinolyloxy)phenyl}ureas. *J. Med. Chem.* **2005**, *48*, 1359–1366. [CrossRef] [PubMed]

13. Hour, M.-J.; Huang, L.-J.; Kuo, S.-C.; Xia, Y.; Bastow, K.; Nakanishi, Y.; Hamel, E.; Lee, K.-H. 6-Alkylamino- and 2,3-Dihydro-3′-methoxy-2-phenyl-4-quinazolinones and related compounds: Their synthesis, cytotoxicity, and inhibition of tubulin polymerization. *J. Med. Chem.* **2000**, *43*, 4479–4487. [CrossRef] [PubMed]
14. Takase, Y.; Saeki, T.; Watanabe, N.; Adachi, H.; Souda, S.; Saito, I. Cyclic GMP Phosphodiesterase inhibitors. 2. requirement of 6-substitution of quinazoline derivatives for potent and selective inhibitory activity. *J. Med. Chem.* **1994**, *37*, 2106–2111. [CrossRef] [PubMed]
15. Khodarahmi, G.; Jafari, E.; Hakimelahi, G.; Abedi, D.; Rahmani, K.M.; Hassanzadeh, F. Synthesis of some new quinazolinone derivatives and evaluation of their antimicrobial activities. *Iran, J. Pharm. Res.* **2012**, *11*, 789–797.
16. Venkatesh, R.; Kasaboina, S.; Jain, N.; Janardhan, S.; Holagunda, U.D.; Nagarapu, L. Design and synthesis of novel sulphamide tethered quinazolinone hybrids as potential antitumor agents. *J. Mol. Struct.* **2019**, *1181*, 403–411. [CrossRef]
17. Patel, M.B.; Kumar, S.P.; Valand, N.N.; Jasrai, Y.T.; Menon, S.K. Synthesis and biological evaluation of cationic fullerene quinazolinone conjugates and their binding mode with modeled Mycobacterium tuberculosis hypoxanthine-guanine phosphoribosyltransferase enzyme. *J. Mol. Model.* **2013**, *19*, 3201–3217. [CrossRef]
18. Mhaske, S.B.; Argade, N.P. the chemistry of recently isolated naturally occurring quinazolinone alkaloids. *Tetrahedron* **2006**, *62*, 9787–9826. [CrossRef]
19. Song, F.; Ren, B.; Yu, K.; Chen, C.; Guo, H.; Yang, N.; Gao, H.; Liu, X.; Liu, M.; Tong, Y.; et al. Quinazolin-4-one coupled with pyrrolidin-2-iminium alkaloids from marine-derived fungus Penicillium aurantiogriseum. *Mar Drugs.* **2012**, *10*, 1297–1306. [CrossRef]
20. Obafemi, C.A.; Fadare, O.A.; Jasinski, J.P.; Millikan, S.P.; Obuotor, E.M.; Iwalewa, E.O.; Famuyiwa, S.O.; Sanusi, K.; Yilmaz, Y.; Ceylan, Ü. Microwave-assisted synthesis, structural characterization, DFT studies, antibacterial and antioxidant activity of 2-methyl-4-oxo-1,2,3,4- tetrahydroquinazoline-2-carboxylic acid. *J. Mol. Struct.* **2018**, *1155*, 610–622. [CrossRef]
21. Patel, N.B.; Patel, V.N. New 2,3-disubstituted quinazolin-4 (3*H*)-ones as antimicrobial agents. *Ind. J. Heterocycl. Chem.* **2007**, *16*, 247–250.
22. Peet, N.P.; Baugh, L.E.; Sunder, S.; Lewis, J.E.; Matthews, E.H.; Olberding, E.L.; Shah, D.N. 3-(1*H*-Tetrazol-5-yl)-4(3*H*)-quinazolinone sodium salt (MDL 427): A new antiallergic agent. *J. Med. Chem.* **1986**, *29*, 2403–2409. [CrossRef] [PubMed]
23. Patil, A.; Barge, M.; Rashinkar, G.; Salunkhe, R. Aqueous hydrotrope: An efficient and reusable medium for a green one-pot, diversity-oriented synthesis of quinazolinone derivatives. *Mol. Divers.* **2015**, *19*, 435–445. [CrossRef] [PubMed]
24. Khattab, S.N.; Haiba, N.S.; Asal, A.M.; Bekhit, A.A.; Guemei, A.A.; Amer, A.; El-Faham, A. Study of antileishmanial activity of 2-aminobenzoyl amino acid hydrazides and their quinazoline derivatives. *Bioorg. Med. Chem. Lett.* **2017**, *27*, 918–921. [CrossRef] [PubMed]
25. Haghighijoo, Z.; Firuzi, O.; Hemmateenejad, B.; Emami, S.; Edraki, N.; Miri, R. Synthesis and biological evaluation of quinazolinone-based hydrazones with potential use in Alzheimer's disease. *Bioorg. Chem.* **2017**, *74*, 126–133. [CrossRef] [PubMed]
26. Mhaske, S.B.; Argade, N.P. Regioselective quinazolinone-directed ortho lithiation of quinazolinoylquinoline: practical synthesis of naturally occurring human DNA topoisomerase I poison luotonin a and luotonins B and E. *J. Organomet. Chem.* **2004**, *69*, 4563–4566. [CrossRef]
27. Houck, D.R.; Ondeyka, J.; Zink, D.L.; Inamine, E.; Goetz, M.A.; Hensens, O.D. On the biosynthesis of asperlicin and the directed biosynthesis of analogs in Aspergillus alliaceus. *J. Antibiot. (Tokyo)* **1988**, *41*, 882–891. [CrossRef]
28. He, L.; Li, H.; Chen, J.; Wu, X. Recent advances in 4(3*H*)-quinazolinone syntheses. *RSC Adv.* **2014**, *4*, 12065–12077. [CrossRef]
29. Chaudhuri, P.K. Echinozolinone, an alkaloid from Echinops echinatus. *Phytochemistry* **1987**, *26*, 587–589. [CrossRef]
30. Ramanathan, M.; Hsu, M.T.; Liu, S.T. Preparation of 4(3*H*)-quinazolinones from aryldiazonium salt, nitriles and 2-aminobenzoate via a cascade annulation. *Tetrahedron* **2019**, *75*, 791–796. [CrossRef]
31. Sales, Z.S.; Mani, N.S.; Allison, B.D. The synthesis of 2-amino-4(3*H*)-quinazolinones and related heterocycles via a mild electrocyclization of aryl guanidines. *Tetrahedron Lett.* **2018**, *59*, 1623–1626. [CrossRef]

32. Ismail, M.F.; El-sayed, G.A. Dodecanoyl isothiocyanate and *N'*-(2-cyanoacetyl)dodecane- hydrazide as precursors for the synthesis of different heterocyclic compounds with interesting antioxidant and antitumor activity. *Synth. Commun.* **2018**, *48*, 892–905. [CrossRef]
33. Ajani, O.O.; Audu, O.Y.; Aderohunmu, D.V.; Owolabi, F.E.; Olomieja, A.O. Review Article Undeniable Pharmacological Potentials of Quinazoline Motifs in Therapeutic Medicine. *Am. J. Drug Discov. Dev.* **2017**, *7*, 1–24. [CrossRef]
34. Abbas, S.Y.; El-Bayouki, K.A.M.; Basyouni, W.M. Utilization of isatoic anhydride in the syntheses of various types of quinazoline and quinazolinone derivatives. *Synth. Commun.* **2016**, *46*, 993–1035. [CrossRef]
35. Maiden, T.M.M.; Harrity, J.P.A. Recent developments in transition metal catalysis for quinazolinone synthesis. *Org. Biomol. Chem.* **2016**, *14*, 8014–8025. [CrossRef]
36. Rohokale, R.S.; Kshirsagar, U.A. Advanced Synthetic Strategies for Constructing Quinazolinone Scaffolds. *Synthesis* **2016**, *48*, 1253–1268. [CrossRef]
37. Youssef, Y.M.; El-Sayed, A.A.; Azab, M.E. Utility of Benzoxazin-4-one and 3-amino- quinazolin-4-one Derivatives as Precursors for Construction of Potent Insecticidal Heterocycles. *J. Heterocyclic Chem.* **2019**. [CrossRef]
38. Park, W.J.; Ma, E. Inhibition of PCAF histone acetyltransferase and cytotoxic effect of *N*-acylanthranilic acids. *Pharmacal. Res.* **2012**, *35*, 1379–1386. [CrossRef]
39. Li, W.; Wu, X.-F. Palladium-catalyzed carbonylative synthesis of benzoxazinones from *N*-(*o*-Bromoaryl)amides using paraformaldehyde as the carbonyl source. *J. Org. Chem.* **2014**, *79*, 10410–10416. [CrossRef]
40. Mahindroo, N.; Ahmed, Z.; Bhagat, A.; Bedi, K.L.; Khajuria, R.K.; Kapoor, V.K.; Dhar, K.L. Synthesis and structure-activity relationships of vasicine analogues as bronchodilatory agents. *Med. Chem. Res.* **2006**, *14*, 347–368. [CrossRef]
41. Zhang, W.; Meng, C.; Liu, Y.; Tang, Y.; Li, F. Auto-tandem catalysis with ruthenium: From o-aminobenzamides and allylic alcohols to quinazolinones via redox isomerization/acceptorless dehydrogenation. *Adv. Synth. Catal.* **2018**, *360*, 3751–3759. [CrossRef]
42. Mosmann, T. Rapid colorimetric assay for cellular growth and survival: application to proliferation and cytotoxicity assays. *J. Immunol. Methods* **1983**, *65*, 55–63. [CrossRef]
43. Denizot, F.; Lang, R. Rapid colorimetric assay for cell growth and survival. Modifications to the tetrazolium dye procedure giving improved sensitivity and reliability. *J. Immunol. Methods* **1986**, *89*, 271–277. [CrossRef]
44. He, D.; Wang, M.; Zhao, S.; Shu, Y.; Zeng, H.; Xiao, C.; Lu, C.; Liu, Y. Pharmaceutical prospects of naturally occurring quinazolinone and its derivatives. *Fitoterapia* **2017**, *119*, 136–149. [CrossRef] [PubMed]
45. Karunakaran, V.; Balachandran, V. FT-IR, FT-Raman spectra, NBO, HOMO-LUMO and thermodynamic functions of 4-chloro-3-nitrobenzaldehyde based on ab initio HF and DFT calculations. *Spectrochim. Acta A* **2012**, *98*, 229–239. [CrossRef] [PubMed]
46. Ayyamperumal, N.; Balachandran, V.; Thangavel, K. Molecular structure, vibrational spectra, first hyperpolarizability and HOMO-LUMO analysis of p-acetylbenzonitrile using quantum chemical calculation. *J. Mol. Struct.* **2013**, *1038*, 134–144. [CrossRef]
47. Prashanth, J.; Ramesh, G.; Naik, J.L.; Ojha, J.K.; Reddy, B.V. Molecular geometry, NBO analysis, Hyperpolarizability and HOMO-LUMO energies of 2-azido-1-phenylethanone using Quantum chemical calculations. *Mater. Today Proc.* **2016**, *3*, 3761–3769. [CrossRef]
48. Al-Omary, F.A.M.; Mary, Y.S.; Panicker, C.Y.; El-Emam, A.A.; Al-Swaidan, I.A.; Al-Saadi, A.A.; Alsenoy, C.V. Spectroscopic investigations, NBO, HOMO-LUMO, NLO analysis molecular docking of 5-(adamantan-1-yl)-3anilinomethyl-2,3-dihydro-1,3,4-oxadiazole-2-thione, a potential bioactive agent. *J. Mol. Struct.* **2015**, *1096*, 1–14. [CrossRef]
49. Koparir, M.; Orek, C.; Koparir, P.; Sarac, K. Synthesis, experimental, theoretical characterization and biological activities of4-ethyl-5-(2-hydroxyphenyl)-2*H*-1,2,4-triazole- 3(4*H*)-thione. *Spectrochim. Acta, Part A* **2013**, *105*, 522–531. [CrossRef]
50. Fleming, I. *Frontier Orbitals and Organic Chemical Reactions*; John Wiley & Sons: New York, NY, USA, 1976.
51. Şahin, Z.S.; Kantar, G.K.; Şaşmaz, S.; Büyükgüngör, O. Synthesis, molecular structure, spectroscopic analysis, thermodynamic parameters and molecular modeling studies of (2-methoxyphenyl)oxalate. *J. Mol. Struct.* **2015**, *1087*, 104–112. [CrossRef]
52. Koopmans, T. Über die Zuordnung von Wellenfunktionen und Eigenwerten zu den Einzelnen Elektronen Eines Atoms. *Physica* **1934**, *1*, 104–113. [CrossRef]

53. Pearson, R.G. Absolute electronegativity and hardness correlated with molecular orbital theory. *Proc. Natl. Acad. Sci. USA.* **1986**, *83*, 8440–8441. [CrossRef] [PubMed]
54. Ismail, M.F.; El-sayed, A.A. Synthesis and in-vitro antioxidant and antitumor evaluation of novel pyrazole-based heterocycles. *J. Iran. Chem. Soc.* **2019**, *16*, 921–937. [CrossRef]
55. Lissi, E.A.; Modak, B.; Torres, R.; Escobar, J.; Urzua, A. Total antioxidant potential of resinous exudates from Heliotropium species, and a comparison of the ABTS and DPPH methods. *Free Radic. Res.* **1999**, *30*, 471. [CrossRef] [PubMed]
56. Brand-Williams, W.; Cuvelier, M.E.; Berset, C. use of a free radical method to evaluate antioxidant activity. *Lebensm. Wiss. Technol.* **1995**, *28*, 25–30. [CrossRef]
57. Mensor, L.L.; Menezes, F.S.; Leitao, G.G.; Reis, A.S.; dos Santos, T.C.; Coube, C.S.; Leitão, S.G. Screening of Brazilian plant extracts for antioxidant activity by the use of DPPH free radical method. *Phytother. Res.* **2001**, *15*, 127–130. [CrossRef]
58. Frisch, M.J.; Trucks, G.W.; Schlegel, H.B.; Scuseria, G.E.; Robb, M.A.; Cheeseman, J.R.; Scalmani, G.; Barone, V.; Mennucci, B.; Petersson, G.A.; et al. *Gaussian 09, Revision D.01*; Gaussian Inc.: Wallingford, CT, USA, 2009.
59. Becke, A.D. Density-functional exchange-energy approximation with correct asymptotic behavior. *Phys. Rev. A* **1988**, *38*, 3098–3100. [CrossRef]
60. Lee, C.; Yang, W.; Parr, R.G. Development of the Colle-Salvetti correlation-energy formula into a functional of the electron density. *Phys. Rev. B* **1988**, *37*, 785–789. [CrossRef]

9

Anti-Cancer Effect of 3-Hydroxy-β-Ionone Identified from *Moringa oleifera* Lam. Leaf on Human Squamous Cell Carcinoma 15 Cell Line

Thitiya Luetragoon [1,2], Rungnapa Pankla Sranujit [3], Chanai Noysang [3], Yordhathai Thongsri [1], Pachuen Potup [1], Nungruthai Suphrom [4], Nitra Nuengchamnong [5] and Kanchana Usuwanthim [1,*]

1 Cellular and Molecular Immunology Research Unit, Faculty of Allied Health Sciences, Naresuan University, Phitsanulok 65000, Thailand; nok.hong.yok49@gmail.com (T.L.); yordhathai.k@gmail.com (Y.T.); pachuenp@nu.ac.th (P.P.)

2 Faculty of Medicine, School of Human Development and Health, University of Southampton, Southampton SO16 6YD, UK

3 Thai Traditional Medicine College, Rajamangala University of Technology Thanyaburi, Pathum Thani 12130, Thailand; rungnapa_s@rmutt.ac.th (R.P.S.); chanai_n@rmutt.ac.th (C.N.)

4 Department of Chemistry, Faculty of Science and Center of Excellence for Innovation in Chemistry, Naresuan University, Phitsanulok 65000, Thailand; suphrom.n1@gmail.com

5 Science Laboratory Centre, Faculty of Science, Naresuan University, Phitsanulok 65000, Thailand; Nitran@nu.ac.th

* Correspondence: kanchanau@nu.ac.th;

Academic Editors: José Antonio Lupiáñez, Amalia Pérez-Jiménez, Eva E. Rufino-Palomares and José Rubén Tormo

Abstract: Squamous cell carcinoma is the most common type of head and neck cancer worldwide. Radiation and chemotherapy are general treatments for patients; however, these remedies can have adverse side effects and tumours develop drug resistance. Effective treatments still require improvement for cancer patients. Here, we investigated the anti-cancer effect of *Moringa oleifera* (MO) Lam. leaf extracts and their fractions, 3-hydroxy-β-ionone on SCC15 cell line. SCC15 were treated with and without MO leaf extracts and their fractions. MTT assay was used to determine cell viability on SCC15. Cell cycle and apoptosis were evaluated by the Muse™ Cell Analyser. Colony formation and wound closure analysis of SCC15 were performed in 6-well plates. Apoptosis markers were evaluated by immunoblotting. We found that Moringa extracts and 3-HBI significantly inhibited proliferation of SCC15. Moreover, they induced apoptosis and cell cycle arrest at G2/M phase in SCC15 compared to the untreated control. MO extracts and 3-HBI also inhibited colony formation and cell migration of SCC15. Furthermore, we observed the upregulation of cleaved caspase-3 and Bax with downregulation of anti-apoptotic Bcl-2, indicating the induction of cancer cell apoptosis. Our results revealed that MO extracts and 3-HBI provided anti-cancer properties by inhibiting progression and inducing apoptosis of SCC15.

Keywords: squamous cell carcinoma; *Moringa oleifera*; anti-cancer; 3-hydroxy-β-ionone

---

1. Introduction

Cancer is a noncommunicable disease and the leading cause of death worldwide. Around 18.1 million new cases of cancer and 9.6 million deaths from the disease were reported in 2018 [1]. Global incidences of head and neck squamous cell carcinoma (HNSCC) were reported at more than 830,000 cases with 430,000 deaths each year [2]. Major risk factors of HNSCC are high smoking levels and alcohol consumption [3]. HNSCC arises from the mucosal surfaces at various sites including skin, nasal cavity, paranasal sinuses, oral cavity, salivary glands, pharynx and larynx [4]. Treatment for HNSCC usually involves therapy with surgery, radiation, chemotherapy, targeted therapy, immunotherapy and combination therapy [2]. Nevertheless, these treatments result in adverse effects including nausea, vomiting, fatigue, mucositis, dysphagia and dermatitis [5]. Major hallmarks during cancer development include the ability to proliferate, evade apoptosis, uncontrolled replicative potential, induction of angiogenesis and tissue invasion and metastasis to other organs. Hence, many drugs and treatment methods have been developed to interfere with each step and impede tumour growth and progression [6]. The goal of medical scientists and researchers is to improve the best treatment for good quality of life for cancer patients. Therefore, targeted therapy and alternative low toxic treatments have received intense focus. Several studies have examined the effects of natural products against tumours by inducing apoptosis via the P53 tumour suppressor and reactive oxygen species production [7–9].

Moringa oleifera Lam. (MO) is known as the miracle tree and is widely cultivated in Asia and Africa. All the different parts of MO have been reported to have medicinal use [10]. The leaves of this plant have been intensively studied and contain high amounts of vitamins, carotenoids, polyphenols, phenolic acids, flavonoids, alkaloids, glucosinolates, isothiocyanates, tannins and saponins [11]. Many studies have reported on the biological activities of Moringa leaf such as antidiabetic [12], antioxidant [13], antibacterial [14] and kidney and hepatic protective effect [15,16]. Our previous study demonstrated that MO leaf extract provides anti-inflammatory potential by reducing the production of pro-inflammatory mediators such as interleukin-6, tumour necrosis factor-α and cyclooxygenase-2 via inactivation of NF-κB, inhibiting both IκB-α degradation and nuclear translocation of p65 [17,18]. 3-hydroxy-β-ionone (3-HBI) derived from MO leaf extract (Figure 1) had potent anti-inflammatory effects [17], while *in vitro* studies showed that soluble extract from MO leaf induced apoptosis and inhibited tumour cell growth in human non-small cell lung cancer A549 and human hepatocellular carcinoma HepG2 cells [19,20]. Another *in vitro* study reported that MO leaf extract and its compounds including eugenol, isopropyl isothiocyanate, D-allose and hexadeconoic acid ethyl ester decreased cell motility and colony formation, inhibited cell growth and triggered cell apoptosis against breast cancer and colorectal cancer cell lines [21]. Astragalin and isoquercetin from bioactive fractions of *M. oleifera* leaf extract suppressed proliferation of HCT116 colon cancer cells by downregulation of ERK1/2 phosphorylation [22]. In addition, glucomoringin from *Moringa oleifera* induced oxidative stress and apoptosis via p53 and Bax activation and Bcl-2 inhibition in human astrocytoma grade IV CCF-STTG1 cells [23], and also promoted apoptosis of SH-SY5Y human neuroblastoma cells through the modulation of NF-κB and apoptotic factors [24]. However, the effect of MO leaf extract on squamous cell carcinoma (SCC) 15 cell line remains unknown.

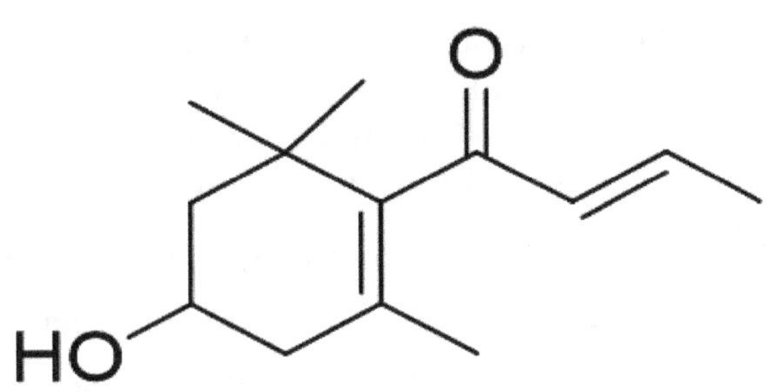

Figure 1. Structure of 3-hydroxy-β-ionone.

In this study, crude EtOAc extracts and MO-derived fractions were tested for anti-SCC15 activities. Active MO-derived fractions were fraction no. 6, sub-fraction no. 6.17.2, LC-MS base peak chromatogram no. 6 identified as 3-HBI (BPC6) and 3-HBI. Our findings revealed that MO leaf extract and its active compound, 3-HBI strongly inhibited tumour cell growth and triggered apoptosis via over-expression of cleaved caspase-3 and Bax, while down-regulating the anti-apoptotic Bcl-2.

2. Results

2.1. Cellular Cytotoxicity of MO Extract, Fraction, and Sub-Fraction on Human Monocyte-Derived Macrophages and SCC15

MTT was developed to evaluate the optimal concentration of antiproliferative effect of Moringa extracts, compound, and drugs. Human monocyte-derived macrophages (MDMs) and SCC15 were treated with different concentrations of extracts, compound, and cisplatin for 24 h. The half maximal inhibitory concentrations (IC_{50}) values of Moringa extracts, compound and drug are shown in Figure 2A,B. A five percent inhibitory concentration (IC_5) results of 3-HBI and cisplatin on MDMs were 18.46 µg/mL and 5.32 µg/mL, respectively (Figure 2A). While IC_5 of crude ethyl acetate (EtOAc) and fraction no. 6 were 26.84 µg/mL and 84.89 µg/mL [17]. These concentrations were used as the non-toxic optimal concentration for cell culture treatment. IC_{50} values of 3-HBI and cisplatin were 487.53 µg/mL and 21.33 µg/mL, respectively (Figure 2A). The IC_{50} values of crude EtOAc, fraction no. 6, 3-HBI and cisplatin on SCC15 cell line were 214.28, 114.55, 243.22 and 28.44 µg/mL, respectively (Figure 2B). Crude EtOAc, fraction no. 6 and 3-HBI showed a strong effect in inhibiting the proliferation of SCC15 cancer cells with lower IC_{50} values compared to primary MDM.

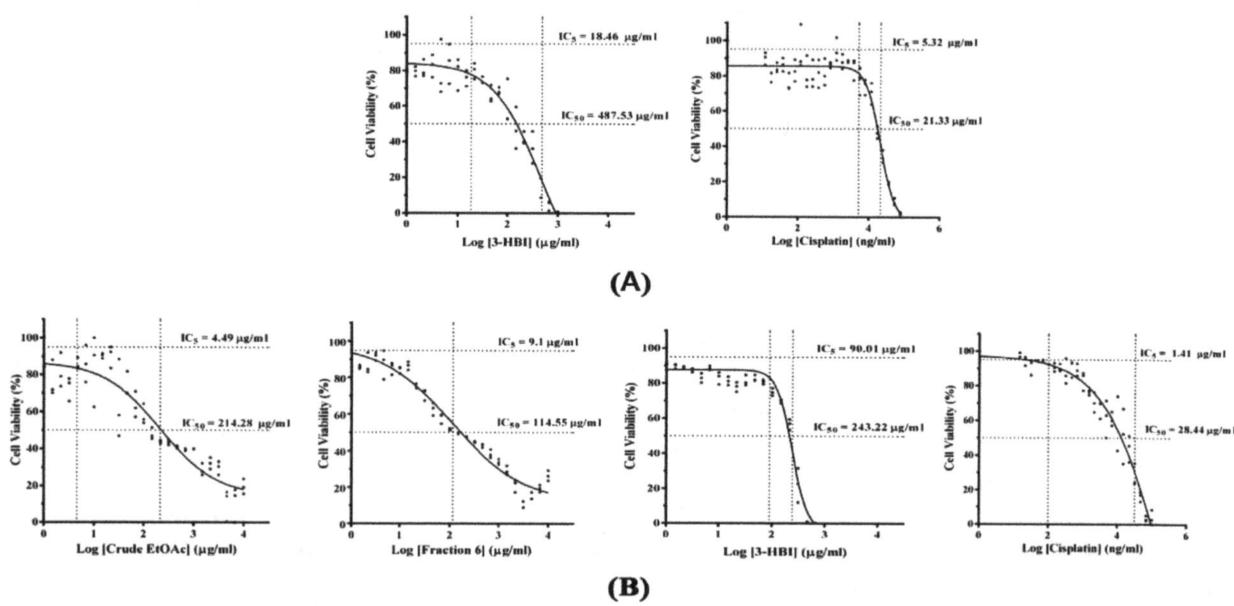

Figure 2. Investigation of the effect of MO crude extracts, fraction no. 6, 3-HBI and cisplatin on cell viability of MDMs and SCC15 cell lines. MTT assay was performed after cell treatment for 24 h. (**A**) IC_5 and IC_{50} results of MDMs after treatment with different concentrations of crude extract, fraction no. 6, 3-HBI and cisplatin. (**B**) IC_{50} results for antiproliferative effect of crude extract, fraction no.6, 3-HBI and cisplatin on SCC15. IC: inhibitory concentration; 3-HBI: 3-hydroxy-β-ionone.

2.2. Effect of MO Extract, Fraction, and Sub-Fraction on Cell Cycle of SCC15

Cell cycle assay was assessed using Muse™ Cell Cycle Kit. The nuclear DNA of the cell line was intercalated with propidium iodide (PI). Cells were discriminated at different phases of the cell cycle based on differential DNA content including G0/G1, S and G2/M phase. To investigate the effect of cisplatin, crude MO extract, fraction no. 6, sub-fraction no. 6.17.2, BPC6 (LC-MS base peak chromatogram no. 6 identified as 3-HBI), and 3-HBI on cell cycle progression, both untreated and treated SCC15 were investigated by Muse™ Cell Analyser. Figure 3A shows the DNA content index histogram of the control and treated cells in each cell cycle phase (G0/G1, S and G2/M). The bar graphs demonstrate that the percentage of cells in G2/M stages. After treatment with cisplatin, crude EtOAc, fraction no. 6, sub-fraction no. 6.17.2, BPC6, and 3-HBI, the G2/M enrichment phase significantly increased in SCC15 compared to the untreated control (Figure 3B). This result indicates that crude

EtOAc, fraction no. 6, sub-fraction no. 6.17.2, BPC6, and 3-HBI significantly increased cell cycle arrest at G2/M phase in SCC15.

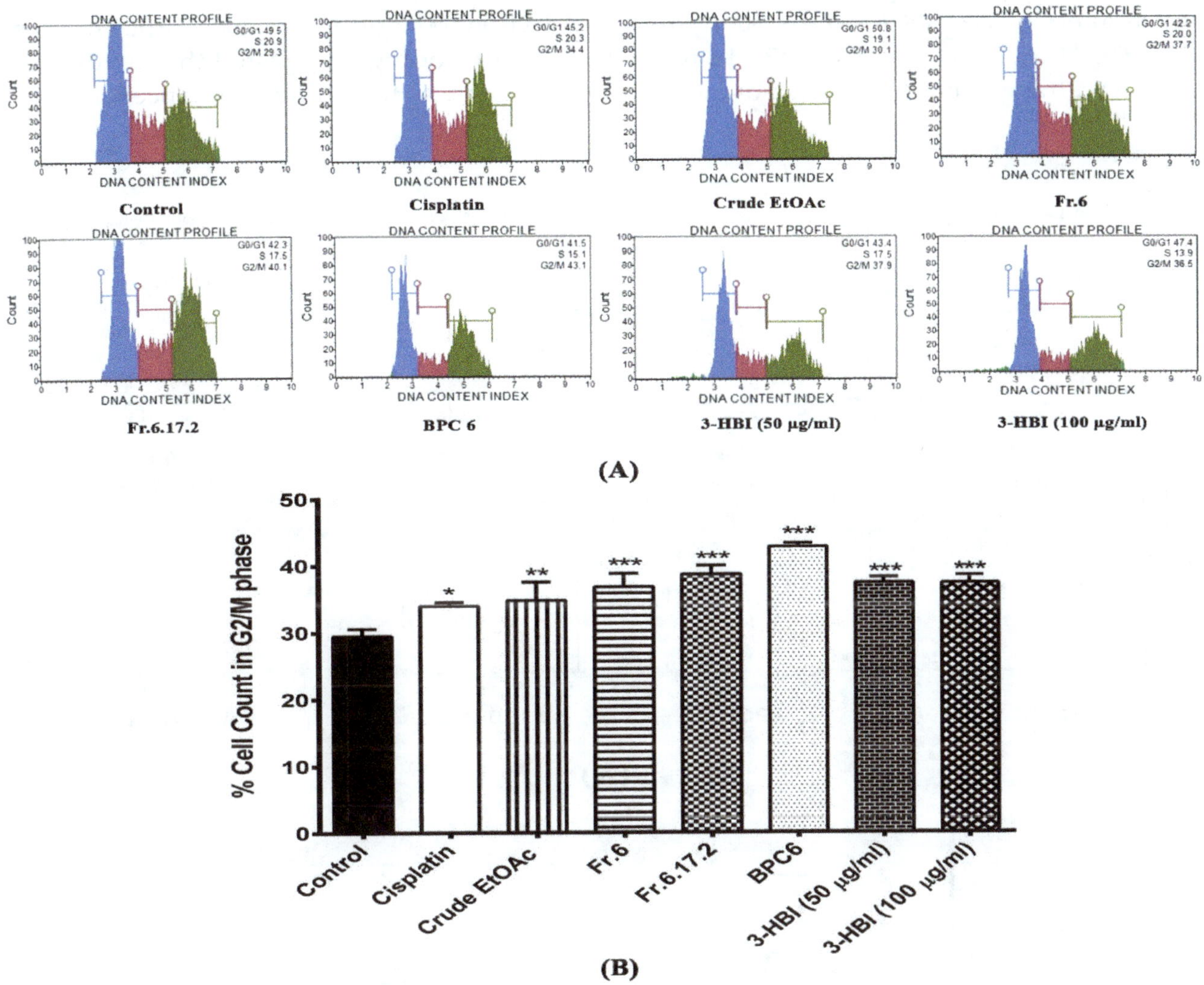

Figure 3. Efficacy of MO extract, fraction no. 6, sub-fraction no. 6.17.2, BPC6, and 3-HBI on distribution of SCC15 in the cell cycle analysed by Muse™ Cell Analyser. (**A**) DNA content index histogram of cell populations in each phase of the cell cycle in SCC15 cell line after treatment with cisplatin, crude EtOAc, Fr.6, Fr.6.17.2, BPC6, and 3-HBI for 24 h. (**B**) Bar graphs of percentage of cell in G2/M phase for SCC15 cell line. Data are presented as means ± SEM. * $p \leq 0.05$, ** $p \leq 0.01$, and *** $p \leq 0.001$ compared to control. Control: untreated SCC15; crude EtOAc: crude ethyl acetate; Fr.6: fraction no. 6; Fr.6.17.2: sub-fraction no. 6.17.2; BPC6: base peak chromatogram no. 6; 3-HBI: 3-hydroxy-β-ionone.

2.3. MO Extract, Fraction, and Sub-Fraction Induce Apoptosis in SCC15

We next evaluated the induction of apoptosis in SCC15 cell line after 24 h of treatment with MO extract, fraction no. 6, sub-fraction no. 6.17.2, BPC6, and 3-HBI. Apoptosis assay was performed by Muse™ Cell Analyser using the Muse™ Annexin V & Dead Cell Kit procedure with dot plots of SCC15 cell line stained with annexin V and 7-AAD (7-amino-actinomycin D). The first and second quadrants represent dead cells and late apoptotic cells, respectively, while the third and fourth quadrants represent live cells and early apoptotic cells, respectively, as shown in Figure 4A. These dot plots reveal that crude EtOAc, fraction no. 6 and sub-fraction no. 6.17.2 triggered late apoptosis and cell death in SCC15 cell line. Interestingly, BPC6 and 3-HBI induced early and late apoptotic cells similar to cisplatin. Figure 4B shows the statistical analysis of total apoptotic cells represented in the form of bar graphs. We observed a significantly increased percentage of total apoptotic cells (early and late apoptosis) after treatment with crude EtOAc, fraction no. 6, sub-fraction no. 6.17.2, BPC6, and 3-HBI compared to the untreated control ($p < 0.001$). The average percentage of total apoptotic cells increased from 4.41% in the control to 31.62% in cisplatin treatment. Moreover, treatment with crude EtOAc, fraction no. 6, sub-fraction no. 6.17.2, BPC6, 3-HBI (50 μg/mL), and 3-HBI (100 μg/mL) enhanced apoptotic cells to 17.85, 26.69, 21.08, 27.60, 14.76 and 17.0%, respectively. Our findings suggested that treatment with crude EtOAc, fraction no. 6, sub-fraction no. 6.17.2, BPC6, and 3-HBI strongly enhanced apoptosis in SCC15 cell line.

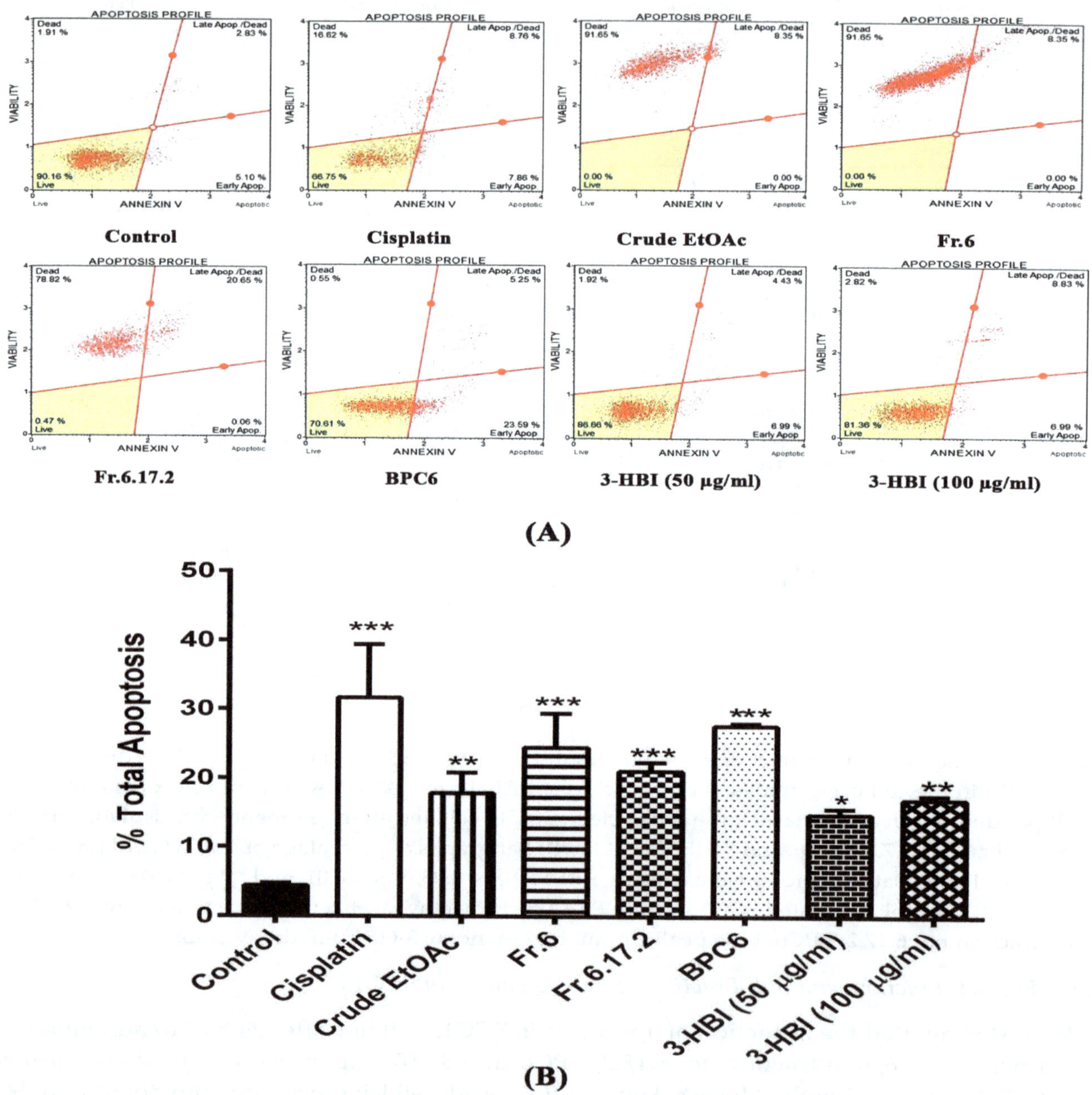

Figure 4. Determination of apoptosis in SCC15 cell line after treatment with MO extract, fraction no. 6, sub-fraction no. 6.17.2 BPC6, and 3-HBI for 24 h. (**A**) Dot plots of annexin V and 7-AAD dual staining showing the percentage of cell populations in each of the four quadrants. (**B**) Bar graphs showing quantitative data of percentage of total apoptotic cells. Results are presented as means ± SEM. * $p \leq 0.05$, ** $p \leq 0.01$, and *** $p \leq 0.001$ compared to control. Control: untreated SCC15; crude EtOAc: crude ethyl acetate; Fr.6: fraction no. 6; Fr.6.17.2: sub-fraction no. 6.17.2; BPC6: base peak chromatogram no. 6; 3-HBI: 3-hydroxy-β-ionone.

2.4. MO Extract and 3-HBI Inhibit Colony Formation of SCC15

The ability of SCC15 cell line to form colonies in the presence or absence of MO extract, fraction no. 6, sub-fraction no. 6.17.2, BPC 6 and 3-HBI for 24 h was studied. SCC15 cell lines were seeded into 6-well plates and incubated for one week. Cells were fixed and stained with 0.5% crystal violet. We found that MO extract, fraction no. 6 and sub-fraction no. 6.17.2 strongly inhibited colony formation of SCC15, similar to cisplatin treatment (Figure 5A,B). Furthermore, colony formation was significantly reduced in a concentration-dependent manner by 3-HBI compared to the control, as shown in Figure 5B. A similar result was observed in SCC15 treated with BPC6. These data confirmed that MO extract, fraction no. 6, sub-fraction no. 6.17.2, BPC6 and 3-HBI showed potential to inhibit the formation of colonies in SCC15 cell lines as an important factor in cancer survival and progression.

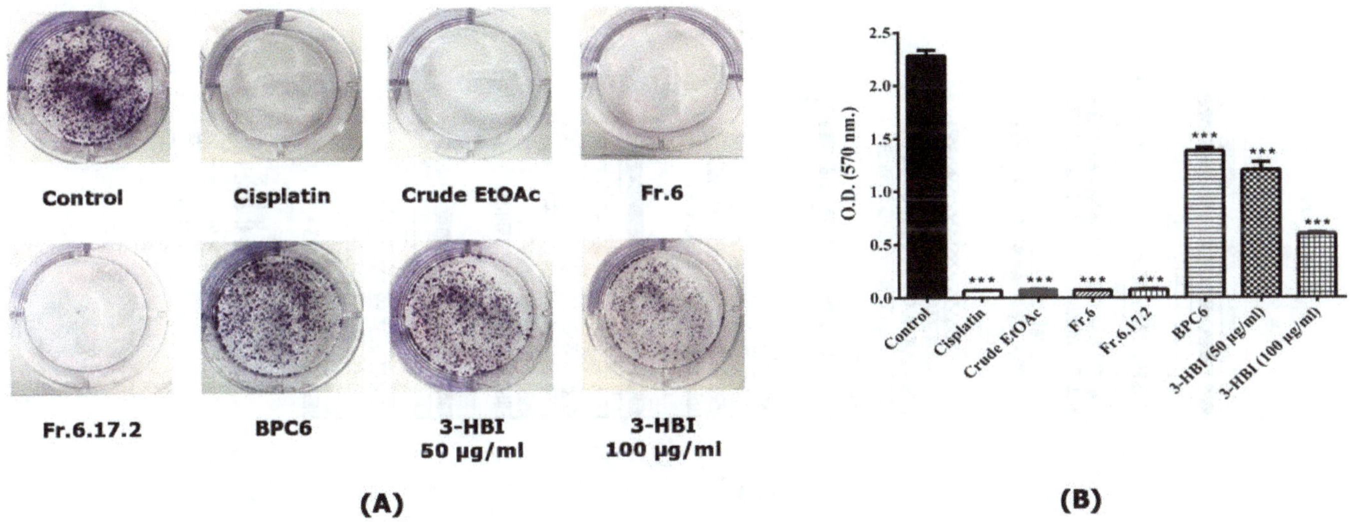

Figure 5. Colony formation of SCC15 cell line performed in 6-well plates with cells stained by crystal violet. (**A**) Untreated control and cells treated with MO extract, fraction no. 6, sub-fraction no. 6.17.2, BPC 6 and 3-HBI for 24 h. (**B**) Colony quantification measured by a microplate reader at OD 570 nm. Data are presented as means ± SEM. *** $p \leq 0.001$, compared to control. Control: untreated SCC15; crude EtOAc: crude ethyl acetate; Fr.6: fraction no. 6; Fr.6.17.2: sub-fraction no. 6.17.2; BPC6: base peak chromatogram no. 6; 3-HBI: 3-hydroxy-β-ionone.

2.5. MO Extract and 3-HBI Inhibit Migration of SCC15

Wound closure assay is a method of *in vitro* study for analysing the migration of cell populations. We evaluated the migrative ability of SCC15 cell line after treatment with and without MO extract, fraction no. 6, sub-fraction no. 6.17.2, BPC6 and 3-HBI for 36 h. Cell monolayers were scratched with a similar size at baseline. We observed a significant inhibition of cell migration after treatment for 6 h. The percentage of wound area for cells treated with cisplatin, crude extract, fraction no. 6, sub-fraction no. 6.17.2, BPC6 and 3-HBI was significantly higher when compared to the control. At 36 h after wound induction, the wound area of the untreated control was almost closed. On the other hand, for the wound areas of cells treated with drugs, all extracts and compounds were still widely open (Figure 6A,B).

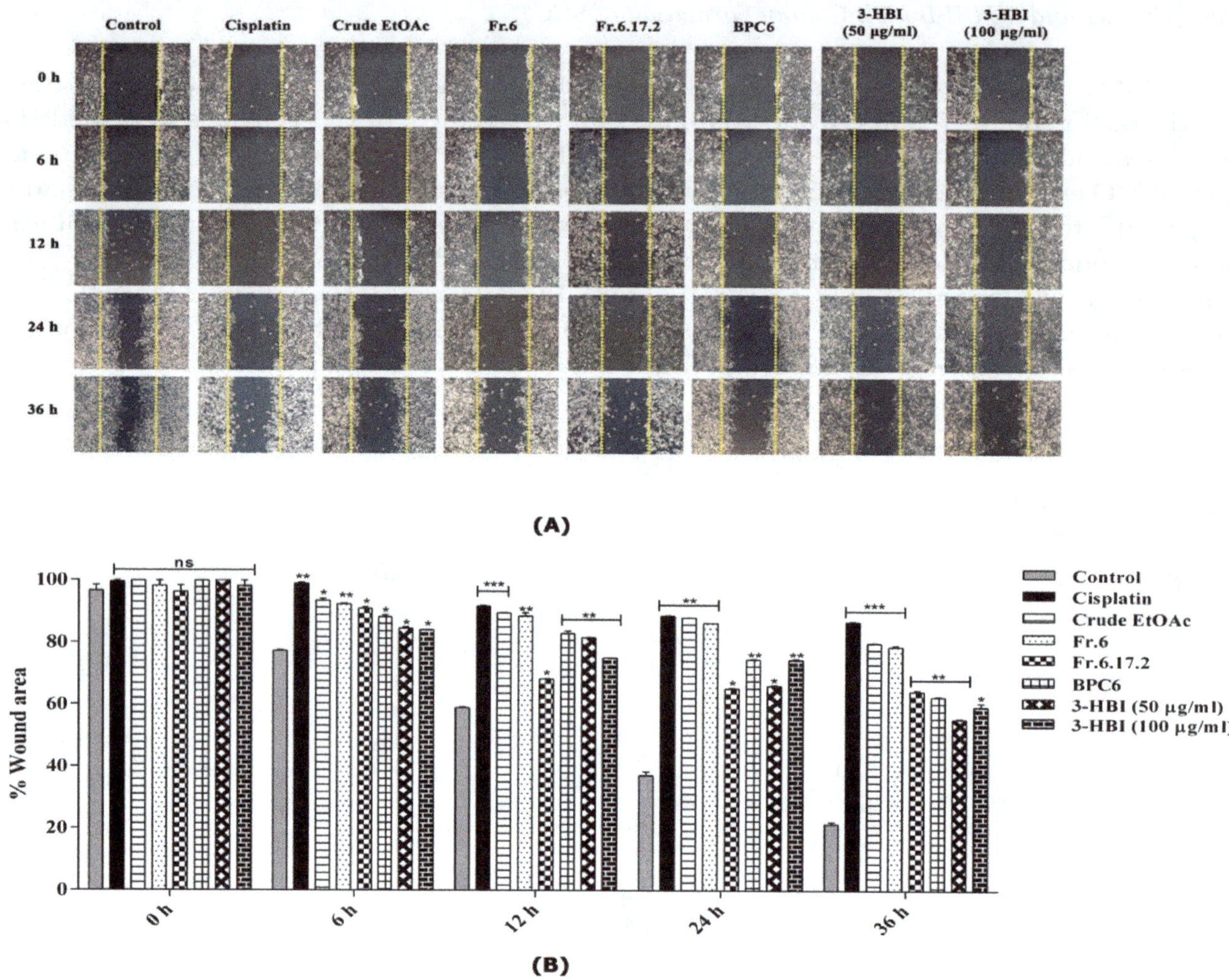

Figure 6. Wound closure analysis of SCC15 cell line for untreated control and cells treated with MO extract, fraction no. 6, sub-fraction no. 6.17.2, BPC 6 and 3-HBI for 36 h. (**A**) Pictures of wound area were taken at 0, 6, 12, 24 and 36 h with an inverted microscope. (**B**) Size of wound area was measured using ImageJ system software. Percentage of wound area was calculated, and bar graphs were represented as means ± SEM. ns = not significant, * $p \leq 0.05$, ** $p \leq 0.01$, and *** $p \leq 0.001$ compared to control. Control: untreated SCC15; crude EtOAc: crude ethyl acetate; Fr.6: fraction no. 6; Fr.6.17.2: sub-fraction no. 6.17.2; BPC6: base peak chromatogram no. 6; 3-HBI: 3-hydroxy-β-ionone.

2.6. *Effect of MO Extracts and Their Fractions on Apoptosis Signaling Pathway in SCC15 Cell Line*

Western blotting was performed to evaluate apoptosis in SCC15 cells after treatment with MO extract and its fractions. The expression of housekeeping protein β-actin was considered as an equal amount of protein was loaded. The pro-apoptotic Bax was significantly upregulated by treatment with cisplatin, MO crude extract, fraction no. 6, sub-fraction no. 6.17.2, BPC6 and 3-HBI. Moreover, they significantly decreased anti-apoptotic Bcl-2 compared to the control ($p \leq 0.001$). Interestingly, MO extracts and their fractions reduced pro-caspase-3 expression, as well as significantly inducing the activation of cleaved caspase-3 (Figure 7A–E). Our results demonstrated that MO extracts and their fractions showed the potential to induce apoptosis of SCC15 cell line by inducing the activation of cleaved caspase-3 and Bax. Furthermore, these extracts and compound significantly decreased anti-apoptotic Bcl-2, which showed strong efficacy similar to the positive drug control.

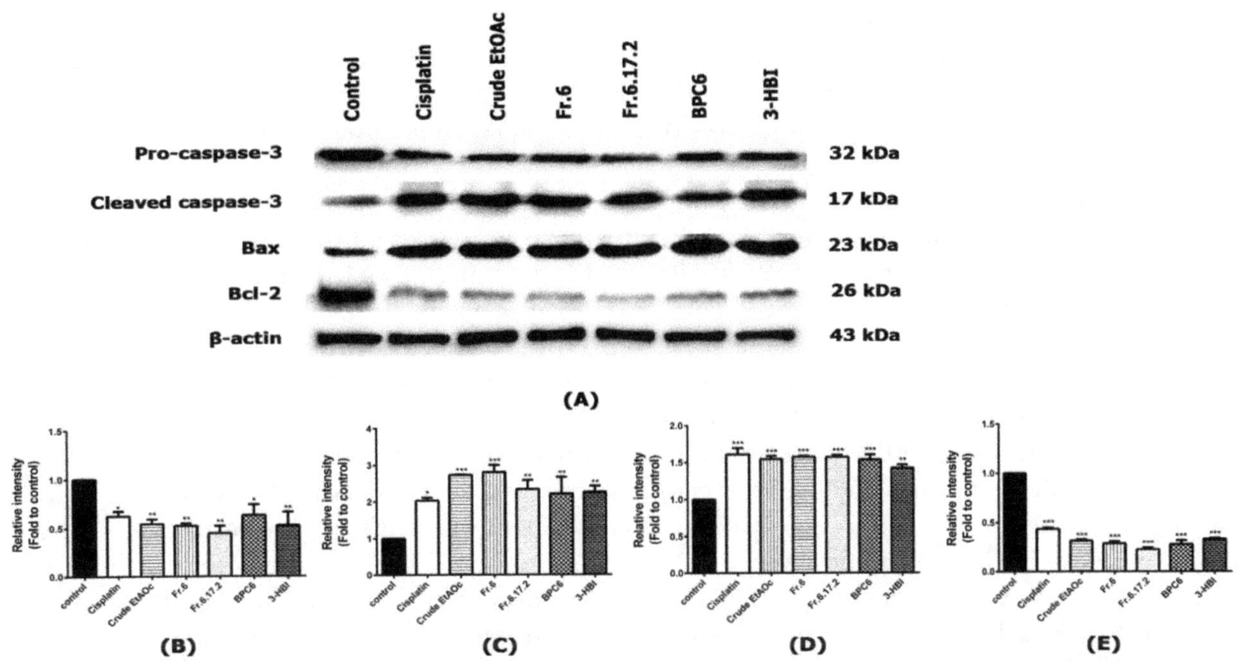

Figure 7. The inhibitory effect of MO extract, fraction no. 6, sub-fraction no. 6.17.2, BPC 6 and 3-HBI on the protein expressions of SCC15 cell line. Cells were treated under different conditions for 24 h. Total proteins were extracted and determined by Western blot analysis. (**A**) Band intensity of total protein levels of pro-caspase-3, cleaved caspase-3, Bax and Bcl-2. β-actin was used as a loading control. (**B**) Relative intensity of pro-caspase-3, (**C**) cleaved caspase-3, (**D**) Bax and (**E**) Bcl-2 were quantified by scanning densitometry and normalised to control. Data are shown as mean ± SEM. * $p \leq 0.05$, ** $p \leq 0.01$, and *** $p \leq 0.001$ compared to control. Control: untreated SCC15; Crude EtOAc: crude ethyl acetate; Fr.6: fraction no. 6; Fr.6.17.2: sub-fraction no. 6.17.2; BPC6: base peak chromatogram no. 6; 3-HBI: 3-hydroxy-β-ionone.

3. Discussion

Cancer cells lack a regulatory system that prevents cell overgrowth. Cancer progression involves a multi-step process including self-sufficiency in proliferative signalling, uncontrolled growth, evading programmed cell death, induction of angiogenesis and inducing invasion and metastasis [6]. Several studies have examined the effects of natural compounds against tumours by inhibiting cancer proliferation and inducing apoptosis. Chikusetsu isolated from *Aralia taibaiensis* induced apoptosis in human prostate cancer [7]. Capsaicin (trans-8-methyl-N-vanillyl-6-nonenamide) is a derivative from chili peppers inhibited the migration of cholangiocarcinoma cells by downregulating metalloproteinase-9 expression [25] and promoting apoptosis by stimulated p53 and Bax expression in HCT116 human colon carcinomas [26]. Arabinogalactan and curcumin have been extensively studied for their anti-cancer properties and both natural products decreased cell growth and significantly increased Bax/Bcl2 ratio as well as cleaved-caspase3 level in MDA-MB-231 human breast cancer cells [8]. Aloe-emodin derived from *Rheum undulatum* L. inhibited proliferation and induced apoptosis via activation of caspase-9 and caspase-3 in SCC15 cells [27]. Our results showed that 3-HBI derived from MO leaf extract inhibited SCC15 cell growth and triggered apoptosis via over-expression of cleaved caspase-3 and Bax, which down-regulated the anti-apoptotic Bcl-2. Additionally, our previous finding indicated that 3-HBI of MO leaf had potent biological anti-inflammatory effects by inhibiting NF-κB translocation in LPS-treated MDMs, leading to down-regulation of pro-inflammatory mediators [17,18]. Thus, 3-HBI exhibited both anti-cancer and anti-inflammatory activities and might be a novel effective therapeutic drug for head and neck cancer since NF-κB signalling pathways are targeted for therapeutic applications in many cancers including HNSCC. Accordingly, the major class of cellular targets controlling NF-κB consists of chemokines, regulators of apoptosis, cell proliferation and cell cycle regulators [28–30]. Curcumin has also been shown to inhibit NF-κB. This regulates several cellular processes including cell growth and survival by suppressing Bcl-2 and cyclin D1, IL-6, COX-2, and MMP-9 protein expression in HNSCC [31]. Erlotinib and EGCG of green tea extract synergistically inhibited HNSCC growth via inhibiting NF-κB in a p53-dependent manner [32].

MO leaf has various medicinal properties including antioxidant, anti-inflammatory, antiulcer, hepatoprotective activities, antibacterial and antifungal activities [33]. Cancer research involving Moringa leaf has been conducted in both *in vitro* and *in vivo* such as Moringa in MDA-MB-231 breast cancer cells, human HCT8 colon cancer cells and mouse melanoma [19,21,34]. This study evaluated the anti-cancer properties of Moringa leaf extract and 3-HBI bioactive compound including cell viability, cell cycle, apoptosis, migration, and colony formation of SCC15 cell line. The MTT assay was performed to evaluate cell viability of human MDMs and SCC15 cell line in the presence of MO leaf extract and its fractions. Our results showed that concentrations of the extract and compound caused cytotoxicity of SCC15 but non-toxicity in normal cells. Interestingly, this result concurred with our findings, indicating cell cycle arrest and an increase in cell apoptosis. We found that MO extracts and fractions caused a significant increase in cell population at the G2/M phase compared to the untreated control ($p \leq 0.001$). A previous study by Al-Asmari et al. (2015), showed similar findings with cell cycle arrest at the G2/M phase in MDA-MB-231 and HCT-8 cancer cell lines after treatment with Moringa leaf extract [21]. Cell migration and colony formation are hallmarks of tumour progression. Wound closure assays allow the observation of cell migration in confluent monolayer cell cultures, while colony formation assay is an *in vitro* technique for studying the survival and proliferation of cancer cells based on the ability of single cells to grow into colonies [35]. In this study, MO leaf fractions were able to significantly inhibit colony formation and cell migration of SCC15 cell line.

Apoptosis is programmed cell death that generally occurs in tissue during development as a homeostatic mechanism. Apoptosis is activated via two pathways, commonly known as intrinsic and extrinsic. The intrinsic pathway is initiated by pro-apoptotic proteins such as Bax and Bad that damage the mitochondrial membrane, leading to release of cytochrome C. Then, the formation of apoptosome complex activates procaspase-9 and stimulates caspase 3-6-7, resulting in apoptosis. The extrinsic pathway is initiated by death receptors at the cell surface to the intracellular signalling pathways. Then, caspase 8 is activated leading to stimulate downstream caspase 3-6-7 [36,37]. In various tumours, pro-apoptotic members are normally downregulated while anti-apoptotic factors are upregulated [6]. Our study showed that cell apoptosis in SCC15 cell line was strongly induced by MO leaf extracts and their fractions. Our results were further confirmed through activating the apoptosis signalling pathway by significantly increasing pro-apoptotic (BAX) and cleaved caspase-3 while suppressing the expression of anti-apoptotic protein Bcl-2 compared to the untreated control. These results indicated that 3-HBI bioactive compound of MO leaf showed strong anti-cancer activity by inducing apoptosis in SCC15 cell line via a caspase-dependent mechanism.

4. Materials and Methods

4.1. *Preparation of Moringa Oleifera Leaf Extracts and Compound Identification*

Moringa leaves were ground to a powder and extracted at room temperature with EtOAc as described in our previous study [17]. Then, 128 g of crude EtOAc extract was obtained after evaporation of the solvent. Fractions and sub-fractions were separated from the crude extract using flash column chromatography (Merck, Darmstadt, Germany). Gradient elution was performed by solvent system with increasing the polarity gradually including hexane, hexane-EtOAc and EtOAc-Methanol (MeOH). Apocarotenoid monoterpene namely 3-hydroxy-β-ionone, an active compound was identified from the Moringa sub-fraction by LC-ESI-QTOF-MS/MS (Agilent Technologies, Inc., Singapore). The crude EtOAc extracts and MO-derived fractions (fraction no.6, sub-fraction no. 6.17.2, BPC6 and 3-HBI) were tested for anti-cancer activities.

4.2. Monocyte Isolation

Human MDMs were used as a primary normal cell control. Buffy coat was obtained from the Blood Bank, Naresuan University Hospital, Phitsanulok, Thailand. Ethics approval was obtained from the Human Ethics Committee of Naresuan University (IRB no. 1013/60). Buffy coat was diluted with Hank's balanced salt solution (HBSS) and then overlaid on 5 mL Lymphoprep (Stemcell Technologies, Singapore) and centrifuged at 2000 rpm for 30 min. The mononuclear cell layer was collected and washed twice with HBSS buffer. Peripheral blood mononuclear cells (PBMCs) were collected and suspended in 5 mL of RPMI medium. Then, the monocytes were separated by size sedimentation centrifugation using Percoll (GE Healthcare Bio-Sciences AB, Uppsala, Sweden). The PBMC suspension was carefully overlaid on 10 mL of 46% Percoll solution and centrifuged for 30 min at 2000 rpm. Monocytes between Percoll were collected and washed with HBSS, followed by centrifugation for 10 min at 1300 rpm. Isolated monocytes were cultured in RPMI 1640 and supplemented with 10% fetal bovine serum (FBS) and 1% Antibiotic-Antimycotic purchased from Gibco™ (Thermo Fisher Scientific, Inc., New York, NY, USA). Cells were incubated at 37 °C with 5% CO_2 for 2 weeks with media replacement every 3 days.

4.3. Cell Line and Culture Conditions

Squamous cell carcinoma 15 (ATCC® CRL-1623™) was purchased from ATCC. Cells were cultured in Dulbecco's modified Eagle's medium (DMEM) and Ham's F12 medium (Caisson Labs Inc., Smithfield, UT, USA) containing 10% FBS. Cells were incubated at 37 °C with 5% CO_2 with medium renewal every 2–3 days. SCC15 cells were seeded in 24-well plates at a density of 5×10^4 cells/well and incubated for 24 h. The cells were treated with MO crude extracts, their fractions and 3-HBI (Santa Cruz Biotechnology, Inc., Dallas, TX, USA) for 24 h. Untreated and Cisplatin (Sigma-Aldrich, St. Louis, MO, USA) treated SCC15 cells were used as control conditions.

4.4. Cell Viability Assay

MTT assay was used to determine the growth inhibitory role of MO leaf extract. MDMs and SCC15 were seeded in a 96-well plate at a density of 1×10^4 cells/well and treated with various concentrations of extract, compound, and cisplatin. Cells were incubated at 37 °C for 24 h. Then, 50 μL of MTT (0.5 mg/mL) (Invitrogen, Carlsbad, CA, USA) in medium-free serum was added in all samples and they were incubated at 37 °C for 3 h. MTT reagent was removed and formazan crystals were dissolved in 100 μL of DMSO. The absorbance of formazan solution was measured at 590 nm by a microplate reader (PerkinElmer, Inc., Waltham, MA, USA). This method followed previous protocol [38]. IC_{50} of cisplatin, crude EtOAc extract and 3-HBI were calculated by concentration response relationships/sigmoidal curve fitting analysis. IC_5 was selected as non-toxic for cellular experiments.

4.5. Cell Cycle Analysis

To confirm the growth inhibitory role of MO extracts and derivative compounds, cell cycle assay was analysed using Muse™ Cell Cycle Kit (Merck, Darmstadt, Germany) following the manufacturer's protocol. Experimental conditions of SCC15 were harvested using trypsin/EDTA solution (Thermo Fisher Scientific) and incubated at 37 °C for 5 min. Then, 200 μL of completed DMEM HamF12 were added to stop the reaction of trypsin. Cells were aspirated and centrifuged at 1500 rpm for 5 min, then fixed with 70% ethanol and incubated for at least 3 h at −20 °C. Cells were washed twice with cold PBS (phosphate buffer saline), resuspended in 200 μL of Muse™ Cell cycle reagent, mixed gently and incubated for 30 min at room temperature in the dark. Cell cycle stage was then analysed by Muse™ Cell Analyser.

4.6. Cell Apoptosis Analysis

Muse™ Annexin V & Dead Cell Kit (Merck, Darmstadt, Germany) was used for the apoptosis study. SCC15 cells from all experimental conditions were harvested by trypsin/EDTA solution as described in cell cycle assay. Cells were washed in PBS and resuspended in medium with 1% FBS. Then, 100 μL of Muse™ Annexin V & Dead Cell Reagent were added, mixed gently, and incubated for 20 min at room temperature in the dark. Cell apoptosis was measured using Muse™ Cell Analyser following the manufacturer's protocol.

4.7. Colony Formation Assay

Colony formation assay was used to study the potentiality of a single cell forming colonies. This assay followed the previous description [35]. SCC15 cell line was seeded into 6-well plates at a density of 500 cells/well and incubated for 24 h in standard culture conditions at 37 °C. Cells were then treated with drugs and Moringa extracts including crude EtOAc, fraction no. 6, sub-fraction no. 6.17.2, BPC6 and 3-HBI for 24 h. Cells were incubated for 1 week with media replacement every 3 days and then fixed with 10% neutral buffer formalin solution for 30 min. The fixative reagent was removed, and the cells were stained with 2 mL of 0.5% crystal violet and incubated for 60 min at room temperature on a rotator. Cells were washed 4 times in a stream of tap water and the plate was air dried for at least 2 h at room temperature. Then, 2 mL of methanol were added to each well and the plate was incubated for 20 min at room temperature on a rotator. Optical density of each well was measured at 570 nm with a microplate reader (PerkinElmer, Inc.).

4.8. Wound Closure Assay

Cell migration of SCC15 cell line was evaluated by wound closure assay modified from a previous method [39]. SCC15 cells were seeded into 6-well plates at a density of 1×10^6 cells/mL and incubated at 37 °C until reaching 80% confluence as a monolayer. The cell monolayer was scraped in a straight line with a SPLScar Scratcher (SPL Life Sciences, Gyeonggi-do, Korea). Detached cells were removed and washed twice with 1 mL of medium. Cells were treated as described in the colony formation assay and incubated for 36 h. Snapshots were taken of the experimental cell plates at several time points including 6, 12, 24 and 36 h using an inverted microscope (Carl Zeiss Microscopy GmbH, Jena, Germany). The distance of the wound area was analysed by ImageJ system software.

4.9. SDS-PAGE and WESTERN BLOT ANALYSIS

Total proteins of SCC15 cell line from each condition were extracted by ice-cold RIPA lysis buffer (Bio Basic Inc., New York, NY, USA) in the presence of Halt Protease/Phosphatase Inhibitor Cocktails (Thermo Fisher Scientific) and centrifuged at 12,000 rpm for 15 min at 4 °C. Quantification of total protein concentration was performed by Bradford Coomassie-binding, colourimetric method. Protein extract was mixed with an equal volume of 4X Laemmli loading buffer and heated to denature at 95 °C for 5 min. Samples were loaded into wells of 12% SDS-polyacrylamide gel electrophoresis (PAGE) with proteins separated according to molecular weight and transferred to a polyvinylidene fluoride membrane (Bio-Rad Laboratories, Inc., Hercules, CA, USA). For Western blot analysis, the membrane was blocked for 2 h at room temperature with blocking buffer containing 5% bovine serum albumin (Capricorn Scientific GmbH, Ebsdorfergrund, Germany) in Tris-buffered saline with Tween 20 (TBST) buffer. The membrane was blotted using primary antibodies specific to cleaved-caspase 3 (Asp175, p17) (Affinity Biosciences, Cincinnati, OH, USA), β-actin, pro-caspase 3, Bax and Bcl-2 (Santa Cruz Biotechnology, Inc., Dallas, TX, USA) overnight at 4 °C on a rotator. The membrane was washed with TBST and incubated with horseradish peroxidase-conjugated goat anti-mouse IgG (H + L) secondary antibody (Thermo Fisher Scientific) for one hour at room temperature. The membrane was observed by soaking in chemiluminescence substrate for 5 min and placed in a ChemiDoc XRS+

Imaging System (Bio-Rad Laboratories, Inc., Hercules, CA, USA). The chemiluminescence signal of the blotted membrane was detected by Image Studio Lite software (LI-COR Corporate, Lincoln, NE, USA).

4.10. Statistical Analysis

All experiments were performed in three independent batches of experiments to provide accurate results. One-way ANOVA and the Bonferroni multiple comparisons test were used for data analysis with GraphPad Prism software. A confidence interval of 95% ($p = 0.05$) was used in all statistical analyses.

5. Conclusions

Moringa extract and its compound, 3-HBI suppressed cell proliferation and induced apoptosis in SCC15 cell line through the activation of cleaved caspase-3 and Bax as well as suppressing anti-apoptotic factor, Bcl-2. Moreover, treatment with MO extract and 3-HBI significantly increased the G2/M phase arrest of cell cycle progression in SCC15 (Figure 8). We observed a significant inhibition of cell migration as well as colony formation in SCC15 cells after treatment with crude extract and 3-HBI. Our findings suggest that MO extract and 3-HBI have potential as an anti-cancer treatment. This is the first report concerning MO extract and 3-HBI activity against SCC15 cell line.

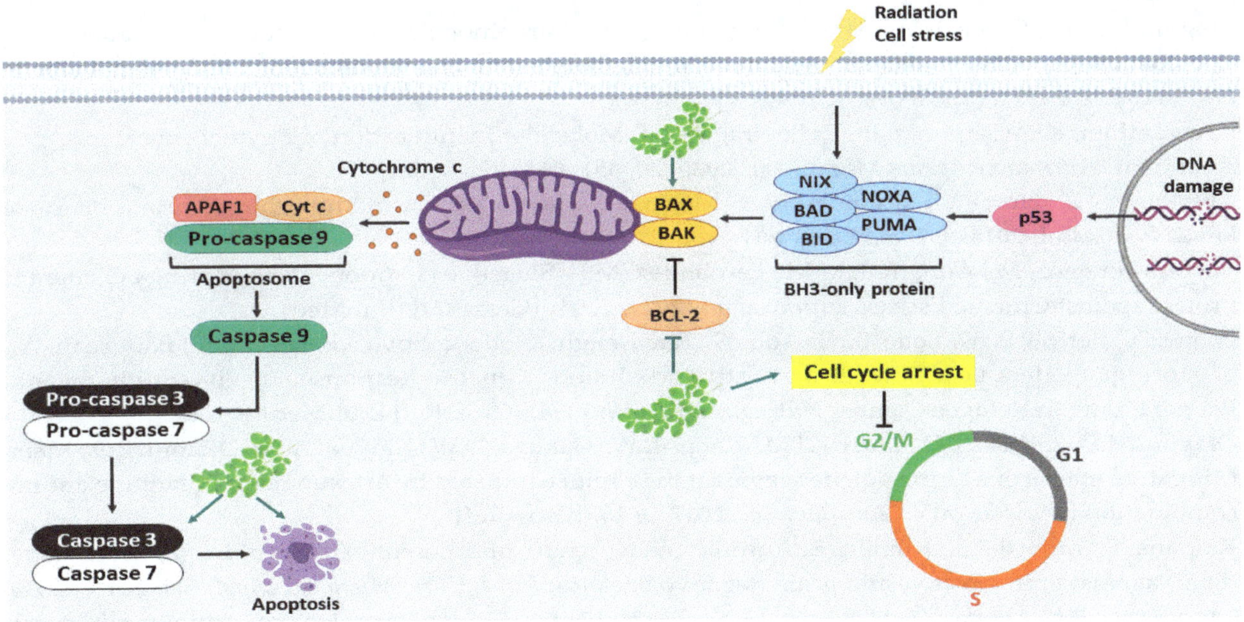

Figure 8. Apoptosis signalling pathway and cell cycle arrest in response to Moringa extract and 3-HBI. MO crude extract and 3-HBI induced G2/M cell cycle arrest and apoptosis in SCC15 cell line by increasing the Bax and cleaved caspase-3 expression and downregulating the levels of Bcl-2.

Author Contributions: This research was contributed by authors "conceptualization, K.U., R.P.S., C.N. and Y.T.; methodology, T.L. and K.U.; software, N.S., N.N. and T.L.; validation, P.P. and K.U.; formal analysis, T.L.; investigation, T.L.; resources, N.S. and N.N.; data curation, K.U., R.P.S. and Y.T.; writing—original draft preparation, T.L.; writing—review and editing, K.U., R.P.S., C.N., N.S. and N.N.; visualization, K.U. and T.L.; supervision, K.U.; project administration, K.U.; funding acquisition, K.U., R.P.S., C.N., Y.T. and P.P." All authors have read and agreed to the published version of the manuscript.

Acknowledgments: We would like to thank Khaolaor Laboratories Co., Ltd., Samutprakan, Thailand for providing *Moringa oleifera* dried powder, Assoc. Prof Kornkanok Ingkaninan from Bioscreening Unit, Faculty of Pharmaceutical Sciences and Center of Excellence for Innovation in Chemistry, Naresuan University and Assoc. Prof Chavi Yenjai from Natural Products Research Unit, Department of Chemistry and Center of Excellence for Innovation in Chemistry, Faculty of Science, Khon Kaen University, Thailand for helpful giving reagents and suggestions.

References

1. Bray, F.; Ferlay, J.; Soerjomataram, I.; Siegel, R.L.; Torre, L.A.; Jemal, A. Global cancer statistics 2018: GLOBOCAN estimates of incidence and mortality worldwide for 36 cancers in 185 countries. *CA Cancer J. Clin.* **2018**, *68*, 394–424. [CrossRef]
2. Cramer, J.D.; Burtness, B.; Le, Q.T.; Ferris, R.L. The changing therapeutic landscape of head and neck cancer. *Nat. Rev. Clin. Oncol.* **2019**, *16*, 669–683. [CrossRef]
3. Castellanos, M.R.; Pan, Q. Novel p53 therapies for head and neck cancer. *World J. Otorhinolaryngol. Head Neck Surg.* **2016**, *2*, 68–75. [CrossRef] [PubMed]
4. Walden, M.J.; Aygun, N. Head and neck cancer. *Semin. Roentgenol.* **2013**, *48*, 75–86. [CrossRef] [PubMed]
5. Cooper, J.S.; Pajak, T.F.; Forastiere, A.A.; Jacobs, J.; Campbell, B.H.; Saxman, S.B.; Kish, J.A.; Kim, H.E.; Cmelak, A.J.; Rotman, M.; et al. Postoperative concurrent radiotherapy and chemotherapy for high-risk squamous-cell carcinoma of the head and neck. *N. Engl. J. Med.* **2004**, *350*, 1937–1944. [CrossRef] [PubMed]
6. Hanahan, D.; Weinberg, R.A. Hallmarks of cancer: The next generation. *Cell* **2011**, *144*, 646–674. [CrossRef] [PubMed]
7. Zhu, W.B.; Tian, F.J.; Liu, L.Q. Chikusetsu (CHI) triggers mitochondria-regulated apoptosis in human prostate cancer via reactive oxygen species (ROS) production. *Biomed. Pharmacother.* **2017**, *90*, 446–454. [CrossRef] [PubMed]
8. Moghtaderi, H.; Sepehri, H.; Attari, F. Combination of arabinogalactan and curcumin induces apoptosis in breast cancer cells in vitro and inhibits tumor growth via overexpression of p53 level in vivo. *Biomed. Pharmacother.* **2017**, *88*, 582–594. [CrossRef]
9. Usuwanthim, K.; Wisitpongpun, P.; Luetragoon, T. Molecular Identification of Phytochemical for Anticancer Treatment. *Anticancer Agents Med. Chem.* **2020**, *20*, 651–666. [CrossRef]
10. Abd Rani, N.Z.; Husain, K.; Kumolosasi, E. Moringa Genus: A Review of Phytochemistry and Pharmacology. *Front. Pharmacol.* **2018**, *9*, 108. [CrossRef]
11. Vergara-Jimenez, M.; Almatrafi, M.M.; Fernandez, M.L. Bioactive Components in Moringa Oleifera Leaves Protect against Chronic Disease. *Antioxidants* **2017**, *6*, 91. [CrossRef] [PubMed]
12. Leone, A.; Bertoli, S.; Di Lello, S.; Bassoli, A.; Ravasenghi, S.; Borgonovo, G.; Forlani, F.; Battezzati, A. Effect of Moringa oleifera Leaf Powder on Postprandial Blood Glucose Response: In Vivo Study on Saharawi People Living in Refugee Camps. *Nutrients* **2018**, *10*, 1494. [CrossRef] [PubMed]
13. Okumu, M.O.; Ochola, F.O.; Mbaria, J.M.; Kanja, L.W.; Gakuya, D.W.; Kinyua, A.W.; Okumu, P.O.; Kiama, S.G. Mitigative effects of Moringa oleifera against liver injury induced by artesunateamodiaquine antimalarial combination in wistar rats. *Clin. Phytosci.* **2017**, *3*, 18. [CrossRef]
14. Kalpana, S.; Moorthi, S.; Kumari, S. Antimicrobial activity of different extracts of leaf of Moringa oleifera (Lam) against gram positive and gram negative bacteria. *Int. J. Curr. Microbiol. Appl. Sci.* **2013**, *2*, 514–518.
15. Omodanisi, E.I.; Aboua, Y.G.; Chegou, N.N.; Oguntibeju, O.O. Hepatoprotective, Antihyperlipidemic, and Anti-inflammatory Activity of Moringa oleifera in Diabetic-induced Damage in Male Wistar Rats. *Pharmacogn. Res.* **2017**, *9*, 182–187.
16. Adeyemi, O.S.; Elebiyo, T.C. Moringa oleifera Supplemented Diets Prevented Nickel-Induced Nephrotoxicity in Wistar Rats. *J. Nutr. Metab.* **2014**, *2014*, 958621. [CrossRef]
17. Luetragoon, T.; Pankla Sranujit, R.; Noysang, C.; Thongsri, Y.; Potup, P.; Suphrom, N.; Nuengchamnong, N.; Usuwanthim, K. Bioactive Compounds in Moringa oleifera Lam. Leaves Inhibit the Pro-Inflammatory Mediators in Lipopolysaccharide-Induced Human Monocyte-Derived Macrophages. *Molecules* **2020**, *25*, 191. [CrossRef]
18. Kooltheat, N.; Sranujit, R.P.; Chumark, P.; Potup, P.; Laytragoon-Lewin, N.; Usuwanthim, K. An ethyl acetate fraction of Moringa oleifera Lam. Inhibits human macrophage cytokine production induced by cigarette smoke. *Nutrients* **2014**, *6*, 697–710. [CrossRef]
19. Jung, I.L. Soluble extract from Moringa oleifera leaves with a new anticancer activity. *PLoS ONE* **2014**, *9*, e95492. [CrossRef]
20. Jung, I.L.; Lee, J.H.; Kang, S.C. A potential oral anticancer drug candidate, Moringa oleifera leaf extract, induces the apoptosis of human hepatocellular carcinoma cells. *Oncol. Lett.* **2015**, *10*, 1597–1604. [CrossRef]

21. Al-Asmari, A.K.; Albalawi, S.M.; Athar, M.T.; Khan, A.Q.; Al-Shahrani, H.; Islam, M. Moringa oleifera as an Anti-Cancer Agent against Breast and Colorectal Cancer Cell Lines. *PLoS ONE* **2015**, *10*, e0135814. [CrossRef]
22. Tragulpakseerojn, J.; Yamaguchi, N.; Pamonsinlapatham, P.; Wetwitayaklung, P.; Yoneyama, T.; Ishikawa, N.; Ishibashi, M.; Apirakaramwong, A. Anti-proliferative effect of Moringa oleifera Lam (Moringaceae) leaf extract on human colon cancer HCT116 cell line. *Trop. J. Pharm. Res.* **2017**, *16*, 371–378. [CrossRef]
23. Rajan, T.S.; De Nicola, G.R.; Iori, R.; Rollin, P.; Bramanti, P.; Mazzon, E. Anticancer activity of glucomoringin isothiocyanate in human malignant astrocytoma cells. *Fitoterapia* **2016**, *110*, 1–7. [CrossRef]
24. Cirmi, S.; Ferlazzo, N.; Gugliandolo, A.; Musumeci, L.; Mazzon, E.; Bramanti, A.; Navarra, M. Moringin from Moringa Oleifera Seeds Inhibits Growth, Arrests Cell-Cycle, and Induces Apoptosis of SH-SY5Y Human Neuroblastoma Cells through the Modulation of NF-kappaB and Apoptotic Related Factors. *Int. J. Mol. Sci.* **2019**, *20*, 1930. [CrossRef]
25. Lee, G.R.; Jang, S.H.; Kim, C.J.; Kim, A.R.; Yoon, D.J.; Park, N.H.; Han, I.S. Capsaicin suppresses the migration of cholangiocarcinoma cells by down-regulating matrix metalloproteinase-9 expression via the AMPK-NF-kappaB signaling pathway. *Clin. Exp. Metastasis* **2014**, *31*, 897–907. [CrossRef] [PubMed]
26. Kim, M.Y.; Trudel, L.J.; Wogan, G.N. Apoptosis induced by capsaicin and resveratrol in colon carcinoma cells requires nitric oxide production and caspase activation. *Anticancer Res.* **2009**, *29*, 3733–3740. [PubMed]
27. Li, Q.; Wen, J.; Yu, K.; Shu, Y.; He, W.; Chu, H.; Zhang, B.; Ge, C. Aloe-emodin induces apoptosis in human oral squamous cell carcinoma SCC15 cells. *BMC Complement. Altern. Med.* **2018**, *18*, 296. [CrossRef]
28. Rahman, M.A.; Amin, A.R.; Shin, D.M. Chemopreventive potential of natural compounds in head and neck cancer. *Nutr. Cancer* **2010**, *62*, 973–987. [CrossRef]
29. Perkins, N.D. Integrating cell-signalling pathways with NF-kappaB and IKK function. *Nat. Rev. Mol. Cell Biol.* **2007**, *8*, 49–62. [CrossRef]
30. Tergaonkar, V. NFkappaB pathway: A good signaling paradigm and therapeutic target. *Int. J. Biochem. Cell Biol.* **2006**, *38*, 1647–1653. [CrossRef]
31. Aggarwal, S.; Takada, Y.; Singh, S.; Myers, J.N.; Aggarwal, B.B. Inhibition of growth and survival of human head and neck squamous cell carcinoma cells by curcumin via modulation of nuclear factor-kappaB signaling. *Int. J. Cancer* **2004**, *111*, 679–692. [CrossRef] [PubMed]
32. Amin, A.R.; Khuri, F.R.; Chen, Z.G.; Shin, D.M. Synergistic growth inhibition of squamous cell carcinoma of the head and neck by erlotinib and epigallocatechin-3-gallate: The role of p53-dependent inhibition of nuclear factor-kappaB. *Cancer Prev. Res.* **2009**, *2*, 538–545. [CrossRef] [PubMed]
33. Anwar, F.; Latif, S.; Ashraf, M.; Gilani, A.H. Moringa oleifera: A food plant with multiple medicinal uses. *Phytother. Res.* **2007**, *21*, 17–25. [CrossRef] [PubMed]
34. Purwal, L.; Pathak, A.K.; Jain, U.K. In vivo anticancer activity of the leaves and fruits of moringa oleifera on mouse melanoma. *Pharmacologyonline* **2010**, *1*, 655–665.
35. Franken, N.A.; Rodermond, H.M.; Stap, J.; Haveman, J.; van Bree, C. Clonogenic assay of cells in vitro. *Nat. Protoc.* **2006**, *1*, 2315–2319. [CrossRef] [PubMed]
36. Elmore, S. Apoptosis: A review of programmed cell death. *Toxicol. Pathol.* **2007**, *35*, 495–516. [CrossRef]
37. Creagh, E.M. Caspase crosstalk: Integration of apoptotic and innate immune signalling pathways. *Trends Immunol.* **2014**, *35*, 631–640. [CrossRef]
38. van Meerloo, J.; Kaspers, G.J.; Cloos, J. Cell sensitivity assays: The MTT assay. *Methods Mol. Biol.* **2011**, *731*, 237–245.
39. Liang, C.C.; Park, A.Y.; Guan, J.L. In vitro scratch assay: A convenient and inexpensive method for analysis of cell migration in vitro. *Nat. Protoc.* **2007**, *2*, 329–333. [CrossRef]

10

Antiproliferative and Pro-Apoptotic Effect of Uvaol in Human Hepatocarcinoma HepG2 Cells by Affecting G_0/G_1 Cell Cycle Arrest, ROS Production and AKT/PI3K Signaling Pathway

Gloria C. Bonel-Pérez [1,†], Amalia Pérez-Jiménez [2,†], Isabel Gris-Cárdenas [1], Alberto M. Parra-Pérez [1], José Antonio Lupiáñez [1], Fernando J. Reyes-Zurita [1], Eva Siles [3], René Csuk [4], Juan Peragón [3,*] and Eva E. Rufino-Palomares [1,*]

1 Department of Biochemistry and Molecular Biology I, Faculty of Sciences, University of Granada, Avenida Fuentenueva, 1, 18071 Granada, Spain; gloria1797@correo.ugr.es (G.C.B.-P.); isagc@ugr.es (I.G.-C.); ampperez@correo.ugr.es (A.M.P.-P.); jlcara@ugr.es (J.A.L.); ferjes@ugr.es (F.J.R.-Z.)

2 Department of Zoology, Faculty of Sciences, University of Granada, Avenida Fuentenueva, 1, 18071 Granada, Spain; calaya@ugr.es

3 Department of Experimental Biology, University of Jaen, Campus Las Lagunillas s/n. 23071 Jaén, Spain; esiles@ujaen.es

4 Berreich Organische Chemie, Martin Luther University Halle-Wittenberg, 06120 Halle (Saale), Germany; rene.csuk@chemie.uni-halle.de

* Correspondence: jperagon@ujaen.es (J.P.); evaevae@ugr.es (E.E.R.-P.);

† These authors contributed equally to this work.

Academic Editors: Enrique Barrajon-Catalan and Wolfgang Weigand

Abstract: Natural products have a significant role in the development of new drugs, being relevant the pentacyclic triterpenes extracted from *Olea europaea L.* Anticancer effect of uvaol, a natural triterpene, has been scarcely studied. The aim of this study was to understand the anticancer mechanism of uvaol in the HepG2 cell line. Cytotoxicity results showed a selectivity effect of uvaol with higher influence in HepG2 than WRL68 cells used as control. Our results show that uvaol has a clear and selective anticancer activity in HepG2 cells supported by a significant anti-migratory capacity and a significant increase in the expression of HSP-60. Furthermore, the administration of this triterpene induces cell arrest in the G_0/G_1 phase, as well as an increase in the rate of cell apoptosis. These results are supported by a decrease in the expression of the anti-apoptotic protein Bcl2, an increase in the expression of the pro-apoptotic protein Bax, together with a down-regulation of the AKT/PI3K signaling pathway. A reduction in reactive oxygen species (ROS) levels in HepG2 cells was also observed. Altogether, results showed anti-proliferative and pro-apoptotic effect of uvaol on hepatocellular carcinoma, constituting an interesting challenge in the development of new treatments against this type of cancer.

Keywords: AKT/PI3K signaling pathway; apoptosis; human hepatocarcinoma HepG2 cells; migration activity; proliferation; oxidative stress; ROS level; uvaol

1. Introduction

Cancer is one of the leading causes of mortality worldwide, especially in developed countries, on account of the aging of the population [1]. Liver cancer is the fifth most common type, as well as the second type of tumor that causes more deaths globally. Specifically, hepatocellular carcinoma (HCC) accounts for 90% of primary liver neoplasms, whose incidence increases progressively with ageing, according to the EASL (European Association for the Study of the Liver) [2].

Hepatocarcinogenesis is a process initiated by different external stimuli that induce genetic changes in hepatocytes or hepatic stem cells, which can cause alterations in the processes of proliferation and apoptosis, by dysfunctions in the cell cycle and its regulation, which eventually lead to tissue dysplasia and can cause a neoplasm [3]. In response to this DNA damage, different control points can be activated throughout the cell cycle phases. Among all the proteins that regulate this process, p53 stands out [4]. The activity blockage of protein kinases regulated by p53 produces an inhibition of cell cycle progression, due to an arrest in G_1 phase [5]. It is known that p53 is frequently mutated in HCC, disrupting the correct role of this protein [6].

Another important pathway involved in hepatocarcinogenesis is the one controlled by c-*Myc* proto-oncogene. The elements of the *Myc* proto-oncogenes family have a role as strong transcription factors of other proteins that take part in the control of cell differentiation and proliferation, oncogenesis and apoptosis [7]. Studies show that c-*Myc* is overexpressed in HCC, in comparison with healthy patients [8].

One of the main characteristics of tumor cells is their resistance to cell death, so the apoptosis process is one of the most studied pathways. This programmed cell death can occur through two pathways: the mitochondrial or intrinsic and the one that involves death receptors, also named extrinsic. In response to various external stimuli, the mitochondria increases its permeability, releasing apoptotic mediators, among which proteins from the Bcl-2 family and cytochrome c stand out [9].

It is well established that NADPH molecules are essential in anabolic processes related to membranogenesis, as well as in nucleotide metabolism through ribose phosphate formation [10], and also plays a decisive role as a modulator of protein synthesis [11]. Therefore, the participation of NADPH in both metabolic aspects makes it especially important for growth and cell differentiation [12]. For these reasons, the regulation of NADPH levels is essential to understand the behavior of numerous physiological processes and, in this sense, nutritional conditions [13–16]; the presence of triterpenes [17,18]; and the redox state [19] modify significantly the levels of those reduction equivalents.

Reactive oxygen species (ROS) in non-pathological concentrations act as second messengers involved in several signal transduction pathways that regulate processes such as cell growth, proliferation and differentiation [20]. Therefore, cells have detoxification mechanisms that maintain a redox balance since, if they are altered, excessive production of ROS can lead to a situation of oxidative stress, which plays an important role in apoptosis and in the beginning of neoplasia development. Within these detoxification mechanisms, several enzymes stand out, such as superoxide dismutase (SOD), catalase (CAT) or glutathione peroxidase (GPX) [21].

Some pharmacological compounds used as HCC treatments, such as Sorafenib, inhibit VEGF angiogenic factor and MAPK pathway [22]. Since the efficacy of current therapies is low when advanced stages of HCC are considered, it is necessary to seek alternative treatments that could offer a better prognosis for patients [23]. Traditional medicine occupies an important place in the development of new drugs, since natural compounds are a recurrent source of molecules with bioactive properties [24].

The Mediterranean diet presents olive oil as its main exponent, which is obtained from the fruit of the *Olea europaea L.*. Its consumption is associated with various health benefits [24], among which there are a lower incidence of cardiovascular diseases, a lower production of ROS and even a reduction in the risk of cancer [25–27]. These properties are associated with their high content of monounsaturated fatty acids, with oleic acid being the most abundant, in addition to other minor compounds, such as tocopherols, polyphenols, triterpenes and squalene [28].

Uvaol (urs-12-ene-3,28-diol) is a natural alcohol pentacyclic triterpene whose formula and molecular weight is $C_{30}H_{50}O_2$ and 442.73 g/mol, respectively. It has a structural isomer, erythrodiol, from which it only differs in the position of a methyl group, since it is located in carbon 19, while uvaol presents it in carbon 20. The most notable feature of this compound is that it exhibits two hydroxyl groups in remote positions, specifically in carbons 3 and 28 (Figure 1A) [29]. Among the described set of triterpenes present in olive oil, uvaol has the lowest characterization of its bioactive properties [30]. Martín et al. [31] studied the effect of uvaol on the 1321N1 cell line and found that uvaol increased the rate of apoptotic cells, as well as producing an activation of the JNK. Allouche et al. [32] studied the effects of uvaol on MCF-7 cells observing a decrease in ROS production and cell viability.

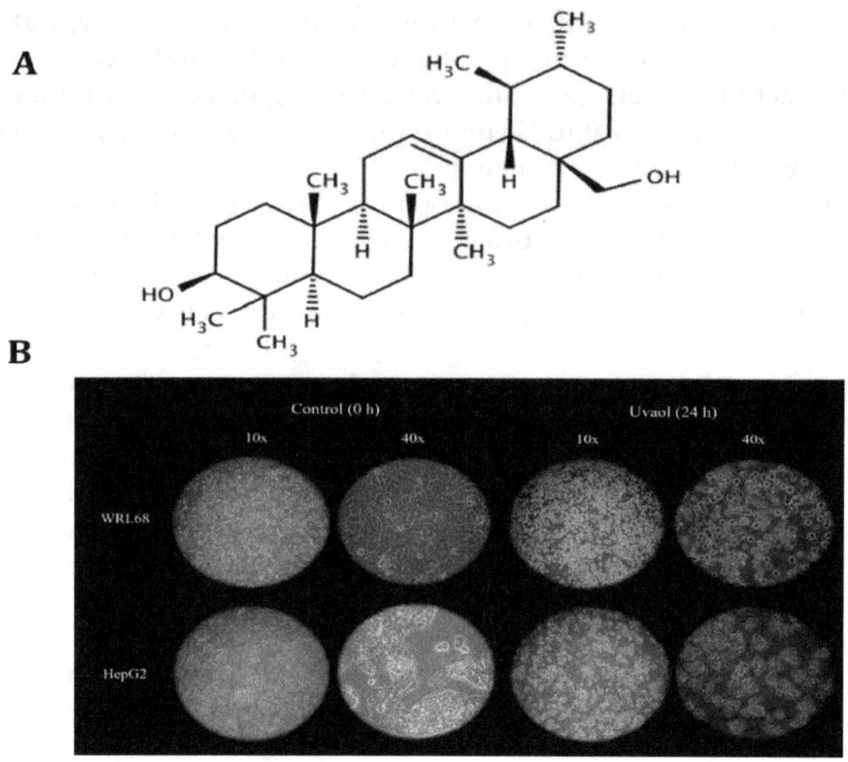

Figure 1. Chemical structure of uvaol (PubChem) (**A**). Morphological changes in response to uvaol treatment incubated at IC_{50} after 24 h in the WRL68 (IC_{50}: 54.3 μg/mL) and HepG2 (IC_{50}: 25.2 μg/mL) cell lines (**B**).

Due to the promising results shown by the few studies carried out to date on the anticancer potential of uvaol, the aim of the present work was to evaluate its cytotoxic capacity, as well as its effect on proliferation, migration, morphology, cell cycle, apoptosis, oxidative stress, dual PI3K/MAPK signaling pathway and expression of protein markers involved in the processes described on the human control liver cell line WRL68 and the human hepatocellular carcinoma line HepG2.

2. Results

2.1. Uvaol Produces Morphological Changes in HepG2 Cells

Uvaol effect on cell morphology was analyzed using the IC_{50} concentration of each cell line for 24 h. The images taken at 10 and 40 magnifications of the four experimental conditions described are shown in Figure 1B. Referring to the WRL68 line, we can observe that its growth on the support is homogeneous, with the cells being initially separated from each other and presenting a fusiform morphology at 10 magnifications. When the treatment described is applied, the cells undergo a structure change, since they become rounded and have cytoplasmic projections towards the environment, due to cell death induced by the administration of uvaol. In addition, this causes them to rise from the support on which they grow.

The morphology of HepG2 cells in a control situation is triangular and shows an islet-shaped growth, each of them being well delimited with respect to the rest of the surrounding islets. Additionally, its cytoplasm is much more irregular than the presented by WRL68 cells. After the compound's administration, as in the previous case, its characteristic morphology is blurred, becoming slightly more rounded, with very sharp projections and a loss of adhesion to the support.

2.2. *Uvaol Has a Selectivity Cytotoxic Effect on the HepG2 Cell Lines*

Uvaol effect was evaluated by the MTT assay on the WRL68 and HepG2 cell lines. The viability results obtained were represented in percentage (%) with respect to the different concentrations of compound administered (in μg/mL) for each cell line at 24, 48 and 72 h of exposure, showed using a sigmoidal adjustment (Figure 2A,B). Similarly, the IC_{20}, IC_{50} and IC_{80} values were calculated in the three times lapses described (Figure 2C). Figure 2A shows that, for the WRL68 line, uvaol reduced cell viability in a dose and time-dependent way, since the IC_{20}, IC_{50} and IC_{80} values decreased with this treatment in a progressive form for the three studied time lapses.

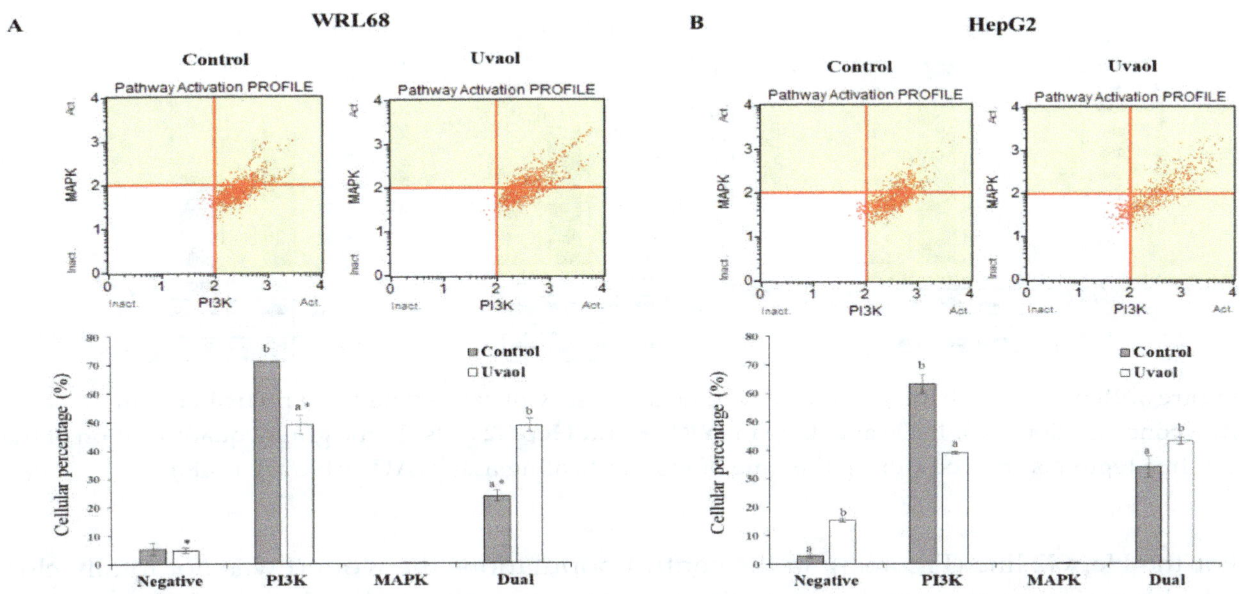

Figure 2. Cytotoxicity curves of uvaol during 24, 48 and 72 h in WRL68 (**A**) and HepG2 cells (**B**). IC_{20}, IC_{50} and IC_{80} values for the WRL68 and HepG2 lines after 24, 48 and 72 h of incubation with uvaol (**C**). These values are represented by mean ± SEM (n = 9).

In the HepG2 line there is also a progressive decrease in cell viability according to concentration and exposure time (Figure 2B). The IC_{50} value obtained was 54.3 μg/mL (12.3 μM) for the WRL68 line and 25.2 μg/mL (5.7 μM) for the HepG2 line after 24 h of uvaol exposure (Figure 2C). Therefore, the concentration needed to inhibit cell proliferation in tumor cells was half that the needed for the same purpose on the control line. Following tests were carried out using the mentioned IC_{50} concentrations and a period of 24 h uvaol incubation. Differences between the IC_{50} values of both cell lines at later time points (48 h and 72 h) were diminished, but still statistically significant.

2.3. *Anti-Migratory Activity of Uvaol in HepG2 Cells*

The wound healing assay (or scratch assay) aims to assess the ability of cancer cells to migrate in vitro. Figure 3 collects the several images taken and quantified in each experimental condition at 10 magnifications for 0, 6, 18, 30 and 42 h after the wound was made. Data in quantification for the WRL68 cell line (Figure 3) showed a progressive wound healing, occurring at 18 h, in the control situation, the junction of the separated areas. The complete closure occurred at 42 h. In the treated populations, the behavior of cells was different, since wound healing was maintained during more hours than the control group.

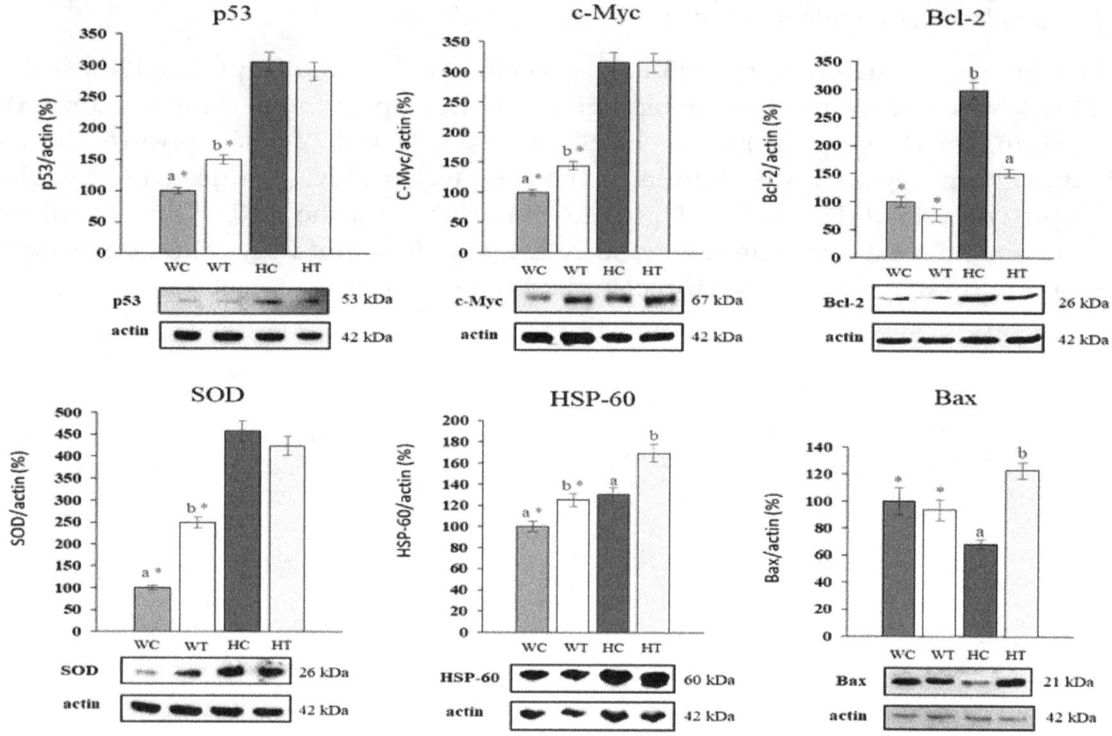

Figure 3. Representative image from wound healing assay of cells treated and no treated with uvaol at IC_{50} concentration (0, 6, 18, 30 and 42 h) in **WRL68** and **HepG2** cells. In the graph, quantification of the cell-free region is showed during the time of wound healing assay (AU: arbitrary units).

For the HepG2 line (Figure 3), in the control populations the wound was not totally closed at the end, although the values of the quantification showed a progressive closure of the wound. In the treated populations, the wound remains until the end of the trial.

2.4. *Uvaol Induces G_0/G_1 Arrest in HepG2 Cells*

In order to analyze the possible effect of uvaol in the cell cycle for each line studied, the proportion of cells that were in each phase of the cycle (G_0/G_1, S and G_2/M) were measured in control and uvaol-incubation conditions. Figure 4 shows the images and quantifications of the cell cycle assay generated by the flow cytometer during its analysis for each experimental condition.

Uvaol produced a significant decrease in the percentage of cells in phase G_0/G_1 and phase S, while, on the contrary, induced an increase in the G_2/M phase for the WRL68 line (Figure 4A). In the case of the HepG2 cell line (Figure 4B), treatment with uvaol resulted in a statistically significant increase in the percentage of cells that were in the G_0/G_1 phase, while causing an equally significant reduction of cells in G_2/M phase. No differences were found in the S phase. When statistically comparing the results obtained between both lines, significant differences were observed in the behavior shown in each phase of the cell cycle after treatment with uvaol.

2.5. *Apoptosis Is Enhanced in HepG2 Cells by Uvaol*

Apoptosis assay provides information about the type of cell death that occurs in each line and for each situation studied: negative control, positive control (treatment with staurosporine with a 1 μg/mL concentration for 2 h) and treatment with uvaol. Figure 5 includes the images of each experimental condition generated by the flow cytometer during its analysis. The data obtained reflect the percentage of viable cells, those that suffer apoptosis and those presenting necrosis (Figure 5).

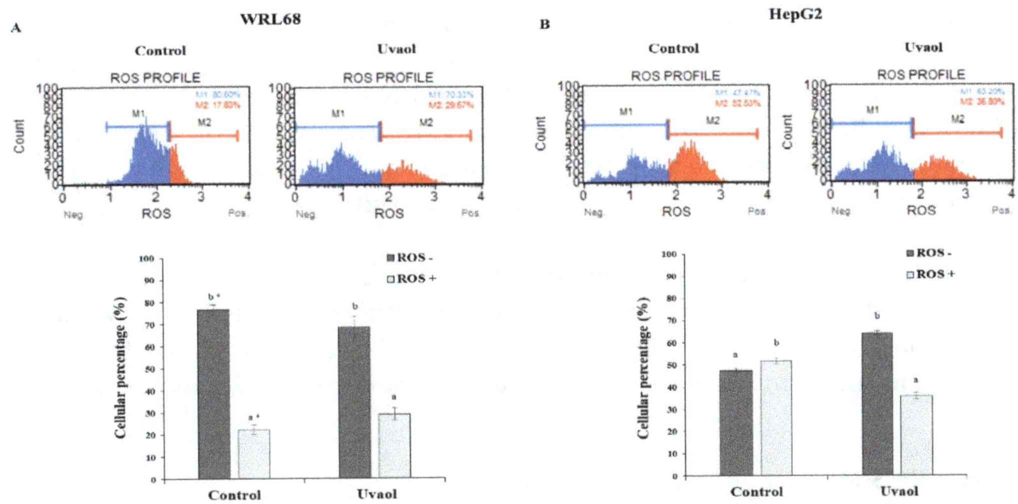

Figure 4. Cell cycle analysis obtained according to the Muse™ cell cycle kit. Panel (**A**) correspond to WRL68 cells and panel (**B**) to HepG2 cells. The cells were treated with IC_{50} of uvaol for 24 h. Top: histograms from a representative experiment show the effect of uvaol on cell cycle profile. Bottom: percentage of cells in each cellular cycle phase. Values are expressed as mean ± SEM (n = 12). Different letters indicate significant differences ($p < 0.05$) between control and uvaol treatment within each phases of the cell cycle for WRL168 or HepG2 cells. The inclusion of asterisks indicates significant differences ($p < 0.05$) between the different cells lines (WRL168 vs. HepG2), under the same treatment (control or uvaol) and phase of cell cycle.

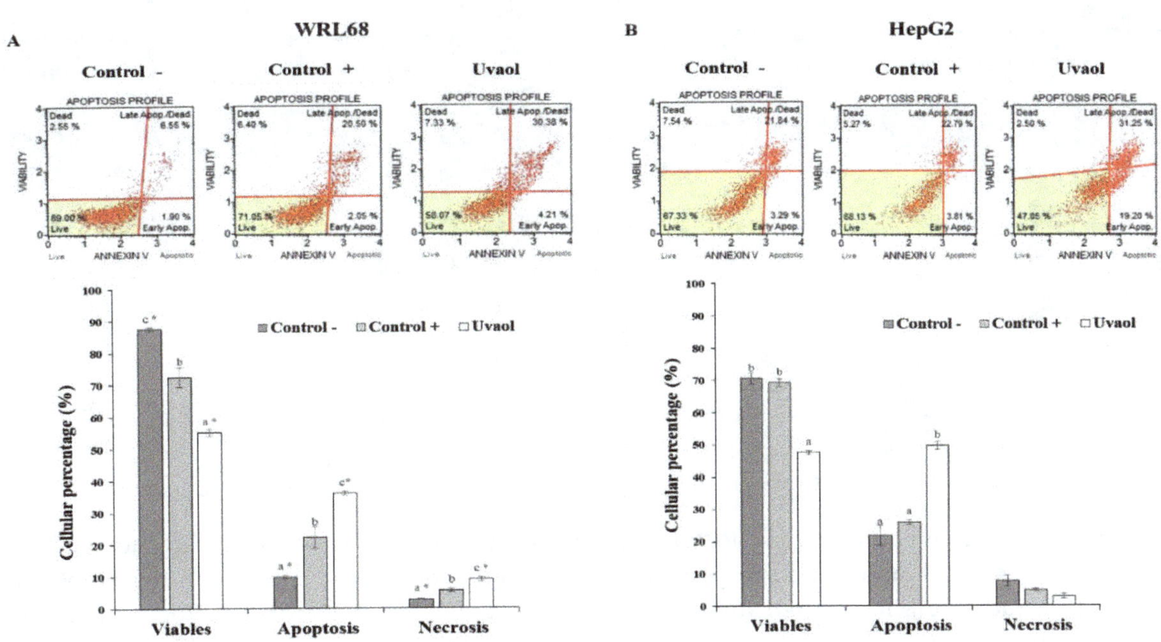

Figure 5. Apoptosis analysis obtained according to the Muse™ apoptosis kit. Panel (**A**) corresponds to the WRL68 cells and panel (**B**) to the HepG2 cells. Treatments included cells not treated (negative control) and cells incubated with staurosporine (1 μg/mL, positive control) or IC_{50} of uvaol for 24 h. Top: dot plots show a representative experiment of the different treatments. Bottom: percentage of lived, apoptotic and necrotic cells for each treatment. Values are expressed as mean ± SEM (n = 12). Different letters indicate significant differences ($p < 0.05$) between control and uvaol treatment within apoptosis stage (viable, apoptosis or necrosis) for WRL168 or HepG2 cells. The inclusion of asterisks indicates significant differences ($p < 0.05$) between different cells lines (WRL168 vs. HepG2), under the same treatment (control or uvaol) and apoptosis stage.

Figure 5A shows how both the addition of staurosporine (control +) and uvaol produced a significant decrease in the number of viable cells in the WRL68 line, which was accompanied by an equally significant increase in the number of apoptotic and necrotic cells in each situation with respect to control. In HepG2 cells (Figure 5B), treatment with staurosporine did not lead to an increase in apoptotic cells, while uvaol did induce a significant reduction in the percentage of viable cells, therefore, increasing the proportion of apoptotic cells. In none of the situations studied, changes in the rate of necrotic cells were generated.

When statistically comparing the results in both cell lines, significant differences were found in the death rate generated by uvaol in each case. The percentage of cells in apoptosis is higher in the HepG2 line, while, on the contrary, a higher rate of necrosis occurred in the WRL68 line, although significantly lower than the number of cells in apoptosis. Therefore, uvaol exerts a pro-apoptotic effect on both lines.

2.6. Uvaol Decreases ROS Production in HepG2 Cells

Intracellular ROS levels were measured by FACS under the four generic test conditions described above. Figure 6 includes the images of each experimental condition generated by the flow cytometer during its analysis. The results show the percentage of cells in each situation studied that express ROS (ROS+) and those that do not express them (ROS−).

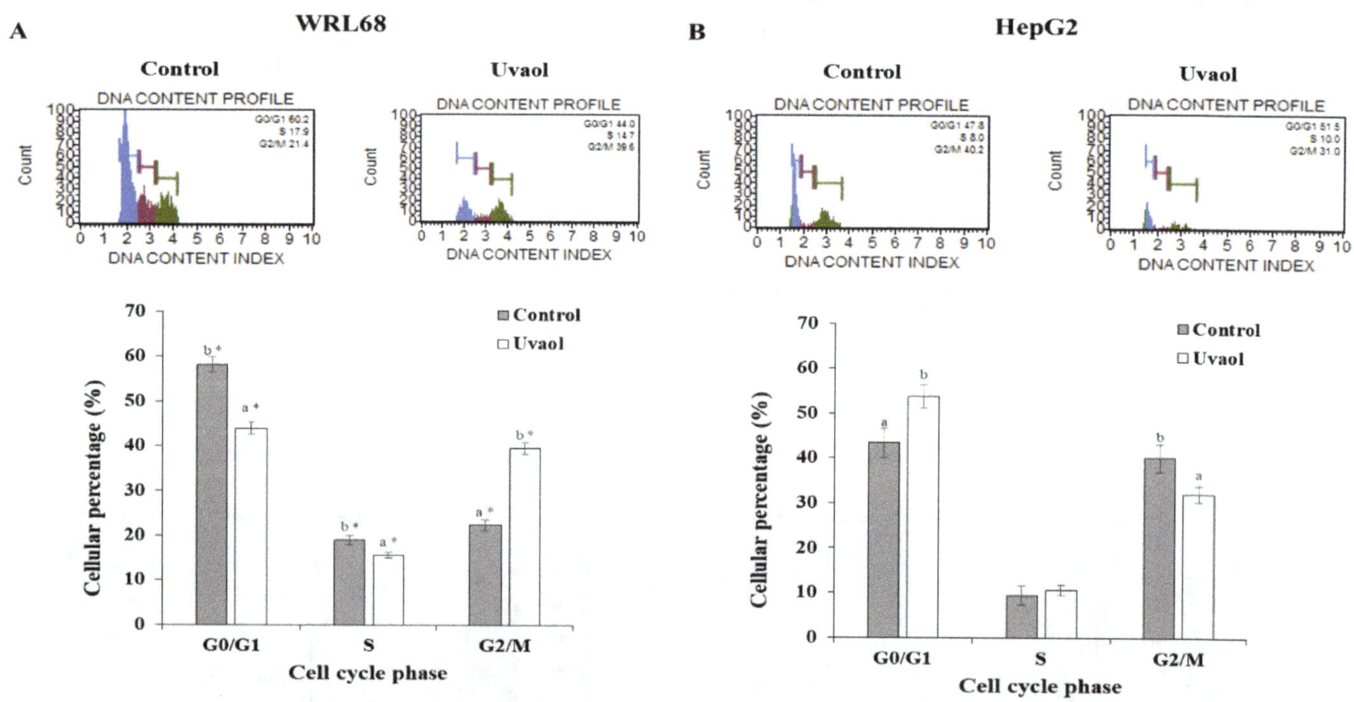

Figure 6. Reactive oxygen species (ROS) quantification was performed according to the Muse™ Oxidative stress kit. Panel (**A**) corresponds to the WRL68 cells and panel (**B**) to the HepG2 cells. Treatments included cells not treated and cells incubated with IC_{50} of uvaol for 24 h. Top: dot plots show a representative experiment of the different treatments. Bottom: percentage of ROS negative (ROS−) and ROS positive (ROS+) values observed for each treatment. Values are expressed as mean ± SEM (n = 12). Different letters indicate significant differences between ROS levels for each treatment and an asterisk indicates significant differences between cell lines for each treatment and ROS levels ($p < 0.05$).

Uvaol treatment maintained the ROS levels produced by the WRL68 cell line without significant differences with respect to the control situation (Figure 6A). The highest levels of ROS were produced in the control situation in the HepG2 cell line (Figure 6B). When treated with uvaol, a significant decrease in the percentage of cells expressing this type of reactive species was observed. When statistically comparing the results in both cell lines, no significant differences in ROS levels between the WRL68 and HepG2 lines after treatment were found. In control situation, significant differences were observed in ROS production levels, since HepG2 express higher levels of radicals.

2.7. *Uvaol Produces Up and Down-Regulation of Target Proteins in HepG2 Cells*

The expression of p53, c-Myc, Bcl-2, SOD, HSP-60 and Bax proteins for the WRL68 and HepG2 cell lines, in control situation and after treatment with the corresponding IC_{50} concentration of uvaol for 24 h, was measured through the Western blot technique. The level of expression obtained in each case was normalized with respect to the expression of actin (constitutive protein) and subsequently referred to that obtained in the control situation for the WRL68 line (Figure 7).

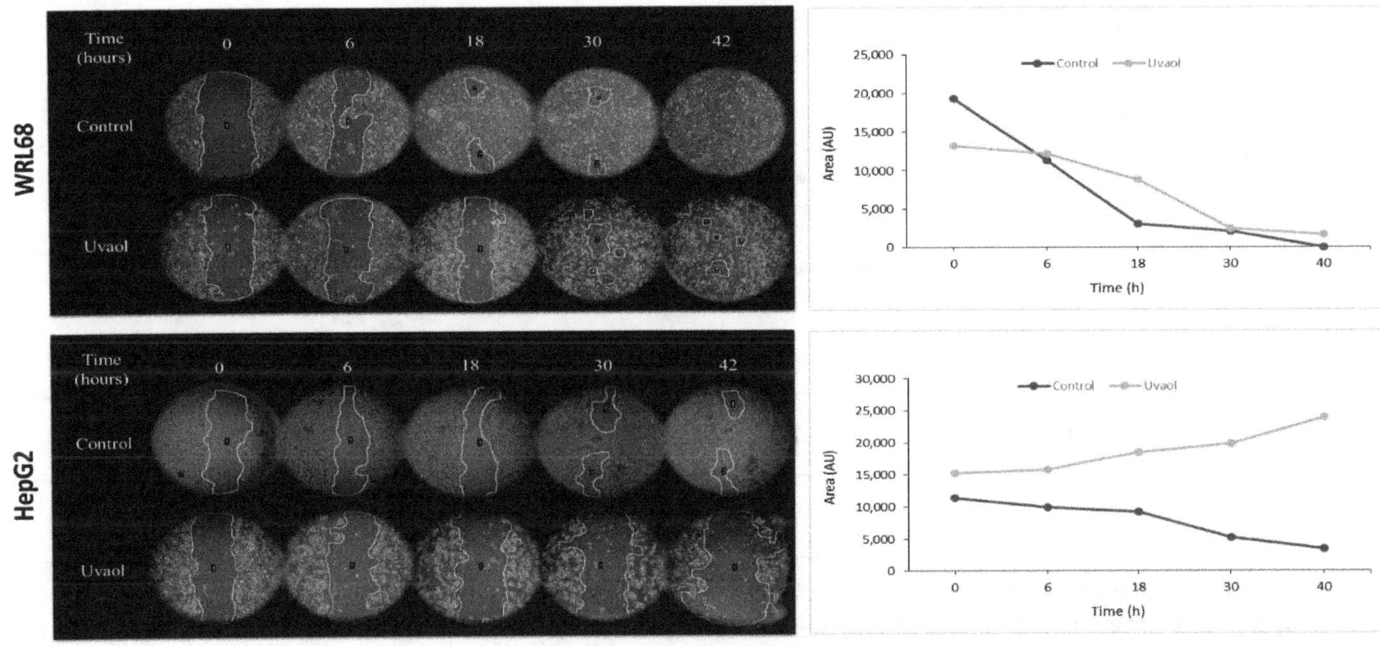

Figure 7. Western-blot analysis of **p53, c-Myc, Bcl-2, SOD, HSP-60** and **Bax** protein levels in WRL68 and HepG2 cells, untreated (WC and HC) and exposed to IC_{50} of uvaol for 24 h (WT and HT). The quantification of protein levels by densitometric analysis is shown in bar graphs. The results are the means ± SEM (n = 9) and are expressed as percentage of expression compared to actin. WRL68 values were used as 100% of expression and the rest of treatments were referred to them. Different letters indicate significant differences between treatments for each cell line and an asterisk indicates significant differences between cell lines for each treatment ($p < 0.05$).

The expression of p53 increased in the WRL68 line after treatment with uvaol regarding control, but remained unchanged in HepG2 cells, a situation that is repeated for SOD. In both cases, the percentage of control expression and after treatment for the HepG2 line was higher, with respect to expression after treatment in WRL68. In the case of c-Myc, an increase in its expression was observed in WRL68 with respect to the control, while it was maintained in HepG2. C-Myc levels in the control situation in HepG2 cells were higher than its expression after treatment in WRL68. The expression of HSP-60 increased in both lines when applying the treatment, being the percentage of expression after the addition of uvaol in WRL68 equal to the control situation in HepG2. Finally, the treatment did not produce changes in the expression of Bcl-2 either Bax in WRL68 cells, while their expression levels decreased and increased in HepG2 cells, respectively. In all the cases, the protein expressions were higher in the HepG2 cells than in the WRL68 cells when compared under the same experimental conditions.

2.8. *Uvaol Modulate Dual PI3K/MAPK Signaling Pathway in HepG2 Cells*

To analyze the mechanism by which uvaol exerts its anticancer activity, we studied whether such effect could be produced through the dual PI3K/MAPK signaling pathway. The results are shown in

Figure 8. Uvaol treatment produced a 22% decrease in cells that only activated the AKT/PI3K pathway, whereas the percentage of cells in which only ERK1/2/MAPK was activated, besides being too low, was not altered in the WRL68 cells. However, an increase of 25% was observed in cells that activated the dual pathway (MAPK and PI3K) (Figure 8A). When a net balance of activated signaling pathways is considered, no modification of the PI3K pathway was observed, but an activation of 25% took place in the ERK1/2/MAPK signaling pathway.

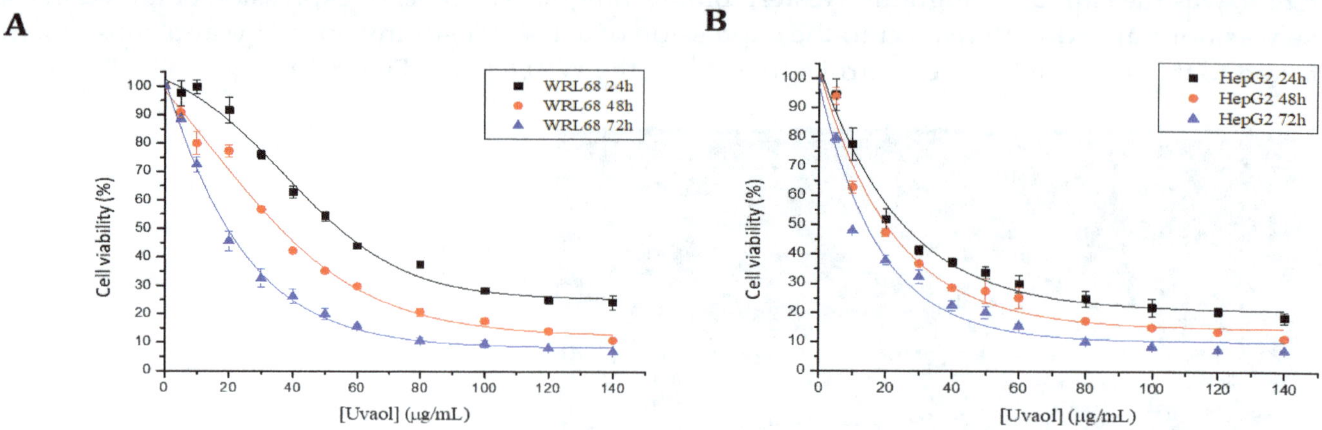

C

Cells	Inhibitory Concentration	Times of exposure of uvaol (μg/mL)		
		24h	48h	72h
WRL68	IC_{20}	27.6 ± 2.9^{a}	13.3 ± 0.8^{b}	6.8 ± 0.6^{c}
	IC_{50}	54.3 ± 1.0^{a}	35.9 ± 0.7^{b}	19.5 ± 1.1^{c}
	IC_{80}	--	79.8 ± 0.6^{a}	47.2 ± 4.3^{b}
Hep68	IC_{20}	8.2 ± 1.8^{a}	6.4 ± 0.4^{ab}	4.0 ± 0.2^{b}
	IC_{50}	25.2 ± 2.4^{a}	20.0 ± 0.3^{a}	14.1 ± 1.0^{b}
	IC_{80}	--	61.7 ± 5.3^{a}	39.2 ± 2.4^{b}

Figure 8. AKT/PI3K and ERK/1/2/MAPK dual pathway determination was performed according to the Muse™ PI3K/MAPK Dual Pathway activation kit. Panel (**A**) correspond to WRL68 cells and panel (**B**) to HepG2 cells. Treatments included cells not treated and cells incubated with IC_{50} of uvaol for 24 h. Top: dot plots show a representative experiment of the different treatments. Bottom: percentage of non-activated cells and cells with PI3K, MAPK and Dual pathway activated for each treatment. Values are expressed as mean ± SEM (n = 12). Different letters indicate significant differences between treatments for each activated pathway and an asterisk indicates significant differences between cell lines for each treatment and activated pathway ($p < 0.05$).

In HepG2 cells, uvaol effect on the percentage of cells that only activated AKT/PI3K induced a decrease of 25%. Similar to WRL68 cells, the percentage of cells that only activated ERK1/2/MAPK, besides being too low, was not altered in HepG2 cells. Regarding the activated dual pathway (MAPK and PI3K), uvaol only produced a 9% increase (Figure 8B). The net balance, in HepG2 cells, resulted in an inhibition of 16% in AKT/PI3K signaling pathway, whereas ERK1/2/MAPK signaling pathway was only increased in 9%.

3. Discussion

The Mediterranean diet is mainly characterized by the regular intake of olive oil, which presents in its composition different molecules with beneficial properties for health. Among them, pentacyclic triterpenes, such as uvaol, have been shown to have an anti-parasitic, anti-oxidant, anti-inflammatory and hepatoprotective activity, especially highlighting their potential as anticancer molecules [18]. Due to the lack of effective treatments against cellular hepatocarcinoma in advanced stages [33], and the fact that no researches about effect of uvaol have been performed in these type of cancer, this study was intended to characterize the anticancer activity of uvaol in the human cell lines WRL68 (hepatic control) and HepG2 (cellular hepatocarcinoma). For this purpose, its effect on the proliferation, migration, morphology, cell cycle, apoptosis, oxidative stress levels and protein markers of the processes described on the liver lines mentioned were determined.

The cytotoxicity assay is a useful test to preliminarily detect compounds that can affect the number of healthy cells in a total population. This trial showed that uvaol exerts an inhibition of cell proliferation in a dose and time dependent manner. Especially noteworthy is the result obtained for the 24 h IC_{50} concentration in both cell lines, being 25.2 μg/mL and 54.3 μg/mL for the HepG2 and WRL68 lines, respectively. As it can be seen, the concentration required to inhibit 50% of proliferation in control cells was more than twice the one used to inhibit the proliferation of tumor cells at the same rate, indicating greater susceptibility and specificity to the compound by hepatocarcinoma cells. To our knowledge, studies of the uvaol in cancer cells are limited. In this sense, similar results were observed in the human mammary tumor line MCF-7 in which uvaol produced anti-proliferative effects in a dose and time-dependent manner with values IC_{50}11.06 μg/mL and 44.27 μg/mL [32]. Other triterpenes olive derived, such as maslinic acid, have been tested in HepG2 cells, in which the cytotoxic effect was lower to that observed in this study, with a IC_{50} of 47 μg/mL at 72 h [34]. These values demonstrate a greater cytotoxic effect of uvaol than maslinic acid. Moreover, oleanolic-type saponins lowered the growth and proliferation of HepG2 in transplanted tumor in mice [35].

Triterpenes present in olive oil, such as ursolic acid or oleanolic acid have demonstrated anti-migratory and anti-angiogenic activities on several tumor lines [18]. To study if uvaol also had this effect, a wound healing assay was performed in the HepG2 cell line, confirming that this compound has an anti-migratory effect. Moreover, this effect was corroborated by a simultaneous morphological characterization, since it was observed that, after the addition of the compound, cells presented alterations in their structure and adhesion ability. Uvaol induced these same changes on the human astrocytoma line 1321N1, making cells show a loss of adhesion [31]. Furthermore, the administration of oleanolic acid in HepG2 caused a cellular retraction and the appearance of cytoplasmic extensions characteristic of the apoptosis process [36].

Some natural triterpenes exert anti-proliferative effects, due to their interference with the progression of the cell cycle or by the induction of cell death through apoptosis [30]. The arrest of the cycle in some of its phases constitutes a defense mechanism that allows damage repair in DNA, characteristic of tumoral cells [4]. Likewise, apoptosis is an essential process in organisms, since it allows for the elimination of cells, in a controlled manner, whose behavior or characteristics are away from homeostasis [5]. For this reason, flow cytometry studies were conducted to determine the process involved in the cytotoxic effect of uvaol on the cell lines under study. The results obtained showed that this triterpene was capable of inducing cell death through apoptosis with the corresponding concentration of IC_{50} in both cell lines. Similar results were found in lymphoma cells (U937), in which 10 and 100 μM of uvaol induced apoptosis [32]. Notwithstanding, the same concentrations of uvaol did not show this effect in MDA-MB-231 (triple negative breast cancer) or in MCF-7 cells [32]. Uvaol-induced cell cycle arrest occurred in the G_0/G_1 phase for HepG2 cells, while in WRL68 it was in the G_2/M phase. The use of uvaol on the MDA-MB-231 line did not produce changes in the progression of the cycle [29], while a concentration of 44.27 μg/mL of uvaol on the MCF-7 line and of 22.11 μg/mL of oleanolic acid on the HepG2 line resulted in an arrest in the same phase of the cycle [32,36], results that match with those obtained. Therefore, the anti-proliferative effect of uvaol on HepG2 cells is due to, simultaneously, the induction of apoptosis and an arrest in the G_0/G_1 phase of the cell cycle.

In cancer initiation, ROS levels are usually increased, due to the generation of a pro-oxidant environment maintained over time. This situation of oxidative stress, generally induced by an exacerbated production of free radicals, or by an imbalance in endogenous cellular antioxidant systems, can lead to the production of DNA damage, an initial step in neoplastic development [21]. For this reason, controlling ROS levels inside a cancer cell could be a good strategy to mitigate the genetic material damage, or even prevent to it. Triterpenes are characterized by having an antioxidant activity [18], a quality manifested in the HepG2 results obtained in the present study. Similar results were obtained in the MCF-7 and MDA-MB-231 lines for uvaol and erythrodiol [29,32]. However, these compounds produced an increase in the intracellular levels of ROS in 1321N1 cells, which also resulted in the reduction of mitochondrial potential and in an induction of apoptosis via the JNK kinase pathway [31]. Therefore, the action of uvaol on the oxidative state of cells is specific to each tumor cell line. Nevertheless, during normal detoxification process of any foreign compound, such as uvaol inside the cell, ROS can be also produced [37]. An augmentation of ROS levels in response to uvaol treatment did not occur in WRL68 cells, probably due to the increase of SOD expression found in the present study.

p53 and c-Myc proteins are directly involved in the regulation of cell proliferation, as well as in the succession of the different phases of the cell cycle and in the apoptosis process [5,7]. For this reason, the expression profile of the mentioned proteins was characterized in the WRL68 and HepG2 cell lines. Contrary to expectations, p53 levels were higher in the HepG2 than in WRL68 cells. This may be due to the fact that, despite being described a decrease in p53 expression in patients with HCC, due to mutations at different points of the gene that encodes it (TP53) [8], the HepG2 line has this gene intact, being probably induced its expression by situations far from homeostasis in cancer cells, such as an increase in ROS intracellular levels, appreciated in our results. Due to the cellular arrest observed in the G_0/G_1 phase and the maintenance of p53 expression levels after treatment with uvaol in HepG2 cells, it is possible that the inhibition of cell cycle progression is on account of the alteration of the expression of other proteins involved in this process, such as the family of Cdks or their inhibitors, among which are p15, p16, p21 or p27 [5]. Similarly, the increase in c-Myc expression caused by treatment in the WRL68 line may be related to the higher rate of cells found in the G_2/M phase, since c-Myc presents an important proliferative function. One of the main activities of c-Myc is cell cycle control, since it has been described that c-Myc expression levels tightly correlate to cell proliferation. Indeed, c-Myc is in charge of inducing the expression of several positive regulators of the cell cycle, such as Cdk4/6, E2F, Cyclin E, Cyclin A, Cdk1/2, among other factors. C-Myc also represses several cell cycle inhibitors, such as p15, p16, p21 or p27 [38]. Overall, it can be stated that an overexpression of c-Myc correlates with an increase percentage of proliferating cells, that is, cells in G2/M phase, as observed in treated WRL68 cells. In the case of the HepG2 line, the increase found in the control situation for c-Myc falls within the expected range, since it is a cancer cell with a high proliferation capacity. This same expression profile was found by Koutb et al. [7] when analyzing the gene expression of the c-Myc gene in blood samples obtained from HCC patients.

The family of proteins that share BH domains contribute to the progression of the cell cycle and the induction of apoptosis, since they are involved in survival mechanisms and in pathways that prevent cell proliferation. The most important member of this family is Bcl-2, a protein with anti-apoptotic effects that is generally increased in certain types of neoplasms, among which is HCC, giving them greater invasive ability and a lower response to treatments [39]. In our study, we observed how Bcl-2 levels remained unchanged after treatment with uvaol in the WRL68 line. As expected, its expression was increased in untreated HepG2 cells with respect to the control line. The administration of uvaol produced a decrease in the levels of this anti-apoptotic protein in the cancer line, a result that is consistent with the induction of cell death due to apoptosis, and the arrest in the G_0/G_1 phase obtained in our findings. Other triterpenes have been reported to also induce apoptosis in HepG2 cells through a down-regulation in Bcl-2 [40]. Similar results have been also found in other cancer cell lines, such as HT29 [41]. Moreover, these authors also observed that Bax pro-apoptotic protein expression increased in response to treatment with maslinic acid [41]. These results are in concordance to the results observed in the present study in which uvaol treatment increased Bax in HepG2 cells.

Heat shock proteins (HSP) form a family with a fundamental role in the correct folding and functionalization of proteins synthesized inside the cell. Clinical studies in patients with HCC show that the expression of HSP-60 is diminished in tumor cells with respect to healthy livers. This finding is related to a greater invasive ability of this neoplasm and a lower survival rate in patients. The lower differentiation gives these cells greater mobility, resulting in a high rate of invasion and subsequent metastasis [42]. Our results show that uvaol treatment induces an increase in the expression of HSP-60 in the WRL68 control line, being this rise more acute for the HepG2 line. This effect of uvaol in the HCC lines is a promising result, since it is related to the results obtained by Zhang et al. [42]. These authors observed that after inducing an overexpression of the gene that codes for the HSP-60 in HepG2 cells, these cells developed a phenotype with lower migratory capacity and greater cell differentiation, thus, decreasing their metastatic ability [42]. Together with HSP-60 overexpression, wound healing results obtained in this study confirm the effect of uvaol as a potential anti-migratory compound.

The AKT/PI3K pathway is known to be one of the most important signaling routes, which participates in cell growth, proliferation, cellular apoptosis and cytoskeletal rearrangement [43,44]. AKT is the major downstream target of the AKT/PI3K pathway. In addition to its interaction with Bcl-2 family effectors, the survival signal to cells is transferred by phospho-AKT [45]. Many studies have demonstrated that this pathway is activated in several types of cancer [46]. The results of the present study showed that uvaol significantly decreased AKT/PI3K pathway in HepG2 cells, whereas no changes were observed in the WRL68 line. On the contrary, levels of ERK1/2/MAPK were increased in both lines, although this increment was significantly lower in hepatoma cells. This up-regulation on MAPK pathway was consequence of the down-regulation on PI3K, since PI3K and Ras pathways can intersect by cross-talk among their downstream effectors [47]. In other HCC studies (HepG2, Huh-7, Hep3B, and Sk-Hep-1 cell lines) using triterpenoids, such as ursolic acid or platycodin D, the results also showed an inhibition of AKT/PI3K signaling pathway [48–50]. These results support the hypothesis that apoptosis induced by uvaol is mediated by the modulation of the AKT/PI3K signaling pathway in HepG2 cells.

Considering the promising in vitro preliminary results of uvaol usage as an anticancer compound (anti-proliferative, pro-apoptotic and antioxidant) drawn from the present work, our future research will be focused on testing these same bioactive properties of uvaol in additional HCC cell lines, with the aim to finally move into in vivo preclinical models. Our next objective is to create HCC cell line-derived xenografts (CDX) and patient derived xenografts (PDX), to see if the observed antitumor properties of uvaol are maintained in vivo. These observations could provide enough evidence for considering a future usage of uvaol in humans as a nutraceutical compound in the food industry or even a therapeutic drug in the clinic; current milestones in cancer research.

4. Materials and Methods

4.1. Cell Cultures

The cell lines used were WRL68 (model liver cells) and HepG2 (hepatocellular carcinoma), provided by "*Centro de Instrumentación Científica*" (CIC) of the University of Granada. The cells were grown in Dulbecco's modified Eagle medium (DMEM) and minimum essential medium (MEM), respectively. In both cases, they were supplemented with 10% heat-inactivated foetal bovine serum (FBS) and 1% streptomycin/penicillin antibiotics. They were kept in a CO_2 incubator at 37 °C, 95% relative humidity and 5% CO_2. Cells were passaged at preconfluent densities by the use of a solution containing 0.05% trypsin and 0.5 mM EDTA. The cells were seeded in the culture dishes at the desired density with the appropriate culture medium.

4.2. Uvaol Solution

The compound tested in the experiments performed was uvaol, provided by Sigma® (St. Louis, MO, USA), with a purity greater than 95%. A stock solution of uvaol with a concentration of 1 mg/mL (in 40 μL of DMSO + 960 μL culture medium) was prepared and subsequently diluted in culture medium until reaching the concentrations required for each test.

4.3. Morphological Changes

A morphological characterization of both cell lines in triplicate was carried out in a control situation (cells growing attached in culture medium) and after uvaol treatment corresponding to the

IC_{50} calculated for 24 h. Optical microscopy (Olympus® model CX22LED, Tokyo, Japan) images of the cultures were obtained in the mentioned conditions at 10 and 40 magnifications for the cell line each after 24 h of the treatment's application.

4.4. MTT Assay

MTT assay was performed as described by Pérez-Jiménez et al. [51]. Briefly, samples containing 200 μL cell suspension (1×10^4 cells/well) were cultured in 96 well plates, in triplicate of three populations of the both cell lines. Subsequent to adherence of the cells within 12 h of incubation, Uvaol was added to the wells at a concentration between 0–140 μg/mL and maintained during 24, 48 and 72 h. MTT was dissolved in the medium and added to the wells at a final concentration of 0.5 mg/mL. Following 2 h of incubation, the generated formazan was dissolved in DMSO. Absorbance was measured at 570 nm in a multiplate reader (Bio-tek®, Winooski, VT, USA). The concentrations that caused 20%, 50% and 80% of inhibition of cell viability (IC_{20}, IC_{50} and IC_{80}) were calculated following the formula: % cell viability = (A0 − AT)/A0·100, where A0 is the control absorbance (100% of cell viability) and AT is de absorbance of the incubated cells with the different concentrations of uvaol. OriginPro 8 (OriginLab Corporation, Northampton, MA, USA) was used to performance a dose-response analysis by the following formula:

$$y = A_1 + \frac{A_2 - A_1}{1 + 10^{(Log\ x_0 - x)p}}$$

In which $Logx_0$ is the center of the curve, p the slope, A_1 the lower asymptote and A_2 the upper asymptote in the adjustment model described.

4.5. Scratch Assay

The wound healing or scratch assay was used to assess the migration capacity of the WRL68 and HepG2 cell lines. With this objective, 3×10^5 cells were seeded per well in a 6-well plate in triplicate for each cell line. When the populations reached a confluence of 80–90%, a sterile pipette tip was used to disrupt in a straight line (make a wound) the layer of cells attached to the culture surface. Subsequently, it was washed with PBS to prevent the cells that had been lifted from being able to rejoin. The control and monitoring of cell migration was carried out by imaging with optical microscopy the culture at different times (0 h, 6 h, 18 h, 30 h and 42 h) at 10 magnifications from the realization of the wound, to be able to identify the possible differences between the control cases (growing cells attached in culture medium) and after the addition of the IC_{50} concentration for 24 h in both lines. Quantification of wound healing was performed by using the MRI-Wound Healing Tool for ImageJ software (ImageJ 1.53a version).

4.6. Cell Sorting by Flow Cytometry

A total of 1.5×10^5 cells were seeded per well in 24-well plates for each cell line (quadruplicates for three different populations of each cell line). After 24 hallowing the cells to adhere, they were separated into four different groups: negative control WRL68 and HepG2 populations and WRL68 and HepG2 populations treated with the concentration corresponding to their uvaol IC_{50} for 24 h (in addition to other specific conditions of each test described in the corresponding section). Negative control populations were incubated only with the appropriate culture medium. The samples were analyzed in the Muse™ Cell Analyzer (Merck-Millipore®, Burlington, MA, USA).

4.6.1. Cell Cycle Assay

The method is based on the analysis of the cell cycle through the discrimination of three populations: cells in phase G_0/G_1, S or G_2/M. For this, the Muse™ Cell Cycle Kit purchased from Millipore (Billerica, MA, USA) was used following the specification of manufacturer.

4.6.2. Apoptosis Assay

Phosphatidylserine (PS) is a phospholipid that is usually found in the inner half of the cytoplasmic membrane, but is outsourced when loss of integrity occurs in the apoptosis process. The method is based on the recognition and binding to the PS exposed by annexin V protein, labeled with a fluorescent substance to detect the interaction and quantify it. We used the Muse^{TM} Annexin V & Dead Cell kit purchased from Millipore (Billerica, MA, USA), which provides the percentage of viable cells, apoptotic and affected by necrosis. A positive control was carried out, incubating cells with staurosporine (1 μg/mL), a nonspecific inhibitor of kinase proteins isolated from the *Streptomyces staurosporeus* species, which shows the ability to induce the apoptotic pathway in a large number of tumor lines, being especially characterized this effect on the HepG2 cell line [35].

4.6.3. Measurement of ROS Production

The method is based on the use of dihydroetide (DHE), a reagent capable of crossing the cell membrane and interacting with superoxide anions, a type of ROS. In this process, DHE oxidizes and forms the DNA intercalating agent ethidium bromide, detectable by its fluorescence emission. This allows two cell populations to be distinguished, those that express remarkable levels of ROS (ROS+) and those that do not (ROS−). The Muse^{TM} Oxidative Stress kit purchased from Millipore (Billerica, MA, USA) was used for this purpose.

4.7. Protein Extraction and Western Blot Analysis

Triplicates of three different populations of each cell line, WRL68 and HepG2, were seeded in 6-well plates with a density of 2.5×10^5 cells per well. The corresponding IC_{50} concentration for 24 h was added in the treated populations. For protein extraction, each sample was resuspended in 20 μL of RIPA buffer (150 mM NaCl, 1% Igepal, 0.5% deoxycholic acid, 0.1% SDS, 50 mM Tris HCl pH 7.5, 0.2 M PMSF, 700 mM OV_4 and Thermo Scientific® PierceTM inhibitor cocktail, Waltham, MA, USA), and held on ice for 15 min. They were centrifuged at 15,000× *g* for 10 min at 4 °C, the supernatant was collected and stored at −80 °C for further analysis. The quantification of the protein concentration was carried out through the Bradford method.

The methodology used for Western blot analysis is described by Mokhtari et al. [19]. Brie fly, the initial separation of the extracts was performed by a 12% polyacrylamide gel electrophoresis under denaturing conditions (SDS-PAGE). A standardized load of 30 μg of protein per well was used after denaturing the samples at 95 °C for 5 min and adding the loading buffer (0.25 mM Tris-HCl pH 6.8, 10% SDS, 1 M DTT and glycerol). The proteins were transferred, by the semi-dry transfer method, (60 mA per gel, 1 h) using the TransBlot Turbo system (BioRad®, Berkeley, CA, USA), to a PVDF membrane. The membranes were blocked with blocking buffer (TBS, 0.1% Tween-20 and 3% skimmed milk) for 1 h at room temperature, incubating with the specific primary antibodies against the proteins studied at 4 °C overnight. The primary antibodies (from Santa Cruz Biotechnology®, Dallas, TX, USA) were diluted in blocking buffer. The membranes were washed with TBS-T (TBS, 0.1% Tween-20) for 5 min three times under stirring, and incubated with the corresponding secondary antibody (from Sigma®, St. Louis, MO, USA) (Table 1) for 1 h at room temperature, repeating the previous washing process later. These secondary antibodies have the enzyme horseradish peroxidase (HRP) coupled, which allows chemiluminescence to be detected in the presence of the protein band due to its ability to oxidize the luminol solution (ECL-plus Western-blot detection system, GE Healthcare, Chicago, IL, USA). The reaction produced was captured inside a ChemiDoc Imaging System (Bio-Rad®, Berkely, CA, USA). The program used to analyze the images obtained was Image Lab Software (Bio-Rad®, for PC 6.1 version). The expression of each protein was normalized referring to actin levels and were represented based on the results obtained for the control situation (WRL68 line without treatment) as percentage of expression (%). The expression obtained in each protein was analyzed through the mentioned program in triplicate.

Table 1. Description of the polyclonal antibodies (IgG) used in the Western blot technique.

Protein	Primary Antibody	Secondary Antibody
p53	Rabbit anti-p53 antibody (1:500)	Anti-mouse IgG antibody (1:5000)
SOD	Rabbit anti-SOD antibody (1:250)	Anti-rabbit IgG antibody (1:5000)
c-Myc	Goat anti-c-Myc antibody (1:500)	Anti-goat IgG antibody (1:5000)
HSP-60	Mouse anti-HSP-60 antibody (1:250)	Anti-mouse IgG antibody (1:5000)
Bcl-2	Rabbit anti-Bcl-2 antibody (1:500)	Anti-rabbit IgG antibody (1:5000)
Bax	Mouse anti-Bax antibody (1:500)	Anti-mouse IgG antibody (1:5000)
Actin	Mouse anti-actin antibody (1:1.000)	Anti-mouse IgG antibody (1:5000)

4.8. PI3K/MAPK Dual Pathway Activation Assay

The Muse® PI3K/MAPK Dual Pathway activation kit purchased from Millipore (Billerica, MA, USA) was employed to examine both the PI3K and MAPK signaling pathways simultaneously using the Muse Cell Analyzer (Merck-Millipore®, Burlington, MA, USA). The protocol followed was performed as the manufacturer instructions. The samples (quadruplicates for three different populations of each cell line) were analyzed in the Muse™ Cell Analyzer.

4.9. Statistical Analysis

The results were expressed as mean ± standard error of the mean (SEM). Likewise, the study of the statistical difference between the data groups was carried out through the analysis of the two-way variance (two-way ANOVA). When interactions between the analyzed factors were present, the one-way analysis of the variance (one-way ANOVA) was used followed by the Tukey test. The differences were considered significant for p values < 0.05. Statistical analyses were performed using the IBM SPSS Statistics (IBM®, 22.0 version) software.

5. Conclusions

In conclusion, taken together, the results of this study suggest that uvaol exhibits a potential anti-proliferative effect through G_0/G_1 cell cycle arrest, apoptosis, by inhibition of AKT/PI3K signaling pathway, and decreased ROS levels on the HepG2 human hepatocarcinoma cell line.

Author Contributions: E.E.R.-P., A.P.-J. and J.P. have designed the research plan; G.C.B.-P., A.P.-J., I.G.-C., A.M.P.-P., F.J.R.-Z., E.S., R.C. and E.E.R.-P. have performed the different experiments; E.E.R.-P., J.P., A.P.-J. and J.A.L. have analyzed the data and G.C.B.-P., A.P.-J. and E.E.R.-P. have written the manuscript. All authors have read and agreed to the published version of the manuscript.

References

1. Bray, F.; Ferlay, J.; Soerjomataram, I.; Siegel, R.L.; Torre, L.A.; Jemal, A. Global Cancer Statistics 2018: GLOBOCAN Estimates of incidence and mortality worldwide for 36 cancers in 185 countries. *CA Cancer J. Clin.* **2018**, *68*, 394–424. [CrossRef]
2. European Association for the Study of the Liver. EASL Clinical practice guidelines: Management of hepatocellular carcinoma. *J. Hepatol.* **2018**, *69*, 182–236. [CrossRef] [PubMed]
3. Shin, J.W.; Chung, Y.H. Molecular targeted therapy for hepatocellular carcinoma: Current and future. *World J. Gastroenterol.* **2013**, *19*, 6144–6155. [CrossRef] [PubMed]

4. Justman, Q.A. Looking beyond the stop sign: Cell-cycle checkpoints reconsidered. *Cell Syst.* **2017**, *5*, 438–440. [CrossRef] [PubMed]
5. Chen, J.D. The cell-cycle arrest and apoptotic functions of p53 in tumor initiation and progression. *Csh. Perspect Med.* **2016**, *6*, a026104. [CrossRef] [PubMed]
6. Villanueva, A.; Newell, P.; Chiang, D.Y.; Friedman, S.L.; Llovet, J.M. Genomics and signaling pathways in hepatocellular carcinoma. *Semin. Liver Dis.* **2007**, *27*, 55–76. [CrossRef]
7. Koutb, F.; Abdel-Rahman, S.; Hassona, E.; Haggag, A. Association of C-myc and p53 gene expression and polymorphisms with hepatitis c (HCV) chronic infection, cirrhosis and hepatocellular carcinoma (HCC) stages in Egypt. *Asian Pac. J. Cancer Prev.* **2017**, *18*, 2049–2057. [CrossRef]
8. Merle, P.; Trepo, C. Molecular mechanisms underlying hepatocellular carcinoma. *Viruses Basel* **2009**, *1*, 852–872. [CrossRef]
9. Zhang, X.R.; Chen, Y.L.; Cai, G.S.; Li, X.; Wang, D. Carnosic acid induces apoptosis of hepatocellular carcinoma cells via ROS-mediated mitochondrial pathway. *Chem. Biol. Interact.* **2017**, *277*, 91–100. [CrossRef]
10. Pilz, R.B.; Willis, R.C.; Boss, G.R. The influence of ribose 5-phosphate availability on purine synthesis of cultured human lymphoblasts and mitogen-stimulated lymphocytes. *J. Biol. Chem.* **1984**, *259*, 2927–2935.
11. Kan, B.; London, I.M.; Levin, D.H. Role of reversing factor in the inhibition of protein synthesis initiation by oxidized glutathione. *J. Biol. Chem.* **1988**, *263*, 15652–15656. [PubMed]
12. Lupiáñez, J.A.; Adroher, F.J.; Vargas, A.M.; Osuna, A. Differential behaviour of glucose 6-phosphate dehydrogenase in two morphological forms of *Trypanosoma cruzi*. *Int. J. Biochem.* **1987**, *19*, 1085–1089. [CrossRef] [PubMed]
13. Barroso, J.B.; García-Salguero, L.; Peragón, J.; de la Higuera, M.; Lupiáñez, J.A. The influence of dietary-protein on the kinetics of NADPH production systems in various tissues of rainbow-trout (*Oncorhynchus mykiss*). *Aquaculture* **1994**, *124*, 47–59. [CrossRef]
14. Barroso, J.B.; Peragón, J.; García-Salguero, L.; de la Higuera, M.; Lupiáñez, J.A. Carbohydrate deprivation reduces NADPH-production in fish liver but not in adipose tissue. *Int. J. Biochem. Cell Biol.* **2001**, *33*, 785–796. [CrossRef]
15. Peragón, J.; Barroso, J.B.; García-Salguero, L.; Aranda, F.; de la Higuera, M.; Lupiáñez, J.A. Selective changes in the protein-turnover rates and nature of growth induced in trout liver by long-term starvation followed by re-feeding. *Mol. Cell Biochem.* **1999**, *201*, 1–10. [CrossRef] [PubMed]
16. Peragón, J.; Barroso, J.B.; García-Salguero, L.; de la Higuera, M.; Lupiáñez, J.A. Dietary alterations in protein, carbohydrates and fat increase liver protein-turnover rate and decrease overall growth rate in the rainbow trout (*Oncorhynchus mykiss*). *Mol. Cell Biochem.* **2000**, *209*, 97–104. [CrossRef]
17. Rufino-Palomares, E.; Reyes-Zurita, F.J.; Fuentes-Almagro, C.A.; de la Higuera, M.; Lupiáñez, J.A.; Peragón, J. Proteomics in the liver of gilthead sea bream (*Sparus aurata*) to elucidate the cellular response induced by the intake of maslinic acid. *Proteomics* **2011**, *11*, 3312–3325. [CrossRef]
18. Rufino-Palomares, E.E.; Pérez-Jiménez, A.; Reyes-Zurita, F.J.; García-Salguero, L.; Mokhtari, K.; Herrera-Merchán, A.; Medina, P.P.; Peragón, J.; Lupiáñez, J.A. Anti-cancer and anti-angiogenic properties of various natural pentacyclic tri-terpenoids and some of their chemical derivatives. *Curr. Org. Chem.* **2015**, *19*, 919–947. [CrossRef]
19. Mokhtari, K.; Rufino-Palomares, E.E.; Pérez-Jiménez, A.; Reyes-Zurita, F.J.; Figuera, C.; García-Salguero, L.; Medina, P.P.; Peragón, J.; Lupiáñez, J.A. Maslinic acid, a triterpene from olive, affects the antioxidant and mitochondrial status of B16F10 melanoma cells grown under stressful conditions. *Evid. Based Compl. Alt.* **2015**, *2015*, 272457. [CrossRef]
20. Yuan, X.X.; Wang, B.Y.; Yang, L.; Zhang, Y.L. The role of ROS-induced autophagy in hepatocellular carcinoma. *Clin. Res. Hepatol. Gas* **2018**, *42*, 306–312. [CrossRef]
21. Brieger, K.; Schiavone, S.; Miller, F.J.; Krause, K. H, Reactive oxygen species: From health to disease. *Swiss Med. Wkly.* **2012**, *142*, w13659. [CrossRef]
22. Kulik, L.; El-Serag, H.B. Epidemiology and management of hepatocellular carcinoma. *Gastroenterology* **2019**, *156*, 477–491. [CrossRef] [PubMed]
23. Llovet, J.M.; Villanueva, A.; Lachenmayer, A.; Finn, R.S. Advances in targeted therapies for hepatocellular carcinoma in the genomic era. *Nat. Rev. Clin. Oncol.* **2015**, *12*, 408–424. [CrossRef] [PubMed]
24. Yuan, H.D.; Ma, Q.Q.; Ye, L.; Piao, G.C. The traditional medicine and modern medicine from natural products. *Molecules* **2016**, *21*, 559. [CrossRef] [PubMed]

25. Escrich, E.; Ramírez-Tortosa, M.C.; Sánchez-Rovira, P.; Colomer, R.; Solanas, M.; Gaforio, J.J. Olive oil in cancer prevention and progression. *Nutr. Rev.* **2006**, *64*, S40–S52. [CrossRef]
26. López-García, E.; Rodríguez-Artalejo, F.; Li, T.Y.; Fung, T.T.; Li, S.S.; Willett, W.C.; Rimm, E.B.; Hu, F.B. The mediterranean-style dietary pattern and mortality among men and women with cardiovascular disease. *Am. J. Clin. Nutr.* **2014**, *99*, 172–180. [CrossRef]
27. Yubero-Serrano, E.M.; López-Moreno, J.; Gómez-Delgado, F.; López-Miranda, J. Extra virgin olive oil: More than a healthy fat. *Eur. J. Clin. Nutr.* **2019**, *72*, 8–17. [CrossRef]
28. Preedy, V.R.; Watson, R.R. *Olives and Olive Oil in Health and Disease Prevention*; Academic Press: San Diego, CA, USA, 2010; p. 1520.
29. Sánchez-Quesada, C.; López-Biedma, A.; Gaforio, J.J. The differential localization of a methyl group confers a different anti-breast cancer activity to two triterpenes present in olives. *Food Funct.* **2015**, *6*, 249–256. [CrossRef]
30. Sánchez-Quesada, C.; López-Biedma, A.; Warleta, F.; Campos, M.; Beltrán, G.; Gaforio, J.J. Bioactive properties of the main triterpenes found in olives, virgin olive oil, and leaves of *Olea europaea*. *J. Agric. Food Chem.* **2013**, *61*, 12173–12182. [CrossRef]
31. Martín, R.; Ibeas, E.; Carvalho-Tavares, J.; Hernández, M.; Ruiz-Gutiérrez, V.; Nieto, M.L. Natural triterpenic diols promote apoptosis in astrocytoma cells through ROS-mediated mitochondrial depolarization and JNK activation. *PLoS ONE* **2009**, *4*, e5975. [CrossRef]
32. Allouche, Y.; Warleta, F.; Campos, M.; Sánchez-Quesada, C.; Uceda, M.; Beltrán, G.; Gaforio, J.J. Antioxidant, antiproliferative, and pro-apoptotic capacities of pentacyclic triterpenes found in the skin of olives on MCF-7 human breast cancer cells and their effects on DNA damage. *J. Agric. Food Chem.* **2011**, *59*, 121–130. [CrossRef]
33. Grandhi, M.S.; Kim, A.K.; Ronnekleiv-Kelly, S.M.; Kamel, I.R.; Ghasebeh, M.A.; Pawlik, T.M. Hepatocellular carcinoma: From diagnosis to treatment. *Surg. Oncol.* **2016**, *25*, 74–85. [CrossRef] [PubMed]
34. Peragón, J.; Rufino-Palomares, E.E.; Muñoz-Espada, I.; Reyes-Zurita, F.J.; Lupiáñez, J.A. A new HPLC-MS method for measuring maslinic acid and oleanolic acid in HT29 and HepG2 human cancer cells. *Int. J. Mol. Sci.* **2015**, *16*, 21681–21694. [CrossRef] [PubMed]
35. Wang, X.Y.; Zhang, W.; Gao, K.; Lu, Y.Y.; Tang, H.F.; Sun, X.L. Oleanane-type saponins from *Anemone taipaiensis* and their cytotoxic activities. *Fitoterapia* **2013**, *89*, 224–230. [CrossRef] [PubMed]
36. Zhu, Y.Y.; Huang, H.Y.; Wu, Y.L. Anticancer and apoptotic activities of oleanolic acid are mediated through cell cycle arrest and disruption of mitochondrial membrane potential in HepG2 human hepatocellular carcinoma cells. *Mol. Med. Rep.* **2015**, *12*, 5012–5018. [CrossRef] [PubMed]
37. Halliwell, B.; Gutteridge, J.M.C. *Free Radicals in Biology and Medicine*, 5th ed.; Oxford University Press: New York, NY, USA, 2015.
38. Bretones, G.; Delgado, M.D.; León, J. Myc and cell cycle control. *Biochim. Biophys. Acta* **2015**, *1849*, 506–516. [CrossRef] [PubMed]
39. Frenzel, A.; Grespi, F.; Chmelewskij, W.; Villunger, A. Bcl2 Family proteins in carcinogenesis and the treatment of cancer. *Apoptosis* **2009**, *14*, 584–596. [CrossRef]
40. Wang, J.J.; Han, H.; Chen, X.F.; Yi, Y.H.; Sun, H.X. Cytotoxic and apoptosis-inducing activity of triterpene glycosides from *Holothuria scabra* and *Cucumaria frondosa* against HepG2 cells. *Mar. Drugs* **2014**, *12*, 4274–4290. [CrossRef]
41. Parra, A.; Martín-Fonseca, S.; Rivas, F.; Reyes-Zurita, F.J.; Medina-O'Donnell, M.; Rufino-Palomares, E.E.; Martínez, A.; García-Granados, A.; Lupiáñez, J.A.; Albericio, F. Solid-phase library synthesis of bi-functional derivatives of oleanolic and maslinic acids and their cytotoxicity on three cancer cell lines. *Acs Comb. Sci.* **2014**, *16*, 428–447. [CrossRef]
42. Zhang, J.; Zhou, X.C.; Chang, H.L.; Huang, X.J.; Guo, X.; Du, X.H.; Tian, S.Y.; Wang, L.X.; Lyv, Y.H.; Yuan, P.; et al. Hsp60 exerts a tumor suppressor function by inducing cell differentiation and inhibiting invasion in hepatocellular carcinoma. *Oncotarget* **2016**, *7*, 68976–68989. [CrossRef]
43. Kauffmann-Zeh, A.; Rodríguez-Viciana, P.; Ulrich, E.; Gilbert, C.; Coffer, P.; Downward, J.; Evan, G. Suppression of c-Myc-induced apoptosis by Ras signalling through PI(3)K and PKB. *Nature* **1997**, *385*, 544–548. [CrossRef] [PubMed]
44. Yang, Y.; Yang, L.; You, Q.D.; Nie, F.F.; Gu, H.Y.; Zhao, L.; Wang, X.T.; Guo, Q.L. Differential Apoptotic Induction of gambogic acid, a novel anticancer natural product, on hepatoma cells and normal hepatocytes. *Cancer Lett.* **2007**, *256*, 259–266. [CrossRef] [PubMed]

45. Duronio, V.; Scheid, M.P.; Ettinger, S. Downstream signalling events regulated by phosphatidylinositol 3-kinase activity. *Cell Signal.* **1998**, *10*, 233–239. [CrossRef]
46. Vivanco, I.; Sawyers, C.L. The phosphatidylinositol 3-kinase-AKT pathway in human cancer. *Nat. Rev. Cancer* **2002**, *2*, 489–501. [CrossRef]
47. Moelling, K.; Schad, K.; Bosse, M.; Zimmermann, S.; Schweneker, M. Regulation of Raf-Akt cross-talk. *J. Biol. Chem.* **2002**, *277*, 31099–31106. [CrossRef] [PubMed]
48. Chuang, W.L.; Lin, P.Y.; Lin, H.C.; Chen, Y.L. The apoptotic effect of ursolic acid on SK-Hep-1 cells is regulated by the PI3K/Akt, p38 and JNK MAPK signaling pathways. *Molecules* **2016**, *21*, 460. [CrossRef] [PubMed]
49. Qin, H.; Du, X.Y.; Zhang, Y.; Wang, R. Platycodin D, a triterpenoid saponin from *Platycodon grandiflorum*, induces G2/M arrest and apoptosis in human hepatoma HepG2 cells by modulating the PI3K/Akt pathway. *Tumor Biol.* **2014**, *35*, 1267–1274. [CrossRef]
50. Tang, C.; Lu, Y.H.; Xie, J.H.; Wang, F.; Zou, J.N.; Yang, J.S.; Xing, Y.Y.; Xi, T. Downregulation of survivin and activation of caspase-3 through the PI3K/Akt pathway in ursolic acid-induced HepG2 cell apoptosis. *AntiCancer Drugs* **2009**, *20*, 249–258. [CrossRef]
51. Pérez-Jiménez, A.; Rufino-Palomares, E.E.; Fernández-Gallego, N.; Ortuño-Costela, M.C.; Reyes-Zurita, F.J.; Peragón, J.; García-Salguero, L.; Mokhtari, K.; Medina, P.P.; Lupiáñez, J.A. Target Molecules in 3T3-L1 adipocytes differentiation are regulated by maslinic acid, a natural triterpene from *Olea europaea*. *Phytomedicine* **2016**, *23*, 1301–1311. [CrossRef]

Potent Cytotoxicity of Novel L-Shaped Ortho-Quinone Analogs through Inducing Apoptosis

Sheng-You Li [1,2], Ze-Kun Sun [2,3], Xue-Yi Zeng [2,4], Yue Zhang [2,5], Meng-Ling Wang [2,4], Sheng-Cao Hu [4], Jun-Rong Song [2,4], Jun Luo [4], Chao Chen [2,4,*], Heng Luo [2,4,*] and Wei-Dong Pan [1,2,4,*]

1 College of Pharmacy, Guizhou University, Huaxi Avenue South, Guiyang 550025, China; 13118517665@163.com
2 State Key Laboratory of Functions and Applications of Medicinal Plants, Guizhou Medical University, 3491 Baijin Road, Guiyang 550014, China; xueyizeng@126.com (X.-Y.Z.); menglingwang@yahoo.com (M.-L.W.); 18275365116@163.com (J.-R.S.); 18798628024@163.com (J.L.)
3 School of Medicine, Guizhou University, Huaxi Avenue South, Guiyang 550025, China; zekunsun@163.com
4 The Key Laboratory of Chemistry for Natural Products of Guizhou Province and Chinese Academy of Sciences, 3491 Baijin Road, Guiyang 550014, China; hushengcao0221@163.com
5 College of Agriculture, Guizhou University, Huaxi Avenue South, Guiyang 550025, China; zhangyueinsect@163.com
* Correspondence: cc283818640@163.com (C.C.); luoheng@gzcnp.cn (H.L.); wdpan@163.com (W.D.P.);

Academic Editor: Qiao-Hong Chen

Abstract: Twenty-seven L-shaped ortho-quinone analogs were designed and synthesized using a one pot double-radical synthetic strategy followed by removing methyl at C-3 of the furan ring and introducing a diverse side chain at C-2 of the furan ring. The synthetic derivatives were investigated for their cytotoxicity activities against human leukemia cells K562, prostate cancer cells PC3, and melanoma cells WM9. Compounds **TB1, TB3, TB4, TB6, TC1, TC3, TC5, TC9, TC11, TC12, TC14, TC15, TC16**, and **TC17** exhibited a better broad-spectrum cytotoxicity on three cancer cells. **TB7** and **TC7** selectively displayed potent inhibitory activities on leukemia cells K562 and prostate cancer cells PC3, respectively. Further studies indicated that **TB3, TC1, TC3, TC7**, and **TC17** could significantly induce the apoptosis of PC3 cells. **TC1** and **TC17** significantly induced apoptosis of K562 cells. **TC1, TC11**, and **TC14** induced significant apoptosis of WM9 cells. The structure-activity relationships evaluation showed that removing methyl at C-3 of the furan ring and introducing diverse side chains at C-2 of the furan ring is an effective strategy for improving the anticancer activity of L-shaped ortho-quinone analogs.

Keywords: ortho-quinones; antitumor activity; beta-lapachone; tanshione IIA

---

1. Introduction

Over several decades, cancer continues to be the most awful disease due to its uncontrolled cell growth and the fact that it is a dominate killer of human beings worldwide [1]. Especially in China, millions of deaths have been caused by tumor. The common cancer types in Chinese male, in 2018, were lung, stomach, colorectum, liver, and esophageal cancer. Additionally, breast, lung, colorectum, thyroid, and stomach cancer were the common types in Chinese female [2]. The incidence of colorectal cancer in males and females has increased, however, the incidence of esophageal, stomach, and liver cancer has decreased between 2000 and 2011 [3]. Meanwhile, the incidence and mortality of prostate cancer and bladder cancer in males, together with obesity and hormonal exposure-related cancers, namely thyroid, breast, and ovarian cancer in females have shown a rising trend [3]. However, the standardized treatments of cancer, including surgery, chemotherapy, and radiation therapy, show many limitations, such as severe adverse effects, recurrence, and increasing drug resistance [4].

Currently, phytochemicals have become a valuable source of anticancer drugs. Actually, over 75% of nonbiological anticancer drugs approved are either plant-derived natural products or developed based on these products [5]. Therefore, natural products have continued to be a hot research topic for the development of new antitumor drugs [6–9].

Tanshinone IIA is a natural ortho-quinone isolated from the rhizome of *Salvia miltiorrhiza Bunge* with antineoplastic activity, such as gastric cancer, breast cancer, osteosarcoma, etc. [10–13]. These various properties demonstrate that tanshinone IIA is a potential antitumor drug candidate. Furthermore, beta-lapachone is another natural ortho-quinone which has been reported to selectively kill many human cancer cells [14], however, the pyran ring of beta-lapachone has been found to be unstable during metabolism in the human body, and may led to side effects on normal tissues [15,16]. Recently, studies have revealed that some tanshinone analogs show similar or stronger antitumor activity when the ring-A is removed but the furan ring is retained [17,18]. You et al. [19,20] discovered that the binding site for quinone oxidoreductase-1 (NQO1) substrates was an L-shaped pocket (Figure 1B) which binds well with tanshinone analogs, and showed higher antitumor activities than the planar compound **1** and beta-lapachone. Therefore, we surmise that removing methyl at C-3 of the furan ring is more suitable for the binding site, and we anticipate that a novel L-shaped molecule without methyl at C-3 of the furan ring could provide better antitumor activities. Considering that some nitrogen, oxygen-substituted, and amino acid substrates can improve aqueous solubility and antitumor activities [21–25], we have attempted to introduce a great diversity of oxygen-substituted, nitrogen-containing groups and amino acids. Thus, in this work, we developed quinone-directed agents by removing methyl at C-3 of the furan ring and introducing a diverse side chain at C-2 of the furan ring, culminating in the discovery of a promising scaffold. The inhibitory activity was assessed in vitro using three cell lines including K562, PC3, and WM9.

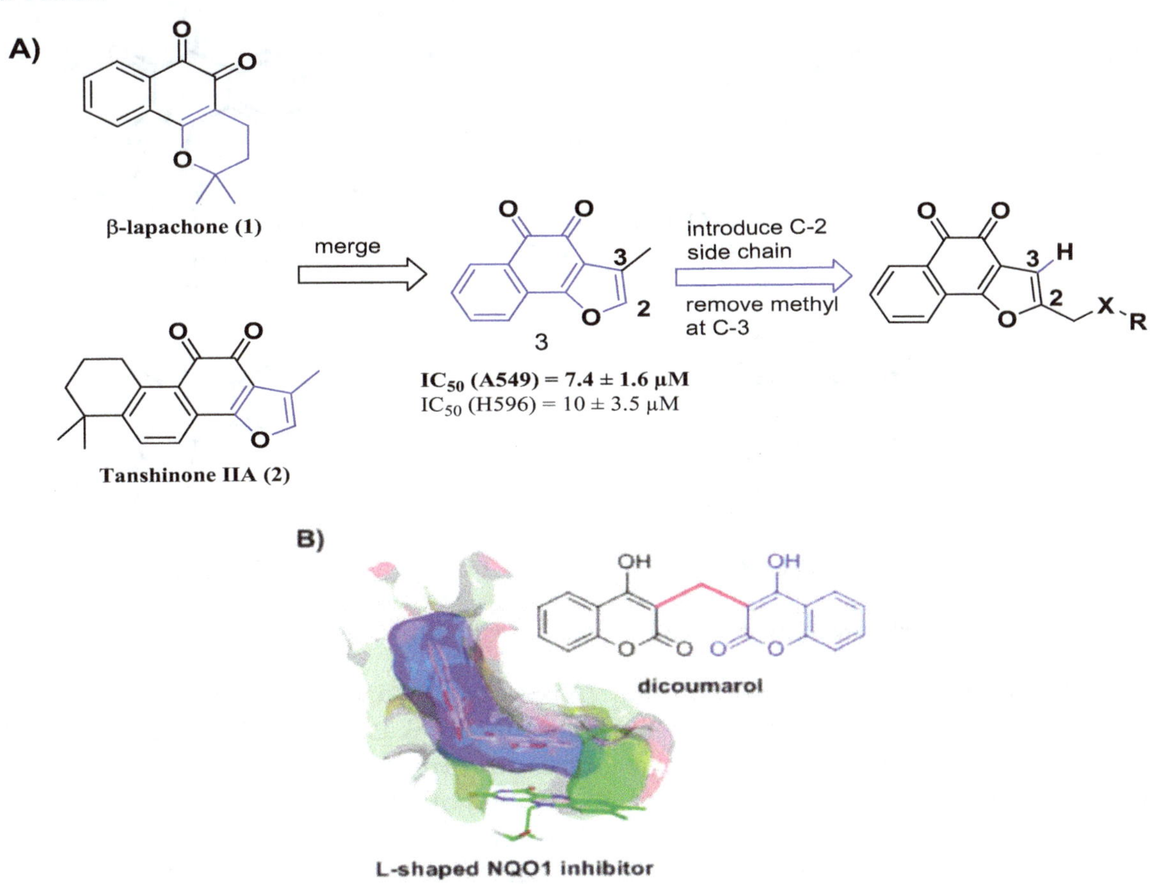

Figure 1. (**A**) Structural design strategy and (**B**) L-shaped pocket. The figure is available in reference [19].

2. Discussion and Results

2.1. Chemistry

The synthesis of two substituted naphtho[1,2-b]furan-4,5-diones is outlined in Scheme 1. Briefly, treatment of lawsone **6** with allyl bromide followed by subsequent Claisen rearrangement afforded **7**, which was then cyclized to get the ortho-quinone **8** by using Lewis acid $NbCl_5$ at room temperature [26].

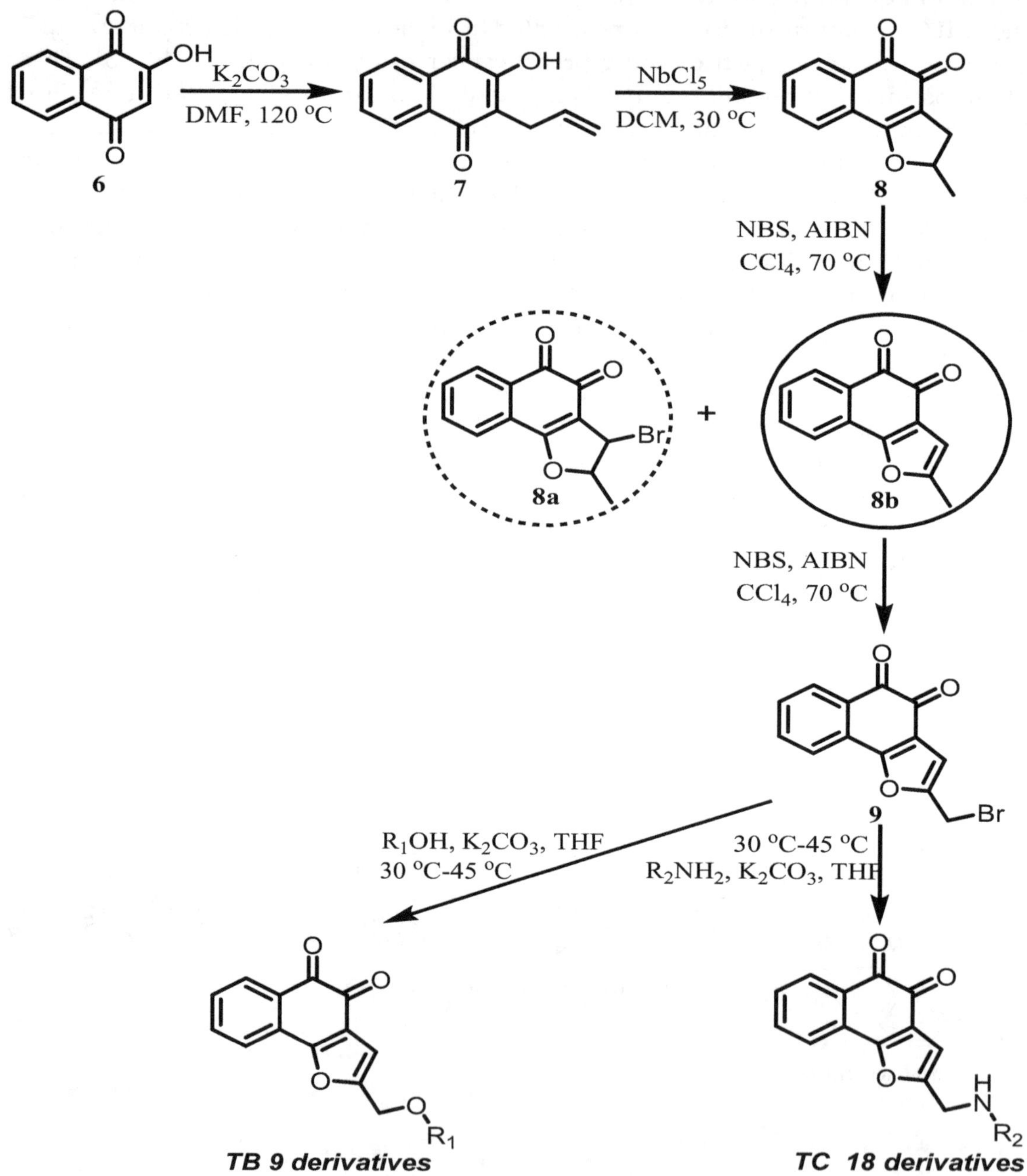

Scheme 1. Synthesis of L-shaped ortho-quinone analogs.

Initially, dealing **8** with *N*-bromosuccinimide (NBS) and 2,2′-azobis(2-methylpropionitrile) (AIBN) afforded only trace amounts of **8a**. Another intermediate, **8b**, was obtained by Nelson's method [27] as shown in Scheme 1. Then, compound **9** was obtained from **8b** through a second radical reaction. Considering the same reaction condition, we successfully got **9** from **8** through a bis-radical reaction. The brominated intermediate **9** was reacted with substituted phenol or amine to provide ortho-quinone derivatives **TB1–TB9** and **TC1–TC18**, respectively. All the structures of ortho-quinone derivatives were identified through ^{1}H, ^{13}C, and HRMS.

In summary, we successfully established an effective synthetic strategy, which removed the methyl at C-3 of the furan ring and introduced diverse side chains at C-2 of the furan ring. In addition, we replaced the bromide of **9** with a variety of oxygen-substituted, nitrogen-containing group, and amino acid by a nucleophilic substitution.

2.2. *In Vitro Cytotoxicity Assay*

The cytotoxic activities of 5 μmol/L of the synthesized L-shaped ortho-quinone analogs were determined by using three cancer cell lines (Table 1). The results revealed that compounds **TB1, TB3, TB4, TB6, TC1, TC3, TC5, TC9, TC11, TC12, TC15, TC16,** and **TC17** showed a broad-spectrum potent inhibitory activity on the proliferation of the cancer cell lines, with a more than 70% inhibition rate, and **TB7** showed better inhibitory activity on K562 cells as compared with other cells. Moreover, we observed that **TC7** inhibited the growth of PC3 cells more efficiently than other cells.

Table 1. The structures and inhibitory rates after treating cancer cell lines with 5 μmol/L of target compounds, respectively. Data was presented as the mean ± SD of three independent experiments.

Compounds	R	Inhibition (%) PC3	K562	WM9
TB1	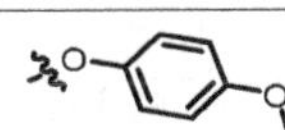	92.078 ± 1.885	88.641 ± 3.055	80.287 ± 6.354
TB2	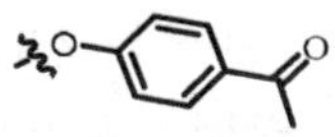	58.700 ± 29.309	20.642 ± 16.695	9.216 ± 2.449
TB3	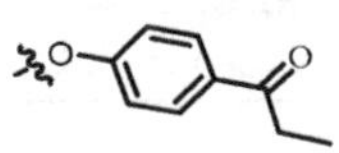	91.861 ± 2.125	83.613 ± 10.448	54.153 ± 3.948
TB4	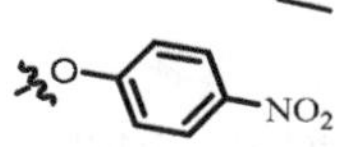	92.224 ± 1.811	91.192 ± 1.479	87.963 ± 2.430
TB5	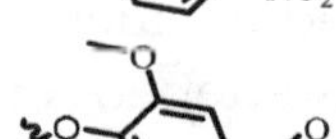	30.673 ± 54.356	49.127 ± 33.985	64.870 ± 2.894
TB6	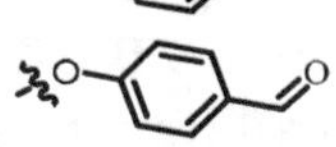	87.165 ± 1.953	82.901 ± 1.484	89.843 ± 2.010
TB7	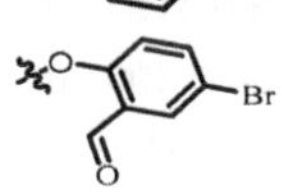	−7.664 ± 10.055	81.835 ± 1.553	31.754 ± 6.422
TB8	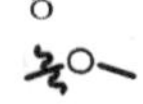	9.692 ± 11.981	7.191 ± 4.705	49.307 ± 3.791
TB9	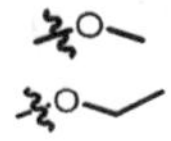	−17.125 ± 11.619	15.334 ± 9.484	−0.591 ± 1.055
TC1	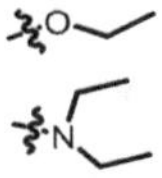	91.027 ± 0.553	83.717 ± 3.469	84.117 ± 2.686
TC2	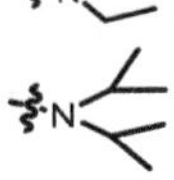	−0.437 ± 1.129	25.032±2.579	16.431±1.583
TC3	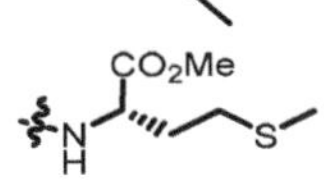	78.849 ± 13.221	83.518 ± 12.045	81.670 ± 0.994
TC4	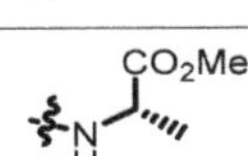	24.242 ± 18.544	0.082 ± 15.067	15.453 ± 1.508
TC5	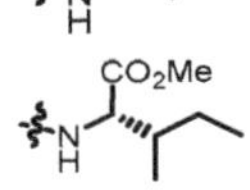	89.676 ± 0.331	81.950 ± 12.469	72.452 ± 8.039
TC6	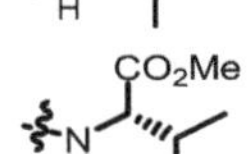	43.133 ± 11.878	31.137 ± 16.045	63.384 ± 8.949
TC7	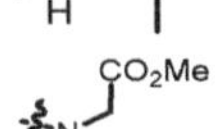	82.402 ± 4.585	30.087 ± 20.307	16.191 ± 2.699
TC8	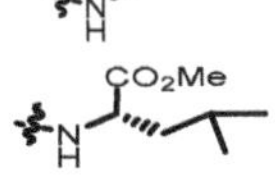	44.842 ± 25.172	28.448 ± 30.220	0.468 ± 5.166

Table 1. *Cont.*

Compounds	R	Inhibition (%) PC3	K562	WM9
TC9	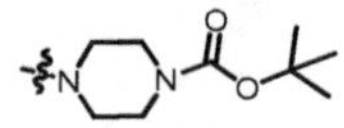	89.869 ± 1.839	81.545 ± 6.968	83.003 ± 2.806
TC10	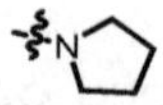	−6.375 ± 8.094	−9.749 ± 17.889	1.005 ± 2.601
TC11	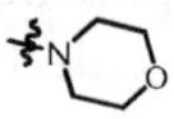	90.214 ± 0.520	85.766 ± 1.737	85.807 ± 3.752
TC12	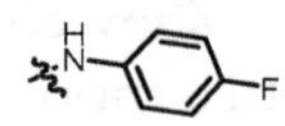	82.522 ± 9.039	83.688 ± 8.252	61.839 ± 3.448
TC13	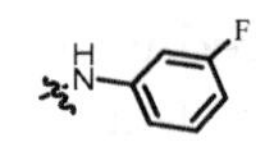	74.681 ± 2.470	84.251 ± 1.430	39.955 ± 6.425
TC14	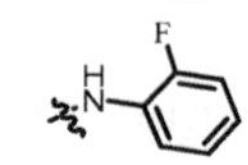	4.453 ± 5.002	84.497 ± 0.876	90.717 ± 1.184
TC15	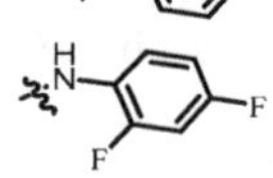	84.916 ± 1.761	84.185 ± 0.419	90.135 ± 1.602
TC16	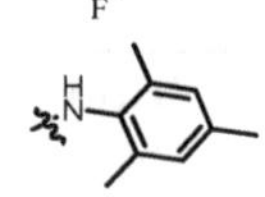	78.720 ± 7.560	84.323 ± 1.273	90.520 ± 2.108
TC17	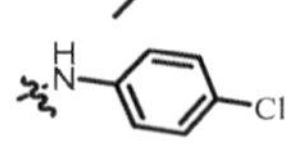	86.637 ± 2.482	83.999 ± 0.943	72.021 ± 6.850
TC18	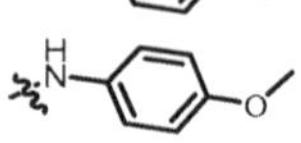	−5.220 ± 13.979	8.854 ± 12.236	1.410 ± 5.093
tanshinone IIA		89.458 ± 1.987	82.215 ± 4.069	85.236 ± 3.654
Paclitaxel		81.589 ± 1.763	91.315 ± 2.467	78.369 ± 6.380

The concentration inhibition curves (Figure 2) were analyzed to calculate the IC_{50} values of the selected active compounds. The results indicated there was a dose-dependent trend of the inhibitory response of all active compounds on three cancer cells for treating 48 h. The IC_{50} values were summarized in Table 2 and show that the cytotoxicity of compounds **TB3, TC1, TC3, TC7, TC9,** and **TC17** on PC3 were better ($P < 0.05$) than that of the positive control (tanshinone IIA and paclitaxel), and another active compound exhibited similar activity to that of the positive control. The inhibition activity of **TC1** against the growth of K562 was better than that of the positive control, paclitaxel, and tanshinone IIA. Compounds **TB6, TC1, TC11, TC14,** and **TC15** inhibited the growth of WM9 better ($P < 0.05$) than that of tanshinone IIA and paclitaxel. In summary, most of novel L-shaped ortho-quinone analogs exhibited relatively better cytotoxicity activity as compared with the two positive controls, which indicated that the analogs containing L-shaped ortho-quinone as the core structure, possessed stronger anticancer activity. This result provided a preliminary biological activity basis for the investigation of anticancer candidate agents.

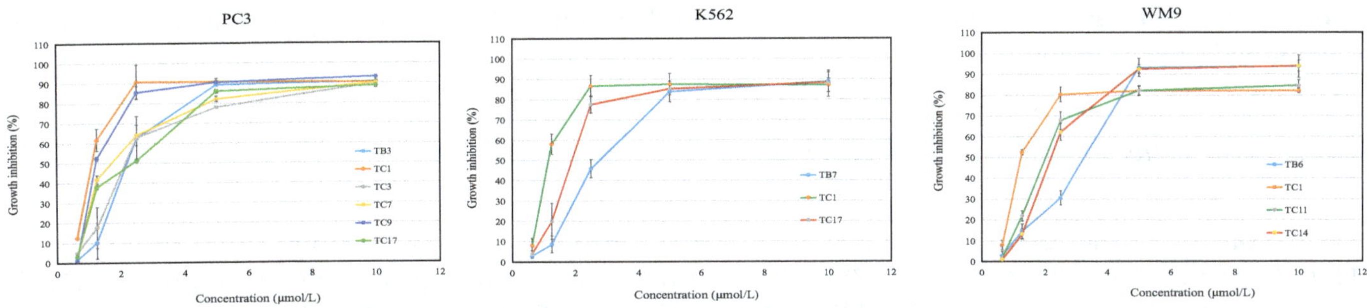

Figure 2. Growth inhibition induced by the active L-shaped ortho-quinone analogs on PC3, K562, and WM9 cells by MTT assay. The IC_{50} values (μM) of the compounds were determined according to these curves at different incubation times. The 100 μL tested compounds were added to 96-well microculture plates and 100 μL cells (a final concentration of 5×10^4/well) were incubated for 48 h at 37 °C. Cell survival was evaluated by MTT assay. The inhibition ratio (%) was calculated as described in the Methods section. Data was presented as mean ± SD of three independent experiments.

Table 2. IC_{50} values of selected compounds in vitro.

Compounds	IC_{50}/μM PC3	K562	WM9
TB1	2.809 ± 0.413	3.157 ± 0.947 **	4.841 ± 0.301
TB3	1.121 ± 0.731 **	2.580 ± 0.285 **	NA [a]
TB4	3.348 ± 0.347	3.103 ± 0.702 **	3.358 ± 0.297
TB6	3.249 ± 0.464	2.964 ± 0.168 *	2.774 ± 0.299 **
TB7	NA	2.981 ± 0.368 **	NA
TC1	0.347 ± 0.290 **	0.379 ± 0.138	0.406 ± 0.117 **
TC3	1.778 ± 0.835 **	4.647 ± 0.647 **	4.990 ± 0.360
TC5	3.018 ± 0.452	3.448 ± 0.224 **	NA
TC7	1.507 ± 0.369 **	NA	NA
TC9	0.469 ± 0.281 **	4.194 ± 0.139 **	4.027 ⊥ 0.341
TC11	2.578 ± 0.957	3.565 ± 0.344 **	2.127 ± 0.582 **
TC12	2.963 ± 0.261	4.157 ± 0.677 **	NA
TC13	3.433 ± 0.444	4.719 ± 0.984	NA
TC14	NA	3.100 ± 0.320 **	2.261 ± 0.111 **
TC15	3.696 ± 0.492	3.644 ± 0.524 **	3.050 ± 0.230 *
TC16	3.874 ± 0.557	2.640 ± 0.642 **	4.324 ± 0.292
TC17	1.914 ± 0.224 **	1.927 ± 0.414	NA
tanshinone IIA	3.162 ± 3.160	4.638 + 1.270	4.261 ± 0.182
Paclitaxel	4.323 ± 0.929	2.149 ± 0.406	4.835 ± 0.359

Note: * represents $p < 0.05$ and ** represents $p < 0.01$, vs. the inhibition of the positive control to the cancer cell lines. The data represented the average of three independent experiments.

2.3. *Structure-Activity Relationships Study*

To obtain two series of analogs, we successfully built an effective synthetic strategy by removing the methyl at C-3 of the furan ring and introducing diverse side chains at C-2 of the furan ring. On the basis of the cytotoxicity results (Tables 1 and 2), a preliminary structure-activity relationships could be established. The TB series molecules bearing electron-withdrawing groups or multi-substituted groups such as compounds **TB3**, **TB4**, and **TB6** showed a better inhibitory effect on PC3 cell lines, K562 cell lines, and WM9 cell lines, whereas the TB series molecules bearing alkane groups at the 2-position showed decreased cytotoxicity in PC3 cell lines, K562 cell lines, and WM9 cell lines, such as compounds **TB9**. The TC series molecules with electron-withdrawing groups, saturate six-membered rings, or multi-substituted groups emerged greater inhibitory effects on three cancer cell lines, such as **TC11**, **TC12**, **TC15**, and **TC16**, whereas the TC series molecules bearing donating groups or alkane groups at the 2-position showed reduced cytotoxicity in three cancer cell lines. The structure-activity relationships evaluation also showed that removing methyl at C-3 of the furan ring and introducing diverse side chains at C-2 of the furan ring were good strategies for improving the anticancer activity of L-shaped ortho-quinone analogs.

2.4. Effects of Active Compounds on Cell Apoptosis

According to the above IC_{50} values of all active compounds, we selected six active compounds (**TB3, TC1, TC3, TC7, TC9,** and **TC17**) for PC3, three active compounds (**TB6, TC1,** and **TC17**) for K562, and four active compounds (**TB6, TC1, TC11,** and **TC14**) for WM9, based on their higher activities than that of the positive control and better selectivity and, then, studied their effects on cell apoptosis by microscope observation (Figure 3) and flow cytometry (Figure 4). The microscopic observations (Figure 3A) showed that the number of PC3 cells was significantly reduced by treatments with 2.5 μmol/L of **TB3, TC1, TC3,** and **TC7**; the apoptotic bodies and cell fragments were significantly observed as compared with the control group. The PC3 cells treated with **TC9** showed that the number of cells were significantly reduced, while fewer cells died and there were no significant apoptotic bodies. The PC3 cells treated with **TC7** showed a significant decrease in the number of cells, meanwhile, some cells died, apoptotic bodies appeared obviously, and the morphology of some cells became an irregular shape of spindle length. Above all, the inhibitory activity of **TB3, TC1, TC3,** and **TC7** may be through inducing apoptosis, another two compounds may be through different types.

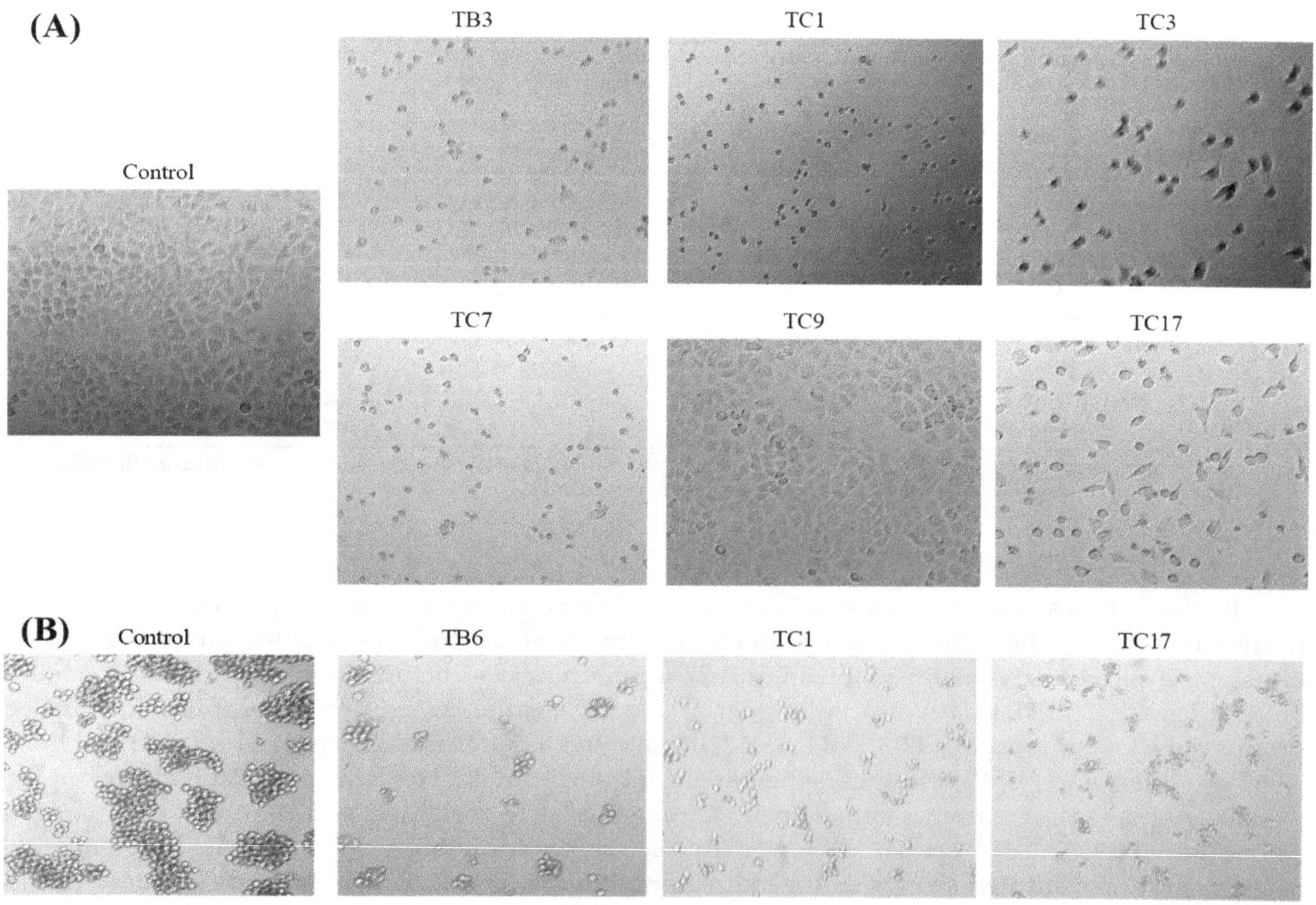

Figure 3. *Cont.*

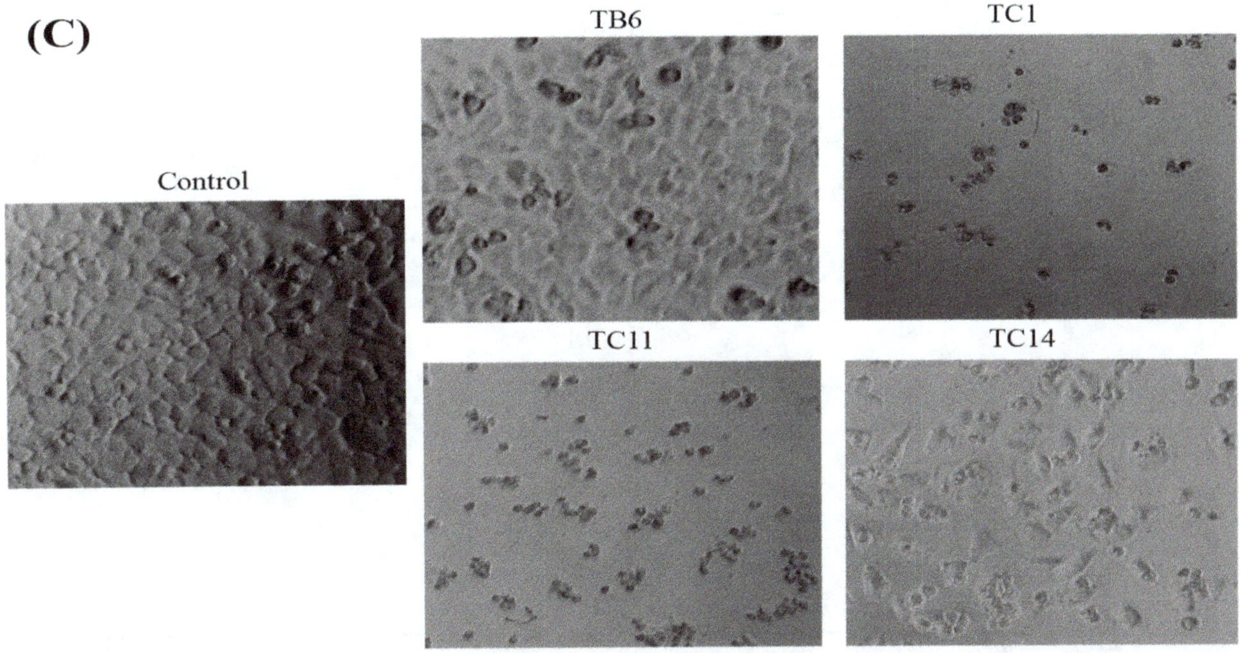

Figure 3. Effects of the active compounds on PC3 (**A**), K562 (**B**), and WM9 (**C**) cell growth and apoptosis. Cell number and morphological appearance of the two types of cell lines treated with 2.5 μmol/L of active compounds, then, it was observed by a fluorescent inverted microscope after 24 h. Scale bar = 100 μM in all images. All experiments were performed in triplicate.

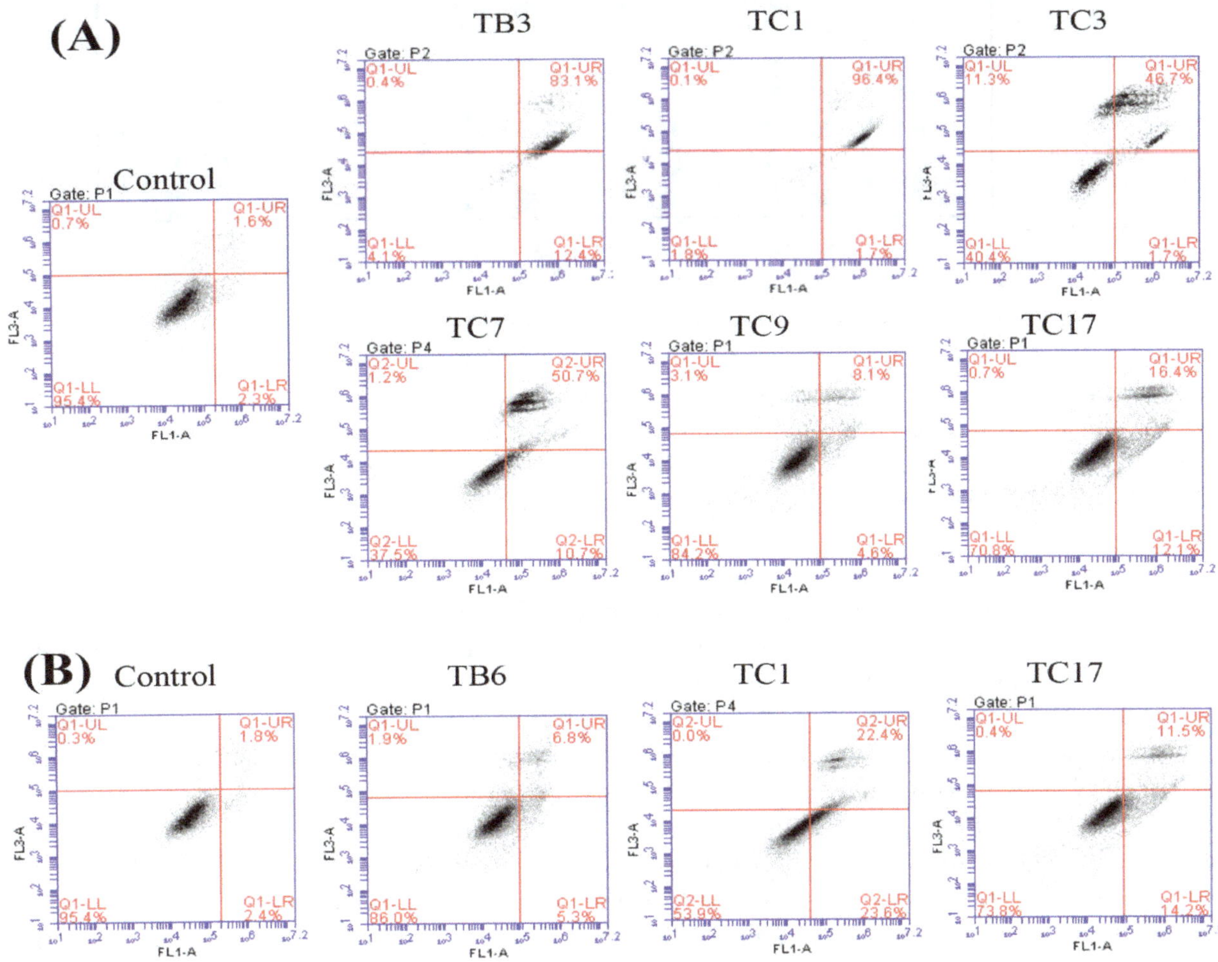

Figure 4. *Cont.*

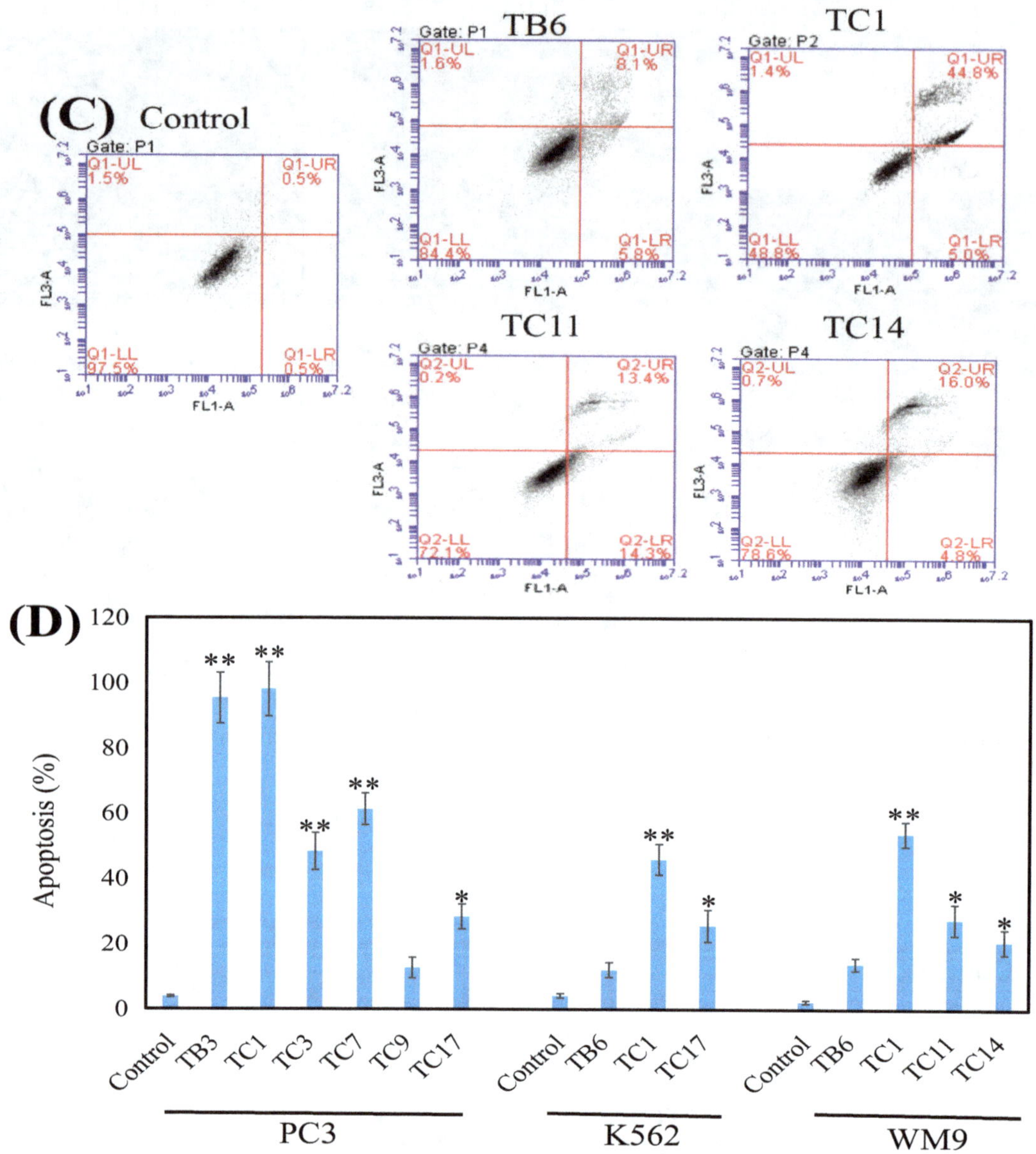

Figure 4. Effects of the active compounds on PC3 (**A**), K562 (**B**), and WM9 (**C**) cell growth and apoptosis. Cell apoptosis induced by the compounds and tested by flow cytometry and the date was analyzed with Origin Pro 9.0 (**D**) and presented as means ± SEM from at least three independent experiments. * $p < 0.05$, ** $p < 0.01$ ($n = 3$) as compared with the control.

The K562 cells treated with **TC1** were obviously dead and dispersed, with the appearance of apoptotic bodies as comparing with the control group (Figure 3B). The cells treated with **TB6** had a significantly reduced number of cells and most cells clumped growth similar to the control cells. For the cells treated with **TC17** we observed both dead cells and fewer clumps of cells. Furthermore, for the WM9 cell lines treated with **TB6**, **TC1**, **TC11**, and **TC14** (Figure 3C), we observed that the cells treated with **TC1** and **TC11** were obviously dead with a large number of apoptotic bodies and dispersed cells; the cells treated with **TB6** showed a significant decrease in the number of cells and fewer dead cells. Observation of the cells treated with **TC14** showed that the number of cells was significantly reduced, while some cells were obviously dead with apoptotic bodies appearing, and the morphology of some cells also became an irregular shape of spindle length. The above results indicated that **TC1** can induce apoptosis for K562 and WM9 cells to inhibit the growth; **TB6**, **TC11**, **TC14**, and **TC17** can jointly inhibit the proliferation of cell through a variety of mechanisms.

Flow cytometry analyzed results (Figure 4) confirmed that **TB3** ($p < 0.01$), **TC1** ($p < 0.01$), **TC3** ($p < 0.01$), **TC7** ($p < 0.01$), and **TC17** ($p < 0.05$) could significantly induce the apoptosis of PC3 cells (Figure 4A), while **TC9** did not. **TC1** ($p < 0.01$) and **TC17** ($p < 0.05$) significantly induced apoptosis of K562 cells (Figure 4B), while **TB6** had no significant effect on apoptosis of K562 and WM9 cells. **TC1** ($p < 0.01$), **TC11** ($p < 0.05$), and **TC14** ($p < 0.01$) could potently induce apoptosis for WM9 cells (Figure 4C).

3. Materials and Methods

3.1. Instruments and Materials

High-resolution mass spectra (HRMS) were obtained on an electrospray ionization (ESI) mode on a Bruker ESI-QTOF mass spectrometry. Nuclear magnetic resonance (NMR) spectra were recorded on a Bruker Avance NEO (^{1}H NMR, 600 MHz; ^{13}C NMR, 150 MHz, Bruker, Switzerland) with TMS as an internal standard. The IR spectra were recorded by using a FTIR Spectrometer (IR 200 Fourier Energy Spectrum Technology Co., Ltd., TianJin, China) and the KBr disk method was adopted. The melting points (mp) were determined on an WRX-4 microscope melting point apparatus. The column chromatography was performed on silica gel (Qingdao, 200–300 mesh) and the thin-layer (0.25 mm) chromatography (TLC) analysis was carried out on silica gel plates (Qingdao, China). Other reagents were analytical grade or guaranteed reagent commercial product and used without further purification, unless otherwise noted.

3.2. Methods of Synthesis

3.2.1. Synthesis of 2-Allyl-3-hydroxy-1,4-naphthoquinone (7)

A mixture of lawsone **6** (10.0 g, 57.42 mmol) and anhydrous K_2CO_3 (7.94 g, 57.42 mmol) in anhydrous DMF (100 mL) were stirred for 15 min at room temperature. Allyl bromide (17.37 g, 143.55 mmol) in DMF (5 mL) was added dropwise and stirred for 15 min at 0 °C. The mixture was refluxed at 120 °C for 3 h and then cooled to room temperature before it was poured into water and extracted with EA. The organic phase was washed with brine, dried over Na_2SO_4, filtered, and concentrated in vacuo. The crude product was purified by column chromatography on silica gel (eluent: petroleum ether/EtOAc 15:1) to afford **7** (7.8 g, 63% yield) as a light yellow solid. Other data was found in reference [26].

3.2.2. Synthesis of 2-Methyl-2,3-dihydrolnaphthol[1,2-*b*]furan-4,5-dione (8)

$NbCl_5$ (18.92 g, 70.02 mmol) was added into **7** (3.0 g, 14.00 mmol) in anhydrous DCM (50 mL) at 0 °C. After stirring for 45 min at 30 °C, the mixture was poured into ice water and extracted with DCM. The organic phase was washed with brine, dried over Na_2SO_4, filtered, and concentrated in vacuo. The crude product was purified by column chromatography on silica gel (eluent: petroleum ether/EtOAc 4:1) to afford **8** (2.16 g, 72% yield) as red solid. Other data was found in reference [26].

3.2.3. Synthesis of 2-Bromomethyl-naphtho[1-*b*]furan-4,5-dione (9)

A mixture of **8** (1.5 g, 7.00 mmol), anhydrous *N*-bromosuccinimide (2.49 g, 1.40mmol), and 2,2′-azobis(2-methylpropionitrile) (114.98 mg, 1.40 mmol) in anhydrous CCl_4 (50 mL) was stirred under argon at 70 °C, until **8** were disappeared. Then, the mixture was cooled to room temperature, and anhydrous N-bromosuccinimide (2.49 g, 1.40 mmol) and 2,2′-azobis(2-methylpropionitrile) (114.98 mg, 1.40 mmol) were added and stirred at 70 °C for 2 h. The mixture was cooled to room temperature, and poured into water, extracted with EA, washed with brine, dried over Na_2SO_4, filtered, and concentrated in vacuo. The crude product was purified by column chromatography on silica gel (eluent: petroleum ether/EtOAc 12:1) to afford **9** (1.0 g, 67% yield) as red solid. Mp: 169–170 °C. ^{1}H NMR (600 MHz, $CDCl_3$) δ 8.09 (d, J = 7.8 Hz, 1H), 7.77 (d, J = 7.6 Hz, 1H), 7.69 (t, J = 7.6 Hz, 1H), 7.51 (t, J = 7.6 Hz, 1H), and 6.83 (s, 1H), 4.55 (s, 2H). ^{13}C NMR (150 MHz, $CDCl_3$) δ 180.06, 174.13, 160.94, 153.46, 135.56, 130.74, 130.69, 129.03, 127.98, 122.69, 122.34, 108.04, and 21.87. IR (ν, cm^{-1}): 3118.33, 2920.28, 2339.32, 1670.84, 1551.16, and 691.42. HRMS (ESI) calcd. for $[M + Na]^+$ $C_{13}H_7O_3BrNa^+$: 312.9471, found 312.9460.

3.2.4. Synthesis of **TB1–9** and **TC1–18**

A mixture of the corresponding amines or alcohols (0.52 mmol), K_2CO_3 (142 mg, 1.03 mmol), and **9** (100 mg, 0.34 mmol) in THF (5 mL) was stirred at 30 °C to 50 °C for 4 h. After cooling, the mixture was poured into water and extracted with EA. The combined organic layer was washed with brine and dried over anhydrous Na_2SO_4, filtered, and concentrated to afford a crude product which was purified through column chromatography on silica gel.

TB1: *2-(((4-methoxyphenyl)oxy)methyl)naphtho[1-b]furan-4,5-dione.* Red solid, yield: 34%. Mp: 112–113 °C. ^{1}H NMR (600 MHz, $CDCl_3$) δ 8.09 (d, J = 7.6 Hz, 1H), 7.75 (d, J = 7.6 Hz, 1H), 7.66 (t, J = 7.5 Hz, 1H), 7.48 (t, J = 7.6 Hz, 1H), 6.94–6.92 (m, 2H), 6.87–6.85 (m, 2H), 6.83 (s, 1H), 5.04 (s, 2H), and 3.78 (s, 3H). ^{13}C NMR (150 MHz, $CDCl_3$) δ 180.34, 174.38, 160.88, 154.72, 153.82, 151.95, 135.47, 130.66, 130.50, 128.98, 128.28, 122.59, 122.12, 116.34, 114.81, 108.37, 63.03, and 55.73. IR (ν, cm^{-1}): 3445.32, 2358.40, 2339.32, 1671.47, 1598.48, 1253.20, 1219.81, 1161.58, and 1057.34. HRMS (ESI) calcd. for $[M + Na]^+$ $C_{20}H_{14}O_5Na^+$: 357.0733, found 357.0723.

TB2: *2-(((4-acetylphenyl)oxy)methyl)naphtho[1,2-b]furan-4,5-dione.* Light orange solid, yield: 40%. Mp: 190–191 °C. ^{1}H NMR (600 MHz, $CDCl_3$) δ 8.13 (d, J = 6.4 Hz, 1H), 8.00 (d, J = 8.9 Hz, 2H), 7.78 (d, J = 9.1 Hz, 1H), 7.69 (t, J = 7.6 Hz, 1H), 7.53 (t, J = 7.6 Hz, 1H), 7.06 (d, J = 8.9 Hz, 2H), 6.94 (s, 1H), 5.19 (s, 2H), and 2.60 (s, 3H). ^{13}C NMR (150 MHz, $CDCl_3$) δ 196.71, 180.20, 174.31, 161.58, 161.10, 152.60, 135.53, 131.28, 130.74, 130.70, 129.02, 128.11, 122.64, 122.08, 114.48, 108.98, 61.92, and 26.43. IR (ν, cm^{-1}): 3445.93, 2358.51, 2341.16, 1671.86, 1599.84, 1249.41, 1217.01, 1178.57, and 1008.47. HRMS (ESI) calcd. for $[M + Na]^+$ $C_{21}H_{14}O_5Na^+$: 369.0733, found 369.0721.

TB3: *2-(((4-propiophenyl)oxy)methyl)naphtho[1,2-b]furan-4,5-dione.* Orange solid, yield: 37%. Mp: 179–180 °C. ^{1}H NMR (600 MHz, $CDCl_3$) δ 8.11 (d, J = 7.6 Hz, 1H), 8.00 (d, J = 8.9 Hz, 2H), 7.77 (d, J = 6.4 Hz, 1H), 7.71–7.68 (m, 1H), 7.53–7.50 (m, 1H), 7.06 (d, J = 8.9 Hz, 2H), 6.93 (s, 1H), 5.18 (s, 2H), 2.99 (q, J = 7.2 Hz, 2H), and 1.24 (t, J = 7.3 Hz, 3H). ^{13}C NMR (150 MHz, $CDCl_3$) δ 199.42, 180.20, 174.30, 161.40, 161.06, 152.68, 135.53, 130.98, 130.72, 130.68, 130.36, 129.01, 128.11, 122.63, 122.08, 114.47, 108.92, 61.90, 31.53, and 8.38. IR (ν, cm^{-1}): 3447.03, 2358.62, 2341.16, 1669.65, 1601.07, 1222.31, 1180.35, and 1002.86. HRMS (ESI) calcd. for $[M + Na]^+$ $C_{22}H_{16}O_5Na^+$: 383.0890, found 383.0876.

TB4: *2-(((4-nitrophenyl)oxy)methyl)naphtho[1,2-b]furan-4,5-dione.* Red solid, yield: 48%. Mp: 205–206 °C. ^{1}H NMR (600 MHz, DMSO-d_6) δ 8.25 (d, J = 9.3 Hz, 2H), 7.96 (d, J = 7.6 Hz, 1H), 7.77–7.74 (m, 2H), 7.59–7.55 (m, 1H), 7.34 (d, J = 9.3 Hz, 2H), 7.18 (s, 1H), and 5.42 (s, 2H). ^{13}C NMR (150 MHz, DMSO-d_6) δ 179.58, 174.56, 163.29, 160.07, 152.42, 141.83, 135.43, 130.84, 130.17, 129.83, 127.89, 126.41, 122.50, 122.36, 115.94, 110.32, and 62.45. IR (ν, cm^{-1}): 3445.75, 2358.70, 2341.16, 1681.37,1592.17, 1507.95, 1384.15, 1340.19, 1277.67, and 1110.13. HRMS (ESI) calcd. for $[M + Na]^+$ $C_{19}H_{11}O_6NNa^+$: 372.0479, found 372.0465.

TB5: *2-(((2-methoxyl-4-formyl)phenyl)oxy)methyl)naphtho[1,2-b]furan-4,5-dione.* Red solid, yield: 34%. Mp: 203–204 °C. ^{1}H NMR (600 MHz, $CDCl_3$) δ 9.91 (s, 1H), 8.13 (d, J = 6.4 Hz, 1H), 7.77 (d, J = 7.6 Hz, 1H), 7.72–7.68 (m, 1H), 7.54–7.48 (m, 3H), 7.15 (d, J = 8.0 Hz, 1H), 6.96 (s, 1H), 5.28 (s, 2H), and 3.97 (s, 3H). ^{13}C NMR (150 MHz, $CDCl_3$) δ 190.88, 180.19, 174.31, 161.15, 152.50, 152.42, 150.30, 135.52, 131.28, 130.75, 129.67, 129.03, 128.10, 122.68, 122.09, 115.30, 112.93, 109.87, 109.40, 62.85, and 56.09. IR (ν, cm^{-1}): 3446.32, 2358.18, 2341.16, 1702.84, 1676.79, 1586.53, 1508.23, 1267.05, 1236.25, 1137.10, and 999.76. HRMS (ESI) calcd. for $[M + Na]^+$ $C_{21}H_{14}O_6Na^+$: 385.0683, found 385.0668.

TB6: *2-(((4-formylphenyl)oxy)methyl)naphtho[1,2-b]furan-4,5-dione.* Orange solid, yield: 30%. Mp: 212–213 °C. ^{1}H NMR (600 MHz, $CDCl_3$) δ 9.95 (s, 1H), 8.13 (d, J = 7.8 Hz, 1H), 7.92 (d, J = 8.9 Hz, 2H), 7.78 (d, J = 7.8 Hz, 1H), 7.73–7.69 (m, 1H), 7.56–7.51 (m, 1H), 7.14 (d, J = 8.7 Hz, 2H), 6.96 (s, 1H), and 5.21 (s, 2H). ^{13}C NMR (150 MHz, $CDCl_3$) δ 190.71, 180.17, 174.30, 162.67, 161.14, 152.36, 135.53, 132.10, 130.82, 130.77, 130.74, 129.05, 128.09, 122.64, 122.08, 115.06, 109.11, and 61.99. IR (ν, cm^{-1}): 3446.21,

2358.24, 2337.30, 1687.41, 1671.45, 1598.48, 1253.19, 1219.95, 1161.49, and 1057.40. HRMS (ESI) calcd. for $[M + Na]^+$ $C_{20}H_{12}O_5Na^+$: 355.0577, found 355.0565.

TB7: *2-(((4-bromo-2-formyl)phenyl)oxy)methyl)naphtho[1,2-b]furan-4,5-dione.* Light orange solid, yield: 33%. Mp: 201–202 °C. ^{1}H NMR (600 MHz, $CDCl_3$) δ 10.43 (s, 1H), 8.14 (d, *J* = 7.6 Hz, 1H), 7.99 (d, *J* = 2.7 Hz, 1H), 7.76 (d, *J* = 7.6 Hz, 1H), 7.73–7.69 (m, 2H), 7.57–7.51 (m, 1H), 7.06 (d, *J* = 8.7 Hz, 1H), 6.96 (s, 1H), and 5.24 (s, 2H). ^{13}C NMR (150 MHz, $CDCl_3$) δ 187.86, 180.06, 174.25, 161.30, 158.94, 151.80, 138.27, 135.59, 131.52, 130.87, 130.82, 129.07, 127.95, 126.84, 122.64, 121.99, 115.01, 114.95, 109.43, and 62.80. IR (ν, cm^{-1}): 3445.63, 2358.34, 2337.30, 1671.90, 1599.56, 1556.29, 1249.42, 1217.50, 1178.60, and 1008.51. HRMS (ESI) calcd. for $[M + Na]^+$ $C_{20}H_{11}O_5BrNa^+$: 432.9682, found 432.9673.

TB8: *2-(methoxymethyl)naphtho[1,2-b]furan-4,5-dione.* Red solid, yield: 12%. Mp: 53–54 °C. ^{1}H NMR (600 MHz, $CDCl_3$) δ 8.11 (dd, *J* = 7.8, 1.5 Hz, 1H), 7.78 (dd, *J* = 7.7, 1.4 Hz, 1H), 7.70–7.66 (m, 1H), 7.52–7.48 (m, 1H), 6.80 (s, 1H), 4.51 (s, 2H), and 3.46 (s, 3H). ^{13}C NMR (150 MHz, $CDCl_3$) δ 180.43, 174.46, 160.91, 154.77, 135.45, 130.64, 130.44, 128.96, 128.34, 122.59, 122.05, 107.97, 66.02, and 58.32. IR (ν, cm^{-1}): 3446.10, 2358.55, 2337.96, 1677.60, 1276.65, 1216.21, 1153.22, and 1082.89. HRMS (ESI) calcd. for $[M + Na]^+$ $C_{14}H_{10}O_4Na^+$: 265.0471, found 265.0463.

TB9: *2-(ethoxymethyl)naphtho[1,2-b]furan-4,5-dione.* Red solid, yield: 11%. Mp: 60–61 °C. ^{1}H NMR (600 MHz, $CDCl_3$) δ 8.10 (dd, *J* = 8.2, 1.3 Hz, 1H), 7.77 (dd, *J* = 7.6, 1.2 Hz, 1H), 7.71–7.65 (m, 1H), 7.52–7.46 (m, 1H), 6.78 (s, 1H), 4.55 (s, 2H), 3.63 (q, *J* = 7.0 Hz, 2H), and 1.29 (t, *J* = 7.0 Hz, 3H). ^{13}C NMR (150 MHz, $CDCl_3$) δ 180.47, 174.45, 160.81, 155.23, 135.45, 130.61, 130.37, 128.90, 128.39, 122.59, 122.08, 107.66, 66.26, 64.25, and 15.10. IR (ν, cm^{-1}): 3446.08, 2358.74, 2342.78, 1681.54, 1275.43, 1215.49, 1159.01, and 1083.47. HRMS (ESI) calcd. for $[M + Na]^+$ $C_{15}H_{12}O_4Na^+$: 279.0628, found 279.0621.

TC1: *2-(diethylaminomethyl)naphtho[1,2-b]furan-4,5-dione.* Red solid, yield: 51%. Mp: 78–79 °C. ^{1}H NMR (600 MHz, $CDCl_3$) δ 8.07 (d, *J* = 7.6 Hz, 1H), 7.72 (d, *J* = 7.6 Hz, 1H), 7.65 (t, *J* = 7.0 Hz, 1H), 7.46 (t, *J* = 7.6 Hz, 1H), 6.66 (s, 1H), 3.77 (s, 2H), 2.62 (q, *J* = 7.2 Hz, 4H), and 1.14 (t, *J* = 7.2 Hz, 6H). ^{13}C NMR (150 MHz, $CDCl_3$) δ 180.65, 174.55, 160.34, 156.44, 135.41, 130.55, 130.12, 128.74, 128.58, 122.45, 122.21, 107.11, 48.69, 47.10, and 12.01. IR (ν, cm^{-1}): 3445.24, 2953.88, 2358.48, 2339.23, 1700.91, 1676.52, 1216.10, and 1111.39. HRMS (ESI) calcd. for $[M + Na]^+$ $C_{17}H_{18}O_3Na^+$: 284.1281, found 284.1271.

TC2: *2-(diisopropylaminomethyl)naphtho[1,2-b]furan-4,5-dione.* Red solid, yield: 18%. Mp: 69–70 °C. ^{1}H NMR (600 MHz, $CDCl_3$) δ 8.06 (d, *J* = 7.8 Hz, 1H), 7.68 (d, *J* = 6.2 Hz, 1H), 7.64 (t, *J* = 7.5 Hz, 1H), 7.44 (t, *J* = 6.7 Hz, 1H), 6.66 (s, 1H), 3.72 (s, 2H), 3.13 (p, *J* = 6.5 Hz, 2H), and 1.08 (d, *J* = 6.7 Hz, 12H). ^{13}C NMR (150 MHz, $CDCl_3$) δ 180.88, 174.66, 161.17, 159.76, 135.37, 130.50, 129.81, 128.91, 128.65, 122.50, 122.09, 105.12, 49.12, 42.36, and 20.81. IR (ν, cm^{-1}): 3445.80, 2966.49, 2358.61, 2337.30, 1676.07, 1558.32, 1215.85, and 1149.51. HRMS (ESI) calcd. for $[M + Na]^+$ $C_{19}H_{22}O_3Na^+$: 312.1594, found 312.1583.

TC3: *2-((L-methionine methyl ester-1-yl)methyl)naphtho[1,2-b]furan-4,5-dione.* Red solid, yield: 12%. Mp: 52–53 °C. ^{1}H NMR (600 MHz, $CDCl_3$) δ 8.08 (d, *J* = 7.8 Hz, 1H), 7.72 (d, *J* = 7.6 Hz, 1H), 7.66 (t, *J* = 7.6 Hz, 1H), 7.47 (t, *J* = 7.6 Hz, 1H), 6.66 (s, 1H), 3.95 (d, *J* = 15.1 Hz, 1H), 3.79 (d, *J* = 15.1 Hz, 1H), 3.74 (s, 3H), 3.52 (dd, *J* = 8.4, 5.0 Hz, 1H), 2.64 (t, *J* = 7.2 Hz, 2H), 2.10 (s, 3H), 2.02–1.97 (m, 1H) and 1.89–1.82 (m, 1H). ^{13}C NMR (150 MHz, $CDCl_3$) δ 180.55, 175.18, 174.44, 160.36, 157.00, 135.44, 130.58, 130.19, 128.80, 128.47, 122.35, 122.17, 106.00, 59.14, 52.14, 44.65, 32.68, 30.48, and 15.38. IR (ν, cm^{-1}): 3446.14, 2923.56, 2358.62, 2335.37, 1698.61, 1670.40, 1215.45, and 1147.65. HRMS (ESI) calcd. for $[M + Na]^+$ $C_{19}H_{19}O_5NSNa^+$: 396.0876, found 396.0865.

TC4: *2-((L-alanine methyl ester-1-yl)methyl)naphtho[1,2-b]furan-4,5-dione.* Red solid, yield: 27%. Mp: 83–84 °C. ^{1}H NMR (600 MHz, $CDCl_3$) δ 8.07 (d, *J* = 6.9 Hz, 1H), 7.73 (d, *J* = 4.9 Hz, 1H), 7.65 (d, *J* = 8.6 Hz, 1H), 7.46 (t, *J* = 6.6 Hz, 1H), 6.66 (s, 1H), 3.94 (d, *J* = 14.1 Hz, 1H), 3.81 (d, *J* = 14.9 Hz, 1H), 3.74 (s, 3H), 3.46 (q, *J* = 6.9 Hz, 1H), and 1.37 (d, *J* = 6.6 Hz, 3H). ^{13}C NMR (150 MHz, $CDCl_3$) δ 180.52, 175.63, 174.42, 160.36, 156.93, 135.40, 130.56, 130.18, 128.80, 128.46, 122.39, 122.18, 105.99, 55.69, 52.05, 44.26, and 19.13. IR (ν, cm^{-1}): 3328.35, 2958.60, 2358.44, 2337.30, 1735.12, 1676.39, 1216.30, and 1139.72. HRMS (ESI) calcd. for $[M + Na]^+$ $C_{17}H_{15}O_5NNa^+$: 336.0842, found 336.0831.

TC5: *2-((L-isoleucinate methyl ester-1-yl)methyl)naphtho[1,2-b]furan-4,5-dione.* Red solid, yield: 39%. Mp: 112–113 °C. ^{1}H NMR (600 MHz, $CDCl_3$) δ 8.07 (d, *J* = 7.7 Hz, 1H), 7.71 (d, *J* = 7.7 Hz, 1H), 7.67–7.62

(m, 1H), 7.48–7.43 (m, 1H), 6.65 (s, 1H), 3.92 (d, J = 15.1 Hz, 1H), 3.72 (d, J = 16.4 Hz, 4H), 3.17 (d, J = 5.8 Hz, 1H), 1.57–1.50 (m, 1H), 1.26–1.16 (m, 2H), and 0.93–0.88 (m, 6H). ^{13}C NMR (150 MHz, $CDCl_3$) δ 180.60, 175.16, 174.46, 160.27, 157.37, 135.45, 130.55, 130.15, 128.78, 128.52, 122.32, 122.19, 105.82, 65.31, 51.64, 45.08, 38.47, 25.39, 15.66, and 11.49. IR (ν, cm^{-1}): 3445.72, 2924.70, 2358.43, 2341.16,1732.42, 1682.86, 1209.15, and 1150.10. HRMS (ESI) calcd. for $[M + Na]^+$ $C_{20}H_{21}O_5NNa^+$: 378.1312, found 378.1299.

TC6: *2-((L-valine methyl ester-1-yl)methyl)naphtho[1,2-b]furan-4,5-dione*. Red solid, yield: 41%. Mp: 54–55 °C. ^{1}H NMR (600 MHz, $CDCl_3$) δ 8.09 (d, J = 6.2 Hz, 1H), 7.73 (d, J = 7.6 Hz, 1H), 7.70–7.64 (m, 1H), 7.50–7.45 (m, 1H), 6.67 (s, 1H), 3.95 (d, J = 15.3 Hz, 1H), 3.77–3.72 (m, 4H), 3.11 (d, J = 5.8 Hz, 1H), 2.02–1.95 (m, 1H), and 0.98 (t, J = 6.3 Hz, 7H). ^{13}C NMR (150 MHz, $CDCl_3$) δ 180.62, 175.22, 174.49, 160.28, 157.39, 135.43, 130.59, 130.14, 128.82, 128.56, 122.32, 122.22, 105.83, 66.36, 51.70, 45.16, 31.75, 19.28, and 18.35. IR (ν, cm^{-1}): 3425.42, 2923,62, 2358.56, 2337.30, 1698.57, 1670.37, 1187.10, and 1118.00. HRMS (ESI) calcd. for $[M + Na]^+$ $C_{19}H_{19}O_5NNa^+$: 364.1155, found 364.1141.

TC7: *2-((L-glycine methyl ester-1-yl)methyl)naphtho[1,2-b]furan-4,5-dione*. Red solid, yield: 17%. Mp: 55–56 °C. ^{1}H NMR (600 MHz, $CDCl_3$) δ 8.06 (d, J = 7.6 Hz, 1H), 7.71 (d, J = 6.4 Hz, 1H), 7.68–7.62 (m, 1H), 7.49–7.43 (m, 1H), 6.67 (s, 1H), 3.93 (s, 2H), 3.75 (s, 3H), and 3.50 (s, 2H). ^{13}C NMR (150 MHz, $CDCl_3$) δ 180.49, 174.42, 172.45, 160.49, 156.62, 135.44, 130.57, 130.25, 128.79, 128.39, 122.41, 122.14, 106.25, 52.03, 49.50, and 45.38. IR (ν, cm^{-1}): 3328.36, 2958.26, 2358.57, 2337.30, 1735.10, 1676.24, 1216.29, and 1180.25. HRMS (ESI) calcd. for $[M + Na]^+$ $C_{16}H_{13}O_5NNa^+$: 322.0686, found 322.0680.

TC8: *2-((L-leucinate methyl ester-1-yl)methyl)naphtho[1,2-b]furan-4,5-dione*. Red solid, yield: 19%. Mp: 54–55 °C. ^{1}H NMR (600 MHz, $CDCl_3$) δ 8.09 (d, J = 7.6 Hz, 1H), 7.73 (d, J = 7.6 Hz, 1H), 7.67 (t, J = 7.6 Hz, 1H), 7.47 (t, J = 7.6 Hz, 1H), 6.66 (s, 1H), 3.94 (d, J = 15.1 Hz, 1H), 3.77 (d, J = 15.1 Hz, 1H), 3.73 (s, 3H), 3.38 (t, J = 7.2 Hz, 1H), 1.82–1.77 (m, 1H), 1.52 (t, J = 7.4 Hz, 2H), 0.95 (d, J = 6.7 Hz, 3H), and 0.90 (d, J = 6.7 Hz, 3H). ^{13}C NMR (150 MHz, $CDCl_3$) δ 180.59, 176.01, 174.47, 160.32, 157.18, 135.42, 130.59, 130.17, 128.84, 128.51, 122.32, 122.20, 105.94, 59.08, 51.88, 44.63, 42.75, 24.89, 22.78, and 22.09. IR (ν, cm^{-1}): 3434.68, 2958.49, 2358.68, 2339.23, 1670.06, 1518.72, 1211.01, and 1107.62. HRMS (ESI) calcd. for $[M + Na]^+$ $C_{20}H_{21}O_5NNa^+$: 378.1312, found 378.1302.

TC9: *2-((4-boc-piperazin-1-yl)methyl)naphtho[1,2-b]furan-4,5-dione*. Red solid, yield: 26%. Mp: 56–57 °C. ^{1}H NMR (600 MHz, $CDCl_3$) δ 8.10 (d, J = 7.4 Hz, 1H), 7.76 (d, J = 7.6 Hz, 1H), 7.67 (t, J = 7.6 Hz, 1H), 7.48 (t, J = 7.6 Hz, 1H), 6.70 (s, 1H), 3.68 (s, 2H), 3.49 (s, 4H), 2.52 (s, 4H), and 1.47 (s, 9H). ^{13}C NMR (150 MHz, $CDCl_3$) δ 180.53, 174.48, 160.57, 155.01, 154.68, 135.44, 130.64, 130.29, 128.81, 128.46, 122.53, 122.17, 107.66, 79.88, 54.60, 52.60, and 28.42. IR (ν, cm^{-1}): 3434.73, 2358.58, 2339.23, 1669.96, 1518.77, 1211.18, and 1107.93. HRMS (ESI) calcd. for $[M + H]^+$ $C_{22}H_{25}O_5N_2^+$: 397.1758, found 397.1751.

TC10: *2-((pyrrolidin-1-yl)methyl)naphtho[1,2-b]furan-4,5-dione*. Red solid, yield: 24%. Mp: 62–63 °C. ^{1}H NMR (600 MHz, $CDCl_3$) δ 8.08 (d, J = 7.8 Hz, 1H), 7.76 (d, J = 7.6 Hz, 1H), 7.65 (t, J = 7.6 Hz, 1H), 7.46 (t, J = 7.6 Hz, 1H), 6.68 (s, 1H), 3.76 (s, 2H), 2.69–2.63 (m, 4H), and 1.89–1.83 (m, 4H). ^{13}C NMR (150 MHz, $CDCl_3$) δ 180.64, 174.54, 160.39, 156.44, 135.40, 130.56, 130.14, 128.80, 128.56, 122.55, 122.24, 106.71, 54.01, 51.84, and 23.53. IR (ν, cm^{-1}): 3388.30, 3110.62, 2358.68, 2337.30, 1660.65, 1510.49, 1222.52, and 1091.51. HRMS (ESI) calcd. for $[M + H]^+$ $C_{17}H_{16}O_3N^+$: 282.1125, found 282.1115.

TC11: *2-(morpholinomethyl)naphtho[1,2-b]furan-4,5-dione*. Red solid, yield: 38%. Mp: 98–99 °C. ^{1}H NMR (600 MHz, $CDCl_3$) δ 8.09 (d, J = 7.6 Hz, 1H), 7.76 (d, J = 7.6 Hz, 1H), 7.69–7.64 (m, 1H), 7.51–7.45 (m, 1H), 6.70 (s, 1H), 3.78–3.74 (m, 4H), 3.66 (s, 2H), and 2.61–2.55 (m, 4H). ^{13}C NMR (150 MHz, $CDCl_3$) δ 180.50, 174.46, 160.50, 155.01, 135.36, 130.59, 130.23, 128.86, 128.47, 122.46, 122.21, 107.64, 66.79, 54.93, and 53.28. IR (ν, cm^{-1}): 3438.84, 2807.27, 2358.54, 2342.76, 1676.47, 1557.77, 1215.99, 1111.32, and 1006.63. HRMS (ESI) calcd. for $[M + Na]^+$ $C_{17}H_{15}O_4NNa^+$: 320.0893, found 320.0886.

TC12: *2-(((4-fluorophenyl)amino)methyl)naphtho[1,2-b]furan-4,5-dione*. Dark red solid, yield: 51%. Mp: 174–175 °C. ^{1}H NMR (600 MHz, DMSO-d_6) δ 7.92 (d, J = 7.3 Hz, 1H), 7.73 (t, J = 7.5 Hz, 1H), 7.65 (d, J = 7.6 Hz, 1H), 7.52 (t, J = 7.5 Hz, 1H), 6.94 (t, J = 8.9 Hz, 2H), 6.74 (s, 1H), 6.73–6.68 (m, 2H), 6.20 (t, J = 6.4 Hz, 1H), and 4.37 (d, J = 6.0 Hz, 2H). ^{13}C NMR (150 MHz, DMSO-d_6) δ 179.86, 174.62, 159.03, 157.32, 155.16 (d, J = 231.0 Hz), 145.06, 135.47, 130.37, 129.85, 129.69, 128.27, 122.42, 122.06, 115.77 (d,

J = 21.0 Hz), 113.88 (d, J = 6.0 Hz), and 105.93. IR (ν, cm^{-1}): 3378.05, 2923.56, 2358.52, 2335.37, 1662.70, 1514.18, 1215.45, and 1161.45. HRMS (ESI) calcd. for $[M + Na]^+$ $C_{19}H_{12}O_3NFNa^+$: 344.0693, found 344.0681.

TC13: *2-(((3-fluorophenyl)amino)methyl)naphtho[1,2-b]furan-4,5-dione*. Dark red solid, yield: 45%. Mp: 169–170 °C. ^{1}H NMR (600 MHz, DMSO-d_6) δ 7.92 (d, J = 7.6 Hz, 1H), 7.74 (t, J = 7.5 Hz, 1H), 7.65 (d, J = 7.6 Hz, 1H), 7.53 (t, J = 7.6 Hz, 1H), 7.10 (q, J = 8.0 Hz, 1H), 6.78 (s, 1H), 6.61 (t, J = 6.3 Hz, 1H), 6.54 (d, J = 8.2 Hz, 1H), 6.50 (d, J = 12.2 Hz, 1H), 6.35 (t, J = 8.4 Hz, 1H), and 4.41 (d, J = 6.2 Hz, 2H). ^{13}C NMR (150 MHz, DMSO-d_6) δ 179.83, 174.63, 163.90 (d, J = 238.5 Hz), 159.09, 156.86, 150.51 (d, J = 10.5 Hz), 135.46, 130.79 (d, J = 9.0 Hz), 130.40, 129.85, 129.73, 128.25, 122.42, 122.04, 109.34, 106.10, 102.99 (d, J = 21.0 Hz), and 99.24 (d, J = 27.0 Hz). IR (ν, cm^{-1}): 3390.68, 3105.83, 2360.44, 2337.30, 1665.28, 1618.38, 1220.09, and 1152.73. HRMS (ESI) calcd. for $[M + Na]^+$ $C_{19}H_{12}O_3NFNa^+$: 344.0693, found 344.0688.

TC14: *2-(((2-fluorophenyl)amino)methyl)naphtho[1,2-b]furan-4,5-dione*. Dark red solid, yield: 46%. Mp: 170–171 °C. ^{1}H NMR (600 MHz, $CDCl_3$) δ 8.08 (d, J = 7.8 Hz, 1H), 7.69 (d, J = 7.4 Hz, 1H), 7.66 (t, J = 7.4 Hz, 1H), 7.47 (t, J = 7.5 Hz, 1H), 7.05–7.00 (m, 2H), 6.79 (t, J = 8.5 Hz, 1H), 6.75–6.72 (m, 1H), 6.71 (s, 1H), and 4.51 (d, J = 6.4 Hz, 2H). ^{13}C NMR (150 MHz, $CDCl_3$) δ 180.39, 174.38, 160.36, 155.98, 151.74 (d, J = 237.0 Hz), 135.45, 135.22 (d, J = 12.0 Hz), 130.63, 130.29, 128.79, 128.36, 124.67 (d, J = 4.5 Hz), 122.26 (d, J = 15.0 Hz), 118.16 (d, J = 6.0 Hz), 114 (d, J = 19.5 Hz), 112.52, 112.50, 106.03, and 40.74. IR (ν, cm^{-1}): 3425.04, 2923.94, 2358.97, 2854,13, 1670.34, 1513.50, 1186.96, and 1117.57. HRMS (ESI) calcd. for $[M + Na]^+$ $C_{19}H_{12}O_3NFNa^+$: 344.0693, found 344.0684.

TC15: *2-(((2,4-difluorophenyl)amino)methyl)naphtho[1,2-b]furan-4,5-dione*. Red solid, yield: 33%. Mp: 154–155 °C. ^{1}H NMR (600 MHz, $CDCl_3$) δ 8.10 (d, J = 7.6 Hz, 1H), 7.71 (d, J = 7.6 Hz, 1H), 7.67 (t, J = 7.4 Hz, 1H), 7.49 (t, J = 7.4 Hz, 1H), 7.14 (t, J = 8.1 Hz, 1H), 6.77 (d, J = 8.0 Hz, 1H), 6.71 (s, 2H), 6.59 (d, J = 8.2 Hz, 1H), and 4.46 (d, J = 6.4 Hz, 2H). ^{13}C NMR (150 MHz, $CDCl_3$) δ 180.36, 174.38, 160.42, 155.83 (d, J = 9.0 Hz), 154.24 (d, J = 10.5 Hz), 151.95 (d, J = 12.0 Hz), 150.34 (d, J = 12.0 Hz), 135.49, 131.73 (d, J = 12.0 Hz), 130.52 (d, J = 46.5 Hz), 129.67, 128.55 (d, J = 73.5 Hz), 122.24 (d, J = 24 Hz), 115.33, 112.73 (dd, J = 12.0 Hz), 110.86 (dd, J = 25.5 Hz), 106.09, 103.90 (dd, J = 49.5 Hz), and 41.22. IR (ν, cm^{-1}): 3434.72, 2358.46, 2337.30, 1689.86, 1518.53, 1210.93, 1107.68, and 957.02. HRMS (ESI) calcd. for $[M + Na]^+$ $C_{19}H_{11}O_3NF_2Na^+$: 362.0599, found 362.0589.

TC16: *2-(((2,4,6-trimethylphenyl)amino)methyl)naphtho[1,2-b]furan-4,5-dione*. Red solid, yield: 33%. Mp: 173–174 °C. ^{1}H NMR (600 MHz, $CDCl_3$) δ 8.10 (d, J = 7.6 Hz, 1H), 7.67 (d, J = 3.8 Hz, 2H), 7.50–7.46 (m, 1H), 6.85 (s, 2H), 6.60 (s, 1H), 4.21 (s, 2H), 2.29 (s, 6H), and 2.25 (s, 3H). ^{13}C NMR (150 MHz, $CDCl_3$) δ 180.53, 174.47, 160.18, 157.50, 141.61, 135.47, 132.42, 130.65, 130.23, 130.13, 129.64, 128.84, 128.47, 122.23, 122.18, 105.72, 44.94, 20.62, and 18.23. IR (ν, cm^{-1}): 3445.76, 2357.38, 2327.66, 1670.28, 1557.44, 1215.32, 1147.47, and 1025.94. HRMS (ESI) calcd. for $[M + Na]^+$ $C_{22}H_{19}O_3NNa^+$: 368.1257, found 368.1250.

TC17: *2-(((4-chlorophenyl)amino)methyl)naphtho[1,2-b]furan-4,5-dione*. Dark red solid, yield: 28%. Mp: 205–206 °C. ^{1}H NMR (600 MHz, DMSO-d_6) δ 7.92 (d, J = 6.8 Hz, 1H), 7.74 (t, J = 7.5 Hz, 1H), 7.65 (d, J = 7.6 Hz, 1H), 7.52 (t, J = 7.1 Hz, 1H), 7.12 (d, J = 8.9 Hz, 2H), 6.75 (s, 1H), 6.72 (d, J = 8.9 Hz, 2H), 6.49 (t, J = 6.3 Hz, 1H), and 4.40 (d, J = 6.2 Hz, 2H). ^{13}C NMR (150 MHz, DMSO-d_6) δ: 179.82, 174.61, 159.06, 156.95, 147.33, 135.46, 130.39, 129.84, 129.72, 129.09, 128.24, 122.41, 122.05, 120.26, 114.42, and 106.08. IR (ν, cm^{-1}): 3388.22, 3110.62, 2358.84, 2342.68, 1660.69, 1510.19, 1222.68 and 1118.65. HRMS (ESI) calcd. for $[M + Na]^+$ $C_{19}H_{12}O_3NClNa^+$, 360.0398, found 360.0384.

TC18: *2-(((4-methoxyphenyl)amino)methyl)naphtho[1,2-b]furan-4,5-dione*. Dark solid, yield: 64%. Mp: 112–113 °C. ^{1}H NMR (600 MHz, $CDCl_3$) δ 8.08 (d, J = 6.4 Hz, 1H), 7.70 (d, J = 7.6 Hz, 1H), 7.69–7.63 (m, 1H), 7.50–7.44 (m, 1H), 6.82 (d, J = 8.9 Hz, 2H), 6.70–6.67 (m, 3H), 4.42 (s, 2H), and 3.77 (s, 3H). ^{13}C NMR (150 MHz, $CDCl_3$) δ 180.49, 174.43, 160.22, 156.83, 152.98, 140.82, 135.43, 130.62, 130.21, 128.77, 128.46, 122.27, 115.00, 114.74, 105.84, 55.77, and 42.13. IR (ν, cm^{-1}): 3370.45, 3105.23, 2358.89, 2337.30, 1660.16, 1514.41, 1234.80, and 1040.25. HRMS (ESI) calcd. for $[M + Na]^+$ $C_{20}H_{15}O_4NNa^+$: 356.0893, found 356.0883.

3.3. *In Vitro Cytotoxicity Assay*

The *human cancer cell lines*, including prostate cancer cells PC3, leukemia cells K562, and melanoma cells WM9, were stored in the biology laboratory of the Key Laboratory of Chemistry for Natural Products of Guizhou Province and Chinese Academy of Sciences (Guiyang, China). All cells were cultured in DMEM supplemented with 10% fetal bovine serum (FBS) and 1% penicillin and streptomycin (Sijiqing, Hangzhou, China) and incubated at 37 °C under 5% CO_2, 95% air, and 95% humidity. Cytotoxicity was evaluated by performing the MTT assay [24]. Briefly, the cells were seeded in 96-well microculture plates at a density from 4×10^3 to 8×10^3 cells/well. Cells were then exposed to different concentrations of the assayed compounds for 48 h. Then, 20 μL of MTT solution (5 mg/mL) was added to each well and incubated at 37 °C for an additional 4 h. The medium was then removed and 200 μL Tris-DMSO solution was added. Plates were lightly shaking up to dissolve the dark blue formazan crystals and the absorbance was measured in an ELISA plate reader at 570 nm.

3.4. *Flow Cytometry Assay*

Cell apoptosis was determined by an inverted fluorescence microscope observation and flow cytometry as describe in our previous study [28]. Briefly, the cancer cells treated with compounds were harvested for centrifugation at 1000 rpm for 5 min at room temperature, washed twice with PBS and resuspended with binding buffer, and then PI (Sigma, St. Louis, MO, USA) was added to a final concentration of 20 mg/mL. The cell lines were analyzed by flow cytometry (Becton Dickinson, Franklin Lakes, NJ, USA).

3.5. *Statistical Analysis*

The IC_{50} values were calculated from the semilogarithmic dose-response curves. The data were analyzed using SPSS 18.0 and reported as mean ± SD of the number of experiments indicated. For all measurements, one-way ANOVA followed by Student's t-test was used to assess the statistical significance of the difference between each group. The LSD method was used to assess the statistical significance of the difference between the two groups. A statistically significant difference was considered at the level of $P < 0.05$. The data are presented as the mean ± SEM of three assays.

4. Conclusions

In this study, 27 novel L-shaped ortho-quinone analogs were synthesized and evaluated for their anti-cancer activities. Compounds **TB1, TB3, TB4, TB6, TC1, TC3, TC5, TC9, TC11, TC12, TC14, TC15, TC16,** and **TC17** possessed broad-spectrum potent cytotoxicity against PC3, K562, and WM9 cells. With more than a 70% inhibitory rate, **TB7** showed better inhibitory activity of K562 cells as compared with other cells. Moreover, we observed that **TC7** inhibited the growth of PC3 cells more efficiently than other cells. Some of the active compounds such as **TB3, TC1, TC3,** and **TC7** inhibited cell proliferation mainly through inducing apoptosis. The structure-activity relationships evaluation showed that removing methyl at C-3 of the furan ring and introducing diverse side chains at C-2 of the furan ring is an effective strategy for improving the anticancer activity of L-shaped ortho-quinone analogs.

Author Contributions: W.-D.P. and H.L. conceived and designed the experiments; S.-Y.L. and X.-Y.Z. performed part of chemical experiment; Z.-K.S., Y.Z., M.-L.W. performed the biology experiment; S.-C.H., J.L., J.-R.S. and C.C. contributed reagents and materials and revised the paper; S.-Y.L. and H.L. wrote the paper.

References

1. Ferlay, J.; Colombet, M.; Soerjomataram, I.; Mathers, C.; Parkin, D.M.; Piñeros, M.; Znaor, A.; Bray, F. Estimating the global cancer incidence and mortality in 2018: GLOBOCAN sources and methods. *Int. J. Cancer* **2019**, *144*, 1941–1953. [CrossRef] [PubMed]
2. Feng, R.M.; Zong, Y.N.; Cao, S.M.; Xu, R.H. Current cancer situation in China: Good or bad news from the 2018 Global Cancer Statistics? *Cancer Commun.* **2019**, *39*, 22. [CrossRef] [PubMed]
3. Chen, W.; Zheng, R.; Baade, P.D.; Zhang, S.; Zeng, H.; Bray, F.; Jemal, A.; Yu, X.Q.; He, J. Cancer statistics in China, 2015. *CA Cancer J. Clin.* **2016**, *66*, 115–132. [CrossRef] [PubMed]
4. Weerink, L.B.; Gant, C.M.; Leeuwen, B.L.V.; De Bock, G.H.; Kouwenhoven, E.A.; Faneyte, I.F. Long-term survival in octogenarians after surgical treatment for colorectal cancer: Prevention of postoperative complications is key. *Ann. Surg. Oncol.* **2018**, *25*, 3874–3882. [CrossRef]
5. Newman, D.J.; Cragg, G.M. Natural products as sources of new drugs over the Last 25 years. *J. Nat. Prod.* **2007**, *70*, 461–477. [CrossRef]
6. Tan, Y.H.; Xiao, X.; Yao, J.N.; Han, F.; Lou, H.Y.; Luo, H.; Liang, G.Y.; Ben-David, Y.; Pan, W.D. Syntheses and Anti-cancer Activities of Glycosylated Derivatives of Diosgenin. *Chem. Res. Chin. Univ.* **2017**, *33*, 80–86. [CrossRef]
7. Lan, J.J.; Huang, L.; Lou, H.Y.; Chen, C.; Liu, T.J.J.; Hu, S.C.; Yao, Y.; Song, J.R.; Luo, J.; Liu, Y.Z.; et al. Design and synthesis of novel C-14-urea-tetrandrine derivatives with potent anti-cancer activity. *Eur. J. Med. Chem.* **2018**, *143*, 1968–1980. [CrossRef]
8. Lan, J.J.; Wang, N.; Huang, L.; Liu, Y.Z.; Ma, X.P.; Lou, H.Y.; Chen, C.; Feng, Y.P.; Pan, W.D. Design and synthesis of novel tetrandrine derivatives as potential anti-tumor agents against human hepatocellular carcinoma. *Eur. J. Med. Chem.* **2019**, *127*, 554–566. [CrossRef]
9. Song, J.R.; Lan, J.J.; Chen, C.; Hu, S.C.; Song, J.L.; Liu, W.L.; Zeng, X.Y.; Lou, H.Y.; Ben-David, Y.; Pan, W.D. Design, synthesis and bioactivity investigation of tetrandrine derivatives as potential anti-cancer agents. *MedChemComm* **2018**, *9*, 1131–1141. [CrossRef]
10. Liu, F.; Yu, G.; Wang, G.; Liu, H.; Wu, X.; Wang, Q.; Liu, M.; Liao, K.; Wu, M.; Cheng, X.; et al. An NQO1-initiated and p53-independent apoptotic pathway determines the anti-tumor effect of tanshinone IIA against non-small cell lung cancer. *PLoS ONE* **2012**, *7*, e42138. [CrossRef]
11. Xu, Z.Y.; Chen, L.; Xiao, Z.G.; Zhu, Y.H.; Jiang, H.; Jin, Y.; Gu, C.; Wu, Y.L.; Wang, L.; Zhang, W.; et al. Potentiation of the anticancer effect of doxorubicinin drug-resistant gastric cancer cells by tanshinone IIA. *Phytomedicine* **2018**, *51*, 58–67. [CrossRef] [PubMed]
12. Lin, C.Y.; Wang, L.; Wang, H.; Yang, L.Q.; Guo, H.J.; Wang, X.J. Tanshinone IIA inhibits breast cancer stem cells growth in vitro and in vivo through attenuation of IL-6/STAT3/NF-kB signaling pathways. *J. Cell Biochem.* **2013**, *114*, 2061–2070. [CrossRef] [PubMed]
13. Huang, S.T.; Huang, C.C.; Huang, W.L.; Lin, T.K.; Liao, P.L.; Wang, P.W.; Liou, C.W.; Chuang, J.H. Tanshinone IIA induces intrinsic apoptosis in osteosarcoma cells both in vivo and in vitro associated with mitochondrial dysfunction. *Sci. Rep.* **2017**, *7*, 40382. [CrossRef] [PubMed]
14. Bentle, M.S.; Reinicke, K.E.; Bey, E.A.; Spitz, D.R.; Boothman, D.A. Calcium-dependent modulation of poly (ADP-ribose) polymerase-1 alters cellular metabolism and DNA repair. *J. Biol. Chem.* **2006**, *281*, 33684–33696. [CrossRef]
15. Bey, E.A.; Bentle, M.S.; Reinicke, K.E.; Dong, Y.; Yang, C.R.; Girard, L.; Minna, J.D.; Bornmann, W.G.; Gao, J.M.; Boothman, D.A. An NQO1- and PARP-1-mediated cell death pathway induced in non-small-cell lung cancer cells by β-lapachone. *Proc. Natl. Acad. Sci. USA* **2007**, *104*, 11832–11837. [CrossRef]
16. Cheng, X.F.; Liu, F.; Yan, T.T.; Zhou, X.Y.; Wu, L.; Liao, K.; Wang, G.J.; Hao, H.P. , Metabolic profile, enzyme kinetics, and reaction phenotyping of β-lapachone metabolism in human liver and intestine in vitro. *Mol. Pharm.* **2012**, *9*, 3476–3485. [CrossRef]
17. Huang, W.G.; Li, J.Y.; Zhang, W.; Zhou, Y.Y.; Xie, C.M.; Luo, Y.; Li, Y.F.; Wang, J.L.; Li, J.; Lu, W. Synthesis of miltirone analogues as inhibitors of Cdc25 phosphatases. *Bioorg. Med. Chem. Lett.* **2006**, *16*, 1905–1908. [CrossRef]
18. Huang, W.G.; Jiang, Y.Y.; Li, Q.; Li, J.; Li, J.Y.; Lu, W.; Cai, J.C. Synthesis and biological evaluation of (±)-cryptotanshinone and its simplified analogues as potent CDC25 inhibitors. *Tetrahedron* **2005**, *61*, 1863–1870. [CrossRef]

19. Bian, J.L.; Deng, B.; Xu, L.L.; Xu, X.L.; Wang, N.; Hu, T.H.; Yao, Z.Y.; Du, J.Y.; Yang, L.; Lei, Y.H.; et al. 2-Substituted 3-methylnaphtho[1,2-*b*]furan-4,5-diones as novel L-shaped ortho-quinone substrates for NAD(P)H: Quinone oxidoreductase (NQO1). *Eur. J. Med. Chem.* **2014**, *82*, 56–67. [CrossRef]
20. Bian, J.L.; Li, X.; Wang, N.; Wu, X.S.; You, Q.D.; Zhang, X.J. Discovery of quinone-directed antitumor agents selectively bioactivated by NQO1 over CPR with improved safety profile. *Eur. J. Med. Chem.* **2017**, *129*, 27–40. [CrossRef]
21. Deniz, N.G.; Ozyurek, M.; Tufan, A.N.; Apak, R. One-pot synthesis, characterization, and antioxidant capacity of sulfur-and oxygen-substituted 1,4-naphthoquinones and a structural study. *Monatshefte für Chemie-Chemical Monthly* **2015**, *146*, 2117–2126. [CrossRef]
22. Arenas, P.; Peña, A.; Rios, D.; Benites, J.; Muccioli, G.G.; Calderon, P.B.; Valderrama, J.A. Eco-friendly synthesis and antiproliferative evaluation of some oxygen substituted diaryl ketones. *Molecules* **2013**, *18*, 9818–9832. [CrossRef]
23. Li, X.; Bian, J.L.; Wang, N.; Qian, X.; Gu, J.; Mu, T.; Fan, J.; Yang, X.W.; Li, S.Z.; Yang, T.T.; et al. Novel naphtho[2,1-*d*]oxazole-4,5-diones as NQO1 substrates with improved aqueous solubility: Design, synthesis, and in vivo antitumor evaluation. *Bioorg. Med. Chem.* **2016**, *24*, 1006–1013. [CrossRef] [PubMed]
24. Jain, M.; Nilsson, R.; Sharma, S.; Madhusudhan, N.; Kitami, T.; Souza, A.L.; Kafri, R.; Kirschner, M.W.; Clish, C.B.; Mootha, V.K. Metabolite profiling identifies a key role for glycine in rapid cancer cell proliferation. *Science* **2012**, *336*, 1040–1044. [CrossRef]
25. Hu, K.Z.; Wang, H.; Huang, T.; Tang, G.; Liang, X.; He, S.; Tang, X. Synthesis and biological evaluation of *N*-(2-[(18)F]Fluoropropionyl)-L-methionine for tumor imaging. *Nucl. Med. Biol.* **2013**, *40*, 926–932. [CrossRef]
26. Kongkathip, N.; Kongkathip, B.; Siripong, P.; Sangma, C.; Luangkamin, S.; Niyomdecha, M.; Pattanapa, S.; Piyaviriyagul, S.; Kongsaeree, P. Potent antitumor activity of synthetic 1,2-Naphthoquinones and 1,4-Naphthoquinones. *Bioorg. Med. Chem.* **2003**, *11*, 3179–3191. [CrossRef]
27. Weerawarna, S.A.; Guha-Biswas, M.; Nelson, W.L. Improved Syntheses of Bufuralol, 7-Ethyl-2-(2-tertbutylamino-1-hydroxyethyl)benzofuran, and 1 Oxobufuralol, 7-Acetyl-2-(2-tert-butylamino-1-hydroxyethyl)benzofuran. *Heterocycl* **1991**, *28*, 1395–1403. [CrossRef]
28. Wen, Z.H.; Zhang, Y.Q.; Wang, X.H.; Zeng, X.P.; Hu, Z.X.; Liu, Y.; Xie, Y.X.; Liang, G.Y.; Zhu, J.G.; Luo, H.; et al. Novel 3′,5′-diprenylated chalcones inhibited the proliferation of cancer cells in vitro by inducing cell apoptosis and arresting cell cycle phase. *Eur. J. Med. Chem.* **2017**, *133*, 227–239. [CrossRef]

12

Synthesis and Cytotoxicity of 7,9-*O*-Linked Macrocyclic C-Seco Taxoids

Yu Zhao [1], Tian-En Wang [1], Alberto Mills [2], Federico Gago [2] and Wei-Shuo Fang [1,*]

1 State Key Laboratory of Bioactive Substances and Functions of Natural Medicines, Institute of Materia Medica, Chinese Academy of Medical Sciences and Peking Union Medical College, 2A Nan Wei Road, Beijing 100050, China; zhaoyu8410@126.com (Y.Z.); wangtianen@imm.ac.cn (T.-E.W.)

2 Department of Biomedical Sciences and "Unidad Asociada IQM-CSIC", School of Medicine and Health Sciences, University of Alcalá, E-28805 Alcalá de Henares, Madrid, Spain; albertomillsfernandez@gmail.com (A.M.); federico.gago@uah.es (F.G.)

* Correspondence: wfang@imm.ac.cn;

Academic Editor: Qiao-Hong Chen

Abstract: A series of novel 7,9-*O*-linked macrocyclic taxoids together with modification at the C2 position were synthesized, and their cytotoxicities against drug-sensitive and P-glycoprotein and βIII-tubulin overexpressed drug-resistant cancer cell lines were evaluated. It is demonstrated that C-seco taxoids conformationally constrained via carbonate containing-linked macrocyclization display increased cytotoxicity on drug-resistant tumors overexpressing both βIII and P-gp, among which compound **22b**, bearing a 2-m-methoxybenzoyl group together with a five-atom linker, was identified as the most potent. Molecular modeling suggested the improved cytotoxicity of **22b** results from enhanced favorable interactions with the T7 loop region of βIII.

Keywords: taxoids; βIII-tubulin; P-glycoprotein; drug resistance

1. Introduction

Antitubulin agent paclitaxel (**1a**, Figure 1) and its semi-synthetic derivative docetaxel (**1b**, Figure 1) are successfully used in the clinic for the treatment of ovarian, breast, and non-small cell lung and prostate cancers and Kaposi's sarcoma.

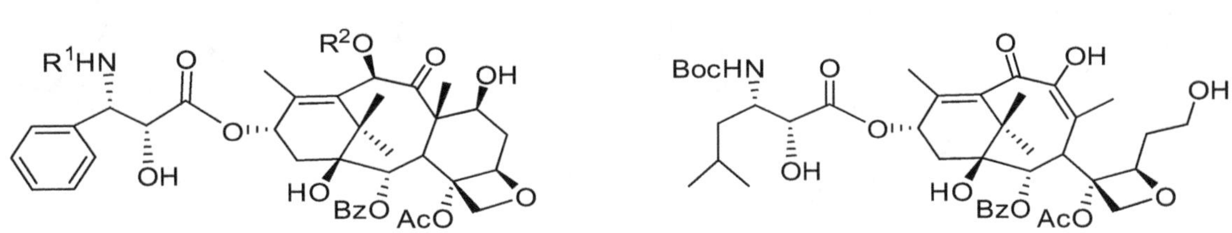

1a R^1 = Bz, R^2 = Ac
1b R^1 = Boc, R^2 = H

2

Figure 1. Structures of paclitaxel (**1a**), docetaxel (**1b**), and IDN5390 (**2**).

However, their clinical uses are severely restricted by drug resistance. Various resistance mechanisms toward taxane-based anticancer drugs have been revealed, among which only overexpression of P-glycoprotein (P-gp) and βIII-tubulin have been confirmed clinically [1–4].

A great deal of effort has been made to overcome multi-drug resistance (MDR) mediated by overexpression of P-gp. Nevertheless, many taxane-based drug candidates targeting P-gp overexpression did not achieve the expected efficacy in clinical trials [5,6].

A correlation between βIII-tubulin overexpression and poor prognosis has been reported in several human tumors, including various advanced malignancies upon treatment of taxanes, such as breast, non-small cell lung, and ovarian cancers [7–10]. It was reported that a C-seco taxane IDN5390 (**2**, Figure 1) is more active than paclitaxel in several paclitaxel-resistant human ovarian adenocarcinoma cell lines (e.g., A2780TC1, A2780TC3, and OVCAR-3), expressing high βIII-tubulin and P-gp levels. However, IDN5390 was nearly 10-fold less active than paclitaxel in paclitaxel-sensitive cells [11].

To find a modified taxane effective against both paclitaxel-sensitive and -resistant tumors, the 7,9-*O*-linked C-seco taxoid **3** (Figure 2) was synthesized in our lab and shown to exhibit significant activity enhancement against drug-sensitive Hela and βIII-tubulin overexpressing HeLa-βIII tumor cells compared to the C-seco paclitaxel derivative **4** (an analog of IDN5390, Figure 2) [12]. Those macrocyclic taxoids provided a successful example for the compromise between structural pre-organization and sufficient flexibility in the C ring of C-seco taxoids to improve the cytotoxicity against tumor cells that overexpress βIII tubulin [12].

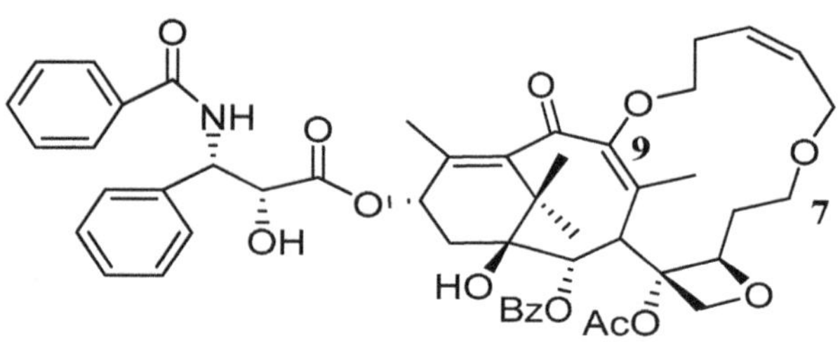

3

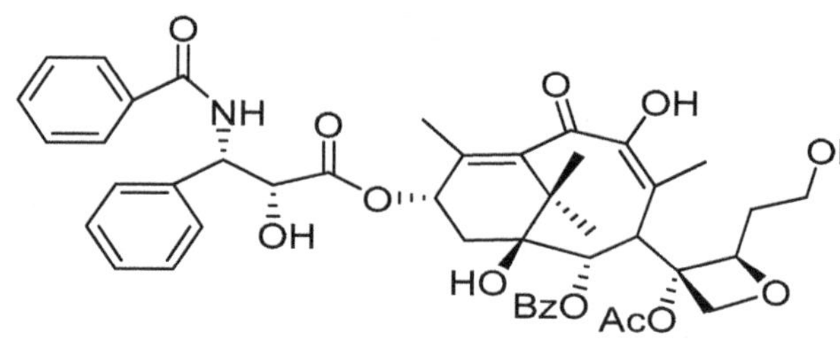

4

Figure 2. Structures of the 7,9-*O*-linked C-seco taxoid **3** and C-seco paclitaxel derivative **4**.

It has long been observed that modification of taxane at the C2 position could play a critical role in its interaction with tubulin. Consistent with this observation, the 7,9-*O*-linked C-seco taxoid with C2 modification **5** (Figure 3) was much more cytotoxic than the C-seco taxoid **6** (Figure 3) in drug-resistant A2780AD and KB-V1 cells (P-gp overexpression) and Hela-βIII (βIII overexpression) [12]. It was demonstrated that the *meta*-substitution (i.e., -OMe, -F, -Cl) of the C2-benzoate moiety of C-seco taxoids derivatives **7a–c** (Figure 3) could increase the interaction of C-seco-taxoids with βIII-tubulin to overcome paclitaxel-resistance [13].

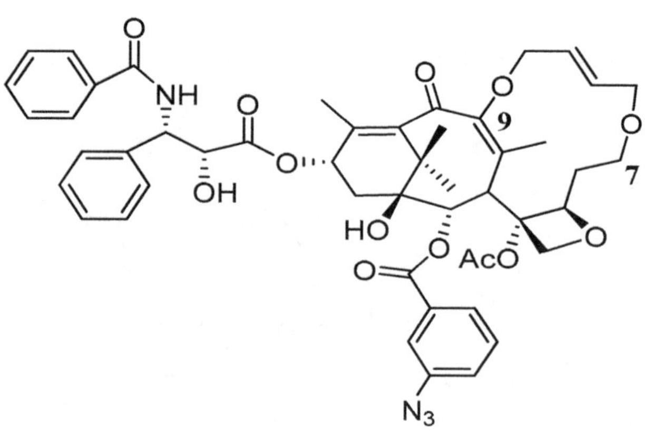

5

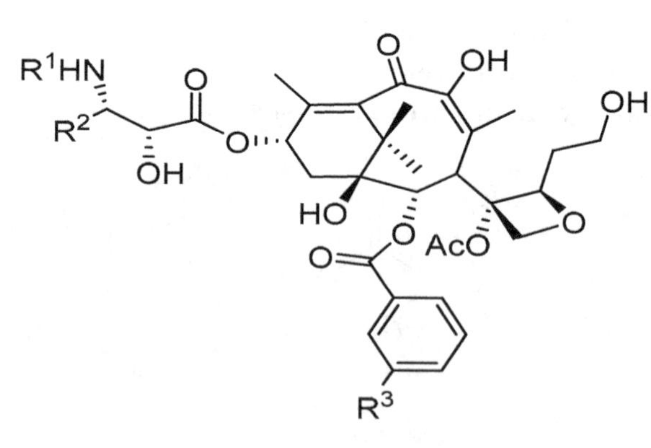

6 $R^1 = Ph$, $R^2 = Ph$, $R^3 = N_3$
7a $R^1 = Boc$, $R^2 = (CH_3)_2CHCH_2$, $R^3 = OCH_3$
7b $R^1 = Boc$, $R^2 = (CH_3)_2CHCH_2$, $R^3 = F$
7c $R^1 = Boc$, $R^2 = (CH_3)_2CHCH_2$, $R^3 = Cl$

Figure 3. Structures of the 7,9-*O*-linked C-seco taxoid **5** and C-seco taxoids **6, 7a–c**.

In order to explore the effect of macrocyclization in a different way from that employed in our previous study (i.e., via the carbonate formation to restrict the conformation), the synthesis and biological activity assessment of a series of 7,9-*O*-linked macrocyclic taxoids together with modification at the C2 position were performed and are reported here.

2. Results and Discussion

2.1. Chemistry

Our synthesis began with the preparation of 2′-*tert*-butyldimethylsilyl-paclitaxel **12a**, which was then converted to 10-deacetylpaclitaxel **13a** upon treatment with hydrazine hydrate in methanol. Synthesis of the analogues **12b–e** of 2′-*tert*-butyldimethylsilyl-paclitaxel with modifications at the C2 positions was then realized by selective C2 debenzoylation and then elaboration with various *m*-substituted benzoyl group. C2-modified 10-deacetylpaclitaxel **13b–e** were afforded in the same manner as compound **13a**. Then the compounds **13a–e** were oxidized by copper (II) diacetate to furnish **14a–e** as a mixture of two epimers. Reductive trapping of the ring C-seco tautomers **15a–e** were obtained by treatment with L-selectride. Subsequent deprotection with pyridine hydrofluoride (HF-pyridine) afforded **16a–e**. The 9-OH in **15a–e** was hydroxylalkylated by 2-bromoethanol or 3-bromo-1-propanol in the presence of potassium carbonate and potassium iodide in *N*,*N*-dimethylformamide (DMF). Cyclization of compounds **17a–e** could be accomplished by treatment with a slight excess of triphosgene, affording the cyclic carbonate analogues **19a–e**. Desilylation of **19a–e** with HF-pyridine afforded macrocyclic analogues **21a–e**. Accordingly, macrocyclic taxoids **22a–e** bearing a linkage with one more carbon atom were synthesized from **18a–e** in a similar manner (Scheme 1).

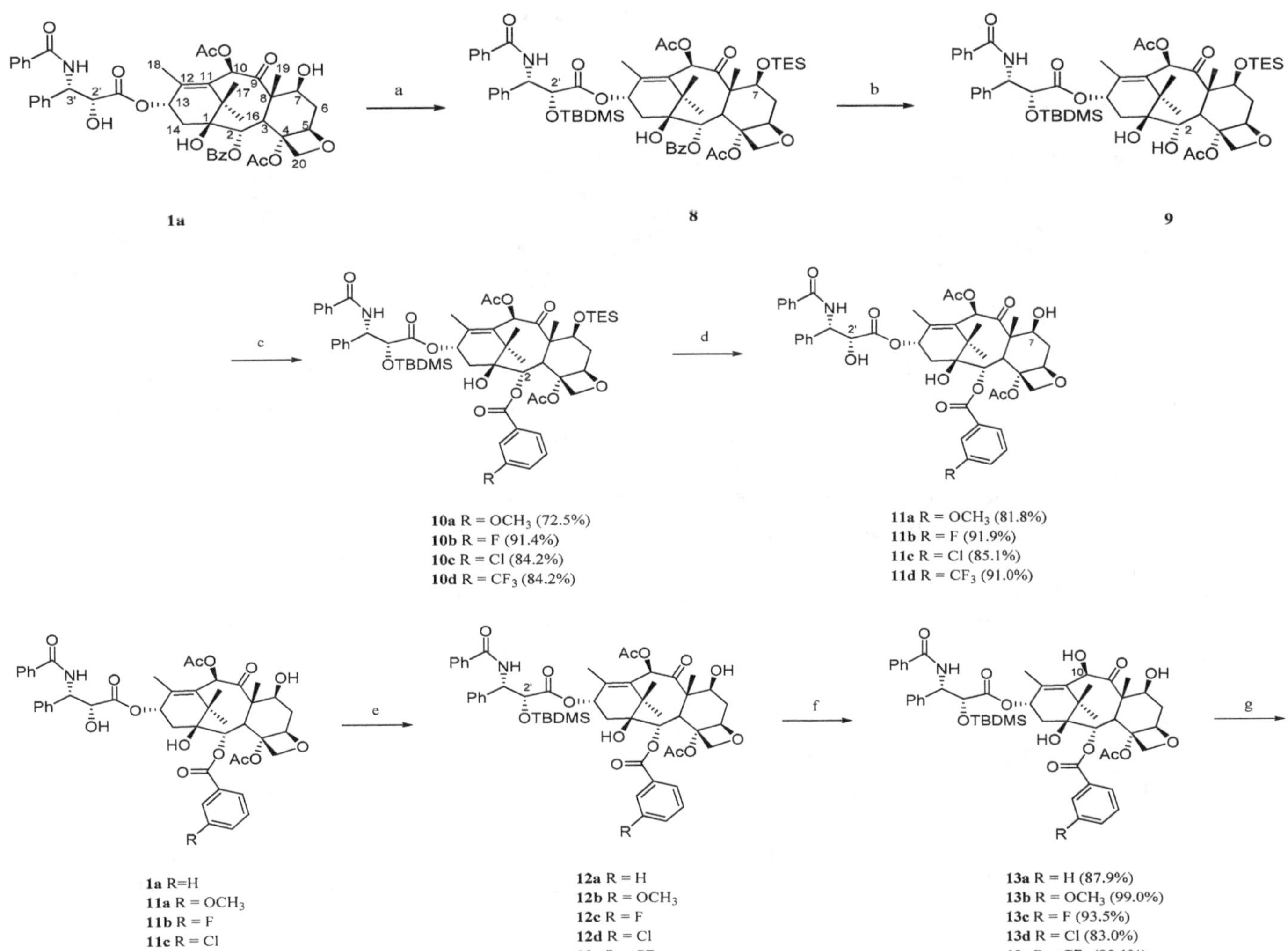

Scheme 1. *Cont.*

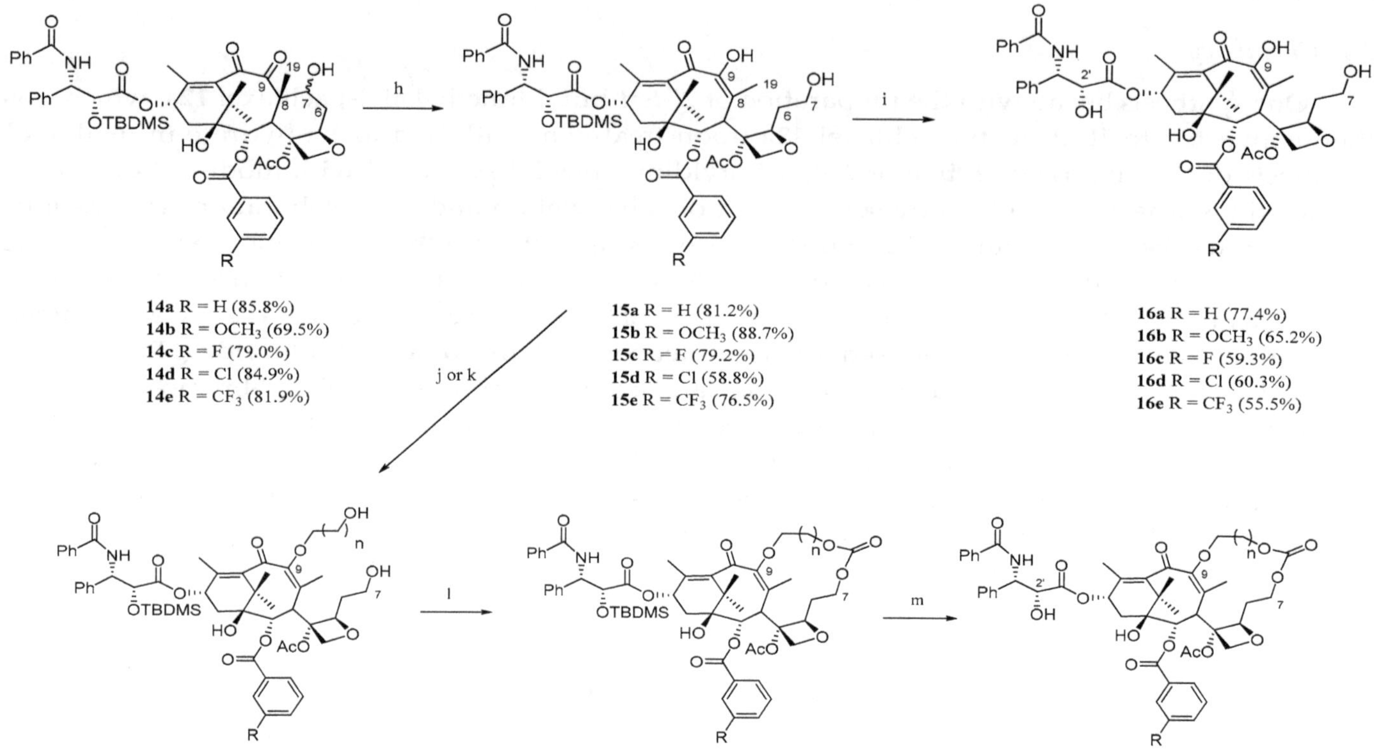

14a R = H (85.8%)
14b R = OCH_3 (69.5%)
14c R = F (79.0%)
14d R = Cl (84.9%)
14e R = CF_3 (81.9%)

15a R = H (81.2%)
15b R = OCH_3 (88.7%)
15c R = F (79.2%)
15d R = Cl (58.8%)
15e R = CF_3 (76.5%)

16a R = H (77.4%)
16b R = OCH_3 (65.2%)
16c R = F (59.3%)
16d R = Cl (60.3%)
16e R = CF_3 (55.5%)

17a n = 1, R = H (52.4%)
17b n = 1, R = OCH_3 (56.1%)
17c n = 1, R = F (53.2%)
17d n = 1, R = Cl (60.9%)
17e n = 1, R = CF_3 (49.9%)
18a n = 2, R = H (72.4%)
18b n = 2, R = OCH_3 (75.3%)
18c n = 2, R = F (69.7%)
18d n = 2, R = Cl (52.6%)
18e n = 2, R = CF_3 (71.8%)

19a n = 1, R = H (15.9%)
19b n = 1, R = OCH_3 (32.7%)
19c n = 1, R = F (32.1%)
19d n = 1, R = Cl (36.1%)
19e n = 1, R = CF_3 (30.5%)
20a n = 2, R = H (24.9%)
20b n = 2, R = OCH_3 (28.6%)
20c n = 2, R = F (27.1%)
20d n = 2, R = Cl (23.6%)
20e n = 2, R = CF_3 (26.7%)

21a n = 1, R = H (46.2%)
21b n = 1, R = OCH_3 (54.1%)
21c n = 1, R = F (52.2%)
21d n = 1, R = Cl (48.7%)
21e n = 1, R = CF_3 (63.7%)
22a n = 2, R = H (51.0%)
22b n = 2, R = OCH_3 (59.2%)
22c n = 2, R = F (51.5%)
22d n = 2, R = Cl (65.4%)
22e n = 2, R = CF_3 (59.5%)

Scheme 1. (a) tert-ButyldiMethylsilyl chloride (TBDMSCl), imidazole, DMF, 2 h, 60 °C, and; triethylchlorosilane (TESCl), imidazole, DMF, overnight, r.t., 90.1%; (b) Triton-B, tetrahydrofuran (THF), 15 min, −40 °C, 47.7%; (c) (**10a**) m-anisic acid, N, N′-diisopropylcarbodiimide (DIC), 4-dimethylaminopyridine (DMAP), toluene, overnight, 60 °C, 72.5%; (**10b**) m-fluorobenzoic acid, DIC, DMAP, toluene, overnight, 60 °C, 91.4%; (**10c**) m-chlorobenzoic acid, DIC, DMAP, toluene, overnight, 60 °C, 84.2%; (**10d**) m-trifluoromethyl acid, DIC, DMAP, toluene, overnight, 60 °C, 84.2%; (d) HF -pyridine, THF, overnight, r.t.; (**11a**) 81.8%; (**11b**) 91.9%; (**11c**) 85.1%; (**11d**) 91.0%; (e) TBDMSCl, imidazole, DMF, 4 h, r.t.; (f) $NH_2NH_2{\cdot}H_2O$, C_2H_5OH, 2 h, r.t. (e and f two steps), (**13a**) 87.9%, (**13b**) 99.0%; (**13c**) 93.5%; (**13d**) 83.0%; (**13e**) 90.1%; (g) $Cu(OAc)_2{\cdot}H_2O$, CH_3OH, overnight, r.t., (**14a**) 85.8%; (**14b**) 69.5%; (**14c**) 79.0%; (**14d**) 84.9%; (**14e**) 81.9%; (h) L-selectride, THF, 15 min, −20 °C, (**15a**) 81.2%; (**15b**) 88.7%; (**15c**) 79.2%; (**15d**) 58.8%; (**15e**) 76.5%; (i) HF/Py, THF, overnight, r.t., (**16a**) 77.4%; (**16b**) 65.2%; (**16c**) 59.3%; (**16d**) 60.3%; (**16e**) 55.5%; (j) 2-bromoethanol, K_2CO_3, KI, DMF, 5–9 h, r.t., (**17a**) 52.4%; (**17b**) 56.1%; (**17c**) 53.2%; (**17d**) 60.9%; (**17e**) 49.9%; (k) 3-bromo-1-propanol, K_2CO_3, KI, DMF, 4–9 h, r.t., (**18a**) 72.4%; (**18b**) 75.3%; (**18c**) 69.7%; (**18d**) 52.6%; (**18e**) 71.8%; (l) triphosgene, pyridine, DCM, 3–5 h, 0 °C to r.t., (**19a**) 15.9%; (**19b**) 32.7%; (**19c**) 32.1%; (**19d**) 36.1%; (**19e**) 30.5%; (**20a**) 24.9%; (**20b**) 28.6%; (**20c**) 27.1%; (**20d**) 23.6%; (**20e**) 26.7%; (m) HF/Py, THF, 30 h, r.t., (**21a**) 46.2%; (**21b**) 54.1%; (**21c**) 52.2%; (**21d**) 48.7%; (**21e**) 63.7%; (**22a**) 51.0%; (**22b**) 59.2%; (**22c**) 51.5%; (**22d**) 65.4%; (**22e**) 59.5%.

2.2. *Bioactivity Evaluation of Taxoids* **21a–e** *and* **22a–e**

Taxoids **21a–e**, **22a–e**, and **16a–e** were evaluated for their in vitro cytotoxicities against cervical carcinoma HeLa cells and their corresponding drug-resistant cell lines (HeLa-βIII).

As shown in Table 1, all the 7,9-*O*-linked macrocyclic analogues (**21a–e, 22a–e**) possessed a remarkably higher potency against HeLa and HeLa-βIII cells than their corresponding C-seco taxoids analogues **16a–e**. The R/S values (IC_{50} in drug resistant cells/IC_{50} in drug sensitive cells) of all macrocyclic analogues were lower than those of their corresponding C-seco taxoids analogues **16a–e**. These findings demonstrate that conformational restraint via carbonate-containing linked macrocyclization can improve the cytotoxicity against human carcinoma cell lines overexpressing βIII tubulin.

Furthermore, all of the 7,9-*O*-linked macrocyclic analogues bearing the four-atom linker (**21a–e**) turned out to be generally more potent against sensitive HeLa cells and HeLa-βIII cells than the corresponding macrocyclic analogues bearing the five-atom linker (**22a–e**). Since the cytotoxicity of **21a–d** was approximately equal to that of paclitaxel, these results suggest that a four-atom tether is optimal in these macrocyclic C-seco taxoids.

For the effect of C2 modifications in these macrocyclic C-seco taxoids, we found similar results as previously reported [12,13]. Pepe et al. studied the cytotoxicity of a series of C-seco taxoids, whereby the introduction of a substituent (-OMe, -F, -Cl) to the *meta*-position of the C2 benzoyl moiety increased potency against the βIII-tubulin-overexpressing, paclitaxel-resistant cell line A2780TC3 [13]. Taxoid **6** bearing a 2-(*m*-azido) benzyloxy group and synthesized in our lab exhibited higher binding affinity for microtubulin (MT) than its corresponding taxoids bearing a 2-benzyloxy group [12]. The 7,9-*O*-linked C-seco taxoid bearing a 2-(*m*-azido) benzyloxy group **5** was significantly more active than **6** on drug-resistant A2780AD, HeLa-βIII, and KB-V1 cells [12].

We investigated this effect in the 7,9-*O*-linked C-seco taxoids **21b–e** and **22b–e** reported here. Thus, introduction of a *meta* substituent (-OMe, -F, -Cl) on derivatives bearing the four-atom linker showed similar cytotoxicity against HeLa sensitive cell lines and Hela-βIII cells lines as their corresponding C-seco taxoid **21a** bearing a 2-benzyloxy group. In contrast, the *meta*-substituted (-OMe, -F, -Cl) derivatives bearing five-atom linker possessed higher potency against HeLa-βIII cells lines than its corresponding C-seco taxoid **22a** (by a factor of 3.1–8.9). Nonetheless, the 2-*m*-CF_3 analogues **21e** and **22e** were considerably less cytotoxic against both drug sensitive and resistant cells by one to two orders of magnitude.

The growth inhibition effects of the 7,9-*O*-linked macrocyclic analogues were also measured on human breast cancer MCF-7 cells and their corresponding P-gp-overexpressing drug-resistant MCF-7/R cells. As shown in Table 1, the 7,9-*O*-linked macrocyclic analogues possessed remarkable potency against MCF-7/R cells compared to their C-seco counterparts, except for the 2-*m*-CF_3 derivatives. Strikingly, macrocyclic taxoids bearing the five-atom linker were almost inactive. The cytotoxicity against MCF-7/R cells of the 7,9-*O*-linked macrocyclic derivatives (-OMe, -F, -Cl) bearing the five-atom linker were slightly higher than that of the compouds bearing the four-atom linker. Compounds **22b–d** (-OMe, -F, -Cl) bearing the five-atom linker and **21a**, **21d** (-H, -Cl) bearing the four-atom linker displayed lower R/S values than that of paclitaxel. All in all, **22b** turned out to be the best compound in the whole series.

Table 1. Cytotoxicity of taxoids **16a–e**, **21a–e**, and **22a–e**.

Compound	Cytotoxicity (IC_{50}, nM)		Ratio	Cytotoxicity (IC_{50}, nM)		Ratio
	HeLa	HeLa-βIII	R/S	MCF-7	MCF-7/R	R/S
21a	5.97 ± 1.13	29.92 ± 2.85	5.01 ± 0.48	11.82 ± 1.10	6291.33 ± 1252.19	532.26 ± 105.94
21b	5.90 ± 1.47	17.61 ± 2.13	3.17 ± 0.25	9.93 ± 2.70	6440.00 ± 1040.85	648.76 ± 104.85
21c	7.82 ± 3.10	22.14 ± 6.36	2.83 ± 0.81	7.70 ± 1.68	6411.67 ± 645.71	832.68 ± 83.86
21d	7.75 ± 2.24	19.02 ± 9.60	2.46 ± 1.24	9.36 ± 1.76	4126.33 ± 91.92	440.85 ± 9.82
21e	186.03 ± 48.30	503.40 ± 132.41	2.61 ± 0.98	159.80 ± 33.91	>10,000	
22a	28.28 ± 0.47	162.33 ± 58.80	5.74 ± 2.08	19.16 ± 2.39	>10,000	
22b	7.97 ± 1.79	18.11 ± 2.91	1.52 ± 1.34	5.15 ± 0.96	2769.00 ± 399.24	538.02 ± 77.57
22c	12.07 ± 0.93	52.40 ± 16.98	4.34 ± 1.41	9.33 ± 1.44	4756.33 ± 443.24	509.79 ± 47.51
22d	11.53 ± 1.98	50.11 ± 16.92	4.35 ± 1.47	14.48 ± 3.37	3704.67 ± 539.43	255.79 ± 37.24
22e	89.71 ± 29.80	267.20 ± 65.38	2.77 ± 0.89	86.00 ± 9.28	>10,000	
16a	149.57 ± 31.70	1423.67 ± 291.75	8.55 ± 1.75	103.53 ± 22.21	>10,000	
16b	13.63 ± 2.09	142.90 ± 5.66	10.48 ± 0.42	7.53 ± 0.19	>10,000	
16c	22.78 ± 2.20	467.13 ± 171.75	20.50 ± 7.54	16.90 ± 4.04	>10,000	
16d	17.73 ± 1.70	181.17 ± 18.92	10.22 ± 1.07	15.08 ± 1.65	>10,000	
16e	110.14 ± 17.40	525.87 ± 88.76	4.77 ± 0.81	110.90 ± 13.25	>10,000	
Paclitaxel	4.59 ± 0.55	12.31 ± 1.27	2.68 ± 0.28	6.21 ± 1.85	3450.00 ± 509.99	555.56 ± 82.12

2.3. Binding Mode of **22b** *and Rationale for the Increased Affinity for the βIII Isotype*

Inspection of the paclitaxel-β-tubulin complex in high-resolution cryo-electron microscopy (cryo-EM) structures of mammalian microtubules reveals a very tight fit between the bulky drug and the taxane-binding site, in which the M-loop is structured as an α-helix [14]. The oxetane ring oxygen of paclitaxel (**1a**) accepts a hydrogen bond from the backbone NH of Thr276, whereas the C-3′ benzamide carbonyl oxygen acts as a hydrogen bond acceptor for N^{ε} of His229. These two hydrogen bonds are likely to be present in the **22b**:β-tubulin complex as well (Figure 4), and definitely contribute to the binding affinity, but these two residues are common to both βIIB and βIII isotypes. In the search for sequence differences that can account for the resistance to taxanes, a lot of emphasis has been placed on the Ser→Ala replacement at position 277, but we believe that the most important replacement in relation to drug resistance possibly involves Cys241→Ser. The reason is that, as a consequence of this substitution, disulfide bond formation with Cys356 is precluded in the βIII isotype and the T7 loop region, which closes over the bound taxane, is likely to be more flexible. By directing the macrocyclic region of **22b** towards this loop, favorable interactions within the taxane-binding site are enhanced and the affinity towards the βIII isotype is improved. We hypothesize that the improved cytotoxicity of **22b** relative to **1a**, and the other taxanes described here, results from enhanced favorable interactions with the T7 loop region of βIII, an isotype in which Cys356 cannot engage in a disulfide bond with the amino acid present at position 241 (Ser).

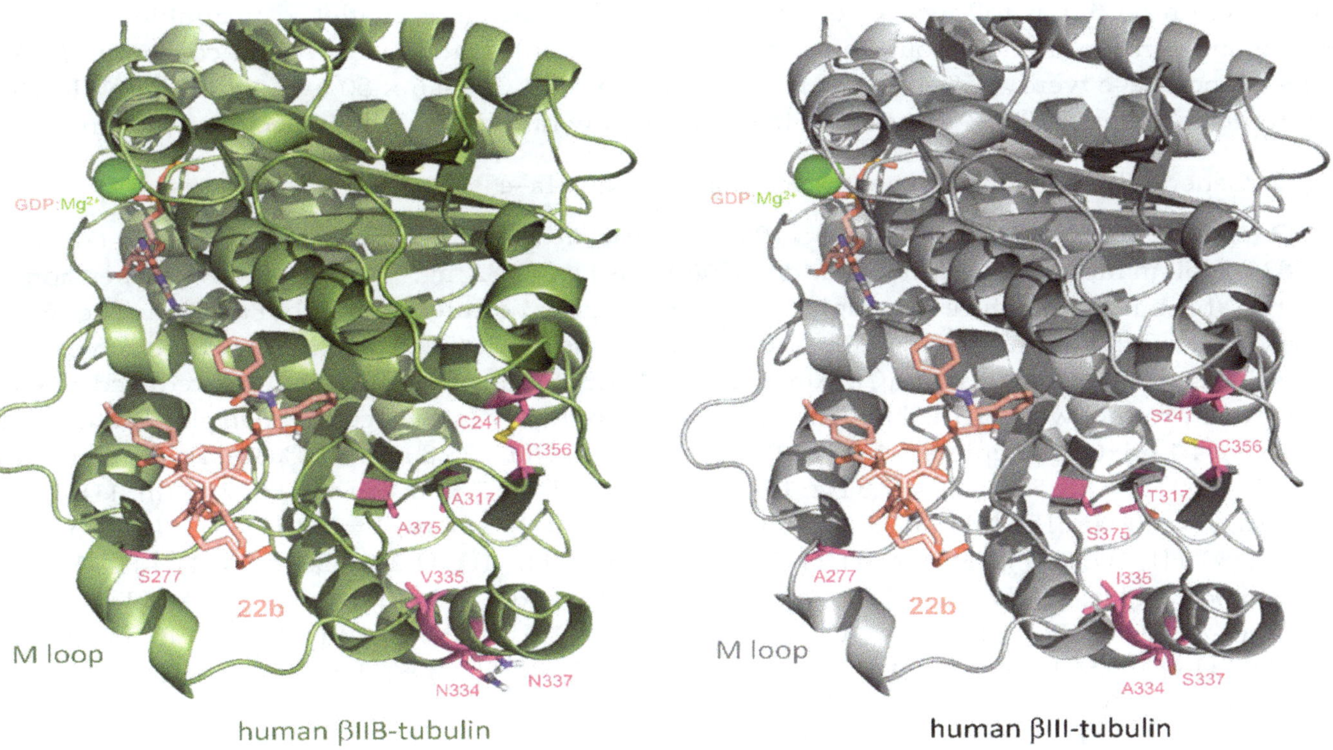

Figure 4. **22b** docked into homology models of human tubulins IIb and III bound to guanosine diphosphate (GDP)-Mg^{2+}. Colored in magenta and labeled are those residues close to the taxane-binding site that differ between these two isotypes.

As shown in this modelling study, the binding of these taxoids to microtubules are similar to that of paclitaxel. Although cyclization does increase the cytotoxicity either in drug-sensitive and -resistant cells in most cases, the 7,9-*O*-linked macrocyclic taxoids only showed comparable cytotoxicity to that of paclitaxel. The enhanced activity is not only arisen from the known C-2 modifications [15,16], but also from the cyclization of the cleaved C-ring of taxane.

3. Experimental

3.1. Chemical Synthesis

3.1.1. General Methods

All chemicals and reagents were purchased from Beijing Innochem Science and Technology Co. Ltd. (Beijing, China), Sinopharm Chemical Reagent Co. Ltd. (Beijing, China), and thin-layer chromatography (TCI). The 200–300 mesh silica gel used for flash column chromatography was purchased from Rushanshi Shuangbang Xincailiao Co. Ltd. (Rushan, Shandong, China). Visualization on TLC (analytical thin layer chromatography) was achieved by the use of UV light (254 nm) and treatment with phosphomolybdic acid or $KMnO_4$ followed by heating. All solvents were purified and dried according to the standard procedures. The purification was performed on flash column chromatography. The high performance liquid chromatography (HPLC)- electrospray ionization (ESI)-mass spectrometry (MS) analysis was carried out in an Agilent 1260 Infinity HPLC system (Agilent Technologies, Waldbronn, Germany) equipped with a reversed phase 4.68 × 50 mm (1.8 um) XDB-C18 Column and consisted of a binary solvent delivery system, an auto sampler, a column temperature controller, and an UV detector. The mass spectra were acquired by a 6120 Quadrupole LC-MS mass spectrometer (Agilent Technologies, Waldbronn, Germany) connected to the HPLC system via an ESI interface. Proton and carbon magnetic resonance spectra (^{1}H-NMR and ^{13}C-NMR) were recorded on a Bruker BioSpin AG 300 or 400 MHz spectrometer or Varian 300, 400, or 600 MHz spectrometer.^{1}H-NMR data were reported as follows: Chemical shifts, multiplicity (s = singlet, d = doublet, t = triplet, q = quartet, m=multiplet), coupling constant(s) in Hz, integration. All tested compounds **16a–e**, **21a–e**, and **22a–e** were ≥95% pure by HPLC (column XDB C18 4.6 × 50 mm 1.8 μm, mobile phase: acetonitrile-water (10:90–100:0 gradient in 4.5 min), flow rate 1.0 mL/min, detected at 220 nm).

3.1.2. General Experimental Procedure for Compounds **14a–e**

2′-O-(tert-Butyldimethylsilyl)-10-dehydro-10-deacetylpaclitaxel (**14a**). To a solution of **13a** (261.3 mg, 0.282 mmol) in methanol (8 mL) was added $Cu(OAc)_2{\cdot}H_2O$ (282 mg, 1.41 mmol). The suspension was stirred at room temperature overnight (open air) and then diluted with ethyl acetate. The organic phase was washed sequentially with saturated aqueous NaCl (50 mL), 2 N NH_3 to remove copper salts and saturated aqueous NH_4Cl. After drying (Na_2SO_4) and evaporation under reduced pressure, the crude product was purified by silica gel chromatography (ethyl acetate: petroleum ether = 1:2) to give a 4:1 mixture of epimers **14a** (14-β-OH and 14-α-OH, 223.8 mg, 85.8% total yield). ^{1}H-NMR ($CDCl_3$, 600 MHz) δ: 8.19 (d, *J* = 7.8 Hz, 1H, Ar-H), 7.73 (d, *J* = 7.8 Hz, 2H, Ar-H), 7.48 (m, 11H, Ar-H), 7.06 (d, *J* = 9.0 Hz, 1H, NH), 6.28 (t, *J* = 8.7 Hz, 1H, H-13), 5.87 (d, *J* = 7.2 Hz, 1H, H-2), 5.79 (dd, *J* = 1.5, 8.7 Hz, 1H, H-3′), 4.93 (m, 1H, H-5), 4.67 (d, *J* = 1.8 Hz, 1H, H-2′), 4.50 (d, *J* = 11.4 Hz, 1H, H-7), 4.44 (d, *J* = 8.4 Hz, 1H, H- 20a), 4.38 (d, *J* = 9.0 Hz, 1H, H-20b), 4.04 (d, *J* = 7.2 Hz, 1H, H-3), 3.88 (m, 1H, OH-7), 2.67 (s, 3H, CH_3), 2.48 (dd, *J* = 9.6, 15.6 Hz, 1H, H-6a), 2.29 (m, 2H, H-14b, H-14a), 2.19 (m, 1H, H-6b), 1.86 (s, 3H, CH_3), 1.75 (s, 3H, CH_3), 1.21 (s, 3H, CH_3), 1.13 (s, 3H, CH_3), 0.79 (s, 9H, $SiC(CH_3)_3$), −0.04 (s, 3H, $Si(CH_3)$), −0.30 (s, 3H, $Si(CH_3)$). (For the chemical characterization refer to http://dx.doi.org/10.1016/j.ejmech.2017.06.001)

2′-O-(tert-Butyldimethylsilyl)-2-debenzoyl-2-(3-methoxybenzoyl)-7-epi-10-dehydro-10-deacetylpaclitaxel (**14b**). 69.5% yield as a 4:1 mixture of two epimers; ^{1}H-NMR ($CDCl_3$, 400 MHz) δ: 7.80 (d, *J* = 7.7 Hz, 1H, Ar-H), 7.74 (d, *J* = 7.2 Hz, 2H, Ar-H), 7.41 (m, 10H, Ar-H), 7.21 (dd, *J* = 2.0, 8.0 Hz, Ar-H), 7.09 (d, *J* = 9.1 Hz, 1H, NH), 6.27 (t, *J* = 8.9 Hz, 1H, H-13), 5.89 (d, *J* = 7.2 Hz, 1H, H-2), 5.79 (dd, *J* = 2.2, 9.4 Hz, 1H, H-3′), 4.94 (m, 1H, H-5), 4.67 (d, *J* = 2.0 Hz, 1H, H-2′), 4.50 (d, *J* = 11.2 Hz, 1H, H-7), 4.47 (d, *J* = 8.8 Hz, 1H, H- 20a), 4.38 (d, *J* = 8.6 Hz, 1H, H-20b), 4.05 (d, *J* = 7.1 Hz, 1H, H-3), 3.90 (s, 3H, OCH_3), 3.88 (m, 1H, OH-7), 2.67 (s, 3H, CH_3), 2.49 (dd, *J* = 9.8, 15.4 Hz, 1H, H-6a), 2.29 (m, 2H, H-14b, H-14a), 1.86 (s, 3H, CH_3), 2.25 (m, 1H, H-6b), 1.75 (s, 3H, CH_3), 1.21(s, 3H, CH_3), 1.13 (s, 3H, CH_3), 0.81 (s, 9H, $SiC(CH_3)_3$), −0.02 (s, 3H, $Si(CH_3)$), −0.26 (s, 3H, $Si(CH_3)$); ^{13}C-NMR ($CDCl_3$, 100 MHz) δ: 207.8, 188.7,

172.2, 170.9, 167.0, 166.9, 159.8, 143.3, 141.1, 138.2, 134.1, 131.9, 130.3, 130.0, 128.8 (2C), 128.1, 127.0, 126.4, 122.7, 120.5, 114.4, 82.7, 81.8, 79.2, 77.4, 75.3, 75.1, 70.7, 57.2, 55.5 (2C), 40.3, 39.4, 36.3, 35.4, 26.9, 26.1, 25.5, 22.9, 18.2, 15.0, 14.4, −5.2, −5.8; LC-MS (ESI, *m/z*): [M + 1], found 954.4, [M + 23], found 976.4, $C_{52}H_{63}NO_{14}Si$: 953.40 (see supplementary materials).

2′-O-(tert-Butyldimethylsilyl)-2-debenzoyl-2-(3-fluorobenzoyl)-7-epi-10-dehydro-10-deacetylpaclitaxel (**14c**). 79.0% yield as a 4:1 mixture of two epimers; ^{1}H-NMR ($CDCl_3$, 400 MHz) δ: 8.02 (d, *J* = 8.0 Hz, 1H, Ar-H), 7.89–7.86 (m, 1H, Ar-H), 7.73 (d, *J* = 7.2 Hz, 2H, Ar-H), 7.59–7.33 (m, 10H, Ar-H), 7.07 (d, *J* = 9.2 Hz, 1H, BzNH), 6.27 (t, *J* = 8.8 Hz, 1H, H-13), 5.86 (d, *J* = 7.2 Hz, 1H, H-2), 5.80 (dd, *J* = 2.0, 9.2 Hz, 1H, H-3′), 4.95 (dd, *J* = 4.0, 8.0 Hz, 1H, H-5), 4.68 (d, *J* = 2.4 Hz, 1H, H-2′), 4.48 (d, *J* = 11.2 Hz, 1H, H-7), 4.44 (d, *J* = 8.8 Hz, 1H, H- 20a), 4.36 (d, *J* = 8.8 Hz, 1H, H-20b), 4.05 (d, *J* = 7.2 Hz, 1H, H-3), 3.92–3.88 (m, 1H, OH-7), 2.68 (s, 3H, $COCH_3$), 2.48 (dd, *J* = 9.6, 15.2 Hz, 1H, H-6a), 2.31–2.29 (m, 2H, H-14b, H-14a), 2.22 (dd, *J* = 8.4, 15.6 Hz, 1H, H-6b), 1.99 (br, 1H, OH), 1.86 (s, 3H, CH_3), 1.76 (s, 3H, CH_3), 1.22 (s, 3H, CH_3), 1.13 (s, 3H, CH_3), 0.81 (s, 9H, $SiC(CH_3)$)), −0.02 (s, 3H, $Si(CH_3)$)), −0.26 (s, 3H, $Si(CH_3)_2$); ^{13}C-NMR ($CDCl_3$, 100 MHz) δ: 207.8, 188.6, 172.3, 171.2, 170.9, 167.0, 165.9 (d, $^{4}J_{C\text{-}F}$ = 2.9 Hz), 162.7 (d, $^{1}J_{C\text{-}F}$ = 246.5 Hz), 143.5, 140.9, 138.2, 134.1, 131.9, 131.3 (d, $^{3}J_{C\text{-}F}$ = 7.3 Hz), 130.7 (d, $^{3}J_{C\text{-}F}$ = 7.6 Hz), 128.83 (2C), 128.77 (2C), 128.1, 127.0 (2C), 126.4 (2C), 126.1 (d, $^{4}J_{C\text{-}F}$ = 3.1 Hz), 120.0 (d, $^{2}J_{C\text{-}F}$ = 21.1 Hz), 117.1 (d, $^{2}J_{C\text{-}F}$ = 23.1 Hz), 82.8, 81.7, 79.4, 75.5, 75.3, 70.6, 57.2, 55.6, 40.3, 39.5, 36.3, 35.4, 26.1, 25.5 (3C), 22.9 (2C), 18.2, 15.0, 14.5, 14.2, −5.2, −5.8; LC-MS (ESI, *m/z*): [M + 1], found 942.4, [M + 23], found 964.3, $C_{51}H_{60}FNO_{13}Si$: 941.38.

2′-O-(tert-Butyldimethylsilyl)-2-debenzoyl-2-(3-chlorobenzoyl)-7-epi-10-dehydro-10-deacetylpaclitaxel (**14d**). 84.9% yield as a 4:1 mixture of two epimers; ^{1}H-NMR ($CDCl_3$, 400 MHz) δ: 8.18 (s, 1H, Ar-H), 8.11 (d, *J* = 7.6 Hz, 1H, Ar-H), 7.73 (d, *J* = 7.6 Hz, 2H, Ar-H), 7.62 (d, *J* = 7.6 Hz, 1H, Ar-H), 7.55–7.50 (m, 2H, Ar-H), 7.44–7.35 (m, 7H, Ar-H), 7.08 (d, *J* = 8.8 Hz, 1H, BzNH), 6.25 (t, *J* = 8.8 Hz, 1H, H-13), 5.84 (d, *J* = 7.2 Hz, 1H, H-2), 5.79 (dd, *J* = 8.8 Hz, 1H, H-3′), 4.96 (m, 1H, H-5), 4.67 (d, *J* = 2.0 Hz, 1H, H-2′), 4.47 (d, *J* = 11.2 Hz, 1H, H-7), 4.44 (d, *J* = 8.4 Hz, 1H, H- 20a), 4.35 (d, *J* = 8.4 Hz, 1H, H-20b), 4.05 (d, *J* = 7.2 Hz, 1H, H-3), 3.89 (m, 1H, OH-7), 2.68 (s, 3H, CH_3), 2.48 (dd, *J* = 10.0, 15.4 Hz, 1H, H-6a), 2.29 (m, 2H, H-14b, H-14a), 2.23 (m, 1H, H-6b), 1.86 (s, 3H, CH_3), 1.76 (s, 3H, CH_3), 1.22 (s, 3H, CH_3), 1.13 (s, 3H, CH_3), 0.82 (s, 9H, $SiC(CH_3)_3$), −0.02 (s, 3H, $Si(CH_3)$)), −0.26 (s, 3H, $Si(CH_3)$)); ^{13}C-NMR ($CDCl_3$, 100 MHz) δ: 207.8, 188.6, 172.2, 170.9, 165.7, 143.5, 140.9, 138.2, 134.9, 134.1, 133.9, 131.9, 130.9, 130.4, 130.3, 128.83 (2C), 128.77 (2C), 128.5, 128.1, 127.0 (2C), 126.5 (2C), 82.7, 81.7, 79.4, 75.4, 75.3, 70.7, 60.4, 57.2, 55.6, 40.2, 39.4, 36.3, 35.3, 29.7, 26.1, 25.5 (2C), 22.9, 22.8, 18.2, 14.9, 14.5, −5.2, −5.8; LC-MS (ESI, *m/z*): [M + 1], found 958.4, [M + 23], found 980.4, $C_{51}H_{60}ClNO_{13}Si$: 957.35.

2′-O-(tert-Butyldimethylsilyl)-2-debenzoyl-2-(3-trifluoromethyl)-7-epi-10-dehydro-10-deacetylpaclitaxel (**14e**). 81.9% yield as a 4:1 mixture of two epimers; ^{1}H-NMR ($CDCl_3$, 400 MHz) δ: 8.50 (s, 1H, Ar-H), 8.43 (d, *J* = 7.6 Hz, 1H, Ar-H), 7.91 (d, *J* = 8.0 Hz, 1H, Ar-H), 7.72 (d, *J* = 7.8 Hz, 3H, Ar-H), 7.51 (m, 1H, Ar-H), 7.41 (m, 7H, Ar-H), 7.06 (d, *J* = 9.2 Hz, 1H, BzNH), 6.24 (t, *J* = 8.6 Hz, 1H, H-13), 5.88 (d, *J* = 7.6 Hz, 1H, H-2), 5.78 (dd, *J* = 1.6, 9.2 Hz, 1H, H-3′), 4.97 (m, 1H, H-5), 4.67 (d, *J* = 2.0 Hz, 1H, H-2′), 4.45 (d, *J* = 11.2 Hz, 1H, H-7), 4.42 (d, *J* = 8.5 Hz, 1H, H-20a), 4.37 (d, *J* = 8.6 Hz, 1H, H-20b), 4.09 (d, *J* = 7.6 Hz, 1H, H-3), 3.90 (m, 1H, OH-7), 2.66 (s, 3H, CH_3), 2.51 (dd, *J* = 9.6, 15.5 Hz, 1H, H-6a), 2.30 (m, 2H, H-14b, H-14a), 2.26 (m, 1H, H-6b), 1.87 (s, 3H, CH_3), 1.77 (s, 3H, CH_3), 1.23 (s, 3H, CH_3), 1.15 (s, 3H, CH_3), 0.83 (s, 9H, $SiC(CH_3)_3$), −0.02 (s, 3H, $Si(CH_3)$)), −0.24 (s, 3H, $Si(CH_3)$)); ^{13}C-NMR ($CDCl_3$, 100 MHz) δ: 207.7, 188.6, 172.1, 171.0, 167.1, 165.6, 143.6, 140.9, 138.3, 134.2, 133.6, 131.9, 131.4 (q, $^{2}J_{C\text{-}F}$ = 33.2 Hz), 130.3 (q, ^{3}J = 3.4 Hz), 130.3, 130.1, 129.9, 128.9, 128.8, 128.1, 127.1 (q, $^{3}J_{C\text{-}F}$ = 4.0 Hz), 127.0, 126.5, 123.7 (q, $^{1}J_{C\text{-}F}$ = 273.6 Hz), 82.8, 81.7, 79.5, 75.6, 75.3, 70.7, 57.2, 55.6, 40.3, 39.5, 36.3, 35.4, 26.1, 25.6, 22.9, 22.7, 18.2, 14.9, 14.5, −5.2, −5.8; LC-MS (ESI, *m/z*): [M + 1], found 992.0, $C_{52}H_{60}F_3NO_{13}Si$: 991.38.

3.1.3. General Experimental Procedure for Compounds **15a–e**

2′-tert-Butyldimethylsilyl-10-dehydro-7-8-seco-10-deacetylpaclitaxel (**15a**). L-selectride (1M solution in THF, 0.8 mL) was added, dropwise, to a solution of **14a** (171.5 mg, 0.186 mmol) in THF (4.1 mL) at −20 °C. After 15 min, the reaction was quenched by addition of cold ethyl acetate (50.0 mL) and 2 N H_2SO_4 (4.0 mL). The reaction mixture was extracted with ethyl acetate and the combined organic phases were washed with a saturated aqueous $NaHCO_3$ and saturated aqueous NH_4Cl. The resulting solution was dried over anhydrous $MgSO_4$ and the solvent evaporated under reduced pressure to give a crude product. The crude product was purified by silica gel chromatography (ethyl acetate: petroleum ether = 1:1) which gave product **15a** (139.5 mg, 81.2% yield) as a white solid

2′-tert-Butyldimethylsilyl-2-debenzoyl-2-(3-methoxybenzoyl)-10-dehydro-7,8-seco-10-deacetylpaclitaxel (**15b**). White solid; yield 88.7%; ^{1}H-NMR ($CDCl_3$, 400 MHz) δ: 7.73–7.70 (m, 3H, Ar-H), 7.55 (s, 1H, Ar-H), 7.42 (m, 10H, Ar-H), 7.14 (dd, J = 2.3, 8.2 Hz, 1H, BzNH), 6.47 (s, 1H, OH-9), 6.29 (t, J = 8.0 Hz, 1H, H-13), 5.91 (d, J = 8.8 Hz, 1H, H-3′), 5.60 (d, J = 9.2 Hz, 1H, H-2), 5.24 (brs, 2H, H-5, H-20a), 4.72 (d, J = 1.6 Hz, 1H, H-2′), 4.29 (d, J = 6.8 Hz, 1H, H-3), 4.20 (brs, 1H, H-7a), 3.96 (brs, 1H, OH), 3.85 (s, 4H, OCH_3, H-7b), 2.82 (brs, 1H, H-6a), 2.71 (brs, 1H, OH), 2.26 (dd, J = 9.6, 15.6 Hz, 2H, H-14a, H-14b), 2.09–2.02 (m, 4H, CH_3, H-6b), 1.87 (brs, 6H, 2 × CH_3), 1.28 (s, 3H, CH_3), 1.10 (s, 3H, CH_3), 0.79 (s, 9H, $SiC(CH_3)_3$), −0.11 (s, 3H, $Si(CH_3)$), −0.28 (s, 3H, $Si(CH_3)$); ^{13}C-NMR ($CDCl_3$, 100 MHz) δ: 191.2, 171.2, 171.1, 168.9, 167.4, 167.2, 159.8, 148.9, 142.1, 138.2, 133.9, 131.9, 130.5, 130.3, 128.7 (4C), 128.0, 127.1 (2C), 126.7 (2C), 124.6, 122.2, 119.5, 115.0, 86.3, 76.1, 75.1, 70.6, 59.2, 55.8, 55.5, 43.1, 36.6, 25.5 (3C), 23.4, 22.2, 21.5, 18.3, 14.8, 14.4, −5.6, −6.0; LC-MS (ESI, *m/z*): [M + 1], found 956.4, [M + 23], found 978.4, $C_{52}H_{65}NO_{14}Si$: 955.42.

2′-tert-Butyldimethylsilyl-2-debenzoyl-2-(3-fluorobenzoyl)-10-dehydro-7,8-seco-10-deacetylpaclitaxel (**15c**). White solid; yield 79.2%; ^{1}H-NMR ($CDCl_3$, 400 MHz) δ: 7.94 (d, J = 7.8 Hz, 1H, Ar-H), 7.76 (d, J = 8.7 Hz, 1H, Ar-H), 7.68 (d, J = 7.4 Hz, 2H, Ar-H), 7.53–7.44 (m, 3H, Ar-H), 7.40–7.30 (m, 8H, NH, Ar-H), 6.48 (s, 1H, OH-9), 6.30 (t, J = 8.0 Hz, 1H, H-13), 5.92 (d, J = 9.0 Hz, 1H, H-3′), 5.60 (d, J = 9.5 Hz, 1H, H-2), 5.25 (brs, 2H, H-5, H-20a), 4.71 (d, J = 2.1 Hz, 1H, H-2′), 4.30 (d, J = 7.8 Hz, 1H, H-3), 4.19 (brs, 1H, H-20b), 3.96 (brs, 1H, H-7a), 3.80 (brs, 1H, H-7b), 2.78 (brs, 1H, H-6a), 2.69 (brs, 1H, H-14a), 2.26 (dd, J = 9.5, 15.6 Hz, 1H, H-14b), 2.10–2.00 (ovelap, 1H, H-6b), 1.90 (s, 3H, CH_3), 1.86 (overlap and brs, 6H, 2 × CH_3), 1.27 (s, 3H, CH_3), 1.10 (s, 3H, CH_3), 0.78 (s, 9H, $SiC(CH_3)_3$), −0.09 (s, 3H, $Si(CH_3)$), −0.29 (s, 3H, $Si(CH_3)$); ^{13}C-NMR ($CDCl_3$, 100 MHz) δ: 191.1, 171.2, 171.0, 168.8, 167.4, 166.4, 131.0 (d, $^1J_{C\text{-}F}$ = 248.1 Hz), 128.8 (2C), 128.1, 127.1, 126.7, 125.8 (d, $^4J_{C\text{-}F}$ = 2.6 Hz), 124.6, 121.1 (d, $^2J_{C\text{-}F}$ = 21.3 Hz), 116.7 (d, $^2J_{C\text{-}F}$ = 22.6 Hz), 86.5, 80.7, 76.1, 75.5, 70.5, 59.0, 55.8, 44.5, 43.2, 36.7, 25.6, 22.3, 21.6, 18.3, 14.9, 14.5, −5.4, −5.9; LC-MS (ESI, *m/z*): [M + 1], found 944.4, [M + 23], found 966.4, $C_{51}H_{62}FNO_{13}Si$: 943.40.

2′-tert-Butyldimethylsilyl-2-debenzoyl-2-(3-chlorobenzoyl)-10-dehydro-7,8-seco-10-deacetylpaclitaxel (**15d**). White solid; yield 58.8%; ^{1}H-NMR ($CDCl_3$, 400 MHz) δ: 8.05 (d, J = 7.6 Hz, 2H, Ar-H), 8.01 (s, 1H, Ar-H), 7.68 (d, J = 7.6 Hz, 2H, Ar-H), 7.57 (d, J = 8.0 Hz, 1H, Ar-H), 7.41–7.31 (m, 9H, NH, Ar-H), 6.49 (s, 1H, OH-9), 6.29 (t, J = 8.4 Hz, 1H, H-13), 5.92 (d, J = 9.3 Hz, 1H, H-3′), 5.59 (d, J = 9.5 Hz, 1H, H-2), 5.23 (brs, 2H, H-5, H-20a), 4.71 (d, J = 1.6 Hz, 1H, H-2′), 4.30 (d, J = 6.9 Hz, 1H, H-3), 4.18 (brs, 1H, H- 20b), 3.98 (brs, 1H, H-7a), 3.83 (brs, 1H, H-7b), 2.78 (brs, 1H, H-6a), 2.67 (brs, 1H, H-14a), 2.25 (dd, J = 9.6, 15.6 Hz, 1H, H-14b), 2.05 (m, 1H, H-6b), 1.89 (s, 3H, CH_3), 1.85 (brs, 6H, 2 × CH_3), 1.26 (s, 3H, CH_3), 1.10 (s, 3H, CH_3), 0.78 (s, 9H, $SiC(CH_3)_3$), −0.11 (s, 3H, $Si(CH_3)$), −0.28 (s, 3H, $Si(CH_3)$); ^{13}C-NMR ($CDCl_3$, 100 MHz) δ: 191.1, 171.0, 168.7, 167.4, 166.3, 148.9, 142.0, 138.0, 137.1, 135.0, 133.9, 131.9, 131.0, 130.6, 129.6, 128.7 (2C), 128.1, 128.0, 127.0 (2C), 126.7 (2C), 124.5, 86.4, 87.0, 80.5, 76.0, 75.4, 70.5, 55.7, 43.1, 36.6, 29.7, 26.9, 25.5 (3C), 22.2, 21.5, 18.3, 14.8, 14.5, −5.5, −6.0; LC-MS (ESI, *m/z*): [M + 1], found 960.0, [M + 23], found 981.9, $C_{51}H_{62}ClNO_{13}Si$: 959.37.

2′-tert-Butyldimethylsilyl-2-debenzoyl-2-(3-trifluoromethylbenzoyl)-10-dehydro-7,8-seco-10-deacetylpaclitaxel (**15e**). White solid; yield 76.5%; ^{1}H-NMR ($CDCl_3$, 400 MHz) δ: 8.38 (d, J = 7.9 Hz, 2H, Ar-H), 7.84 (d, J = 7.9 Hz, 2H, Ar-H), 7.48 (m, 11H, NH, Ar-H), 6.51 (s, 1H, OH-9), 6.29 (t, J = 8.4 Hz, 1H, H-13), 5.89 (d,

J = 9.3 Hz, 1H, H-3′), 5.62 (d, J = 9.4 Hz, 1H, H-2), 5.25 (brs, 2H, H-5, H-20a), 4.72 (brs, 1H, H-2′), 4.32 (d, J = 6.8 Hz, 1H, H-3), 4.24 (brs, 1H, H- 20b), 3.94 (brs, 1H, H-7a), 3.76 (brs, 1H, H-7b), 2.78 (brs, 1H, H-6a), 2.66 (brs, 1H, H-14a), 2.28 (dd, J = 9.5, 15.6 Hz, 1H, H-14b), 2.05 (m, 1H, H-6b), 1.92 (s, 3H, CH_3), 1.85 (brs, 6H, 2 × CH_3), 1.27 (s, 3H, CH_3), 1.11 (s, 3H, CH_3), 0.78 (s, 9H, $SiC(CH_3)_3$), −0.08 (s, 3H, $Si(CH_3)$), −0.29 (s, 3H, $Si(CH_3)$); ^{13}C-NMR ($CDCl_3$, 100 MHz) δ: 191.0, 170.9, 167.5, 166.2, 148.9, 142.1, 137.9, 133.9, 133.1, 131.9, 131.4 (q, $^2J_{C\text{-}F}$ = 33.3 Hz), 130.2, 128.7, 128.0, 126.9, 126.7 (q, $^3J_{C\text{-}F}$ = 4.1 Hz), 126.5, 123.5 (q, $^1J_{C\text{-}F}$ = 273.7 Hz), 87.2, 86.3, 80.6, 75.8, 75.6, 74.5, 70.4, 67.6, 59.0, 55.7, 44.4, 43.2, 38.3, 36.6, 29.7, 29.1, 25.5, 22.1, 21.5, 18.2, 14.8, 14.4, −5.5, −6.0; LC-MS (ESI, *m/z*): [M + 1], found 994.3, [M + 23], found 1016.3, $C_{52}H_{62}F_3NO_{13}Si$: 993.39.

3.1.4. General Experimental Procedure for Compounds **16a–e**

10-Dehydro-7,8-seco-10-deacetylpaclitaxel (**16a**). To a solution of of **15a** (19.8 mg, 0.0214 mmol) in THF (1.4 mL) was added, dropwise, 0.3 mL of HF-pyridine (*v/v* = 1:2) at 0 °C, and the reaction mixture was stirred at room temperature for 30 h. The reaction was quenched with saturated aqueous $NaHCO_3$, diluted with ethyl acetate, washed with saturated NH_4Cl. The organic layer dried over anhydrous Na_2SO_4 and then concentrated under reduced pressure. Purification of the crude product by silica gel chromatography (ethyl acetate: petroleum ether = 2:1) gave product **16a** as a white solid (13.4 mg, 77.4% yield). ^{1}H-NMR ($CDCl_3$, 400 MHz) δ: 8.04 (d, J = 7.6 Hz, 2H, Ar-H), 7.69 (d, J = 7.2 Hz, 2H, Ar-H), 7.57 (t, J = 7.4 Hz, 1H, Ar-H), 7.48–7.44 (m, 5H, Ar-H), 7.38–7.27 (m, 6H, NH, Ar-H), 6.47 (s, 1H, OH-9), 6.16 (t, J = 7.5 Hz, 1H, H-13), 5.86 (dd, J = 2.8, 9.4 Hz, 1H, H-3′), 5.60 (d, J = 9.5 Hz, 1H, H-2), 5.20 (brs, 1H, H-5), 5.16 (d, J = 11.4 Hz, 1H, H-20a), 4.78 (d, J = 3.0 Hz, 1H, H-2′), 4.27 (d, J = 8.1 Hz, 1H, H-3), 4.20 (brs, 1H, H-20b), 3.89 (brs, 1H, H-7a), 3.68 (dt, J = 6.2, 10.1 Hz, 1H, H-7b), 2.77 (brs, 1H, H-6a), 2.61 (brs, 1H, H-14a), 2.38 (dd, J = 9.7, 15.9 Hz, 1H, H-14b), 2.29 (brs, 1H, OH), 2.10–2.07 (m, 1H, H-6b), 1.83 (brs, 6H, 2 × CH_3), 1.75 (s, 3H, CH_3), 1.20 (s, 3H, CH_3), 1.07 (s, 3H, CH_3); ^{13}C-NMR ($CDCl_3$, 100 MHz) δ: 191.0, 172.4, 169.0, 167.3, 167.2, 148.8, 142.2, 138.0, 136.7, 133.8, 133.6, 132.0, 129.7, 129.3, 129.0, 128.8, 128.7, 128.1, 127.1, 127.0, 124.6, 86.9, 86.2, 80.5, 74.8, 73.7, 70.7, 59.6, 54.8, 43.0, 36.6, 29.7, 24.9, 22.1, 21.2, 18.4, 14.6, 14.5; LC-MS (ESI, *m/z*): [M + 1], found 812.0, [M + 23], found 834.0, $C_{45}H_{49}NO_{13}$: 811.32.

2-Debenzoyl-2-(3-methoxybenzoyl)-10-dehydro-7,8-seco-10-deacetylpaclitaxel (**16b**). White solid; yield 65.2%; ^{1}H-NMR ($CDCl_3$, 400 MHz) δ: 7.72 (d, J = 7.6 Hz, 2H, Ar-H), 7.60 (d, J = 7.1 Hz, 1H, Ar-H), 7.47–7.43 (m, 5H, Ar-H), 7.36–7.31 (m, 5H, Ar-H), 7.29–7.25 (m, 1H, Ar-H), 7.10 (d, J = 8.1 Hz, 1H, NH), 6.49 (brs, 1H, OH-9), 6.09 (t, J = 7.4 Hz, 1H, H-13), 5.81 (d, J = 9.2 Hz, 1H, H-3′), 5.58 (d, J = 9.5 Hz, 1H, H-2), 5.20 (brs, 1H, H-5), 5.14 (d, J = 11.3 Hz, 1H, H-20a), 4.73 (brs, 1H, H-2′), 4.24 (d, J = 7.2 Hz, 1H, H-3), 4.19 (brs, 1H, H-20b), 3.87 (brs, 1H, H-7a), 3.79 (s, 3H, OCH_3), 3.65 (brs, 1H, H-7b), 2.74 (brs, 1H, H-6a), 2.56 (brs, 1H, H-14a), 2.40 (dd, J = 9.9, 15.9 Hz, 1H, H-14b), 2.35 (brs, 1H, OH-1), 2.09 (m, 1H, H-6b), 1.83 (brs, 6H, 2 × CH_3), 1.69 (s, 3H, CH_3), 1.17 (s, 3H, CH_3), 1.06 (s, 3H, CH_3); ^{13}C-NMR ($CDCl_3$, 100 MHz) δ: 191.1, 172.4, 169.0, 167.1, 159.8, 148.8, 142.1, 138.1, 136.7, 133.6, 131.9, 130.7, 130.1, 129.0, 128.7, 128.6, 128.2, 128.1, 127.1, 124.5, 121.8, 119.5, 114.8, 86.9, 86.1, 80.4, 74.8, 73.7, 70.5, 59.7, 55.5, 55.0, 44.5, 42.9, 36.6, 29.8, 29.7, 24.9, 22.2, 21.1, 14.6, 14.5; LC-MS (ESI, *m/z*): [M + 1], found 842.4, [M + 23], found 864.3, $C_{46}H_{51}NO_{14}$: 841.33.

2-Debenzoyl-2-(3-fluorobenzoyl)-10-dehydro-7, 8-seco-10-deacetylpaclitaxel (**16c**). White solid; yield 59.3%, ^{1}H-NMR ($CDCl_3$, 300 MHz) δ: 7.90 (d, J = 7.7 Hz, 1H, Ar-H), 7.75–7.68 (m, 3H, Ar-H), 7.48–7.44 (m, 4H, Ar-H), 7.41–7.31 (m, 6H, Ar-H), 7.24 (d, J = 8.0 Hz, 1H, NH), 6.46 (brs, 1H, OH-9), 6.20 (t, J = 7.9Hz, 1H, H-13), 5.88 (d, J = 7.6 Hz, 1H, H-3′), 5.59 (d, J =9.5 Hz, 1H, H-2), 5.19 (overlap, J = 11.5 Hz, 2H, H-20a, H-5), 4.81 (brs, 1H, H-2′), 4.46 (brs, 1H, OH), 4.29 (d, J = 7.9Hz, 1H, H-3), 4.22 (brs, 1H, H-20b), 3.92 (brs, 1H, H-7a), 3.70 (brs, 1H, H-7b), 3.39 (brs, 1H, OH), 2.77 (brs, 1H, H-6a), 2.60 (brs, 1H, H-14a), 2.37 (dd, J = 9.7, 15.8 Hz, 1H, H-14b), 2.09 (m, 1H, H-6b), 1.85 (brs, 6H, 2 × CH_3), 1.78 (s, 3H, CH_3), 1.64 (brs, 1H, OH-1), 1.22 (s, 3H, CH_3), 1.09 (s, 3H, CH_3); ^{13}C-NMR ($CDCl_3$, 75 MHz) δ: 190.9, 172.4, 167.2, 166.2, 162.7 (d, $^1J_{C\text{-}F}$ = 248.7 Hz), 148.9, 142.1, 137.9, 133.6, 132.0, 131.4 (d, $^2J_{C\text{-}F}$ = 7.4 Hz), 130.8 (d, $^3J_{C\text{-}F}$ = 7.9 Hz), 128.9, 128.7, 128.2, 127.0, 126.9, 125.5, 124.4, 121.0 (d, $^2J_{C\text{-}F}$ = 21.2 Hz), 116.5 (d,

$^{2}J_{C-F}$ = 23.5 Hz), 86.8, 86.2, 80.5, 75.2, 74.7, 73.6, 70.7, 59.5, 54.6, 42.9, 36.5, 29.7, 29.3, 24.9, 22.1, 21.2, 14.7, 14.5; LC-MS (ESI, *m/z*): [M + 1], found 830.3, [M + 23], found 852.3, $C_{45}H_{48}FNO_{13}$: 829.31.

2-Debenzoyl-2-(3-chlorobenzoyl)-10-dehydro-7, 8-seco-10-deacetylpaclitaxel (**16d**). White solid; yield 60.3%; ^{1}H-NMR ($CDCl_3$, 400 MHz) δ: 7.98 (d, *J* = 7.5 Hz, 2H, Ar-H), 7.72 (d, *J* = 7.0 Hz, 2H, Ar-H), 7.56 (d, *J* = 8.4 Hz, 1H, Ar-H), 7.47–7.42 (m, 4H, Ar-H), 7.40–7.29 (m, 6H, NH, Ar-H), 6.49 (brs, 1H, OH-9), 6.15 (t, *J* = 7.8 Hz, 1H, H-13), 5.86 (d, *J* = 8.1 Hz, 1H, H-3′), 5.58 (d, *J* = 9.5 Hz, 1H, H-2), 5.21 (brs, 1H, H-5), 5.14 (d, *J* =11.0 Hz, 1H, H-20a), 4.79 (d, *J* = 2.8 Hz, 1H, H-2′), 4.27 (d, *J* =7.8 Hz, 1H, H-3), 4.20 (brs, 1H, H-20b), 3.89 (brs, 1H, H-7a), 3.71–3.67 (m, 1H, H-7b), 2.75 (brs, 1H, H-6a), 2.59 (brs, 1H, H-14a), 2.38 (dd, *J* = 9.7, 15.8 Hz, 1H, H-14b), 2.25 (brs, 1H, OH), 2.09 (m, 1H, H-6b), 2.00 (m, 1H, OH), 1.84 (brs, 6H, 2 × CH_3), 1.74 (s, 3H, CH_3), 1.20 (s, 3H, CH_3), 1.07 (s, 3H, CH_3); ^{13}C-NMR ($CDCl_3$, 100 MHz) δ: 191.0, 172.5, 167.2, 166.0, 148.9, 142.1, 138.1, 135.0, 133.8, 133.7, 132.0, 131.1, 130.4, 129.5, 128.8, 128.7, 128.1, 127.9, 127.0, 124.3, 86.9, 86.2, 80.4, 75.3, 74.7, 73.6, 70.6, 59.6, 54.8, 50.8, 42.9, 36.6, 29.7, 29.5, 29.3, 24.9, 22.2, 21.2, 14.6, 14.5; LC-MS (ESI, *m/z*): [M + 1], found 845.9, [M + 23], found 867.8, $C_{45}H_{48}ClNO_{13}$: 845.28.

2-Debenzoyl-2-(3-trifluoromethylbenzoyl)-10-dehydro-7,8-seco-10-deacetylpaclitaxel (**16e**). White solid; yield 55.5%; ^{1}H-NMR ($CDCl_3$, 400 MHz) δ: 8.33 (d, *J* = 7.7 Hz, 1H, Ar-H), 8.25 (brs, 1H, NH), 7.85 (d, *J* = 7.4 Hz, 1H, Ar-H), 7.68–7.62 (m, 3H, Ar-H), 7.48–7.45 (m, 3H, Ar-H), 7.40–7.29 (m, 6H, Ar-H), 6.47 (brs, 1H, OH-9), 6.18 (t, *J* = 7.9 Hz, 1H, H-13), 5.87 (d, *J* = 7.6 Hz, 1H, H-3′), 5.62 (d, *J* = 9.4 Hz, 1H, H-2), 5.18 (overlap, *J* = 11.5 Hz, 2H, H-20a, H-5), 4.80 (d, *J* = 2.8 Hz, 1H, H-2′), 4.62 (brs, 1H, OH), 4.28 (d, *J* = 7.6 Hz, 1H, H-3), 4.24 (brs, 1H, H-20b), 3.90 (brs, 1H, H-7a), 3.68 (brs, 1H, H-7b), 3.38 (brs, 1H, OH), 2.77 (brs, 1H, H-6a), 2.58 (brs, 1H, H-14a), 2.37 (dd, *J* = 9.7, 15.7 Hz, 1H, H-14b), 2.05 (brs, 1H, OH), 2.03–1.98 (m, 1H, H-6b), 1.84 (brs, 6H, 2 × CH_3), 1.78 (s, 3H, CH_3), 1.22 (s, 3H, CH_3), 1.09 (s, 3H, CH_3); ^{13}C-NMR ($CDCl_3$, 100 MHz) δ: 190.9, 172.4, 167.2, 166.0, 148.9, 142.1, 138.0, 133.7, 133.0, 132.0, 131.7, 130.3, 130.0, 129.7, 128.9, 128.7, 128.2, 127.0 (2C), 126.4, 124.8, 124.2, 122.1, 86.9, 86.2, 80.5, 75.4, 74.7, 73.5, 70.7, 59.6, 54.7, 43.0, 36.6, 31.9, 29.7, 25.5, 22.1, 21.2, 14.6, 14.4; LC-MS (ESI, *m/z*): [M + 1], found 880.0, [M + 23], found 901.9, $C_{46}H_{48}F_3NO_{13}$: 879.31.

3.1.5. General Experimental Procedure for Compounds **17a–e**

2′-O-(tert-Butyldimethylsilyl)-9-O-(2-hydroxyethyl)-10-dehydro-7, 8-seco-10-deacetylpaclitaxel (**17a**). To a mixture of **15a** (50 mg, 0.0540 mmol), potassium carbonate (104 mg, 0.754 mmol), and potassium iodide (18 mg, 0.108 mmol) in DMF (0.9 mL) was added 2-bromoethanol (54 μL 0.762 mmol), dropwise, at 0 °C. The reaction mixture was stirred for 9 h at room temperature and then was diluted with ethyl acetate. The organic phase was washed with saturated aqueous NH_4Cl. The organic layer was dried over anhydrous Na_2SO_4 and then concentrated under reduced pressure. Purification of the crude product by silica gel chromatography (ethyl acetate: petroleum ether = 1:1) gave product **17a** as a white solid (19 mg, 52.4% yield). ^{1}H-NMR ($CDCl_3$, 300 MHz) δ: 8.09 (d, *J* = 7.2 Hz, 2H, Ar-H), 7.62 (d, *J* = 7.2 Hz, 2H, Ar-H), 7.57 (d, *J* = 7.5 Hz, 1H, Ar-H), 7.49 (t, *J* = 7.5 Hz, 2H, Ar-H), 7.36 (m, 8H, Ar-H), 6.30 (t, *J* = 8.4 Hz, 1H, H-13), 5.88 (d, *J* = 9.0 Hz, 1H, H-3′), 5.57 (d, *J* = 9.6 Hz, 1H, H-2), 5.28 (overlap, 2H, H-5, H-20a), 4.69 (d, *J* = 1.8 Hz, 1H, H-2′), 4.26 (d, *J* = 7.8 Hz, 1H, H-3), 4.20 (m, 2H, H-20b, $OCH_2\underline{CH_2}OCO$), 3.94 (m, 1H, $OCH_2\underline{CH_2}OCO$), 3.87 (m, *J* = 1.8, 6.3, 8.7, 12.0 Hz, 1H, H-7a), 3.74 (overlap, 2H, H-7b, $\underline{OCH_2}CH_2OCO$), 3.62 (m, 1H, $\underline{OCH_2}CH_2OCO$), 2.71 (m, 2H, H-6a, H-14a), 2.25 (dd, *J* = 9.3, 15.9 Hz, 2H, H-6b, H-14b), 1.97 (s, 3H, CH_3), 1.92 (s, 3H, CH_3), 1.82 (s, 3H, CH_3), 1.27 (s, 3H, CH_3), 1.16 (s, 3H, CH_3), 0.76 (s, 9H, $SiC(CH_3)_3$), −0.08 (s, 3H, $Si(CH_3)$), −0.33 (s, 3H, $Si(CH_3)$); ^{13}C-NMR ($CDCl_3$, 100 MHz) δ: 192.3, 170.7, 168.7, 167.3, 153.8, 144.0, 139.4, 138.0, 133.7 (2C), 131.8, 129.9 (2C), 128.9 (2C), 128.6 (4C), 127.9, 126.9 (2C), 126.4 (2C), 87.1, 87.7, 85.7, 79.9, 75.6, 75.4, 74.6, 73.8, 70.5, 61.8, 58.7, 55.6, 42.9, 36.6, 25.4 (3C), 22.9, 22.0, 18.1, 15.3, 14.6, −5.5, −6.1; LC-MS (ESI, *m/z*): [M + 1], found 970.5, [M + 23], found 992.4, $C_{53}H_{67}NO_{14}Si$: 969.43.

2′-O-(tert-Butyldimethylsilyl)-2-debenzoyl-2-(3-methoxybenzoyl)-9-O-(2-hydroxyethyl)-10-dehydro-7,8-seco-10-deacetylpaclitaxel (**17b**). White solid; yield 56.1%; ^{1}H-NMR ($CDCl_3$, 400 MHz) δ: 7.72–7.66 (m, 3H, Ar-H), 7.54 (s, 1H, Ar-H), 7.47–7.43 (m, 2H, Ar-H), 7.42–7.29 (m, 8H, Ar-H), 7.12 (dd, *J* = 2.0, 8.4 Hz, 1H, BzNH), 6.29 (t, *J* = 8.5 Hz, 1H, H-13), 5.88 (d, *J* = 9.3 Hz, 1H, H-3′), 5.59 (d, *J* = 9.6 Hz, 1H, H-2), 5.26 (overlap, 2H, H-5, H-20a), 4.72 (s, 1H, H-2′), 4.26 (d, *J* = 6.4 Hz, 1H, H-3), 4.19–4.15 (m, 1H, H-20b), 3.94–3.64 (m, 9H, OCH_3, OCH_2CH_2OH, H-7a, H-7b), 2.61 (br, 2H, H-6b, H-14b), 2.25 (dd, *J* = 9.6, 15.6 Hz, 2H, H-6a, H-14a), 2.03 (s, 3H, OAc), 1.93 (s, 6H, 2 × CH_3), 1.26 (s, 3H, CH_3), 1.16 (s, 3H, CH_3), 0.77 (s, 9H, $SiC(CH_3)_3$), −0.10 (s, 3H, $Si(CH_3)$), −0.30 (s, 3H, $Si(CH_3)$); ^{13}C-NMR ($CDCl_3$, 100 MHz) δ: 192.4, 171.2, 170.9, 168.8, 167.3, 167.0, 162.6, 159.7, 144.1, 138.1, 133.8, 131.8, 130.4, 130.2, 128.6 (2C), 127.9, 127.0 (2C), 126.6 (2C), 122.2, 119.5, 114.9, 85.7, 79.8, 75.8, 74.8, 61.8, 58.9, 55.7, 55.5, 42.9, 36.6, 36.5, 31.9, 31.4, 29.7, 25.5 (3C), 22.9, 22.1, 18.2, 15.2, 14.6, −5.5, −6.1; LC-MS (ESI, *m/z*): [M + 1], found 1000.5, [M + 23], found 1022.5, $C_{54}H_{69}NO_{16}Si$: 999.44.

2′-O-(tert-Butyldimethylsilyl)-2-debenzoyl-2-(3-fluorobenzoyl)-9-O-(2-hydroxyethyl)-10-dehydro-7,8-seco-10-deacetylpaclitaxel (**17c**). White solid; yield 53.2%; ^{1}H-NMR ($CDCl_3$, 400 MHz) δ: 7.93 (d, *J* = 7.8 Hz, 1H, Ar-H), 7.76 (d, *J* = 8.8 Hz, 1H, Ar-H), 7.63 (d, *J* = 7.6 Hz, 2H, Ar-H), 7.52–7.28 (m, 11H, NH, Ar-H), 6.29 (t, *J* = 8.1 Hz, 1H, H-13), 5.89 (d, *J* = 9.2 Hz, 1H, H-3′), 5.58 (d, *J* = 9.6 Hz, 1H, H-2), 5.35–5.15 (overlap, 2H, H-5, H-20a), 4.70 (d, *J* = 1.9 Hz, 1H, H-2′), 4.26 (d, *J* = 7.6 Hz, 1H, H-3), 4.20–4.16 (m, 2H, H-20b, OCH_2CH_2OCO), 3.95 (brs, 1H, OCH_2CH_2OCO), 3.89–3.84 (ddd, *J* = 2.3, 6.8, 8.7, 12.4 Hz, 1H, H-7a), 3.80–3.70 (overlap, 2H, H-7b, OCH_2CH_2OCO), 3.60–3.58 (m, 1H, OCH_2CH_2OCO), 2.71–2.63 (m, 2H, H-6a, H-14a), 2.25 (dd, *J* = 9.6, 15.8 Hz, 2H, H-6b, H-14b), 2.03 (s, 3H, CH_3), 1.91(s, 3H, CH_3), 1.87 (brs, 3H, CH_3), 1.83 (brs, 2H, 2 × OH), 1.26 (s, 3H, CH_3), 1.15 (s, 3H, CH_3), 0.73 (s, 9H, $SiC(CH_3)_3$), −0.08 (s, 3H, $Si(CH_3)$), −0.32 (s, 3H, $Si(CH_3)$); ^{13}C-NMR ($CDCl_3$, 100 MHz) δ: 192.3, 171.2, 170.8, 168.6, 167.4, 166.2, 162.7 (d, $^1J_{C\text{-}F}$ = 248.3 Hz), 144.0, 137.9, 133.9, 131.9, 131.2 (d, $^3J_{C\text{-}F}$ = 7.4 Hz), 131.0 (d, $^3J_{C\text{-}F}$ = 7.7 Hz), 128.7 (2C), 128.0, 127.0, 126.5, 125.8 (d, $^4J_{C\text{-}F}$ = 2.6 Hz), 121.0 (d, $^2J_{C\text{-}F}$ = 21.2 Hz), 116.3 (d, $^2J_{C\text{-}F}$ = 22.9 Hz), 85.8, 80.0, 75.7, 75.2, 70.5, 61.9, 58.7, 55.6, 45.7, 42.9, 36.7, 25.5, 22.9, 22.1, 18.2, 15.3, 14.6, 13.7, −5.4, −6.0; LC-MS (ESI, *m/z*): [M + 1], found 988.0, $C_{53}H_{66}FNO_{14}Si$: 987.42.

2′-O-(tert-Butyldimethylsilyl)-2-debenzoyl-2-(3-chlorobenzoyl)-9-O-(2-hydroxyethyl)-10-dehydro-7,8-seco-10-deacetylpaclitaxel (**17d**). White solid; yield 60.9%; ^{1}H-NMR ($CDCl_3$, 400 MHz) δ: 8.06 (d, *J* = 8.8 Hz, 2H, Ar-H), 7.63 (d, *J* = 7.5 Hz, 2H, Ar-H), 7.57 (d, *J* = 8.2 Hz, 1H, Ar-H), 7.50–7.43 (m, 3H, Ar-H), 7.43–7.33 (m, 8H, Ar-H, BzNH), 6.31 (t, *J* = 8.0 Hz, 1H, H-13), 5.90 (d, *J* = 9.2 Hz, 1H, H-3′), 5.59 (d, *J* = 9.6 Hz, 1H, H-2), 5.32–5.28 (overlap, 2H, H-5, H-20b), 4.71 (d, *J* = 1.9 Hz, 1H, H-2′), 4.28 (d, *J* = 7.6 Hz, 1H, H-3), 4.24–4.20 (m, 2H, H-20a, OCH_2CH_2OH), 3.98–3.95 (m, 1H, OCH_2CH_2OH), 3.93–3.89 (m, 1H, H-7b), 3.78–3.72 (overlap, 2H, H-7a, OCH_2CH_2OH), 3.65 (br, 1H, OCH_2CH_2OH), 2.72–2.68 (m, 2H, H-6b, H-14b), 2.26 (dd, *J* = 7.2, 13.4 Hz, 2H, H-6a, H-14a), 1.98 (s, 3H, CH_3), 1.93 (brs, 1H, OH), 1.85 (brs, 2H, OH), 1.29 (brs, 6H, CH_3), 1.18 (s, 3H, CH_3), 0.78 (s, 9H, $SiC(CH_3)_3$), −0.08 (s, 3H, $Si(CH_3)$), −0.30 (s, 3H, $Si(CH_3)$); ^{13}C-NMR ($CDCl_3$, 100 MHz) δ: 192.3, 170.8, 167.4, 166.3, 144.0, 137.9, 135.0, 133.9 (2C), 132.0, 130.8, 130.7, 129.7, 128.8 (2C), 128.7 (2C), 128.2, 128.1, 127.0 (2C), 126.6 (2C), 85.9, 75.8, 75.3, 70.5, 62.0, 55.6, 43.0, 36.7, 32.0, 29.7, 29.4, 27.3, 25.5 (3C), 23.0, 22.7, 22.2, 18.3, 15.3, 14.7, 14.2, −5.4, −6.0; LC-MS (ESI, *m/z*): [M + 1], found 1004.4, [M + 23], found 1026.4, $C_{53}H_{66}ClNO_{14}Si$: 1003.39.

2′-O-(tert-Butyldimethylsilyl)-2-debenzoyl-2-(3-trifluoromethylbenzoyl)-9-O-(2-hydroxyethyl)-10-dehydro-7,8-seco-10-deacetylpaclitaxel (**17e**). White solid; yield 49.9%; ^{1}H-NMR ($CDCl_3$, 400 MHz) δ: 7.83 (d, *J* = 7.7 Hz, 2H, Ar-H), 7.68 (t, *J* = 7.8 Hz, 1H, Ar-H), 7.58 (d, *J* = 7.3 Hz, 1H, Ar-H), 7.45 (t, *J* = 7.4 Hz, 2H, Ar-H), 7.35 (m, 8H, Ar-H), 6.29 (t, *J* = 8.2 Hz, 1H, H-13), 5.87 (d, *J* = 8.7 Hz, 1H, H-3′), 5.60 (d, *J* = 9.65 Hz, 1H, H-2), 5.26 (overlap, 2H, H-5, H-20a), 4.70 (d, *J* = 1.3 Hz, 1H, H-2′), 4.28 (d, *J* = 6.8 Hz, 1H, H-3), 4.19 (m, 2H, H-20b, OCH_2CH_2OCO), 3.98 (m, 1H, OCH_2CH_2OCO), 3.87 (m, *J* = 1.8, 6.3, 8.7, 12.0 Hz, 1H, H-7a), 3.75 (overlap, 2H, H-7b, OCH_2CH_2OCO), 3.66 (m, 1H, OCH_2CH_2OCO), 2.65 (m, 2H, H-6a, H-14a), 2.24 (dd, *J* = 6.7, 16.3 Hz, 2H, H-6b, H-14b), 1.97 (s, 3H, CH_3), 1.92 (s, 3H, CH_3), 1.82 (s, 3H, CH_3), 1.26 (s, 3H, CH_3), 1.17 (s, 3H, CH_3), 0.77 (s, 9H, $SiC(CH_3)_3$), −0.08 (s, 3H, $Si(CH_3)$), −0.32 (s, 3H, $Si(CH_3)$); ^{13}C-NMR ($CDCl_3$, 100 MHz) δ: 192.3, 170.8, 167.6, 166.1, 144.1, 137.8, 133.9, 133.2,

132.0, 131.4 (q, $^2J_{C\text{-}F}$ = 33.2 Hz), 130.3, 130.2 (q, $^3J_{C\text{-}F}$ = 3.5 Hz), 130.0, 128.8, 128.7, 128.1, 126.9, 126.8 (q, $^3J_{C\text{-}F}$ = 3.6 Hz), 126.5, 123.6 (q, $^1J_{C\text{-}F}$ = 273.8 Hz), 85.8, 75.6, 75.4, 70.5, 62.0, 58.4, 55.6, 43.0, 36.7, 31.9, 29.8, 29.7, 29.6 (2C), 29.3 (2C), 27.2, 25.5, 23.0, 22.7, 22.1, 18.4, 18.2, 15.3, 14.6, 14.1, −5.4, −6.0; LC-MS (ESI, *m/z*): [M + 1], found 1038.4, [M + 23], found 1060.4, $C_{54}H_{66}F_3NO_{14}Si$: 1037.42.

3.1.6. General Experimental Procedure for Compounds **19a–e**

2′-O-(tert-Butyldimethylsilyl)-macrocyclic taxoid (**19a**). To a solution of **17a** (19 mg, 0.0196 mmol) in dichloromethane (4.2 mL) was added, dropwise, pyridine (22 μL, 0.266 mmol) and triphosgene (8.7 mg, 0.0293 mmol) at 0 °C, then the reaction mixture was stirred at room temperature for 5 h. The reaction was diluted with ethyl acetate, washed with saturated NaCl. The organic layer was dried over anhydrous Na_2SO_4 and then concentrated under reduced pressure. Purification of the crude product by silica gel chromatography (ethyl acetate: petroleum ether = 1:3) gave product **19a** as a white solid (3.1 mg, 15.9% yield). ^{1}H-NMR ($CDCl_3$, 400 MHz) δ: 8.17 (d, *J* = 7.2 Hz, 2H, Ar-H), 7.75 (d, *J* = 7.2 Hz, 2H, Ar-H), 7.63 (t, *J* = 7.2 Hz, 1H, Ar-H), 7.54 (t, *J* = 7.6 Hz, 2H, Ar-H), 7.50 (d, *J* = 7.6 Hz, 1H, Ar-H), 7.43 (d, *J* = 7.6 Hz, 2H, Ar-H), 7.39 (t, *J* = 7.2 Hz, 2H, Ar-H), 7.34–7.29 (m, 3H, Ar-H), 7.08 (d, *J* = 9.2 Hz, 1H, NH), 6.27 (t, *J* = 8.8 Hz, 1H, H-13), 5.76 (d, *J* = 8.4 Hz, 1H, H-3′), 5.60 (d, *J* = 7.6 Hz, 1H, H-2), 4.84 (overlap, 2H, H-5, OCH_2CH_2OCO), 4.79 (d, *J* = 7.6 Hz, 1H, H-3), 4.67 (d, *J* = 2.0 Hz, 1H, H-2′), 4.57 (dd, *J* = 6.8, 12.0 Hz, 1H, OCH_2CH_2OCO), 4.49 (dd, *J* = 6.8, 12.0 Hz, 1H, OCH_2CH_2OCO), 4.46 (d, *J* = 8.4 Hz, 1H, H-20a), 4.35 (d, *J* = 8.4 Hz, 1H, H-20b), 4.32 (dd, *J* = 5.2, 13.6 Hz, 1H, OCH_2CH_2OCO), 4.13 (ddd, *J* = 6.4, 10.8, 17.2 Hz, 1H, H-7a), 4.02 (ddd, *J* = 8.8, 11.6, 17.2 Hz, 1H, H-7b), 2.55 (s, 3H, 4-OAc), 2.35 (m, 3H, H-6a, H-6b, H-14a), 2.18 (dd, *J* = 8.8, 15.2 Hz, 1H, H-14b), 1.84 (s, 3H, CH_3), 1.25 (s, 3H, CH_3), 1.24 (s, 3H, CH_3), 1.19 (s, 3H, CH_3), 0.79 (s, 9H, $SiC(CH_3)_3$), −0.03 (s, 3H, $Si(CH_3)$), −0.30 (s, 3H, $Si(CH_3)$); ^{13}C-NMR ($CDCl_3$, 150 MHz) δ: 192.1, 171.0, 169.4, 166.9, 166.8, 152.4, 151.5, 144.5, 139.7, 138.3, 134.6, 134.1, 133.8, 131.8, 130.2 (2C), 129.0, 128.8 (2C), 128.7, 127.9, 127.0 (2C), 126.3 (2C), 89.6, 84.7, 78.6, 76.1, 75.3, 75.2, 71.4, 70.6, 68.9, 65.9, 55.6, 42.9, 42.4, 36.5, 31.0, 26.2, 25.5 (3C), 22.9, 21.6, 18.1, 14.4, 13.6, −5.3, −5.9; LC-MS (ESI, *m/z*): [M + 1], found 996.4, [M + 23], found 1018.4, $C_{54}H_{65}NO_{15}Si$: 995.41.

2′-O-(tert-Butyldimethylsilyl)-2-debenzoyl-2-(3-methoxybenzoyl)-macrocyclic taxoid (**19b**). White solid; yield 32.7%; ^{1}H-NMR ($CDCl_3$, 400 MHz) δ: 7.80 (d, *J* = 1.2, 7.6 Hz, 1H, Ar-H), 7.77 (d, *J* = 6.8 Hz, 2H, Ar-H), 7.67 (dd, *J* = 1.5, 2.5 Hz, 1H, Ar-H), 7.55–7.51 (m, 1H, Ar-H), 7.49–7.39 (m, 3H, Ar-H), 7.40–7.31 (m, 5H, Ar-H), 7.20–7.17 (m, 1H, Ar-H), 7.08 (d, *J* = 9.2 Hz, 1H, BzNH), 6.28 (t, 1H, H-13), 5.76 (dd, *J* = 1.6, 8.9 Hz, H-3′), 5.62 (d, *J* = 7.5 Hz, 1H, H-2), 4.87 (d, *J* = 7.6 Hz, 1H, H-20b), 4.85 (d, *J* = 4.8 Hz, 1H, H-5), 4.81 (d, *J* = 7.5 Hz, 1H, H-20a), 4.68 (d, *J* = 2.0 Hz, 1H, H-2′), 4.60–4.32 (m, 5H, H-7a, H-7b, H-16a, H-16b, H-3), 4.18–4.03 (m, H-15a, H-15b), 3.91 (s, 3H, OCH_3), 2.55 (d, *J* = 1.3 Hz, 6H, 2 × CH_3), 2.41–2.35 (m, 3H, H-14b, H-6a, H-6b), 2.24–2.20 (m, 1H, H-14a), 1.84 (d, *J* = 1.2 Hz, 3H, $COCH_3$), 1.26 (s, 3H, CH_3), 1.21 (s, 3H, CH_3), 0.81 (s, 9H, $SiC(CH_3)_3$), −0.008 (s, 3H, $Si(CH_3)$), −0.28 (s, 3H, $Si(CH_3)$); ^{13}C-NMR ($CDCl_3$, 100 MHz) δ: 192.2, 171.1, 169.4, 166.9, 166.8, 159.8, 152.5, 151.6, 144.6, 139.7, 138.4, 134.7, 134.2, 131.9, 130.4, 130.0, 128.82 (2C), 128.78 (2C), 128.0, 127.0 (2C), 126.4 (2C), 122.6, 120.3, 114.7, 89.6, 84.8, 78.5, 75.4, 75.3, 71.5, 70.7, 69.0, 65.9, 55.6, 43.0, 42.5, 36.5, 31.1, 29.7, 26.3, 25.6 (3C), 22.9, 21.6, 18.2, 14.4, 13.7, −5.2,−5.8; LC-MS (ESI, *m/z*): [M + 1], found 1026.4, [M + 23], found 1048.4, $C_{55}H_{67}NO_{16}Si$: 1025.42.

2′-O-(tert-Butyldimethylsilyl)-2-debenzoyl-2-(3-fluorobenzoyl)-macrocyclic taxoid (**19c**). White solid; yield 32.1%; ^{1}H-NMR ($CDCl_3$, 400 MHz) δ: 8.01(d, *J* = 7.8 Hz, 1H, Ar-H), 7.84–7.87 (m, 1H, Ar-H), 7.75–7.73 (m, 2 H, Ar-H), 7. 56–7.49 (m, 2H, Ar-H), 7.44–7.31 (m, 8H, Ar-H), 7.09 (d, *J* = 9.0 Hz, 1H, NH), 6.28 (t, *J* = 8.8 Hz,1H, H-13), 5.78 (dd, *J* = 1.4, 9.1 Hz, 1H, H-3′), 5.61 (d, *J* = 7.6 Hz, 1H, H-2), 4.87–4.82 (overlap, 2H, OCH_2CH_2OCO, H-5), 4.83 (d, *J* = 7.5 Hz, 1H, H-3), 4.69 (d, *J* = 2.0 Hz, 1H, H-2′), 4.58 (dd, *J* = 6.4, 11.9 Hz, 1H, OCH_2CH_2OCO), 4.51 (dd, *J* = 6.4, 13.7 Hz, 1H, OCH_2CH_2OCO), 4.46 (d, *J* = 8.2 Hz, 1H, H-20a), 4.36–4.30 (overlap, 2H, OCH_2CH_2OCO, H-20b), 4.16–4.09 (m, 1H, H-7a), 4.06–3.99 (m, 17.2 Hz, 1H, H-7b), 2.57 (s, 3H, $COCH_3$), 2.56 (s, 3H, 4-OAc), 2.39–2.31 (m, 3H, H-6a, H-6b, H-14a), 2.18 (dd, *J* = 8.4, 15.4 Hz, 1H, H-14b), 1.90 (brs, 1H, OH), 1.84 (s, 3H, CH_3), 1.23 (s, 3H, CH_3), 1.19 (s, 3H, CH_3), 0.80 (s, 9H, $SiC(CH_3)_3$), −0.29 (s, 3H, $Si(CH_3)$), −0.03 (s, 3H, $Si(CH_3)$); ^{13}C-NMR ($CDCl_3$, 100 MHz) δ: 192.1, 171.1, 169.4, 167.0, 165.7, 162.7 (d, $^1J_{C\text{-}F}$ = 247.8 Hz), 152.5, 151.6, 144.5, 139.8, 138.4, 134.5, 134.2, 131.9, 131.3 (d, $^3J_{C\text{-}F}$ = 7.6Hz), 130.6 (d, $^3J_{C\text{-}F}$ = 7.6 Hz), 128.8 (2C), 128.0, 127.0, 126.5, 126.0 (d, $^4J_{C\text{-}F}$ = 3.0 Hz), 121.0 (d, $^2J_{C\text{-}F}$ = 21.4 Hz), 117.1 (d, $^2J_{C\text{-}F}$ = 23.3 Hz), 89.6, 84.7, 78.6, 76.1, 75.7, 75.3, 71.5, 70.7, 68.9, 65.9, 55.6, 43.0, 42.5, 36.4, 31.0, 26.3, 25.6, 22.8, 21.6, 18.2, 14.4, 13.6, −5.2, −5.8; LC-MS (ESI, *m/z*): [M + 1], found 1014.4, [M + 23], found 1036.4, $C_{54}H_{64}FNO_{15}Si$: 1013.40.

2′-O-(tert-Butyldimethylsilyl)-2-debenzoyl-2-(3-chlorobenzoyl)-macrocyclic taxoid (**19d**). White solid; yield 36.1%; ^{1}H-NMR ($CDCl_3$, 400 MHz) δ: 8.19 (t, *J* = 1.6 Hz, 1H, Ar-H), 8.10–8.07 (m, 1H, Ar-H), 7.77–7.75 (m, 2H, Ar-H), 7.64–7.61 (m, 1H, Ar-H), 7.55–7.49 (m, 2H, Ar-H), 7.46–7.33 (m, 7H, Ar-H), 7.08 (d, *J* = 9.2 Hz, 1H, BzNH), 6.25 (m, 1H, H-13), 5.76 (dd, *J* = 1.6, 9.0 Hz, 1H, H-3′), 5.59 (d, *J* = 7.6 Hz, 1H, H-2), 4.89–4.81 (m, 3H, OCH_2CH_2OCO, H-5, H-3), 4.68 (d, *J* = 2.0 Hz, 1H, H-2′), 4.57 (dd, *J* = 6.6, 11.9 Hz, 1H, OCH_2CH_2OCO), 4.50 (dd, *J* = 6.5, 11.8 Hz, 1H, OCH_2CH_2OCO), 4.44 (d, *J* = 8.0 Hz, 1H, H-20a), 4.38–4.32 (m, 2H, OCH_2CH_2OCO, H-20b), 4.15–4.10 (m, 1H, H-7a), 4.07–4.01 (m, *J* = 17.2 Hz, 1H, H-7b), 2.56 (s, 3H, CH_3), 2.55 (s, 3H, CH_3), 2.41–2.30 (m, 3H, H-6a, H-6b, H-14a), 2.25–2.18 (m, 1H, H-14b), 1.84 (d, *J* = 1.2 Hz, 3H, CH_3), 1.25 (s, 3H, CH_3), 1.20 (s, 3H, CH_3), 0.82 (s, 9H, $SiC(CH_3)_3$), −0.01 (s, 3H, $Si(CH_3)$), −0.26 (s, 3H, $Si(CH_3)$); ^{13}C-NMR ($CDCl_3$, 100 MHz) δ: 192.1, 171.1, 169.4, 165.6, 152.5, 151.7, 144.5, 139.8, 138.4, 134.9, 134.5, 133.6, 131.8, 131.0, 130.3, 128.81 (2C), 128.79 (2C), 128.4, 128.0, 127.0 (2C), 126.5 (2C), 89.6, 84.7, 78.7, 77.3, 75.6, 75.3, 70.8, 69.0, 55.7, 43.0, 42.5, 36.4, 29.7, 26.3, 25.6 (3C), 22.8, 21.6, 18.2, 14.4, 13.6, −5.2, −5.8; LC-MS (ESI, *m/z*): [M + 1], found 1030.4, [M + 23], found 1052.4, $C_{54}H_{64}ClNO_{15}Si$: 1029.37.

2′-O-(tert-Butyldimethylsilyl)-2-debenzoyl-2-(3-trifluoromethylbenzoyl)-macrocyclic taxoid (**19e**). White solid; yield 30.5%; ^{1}H-NMR ($CDCl_3$, 400 MHz) δ: 8.51 (s, 1H, Ar-H), 8.41 (d, *J* = 7.8 Hz, 1H, Ar-H), 7.92 (d, *J* = 7.8 Hz, 1H, Ar-H), 7.76–7.72 (m, 3H, Ar-H), 7.55–7.51 (m, 1H, Ar-H), 7.47–7.40 (m, 4H, Ar-H), 7.37–7.33 (m, 3H, Ar-H), 7.09 (d, *J* = 9.1 Hz, 1H, NH), 6.24 (t, *J* = 8.8 Hz, 1H, H-13), 5.76 (dd, *J* = 1.0, 9.0 Hz, 1H, H-3′), 5.63 (d, *J* = 7.6 Hz, 1H, H-2), 4.91–4.84 (m, 3H, H-3, H-5, OCH_2CH_2OCO), 4.67 (d, *J* = 1.8 Hz, 1H, H-2′), 4.58 (dd, *J* = 6.8, 11.8 Hz, 1H, OCH_2CH_2OCO), 4.52 (dd, *J* = 6.8, 13.7 Hz, 1H, OCH_2CH_2OCO), 4.44 (d, *J* = 8.1 Hz, 1H, H-20a), 4.38–4.33 (m, 2H, OCH_2CH_2OCO, H-20b), 4.11–4.18 (m, 1H, H-7a), 4.09–4.02 (m, *J* = 17.2 Hz, 1H, H-7b), 2.55 (s, 3H, 4-OAc), 2.42–2.36 (m, 3H, H-6a, H-6b, H-14a), 2.29–2.20 (m,1H, H-14b), 1.94 (s, 1H, OH), 1.86 (d, *J* = 1.04 Hz, 3H, CH_3), 1.29 (s, 3H, CH_3), 1.26 (s, 3H, CH_3), 1.22 (s, 3H, CH_3), 0.84 (s, 9H, $SiC(CH_3)_3$), −0.004 (s, 3H, $Si(CH_3)$), −0.24 (s, 3H, $Si(CH_3)$); ^{13}C-NMR ($CDCl_3$, 100 MHz) δ: 192.0, 171.1, 169.3, 167.0, 165.4, 152.5, 151.6, 144.5, 139.8, 138.4, 134.4, 134.3, 133.6, 131.8, 131.4 (q, $^2J_{C\text{-}F}$ = 33.2 Hz), 130.3 (q, $^3J_{C\text{-}F}$ = 3.4 Hz), 130.2, 129.7, 128.8, 128.0, 127.0, 126.9 (q, $^3J_{C\text{-}F}$ = 4.3 Hz), 126.5, 123.7 (q, $^1J_{C\text{-}F}$ = 273.8 Hz), 89.6, 84.7, 78.7, 76.0, 75.8, 75.2, 71.5, 70.8, 69.0, 65.9, 55.7, 43.0, 42.4, 36.4, 31.0, 29.0, 26.3, 25.6, 22.7, 21.6, 18.2, 14.4, 13.6, −5.2,−5.8; LC-MS (ESI, *m/z*): [M + 1], found 1064.4, [M + 23], found 1086.4, $C_{55}H_{64}F_3NO_{15}Si$: 1063.40.

3.1.7. General Procedure for the Syntheses of Compounds **21a–e**

Macrocyclic taxoid (**21a**)

To a solution of of **19a** (32.3 mg, 0.0464 mmol) in THF (8 mL) was added, dropwise, 1.53 mL of HF-pyridine (*v/v* = 1:2) at 0 °C, and the reaction mixture was stirred at room temperature for 30 h. The reaction was quenched with saturated aqueous $NaHCO_3$, diluted with ethyl acetate, and washed with saturated NH_4Cl. The organic layer was dried over anhydrous Na_2SO_4 and then concentrated under reduced pressure. Purification of the crude product by silica gel chromatography (ethyl acetate: petroleum ether = 2:1) gave product **21a** as a white solid (13.2 mg, 46.2% yield). ^{1}H-NMR ($CDCl_3$, 400 MHz) δ: 8.14 (d, *J* = 7.0 Hz, 2H, Ar-H), 7.73 (d, *J* = 8.6 Hz, 2H, Ar-H), 7.62 (t, *J* = 7.5 Hz, 1H, Ar-H), 7.52–7.45 (m, 5H, Ar-H), 7.40–7.30 (m, 5H, Ar-H), 7.22 (d, *J* = 9.1 Hz, 1H, NH), 6.20 (t, *J* = 8.5 Hz, 1H, H-13), 5.78 (dd, *J* = 2.5, 9.1 Hz, 1H, H-3′), 5.58 (d, *J* = 7.5 Hz, 1H, H-2), 4.80–4.74 (overlap, 4H, H-5, H-2′, H-3, OCH_2CH_2OCO), 4.52 (dd, *J* = 6.4, 12.0 Hz, 1H, OCH_2CH_2OCO), 4.45–4.44 (overlap, 2H, H-20a, OCH_2CH_2OCO), 4.31-4.25 (overlap, 2H, H-20b, OCH_2CH_2OCO), 4.07–3.91 (overlap, 2H, H-7b, H-7a),

2.56 (br, 1H, OH-2′), 2.51 (s, 3H, CH_3), 2.35 (s, 3H, CH_3), 2.33–2.25 (overlap, 4H, H-14a, H-14b, H-6a, H-6b), 1.68 (s, 3H, CH_3), 1.18 (s, 3H, CH_3), 1.16 (s, 3H, CH_3); ^{13}C-NMR ($CDCl_3$, 150 MHz) δ: 191.8, 172.4, 169.7, 166.9, 166.8, 152.4, 151.5, 144.8, 138.6, 137.9, 135.0, 133.9, 133.6, 132.0, 130.1 (2C), 129.0 (2C), 128.8 (4C), 128.3, 127.0 (2C), 89.4, 84.7, 78.4, 76.1, 75.1, 73.1, 71.8, 71.5, 68.9, 65.8, 54.8, 42.8, 42.4, 36.4, 30.9, 29.7, 26.3, 22.5, 21.2, 14.0, 13.7; LC-MS (ESI, *m/z*): [M + 1], found 882.8, [M + 23], found 904.4, $C_{48}H_{51}NO_{15}$: 881.33.

2-Debenzoyl-2-(3-methoxybenzoyl)-macrocyclic taxoid (**21b**). White solid; yield 54.1%; ^{1}H-NMR ($CDCl_3$, 400 MHz) δ: 7.76–7.74 (m, 3H, Ar-H), 7.66-7.65 (m, 1H, Ar-H), 7.53–7.46 (m, 8H, Ar-H), 7.36–7.32 (m, 1H, Ar-H), 7.03 (d, J = 8.9 Hz, 1H, NH), 6.17 (t, J = 8.2 Hz, 1H, H-13), 5.79 (dd, J = 2.3, 9.0 Hz, 1H, H-3′), 5.59 (d, J = 7.5 Hz, 1H, H-2), 4.84–4.77 (overlap, 4H, H-5, H-2′, H-3, $O\underline{CH_2}CH_2OCO$), 4.55 (dd, J = 6.5, 11.9 Hz, 1H, $OCH_2\underline{CH_2}OCO$), 4.45 (dd, J = 6.6, 13.2 Hz, 1H, $OCH_2\underline{CH_2}OCO$), 4.43 (d, J = 7.5 Hz, 1H, H-20a), 4.36 (d, J = 8.29 Hz, 1H, H-20b), 4.32 (dd, J = 5.2, 13.8 Hz, 1H, $O\underline{CH_2}CH_2OCO$), 4.12–3.96 (m, 2H, H-7b, H-7a), 3.88 (s, 3H, OAc), 3.62 (brs, 1H, OH-2′), 2.53 (s, 3H, CH_3), 2.36 (s, 3H, CH_3), 2.40–2.27 (overlap, 4H, H-14a, H-14b, H-6a, H-6b), 1.93 (brs, 1H, OH-1), 1.68 (d, 3H, CH_3), 1.23 (s, 3H, CH_3), 1.18 (s, 3H, CH_3); ^{13}C-NMR ($CDCl_3$, 100 MHz) δ: 191.9, 172.4, 169.7, 167.0, 166.7, 159.8, 152.4, 151.5, 144.8, 138.6, 138.0, 135.1, 133.7, 132.0, 130.3 (2C), 130.0, 129.8, 129.7, 129.0 (2C), 128.7 (4C), 128.3, 127.0 (2C), 122.5, 120.0, 115.0, 89.4, 84.7, 78.4, 76.2, 75.3, 73.2, 71.7, 71.5, 68.9, 65.8, 55.5, 54.9, 42.8, 42.4, 36.4, 31.9, 30.9, 29.7, 26.3, 22.5, 21.2, 14.0, 13.7; LC-MS (ESI, *m/z*): [M + 1], found 912.3, [M + 23], found 934.3, $C_{49}H_{53}NO_{16}$: 911.34.

2-Debenzoyl-2-(3-fluorobenzoyl)-macrocyclic taxoid (**21c**). White solid; yield 52.2%; ^{1}H-NMR ($CDCl_3$, 400 MHz) δ: 7.97–7.92 (m, 1H, Ar-H), 7.86–7.83 (ddd, J = 1.5, 2.5, 9.2 Hz, 1H, Ar-H), 7.75–7.72 (m, 2H, Ar-H), 7.54–7.47 (m, 4H, Ar-H), 7.43–7.39 (m, 4 H, Ar-H), 7.37–7.32 (m, 2H, Ar-H), 7.02 (d, J = 9.1 Hz, 1H, NH), 6.17 (dd, J = 7.5, 8.8 Hz, 1H, H-13), 5.79 (dd, J = 2.4, 9.0 Hz, 1H, H-3′), 5.57 (d, J = 7.6 Hz, 1H, H-2), 4.84–4.78 (overlap, 4H, H-5, H-2′, H-3, $O\underline{CH_2}CH_2OCO$), 4.55 (dd, J = 6.4, 11.9 Hz, 1H, $OCH_2\underline{CH_2}OCO$), 4.47–4.40 (m, 2H, H-20b, H-20a), 4.34–4.29 (m, 2H, $OCH_2\underline{CH_2}OCO$), 4.12–3.96 (m, 2H, H-7b, H-7a), 3.62 (d, J = 4.9 Hz, 1H, OH-2′), 2.53 (s, 3H, CH_3), 2.36 (s, 3H, CH_3), 2.35–2.25 (m, 4H, H-14a, H-14b, H-6a, H-6b), 1.93 (brs, 1H, OH-1), 1.68 (d, J = 1.2 Hz, 3H, CH_3), 1.23 (s, 3H, CH_3), 1.18 (s, 3H, CH_3); ^{13}C-NMR ($CDCl_3$, 100 MHz) δ: 191.8, 172.4, 169.6, 167.1, 165.6 (d, $J_{C\text{-}F}$ = 3.2 Hz, CO), 162.4 (d, $^1J_{C\text{-}F}$ = 247.8 Hz), 152.4, 151.6, 144.7, 138.7, 138.0, 134.8, 133.7, 132.0, 131.3 (d, $^3J_{C\text{-}F}$ = 7.6 Hz), 130.5 (d, $^3J_{C\text{-}F}$ = 7.8 Hz), 129.9 (d, $^4J_{C\text{-}F}$ = 3.9 Hz), 129.7, 129.0, 128.7, 128.4, 127.0, 126.0, 121.0 (d, $^2J_{C\text{-}F}$ = 21.3 Hz), 117.0 (d, $^2J_{C\text{-}F}$ = 23.3 Hz), 89.5, 84.7, 78.5, 76.0, 75.5, 73.2, 71.7, 71.5, 68.9, 65.7, 55.0, 42.8, 42.4, 36.3, 30.9, 26.3, 25.5, 22.7, 22.4, 21.2, 14.1, 14.0, 13.6; LC-MS (ESI, *m/z*): [M + 1], found 900.0, [M + 23], found 922.0, $C_{48}H_{50}FNO_{15}$: 899.32.

2-Debenzoyl-2-(3-chlorobenzoyl)-macrocyclic taxoid (**21d**). White solid; yield 48.7%; ^{1}H-NMR ($CDCl_3$, 400 MHz) δ: 8.16 (t, 1H, Ar-H), 8.06–8.03 (m, 1H, Ar-H), 7.75–7.72 (m, 2H, Ar-H), 7.61 (ddd, J = 1.1, 2.1, 8.0 Hz, 1H, Ar-H), 7.53–7.45 (m, 4H, Ar-H), 7.43–7.39 (m, 4 H, Ar-H), 7.36–7.32 (m, 1H, Ar-H), 7.01 (d, J = 9.1 Hz, 1H, NH), 6.17 (td, J =1.3, 8.7 Hz, 1H, H-13), 5.78 (dd, J = 2.3, 9.0 Hz, 1H, H-3′), 5.56 (d, J = 7.6 Hz, 1H, H-2), 4.84–4.78 (overlap,4H, H-5, H-2′, H-3, $O\underline{CH_2}CH_2OCO$), 4.55 (dd, J = 6.4, 11.9 Hz, 1H, $OCH_2\underline{CH_2}OCO$), 4.47–4.38 (m, 2 H, H-20b, H20a), 4.34–4.29 (m, 2H, $O\underline{CH_2}CH_2OCO$), 4.11–3.96 (m, 2H, H-7b, H-7a), 3.62 (brs, 1H, OH-2′), 2.52 (s, 3H, CH_3), 2.37 (s, 3H, CH_3), 2.42–2.27 (overlap, 4H, H-14a, H-14b, H-6a, H-6b), 2.0 (brs, 1H, OH-1), 1.68 (d, J = 1.2 Hz, 3H, CH_3), 1.23 (s, 3H, CH_3), 1.18 (s, 3H, CH_3); ^{13}C-NMR ($CDCl_3$, 100 MHz) δ: 191.8, 172.4, 169.6, 167.1, 165.5, 152.4, 151.6, 144.7, 138.7, 138.0, 134.8 (2C), 133.8, 133.7, 132.0, 130.9, 130.2 (2C), 129.0, 128.7, 128.4 (2C), 127.1, 127.0, 89.4, 84.7, 78.4, 76.0, 75.5, 73.1, 71.7, 71.5, 68.9, 65.7, 55.0, 42.8, 42.4, 36.3, 30.9, 26.2, 22.4, 21.2, 14.0, 13.6; LC-MS (ESI, *m/z*): [M + 1], found 916.3, [M + 23], found 938.3, $C_{48}H_{50}ClNO_{15}$: 915.29.

2-Debenzoyl-2-(3-trifluoromethylbenzoyl)-macrocyclic taxoid (**21e**). White solid; yield 63.7%; ^{1}H-NMR ($CDCl_3$, 400 MHz) δ: 8.47 (s, 1H, Ar-H), 8.36 (d, J = 7.9 Hz, 1H, Ar-H), 7.90 (d, J = 7.8 Hz, 1H, Ar-H), 7.73–7.67 (m, 3H, Ar-H), 7.46–7.52 (m, 3 H, Ar-H), 7.43–7.32 (m, 5H, Ar-H), 6.94 (d, J = 9.0 Hz, 1H,

NH), 6.16 (dd, J = 7.5, 8.8 Hz, 1H, H-13), 5.77 (dd, J = 2.0, 8.9 Hz, 1H, H-3′), 5.60 (d, J = 7.5 Hz, 1H, H-2), 4.85–4.78 (overlap, 4H, H-5, H-2′, H-3, OCH_2CH_2OCO), 4.55 (dd, J = 6.6, 12.0 Hz, 1H, OCH_2CH_2OCO), 4.45 (dd, J = 6.7, 13.6 Hz, 1H, OCH_2CH_2OCO), 4.39 (d, J = 8.0 Hz, 1 H, H-20b), 4.33 (dd, 1H, OCH_2CH_2OCO), 4.31 (d, J = 7.7 Hz, 1H, H-20a),4.12-3.97 (m, 2H, H-7b, H-7a), 3.53 (d, J = 6.9 Hz, 1H, OH-2′), 2.53 (s, 3H, CH_3), 2.34 (s, 3H, CH_3), 2.46–2.28 (m, 4H, H-14a, H-14b, H-6a, H-6b), 1.93 (brs, 1H, OH-1), 1.70 (d, J = 1.2 Hz, 3H, CH_3), 1.24 (s, 3H, CH_3),1.15 (s, 3H, CH_3); ^{13}C-NMR ($CDCl_3$, 100 MHz) δ: 192.0, 171.1, 169.3, 167.0, 165.4, 152.5, 151.6, 144.5, 139.8, 138.4, 134.4, 134.3, 133.6, 131.8, 131.4 (q, $^2J_{C\text{-}F}$ = 33.2 Hz), 130.3 (q, $^3J_{C\text{-}F}$ = 3.4 Hz), 130.2, 129.7, 128.8, 128.0, 127.0, 126.9 (q, $^3J_{C\text{-}F}$ = 4.3 Hz), 126.5, 123.7 (q, $^1J_{C\text{-}F}$ = 273.8 Hz), 89.6, 84.7, 78.7, 76.0, 75.8, 75.2, 71.5, 70.8, 69.0, 65.9, 55.7, 43.0, 42.4, 36.4, 31.0, 29.0, 26.3, 25.6, 22.7, 21.6, 18.2, 14.4, 13.6, −5.2, −5.8; LC-MS (ESI, *m/z*): [M + 1], found 950.3, [M + 23], found 972.3, $C_{49}H_{50}F_3NO_{15}$: 949.31.

3.1.8. General Experimental Procedure for Compounds **18a–e**

2′-O-(tert-Butyldimethylsilyl)-9-O-(3-hydroxyethyl)-10-dehydro-7, 8-seco-10-deacetylpaclitaxel (**18a**). To a mixture of **15a** (65 mg, 0.0703 mmol), potassium carbonate (67.8 mg, 0.491 mmol) and potassium iodide (11.7 mg, 0.0705 mmol) in DMF (0.65 mL) was added 3-bromo-1-propanol (44 μL 0.487 mmol), dropwise, at 0 °C. The reaction mixture was stirred for 4 h at room temperature and then was diluted with ethyl acetate. The organic phase was washed with saturated aqueous NH_4Cl. The organic layer was dried over anhydrous Na_2SO_4 and then concentrated under reduced pressure. Purification of the crude product by silica gel chromatography (ethyl acetate: petroleum ether = 1:1) gave product **18a** as a white solid (50 mg, 72.4% yield). ^{1}H-NMR ($CDCl_3$, 400 MHz) δ: 8.10 (d, J = 7.6 Hz, 2H, Ar-H), 7.62 (d, J = 7.6 Hz, 2H, Ar-H), 7.58 (t, J = 7.2 Hz, 1H, Ar-H), 7.47 (dd, J = 7.6, 14.8 Hz, 2H, Ar-H), 7.43–7.40 (m, 1H, Ar-H), 7.38–7.36 (m, 4H, Ar-H), 7.30–7.29 (m, 3H, Ar-H), 6.30 (t, J = 8.4 Hz, 1H, H-13), 5.88 (d, J = 9.6 Hz, 1H, H-3′), 5.57 (d, J = 9.6 Hz, 1H, H-2), 5.30–5.27 (overlap, 2H, H-5, H-20a), 4.69 (d, J = 2.0 Hz, 1H, H-2′), 4.26 (d, J = 7.6 Hz, 1H, H-3), 4.20 (brs, 1H, H-20b), 4.00-3.95 (m, 2H, $OCH_2CH_2CH_2OCO$), 3.91–3.83 (m, 3H, $OCH_2CH_2CH_2OCO$, H-7a), 3.76 (brs, 1H, H-7b), 2.75–2.64 (m, 2H, H-6a, H-14a), 2.27–2.21 (m, 2H, H-6b, H-14b), 1.92–1.90 (m, 5H, CH_3, $OCH_2CH_2CH_2OCO$), 1.96 (s, 3H, CH_3), 1.81 (brs, 3H, CH_3), 1.27 (s, 3H, CH_3), 1.18 (s, 3H, CH_3), 0.76 (s, 9H, $SiC(CH_3)_3$), −0.08 (s, 3H, $Si(CH_3)$), −0.33 (s, 3H, $Si(CH_3)$); ^{13}C-NMR ($CDCl_3$, 100 MHz) δ: 191.6, 170.7, 168.7, 167.3 (2C), 153.1, 152.8, 144.1, 137.9, 133.8, 133.7, 131.9, 129.9 (2C), 128.9 (2C), 128.7 (4C), 128.6, 127.9 (2C), 126.5 (2C), 82.1, 79.9, 75.7, 74.7, 70.5, 68.8, 60.4, 59.3, 58.8, 55.6, 42.8, 36.6, 32.2, 25.4 (3C), 23.2, 22.1, 18.2, 14.9, 14.2, −5.5, −6.1; LC-MS (ESI, *m/z*): [M + 23], found 1006.0, $C_{54}H_{69}NO_{14}Si$: 983.45.

2′-O-(tert-Butyldimethylsilyl)-2-debenzoyl-2-(3-methoxybenzoyl)-9-O-(3-hydroxyethyl)-10-dehydro-7,8-seco-10-deacetylpaclitaxel (**18b**). White solid; yield 75.3%; ^{1}H-NMR ($CDCl_3$, 400 MHz) δ: 7.71–7.65 (m, 3H, Ar-H), 7.53 (m, 1H, Ar-H), 7.46–7.41 (m, 2H, Ar-H), 7.11 (dd, J = 2.4, 8.0 Hz, 1H, BzNH), 6.28 (t, J = 8.6 Hz, 1H, H-13), 5.87 (d, J = 9.2 Hz, 1H, H-3′), 5.58 (d, J = 9.5 Hz, 1H, H-2), 5.29–5.26 (overlap, 2H, H-5, H-20a), 4.72 (d, J = 2.1 Hz, 1H, H-2′), 4.26 (d, J = 6.6 Hz, 1H, H-3), 4.21 (brs, 1H, H-20b), 4.00-3.95 (m, 2H, $OCH_2CH_2CH_2O$), 3.98–3.86 (m, 3H, $OCH_2CH_2CH_2O$, H-7b), 3.83 (overlap, 4H, OCH_3, H-7a), 2.77–2.66 (m, 2H, H-6b, H-14b), 2.27–2.21 (m, 2H, H-6a, H-14a), 1.96 (s, 3H, CH_3), 1.92 (brs, 2H, $OCH_2CH_2CH_2O$), 1.83 (m, 2H, OH), 1.84 (brs, 3H, CH_3), 1.26 (s, 3H, CH_3), 1.19 (s, 3H, CH_3), 0.78 (s, 9H, $SiC(CH_3)_3$), −0.09 (s, 3H, $Si(CH_3)$), −0.29 (s, 3H, $Si(CH_3)$); ^{13}C-NMR ($CDCl_3$, 100 MHz) δ: 191.6, 171.2, 170.9, 168.9, 167.3, 167.2, 159.8, 144.4, 138.1, 133.8, 131.9, 130.4, 130.3, 128.7 (2C), 128.7 (2C), 128.0, 127.0 (2C), 126.7 (2C), 122.3, 119.6, 114.9, 85.8, 79.9, 75.8, 74.9, 70.7, 68.8, 59.3, 59.0, 55.7, 55.5, 42.8, 36.6, 32.3, 25.5 (3C), 25.2, 23.2, 22.2, 18.2, 14.9, 14.5, −5.5, −6.0; LC-MS (ESI, *m/z*): [M + 1], found 1014.4, [M + 23], found 1036.4, $C_{55}H_{71}NO_{16}Si$: 1013.46.

2′-O-(tert-Butyldimethylsilyl)-2-debenzoyl-2-(3-fluorobenzoyl)-9-O-(3-hydroxyethyl)-10-dehydro-7, 8-seco-10-deacetylpaclitaxel (**18c**). White solid; yield 69.7%; ^{1}H-NMR ($CDCl_3$, 400 MHz) δ: 7.93 (d, J = 7.6 Hz, 1H, Ar-H), 7.75 (d, J = 8.9 Hz, 1H, Ar-H), 7.63 (d, J = 7.5 Hz, 1H, Ar-H), 7.52–7.28 (m, 11H, NH, Ar-H), 6.29 (t, J = 8.1 Hz, 1H, H-13), 5.89 (d, J = 9.2 Hz, 1H, H-3′), 5.57 (d, J = 9.6 Hz, 1H, H-2), 5.28–5.26

(overlap, 2H, H-5, H-20a), 4.70 (d, J = 2.0 Hz, 1H, H-2′), 4.27 (d, J = 8.1 Hz, 1H, H-3), 4.19 (brs, 1H, H-20b), 3.99–3.94 (m, 2H, $OCH_2CH_2\underline{CH_2}OH$), 3.88–3.81 (m, 3H, $O\underline{CH_2}CH_2CH_2OH$, H-7a), 3.76 (brs, 1H, H-7b), 2.72–2.63 (m, 2H, H-6a, H-14a), 2.24 (dd, 1H, J = 9.5, 15.8 Hz, H-14b), 2.06– 1.98 (overlap, 1 H, H-6b), 1.95 (s, 3H, CH_3), 1.93–1.87 (m, 4H, CH_3, $OCH_2\underline{CH_2}CH_2OH$), 1.83 (brs, 3H, CH_3), 1.26 (brs, 3H, CH_3), 1.17 (s, 3H, CH_3), 0.77 (s, 9H, $SiC(CH_3)_3$), −0.09 (s, 3H, $Si(CH_3)$), −0.32 (s, 3H, $Si(CH_3)$); ^{13}C-NMR ($CDCl_3$, 100 MHz) δ: 191.5, 171.2, 170.8, 168.6, 167.4, 166.3, 162.7 (d, $^1J_{C\text{-}F}$ = 248.2 Hz), 144.3, 137.9, 133.9, 131.9, 131.2 (d, $^2J_{C\text{-}F}$ = 7.3 Hz), 131.0 (d, $^3J_{C\text{-}F}$ = 7.7 Hz), 128.8, 128.7, 128.0, 127.0, 126.5, 125.8 (d, $^4J_{C\text{-}F}$ = 2.6 Hz), 121.0 (d, $^2J_{C\text{-}F}$ = 21.2 Hz), 116.6 (d, $^2J_{C\text{-}F}$ = 22.8 Hz), 85.9, 80.0, 75.8, 75.2, 70.5, 68.9, 59.3, 55.6, 42.8, 36.7, 32.3, 25.5, 23.2, 22.1, 18.2, 15.0, 14.5, −5.4, −6.0; LC-MS (ESI, *m/z*): [M + 1], found 1002.0, [M + 23], found 1025.0, $C_{54}H_{68}FNO_{14}Si$: 1001.44.

2′-O-(tert-Butyldimethylsilyl)-2-debenzoyl-2-(3-chlorobenzoyl)-9-O-(3-hydroxyethyl)-10-dehydro-7,8-seco-10-deacetylpaclitaxel (**18d**). White solid; yield 52.6%; ^{1}H-NMR ($CDCl_3$, 400 MHz) δ: 8.03 (d, J = 7.6 Hz, 1H, Ar-H), 8.00–7.96 (m, J = 7.6 Hz, 1H, Ar-H), 7.65 (d, J = 7.6 Hz, 2H, Ar-H), 7.54 (t, J = 7.2 Hz, 1H, Ar-H), 7.48–7.44 (m, 2H, Ar-H), 7.43–7.40 (m, 1H, Ar-H), 7.38–7.36 (m, 4H, Ar-H), 7.39–7.28 (m, 7H, Ar-H), 6.30 (t, J = 8.4 Hz, 1H, H-13), 5.88 (d, J = 9.6 Hz, 1H, H-3′), 5.57 (d, J = 9.6 Hz, 1H, H-2), 5.30–5.27 (overlap, 2H, H-5, H-20a), 4.71 (s, 1H, H-2′), 4.26 (d, J = 7.6 Hz, 1H, H-3), 4.18 (brs, 1H, H-20b), 3.99–3.93 (m, 2H, $OCH_2CH_2\underline{CH_2}O$), 3.79–3.40 (m, 3H, $O\underline{CH_2}CH_2CH_2O$, H-7a), 3.73–3.64 (brs, 1H, H-7b), 2.94 (s, 3H, CH_3), 2.84 (s, 3H, CH_3), 2.66 (br, 2H, H-6a, H-14a), 2.29–2.22 (m, 2H, H-6b, H-14b), 1.93 (s, 3H, CH_3), 1.93–1.86 (m, 5H, CH_3, $OCH_2\underline{CH_2}CH_2O$), 1.82 (brs, 3H, CH_3), 1.24 (s, 3H, CH_3), 1.16 (s, 3H, CH_3), 0.76 (s, 9H, $SiC(CH_3)_3$), −0.11 (s, 3H, $Si(CH_3)$), −0.31 (s, 3H, $Si(CH_3)$); ^{13}C-NMR ($CDCl_3$, 100 MHz) δ: 191.5, 171.1, 170.8, 167.4, 165.9, 162.5, 144.3, 137.9, 134.8, 133.9, 133.7, 131.8, 131.0, 130.6, 129.5, 128.7 (2C), 128.6 (2C), 128.1, 127.9, 126.9 (2C), 126.5 (2C), 85.8, 75.7, 75.2, 70.5, 68.8, 67.9, 60.4, 59.2, 55.6, 42.7, 36.6, 36.4, 32.3, 31.4, 25.4 (3C), 23.2, 22.1, 21.0, 18.2, 14.5, 14.2, −5.5, −6.1; LC-MS (ESI, *m/z*): [M + 1], found 1018.4, [M + 23], found 1040.4, $C_{54}H_{68}ClNO_{14}Si$: 1017.41.

2′-O-(tert-Butyldimethylsilyl)-2-debenzoyl-2-(3-trifluoromethylbenzoyl)-9-O-(3-hydroxyethyl)-10-dehydro-7,8-seco-10-deacetylpaclitaxel (**18e**). White solid; yield 71.8%; ^{1}H-NMR ($CDCl_3$, 400 MHz): δ 8.38 (d, J = 7.8 Hz, 2H, Ar-H), 7.83 (d, J = 7.7 Hz, 2H, Ar-H), 7.68 (t, J = 7.8 Hz, 1H, Ar-H), 7.44 (dd, J = 15.4, 8.0 Hz, 2H, Ar-H), 7.47–7.41 (m, 1H, Ar-H), 7.40–7.36 (m, 4H, Ar-H), 7.30–7.29 (m, 3H, Ar-H), 6.29 (t, J = 8.5 Hz, 1H, H-13), 5.86 (d, J = 8.6 Hz, 1H, H-3′), 5.59 (d, J = 9.5 Hz, 1H, H-2), 5.26 (overlap, 2H, H-5, H-20a), 4.70 (d, J = 2.0 Hz, 1H, H-2′), 4.29 (d, J = 7.3 Hz, 1H, H-3), 4.21 (brs, 1H, H-20b), 4.00–3.96 (m, 2H, $OCH_2CH_2\underline{CH_2}OH$), 3.90–3.87 (m, 3H, $O\underline{CH_2}CH_2CH_2OH$, H-7a), 3.75 (brs, 1H, H-7b), 2.70–2.60 (m, 2H, H-6a, H-14a), 2.28–2.22 (m, 2H, H-6b, H-14b), 1.97 (s, 3H, CH_3), 1.94–1.92 (m, 5H, CH_3, $OCH_2\underline{CH_2}CH_2OH$), 1.81 (brs, 3H, CH_3), 1.27 (s, 3H, CH_3), 1.19 (s, 3H, CH_3), 0.76 (s, 9H, $SiC(CH_3)_3$), −0.08 (s, 3H, $Si(CH_3)$), −0.32 (s, 3H, $Si(CH_3)$); ^{13}C-NMR ($CDCl_3$, 100 MHz) δ: 191.5, 170.8, 167.5, 144.3, 137.9, 133.9, 133.2, 132.0, 131.4 (q, $^2J_{C\text{-}F}$ = 33.3 Hz), 130.2 (q, $^3J_{C\text{-}F}$ = 4.0 Hz), 130.0, 128.8, 128.1, 126.9, 126.8 (q, $^3J_{C\text{-}F}$ = 3.9 Hz), 126.5, 123.6 (q, $^1J_{C\text{-}F}$ = 274.2 Hz), 85.9, 75.6, 75.4, 70.5, 59.4, 55.6, 42.9, 36.7, 32.3, 25.5, 18.2, 14.6, −5.4, −6.0; LC-MS (ESI, *m/z*): [M + 1], found 1052.4, [M + 23], found 1074.4, $C_{55}H_{68}NO_{14}F_3Si$: 1051.44.

3.1.9. General Experimental Procedure for Compounds **20a–e**

2′-O-(tert-Butyldimethylsilyl)-macrocyclic taxoid (**20a**). To a solution of **18a** (26.2 mg, 0.0266 mmol) in dichloromethane (5.7 mL) was added, dropwise, pyridine (11 µL, 0.133 mmol) and triphosgene (8.7 mg, 0.0293 mmol) at 0 °C, then the reaction mixture was stirred at room temperature for 3.5 h. The reaction was diluted with ethyl acetate, then washed with saturated NaCl. The organic layer was dried over anhydrous Na_2SO_4 and then concentrated under reduced pressure. Purification of the crude product by silica gel chromatography (ethyl acetate: petroleum ether = 1:3) gave product **20a** as a white solid (6.7 mg, 24.9% yield). ^{1}H-NMR ($CDCl_3$, 400 MHz) δ: 8.17 (d, J = 8.0 Hz, 2H, Ar-H), 7.75 (d, J = 7.6 Hz, 2H, Ar-H), 7.63 (t, J = 7.2 Hz, 1H, Ar-H), 7.56–7.49 (m, 3H, Ar-H), 7.44–7.29 (m, 7H, Ar-H), 7.09 (d, J = 9.2 Hz, 1H, NH), 6.27 (t, J = 8.8 Hz, 1H, H-13), 5.76 (d, J = 8.8 Hz, 1H, H-3′), 5.60 (d, J = 8.0 Hz, 1H,

H-2), 4.80 (d, J = 7.6 Hz, 2H, H-5, H-3), 4.67 (brs, 1H, H-2′), 4.63 (m, 1H, $O\underline{CH_2}CH_2CH_2OCO$), 4.53 (dd, J = 6.4, 11.6 Hz, 1H, $OCH_2CH_2\underline{CH_2}OCO$), 4.47 (d, J = 8.4 Hz, 1H, H-20a), 4.42 (dd, J = 4.0, 7.2 Hz, 1H, $OCH_2CH_2\underline{CH_2}OCO$), 4.34 (d, J = 8.4 Hz, 1H, H-20b), 4.11 (overlap, 2H, H-7a, $O\underline{CH_2}CH_2CH_2OCO$), 3.98 (dt, J = 6.0, 11.6 Hz, 1H, H-7b), 2.66 (m, 1H, H-6a), 2.56 (s, 3H, CH_3), 2.52 (s, 3H, CH_3), 2.42–2.11 (m, 5H, H-6b, H-14a, H-14b, $OCH_2\underline{CH_2}CH_2O$), 1.82 (s, 3H, CH_3), 1.24 (s, 3H, CH_3), 1.17 (s, 3H, CH_3), 0.79 (s, 9H, $SiC(CH_3)_3$), −0.04 (s, 3H, $Si(CH_3)$), −0.31 (s, 3H, $Si(CH_3)$); ^{13}C-NMR ($CDCl_3$, 150 MHz) δ: 191.6, 170.7, 169.7, 169.3, 166.7, 166.6, 153.6, 152.4, 144.1, 138.8, 138.1, 135.5, 133.6, 131.6, 130.2 (2C), 130.0, 128.7, 128.6, 128.5, 127.7, 126.8 (2C), 126.1 (2C), 90.3, 84.4, 78.4, 76.1, 75.2, 75.0, 70.4, 68.9, 65.8, 64.2, 55.4, 42.6 (2C), 36.4, 30.8, 28.8, 25.9, 25.3 (3C), 22.5, 21.5, 17.9, 14.5, 14.1, −5.5, −6.1; LC-MS (ESI, *m/z*): [M + 23], found 1032.0, $C_{55}H_{67}NO_{15}Si$: 1009.43.

2′-O-(tert-Butyldimethylsilyl)-2-debenzoyl-2-(3-methoxybenzoyl)-macrocyclic taxoid (**20b**). White solid; yield 28.6%; ^{1}H-NMR ($CDCl_3$, 400MHz) δ: 7.79 (d, J = 7.6 Hz, 1H, Ar-H), 7.76 (d, J = 7.2 Hz, 2H, Ar-H), 7.67–7.66 (m, 1H, Ar-H), 7.55–7.50 (m, 1H, Ar-H), 7.48–7.42 (m, 3H, Ar-H), 7.40–7.29 (m, 5H, Ar-H), 7.19–7.16 (m, 1H, Ar-H), 7.09 (d, J = 8.8 Hz, 1H, BzNH), 6.27 (t, J = 8.8 Hz, 1H, H-13), 5.76 (dd, J = 1.5, 9.0 Hz, 1H, H-3′), 5.62 (d, J = 7.64 Hz, 1H, H-2), 4.85–4.82 (m, 2H, H-5, H-3), 4.69–4.63 (m, 2H, H-2′, $O\underline{CH_2}CH_2CH_2OCO$), 4.56–4.51 (m, 1H, $OCH_2CH_2\underline{CH_2}OCO$), 4.48–4.38 (m, 3H, H-20a, H-20b, $OCH_2CH_2\underline{CH_2}OCO$), 4.16–4.07 (m, 2H, H-7a, $O\underline{CH_2}CH_2CH_2OCO$), 4.01–3.96 (m, 1H, H-7b), 3.90 (s, 3H, OCH_3), 2.72–2.62 (m, 1H, H-6a), 2.57 (s, 3H, CH_3), 2.53 (s, 3H, CH_3), 2.43–2.36 (m, 1H, H-6b), 2.35–2.28 (m, 1H, H-14a), 2.16–2.14 (m, 2H, H-14b, $OCH_2\underline{CH_2}CH_2O$), 1.82 (d, J = 1.1 Hz, 3H, CH_3), 1.25 (s, 3H, CH_3), 1.18 (s, 3H, CH_3), 0.88 (s, 9H, $SiC(CH_3)_3$), −0.014 (s, 3H, $Si(CH_3)$), −0.29 (s, 3H, $Si(CH_3)$); ^{13}C-NMR ($CDCl_3$, 100 MHz) δ: 190.8, 171.3, 171.2, 169.2, 166.9, 166.8, 159.8, 144.8, 138.3, 134.2, 131.8, 130.6, 130.1, 128.8 (2C), 128.7 (2C), 128.0, 127.0 (2C), 126.6 (2C), 122.3, 120.0, 114.5, 85.1, 77.4, 77.3, 76.8, 75.3, 74.9, 70.8, 67.8, 60.4, 55.8, 55.5, 42.8, 41.6, 40.4, 36.6, 33.0, 29.7, 25.5 (3C), 23.2, 22.4, 21.0, 18.2, 14.5, 14.2, −5.3,−5.8; LC-MS (ESI, *m/z*): [M + 1], found 1040.5, [M + 23], found 1062.5, $C_{56}H_{69}NO_{16}Si$: 1039.44.

2′-O-(tert-Butyldimethylsilyl)-2-debenzoyl-2-(3-fluorobenzoyl)-macrocyclic taxoid (**20c**). White solid; yield 27.1%; ^{1}H-NMR ($CDCl_3$, 400 MHz) δ: 8.00 (d, J = 7.7 Hz, 1H, Ar-H), 7.87 (d, J = 8.8 Hz, 1H, Ar-H), 7.77 (d, J = 7.32 Hz, 1H, Ar-H), 7.57–7.51 (m, 2H, Ar-H), 7.46–7.33 (m, 8H, Ar-H), 7.10 (d, J = 9.0 Hz, 1H, NH), 6.26 (t, J = 8.5 Hz, 1H, H-13), 5.78 (d, J = 8.5 Hz, 1H, H-3′), 5.60 (d, J = 7.7 Hz, 1H, H-2), 4.85–4.82 (overlap, 2H, H-5, H-3), 4.72–4.63 (overlap, 2H, $O\underline{CH_2}CH_2CH_2OCO$, H-2′), 4.55 (dt, J = 5.5, 10.3 Hz, 1H, $OCH_2CH_2\underline{CH_2}OCO$), 4.47–4.42 (overlap, 2H, $OCH_2CH_2\underline{CH_2}OCO$, H-20a), 4.37 (d, J = 8.2 Hz, 1H, H-20b), 4.14–4.10 (overlap, 2H, H-7a, $O\underline{CH_2}CH_2CH_2OCO$), 3.99 (dt, J = 6.4, 11.3 Hz, 1H, H-7b), 2.73–2.64 (m, 1H, H-6a), 2.57 (s, 3H, CH_3), 2.54 (s, 3H, CH_3), 2.42–2.18 (m, 5H, H-6b, H-14a, H-14b, $OCH_2\underline{CH_2}CH_2O$), 2.10 (brs, 1H, OH), 1.83 (s, 3H, CH_3), 1.25 (s, 3H, CH_3), 1.18 (s, 3H, CH_3), 0.82 (s, 9H, $SiC(CH_3)_3$), −0.008 (s, 3H, $Si(CH_3)$), −0.27 (s, 3H, $Si(CH_3)$); ^{13}C-NMR ($CDCl_3$, 100 MHz) δ: 191.8, 171.0, 169.5, 166.9, 165.7 (d, $^5J_{C\text{-}F}$ = 3.0 Hz, ArCO), 162.6 (d, $^1J_{C\text{-}F}$ = 247.8 Hz), 153.8, 152.6, 144.3, 139.1, 138.4, 135.5, 134.2, 131.8, 131.3 (d, $^3J_{C\text{-}F}$ = 7.5 Hz), 130.6 (d, $^3J_{C\text{-}F}$ = 7.7 Hz), 128.8, 128.7, 127.9, 127.0, 126.4, 126.0 (d, $^4J_{C\text{-}F}$ = 2.6 Hz), 120.9 (d, $^2J_{C\text{-}F}$ = 21.1 Hz), 117.0 (d, $^2J_{C\text{-}F}$ = 23.2 Hz), 90.6, 84.6, 78.6, 77.4, 77.1, 76.7, 76.2, 75.8, 75.3, 70.6, 69.2, 66.0, 64.4, 55.6, 42.8 (2C), 36.5, 31.0, 29.0, 26.1, 25.5 (3C), 22.7, 21.7, 18.2, 14.7, 14.4, −5.2, −5.8; LC-MS (ESI, *m/z*): [M + 1], found 1028.4, [M + 23], found 1050.4, $C_{55}H_{66}FNO_{15}Si$: 1027.42.

2′-O-(tert-Butyldimethylsilyl)-2-debenzoyl-2-(3-chlorobenzoyl)-macrocyclic taxoid (**20d**). White solid; yield 23.6%; ^{1}H-NMR ($CDCl_3$, 400 MHz) δ: 8.20 (t, J = 1.6 Hz, 1H, Ar-H), 8.12–8.09 (m, 1H, Ar-H), 7.77 (d, J = 7.2 Hz, 1H, Ar-H), 7.65–7.62 (m, 1H, Ar-H), 7.56–7.51 (m, 2H, Ar-H), 7.47–7.33 (m, 7H, Ar-H), 7.09 (d, J = 9.0 Hz, 1H, BzNH), 6.26 (t, J = 8.8 Hz, 1H, H-13), 5.77 (dd, J = 1.5, 8.98 Hz, 1H, H-3′), 5.60 (d, J = 7.8 Hz, 1H, H-2), 4.85–4.82 (dd, J = 3.5, 11.0 Hz, 2H, H-5, H-17b), 4.72–4.64 (m, 2H, $O\underline{CH_2}CH_2CH_2OCO$, H-2′), 4.59–4.53 (m, 1H, $OCH_2CH_2\underline{CH_2}OCO$), 4.49–4.43 (m, 2H, $OCH_2CH_2\underline{CH_2}OCO$, H-20a), 4.38 (d, J = 8.4 Hz, 1H, H-20b), 4.15–4.10 (m, 2H, $OCH_2CH_2\underline{CH_2}OCO$, H-20a), 4.02–3.96 (m, 1H, H-7b), 2.74–2.65 (m, 1H, H-6a), 2.57 (s, 3H, CH_3), 2.55 (s, 3H, CH_3), 2.42–2.20 (m, 5H, H-6b, H-14a, H-14b, $OCH_2\underline{CH_2}CH_2O$), 1.84 (d, J = 1.0 Hz, 3H, CH_3), 1.26 (s, 3H, CH_3), 1.19 (s, 3H, CH_3), 0.83 (s, 9H,

$SiC(CH_3)_3$), −0.005 (s, 3H, $Si(CH_3)$), −0.26 (s, 3H, $Si(CH_3)$); ^{13}C-NMR ($CDCl_3$, 100 MHz) δ: 190.7, 171.2, 169.1, 167.0, 165.7, 144.8, 138.3, 135.5, 135.0, 134.3, 133.9, 131.8, 131.1, 130.5, 129.9, 128.8 (2C), 128.7 (2C), 128.2, 128.0, 127.0 (2C), 126.7 (2C), 90.6, 84.6, 78.7, 76.2, 75.8, 75.3, 70.7, 67.8, 55.7, 42.8, 41.6, 36.5, 34.7, 31.6, 29.7, 25.6 (3C), 22.7, 22.4, 18.2, 14.5, 14.1, −5.3, −5.8; LC-MS (ESI, *m/z*): [M + 1], found 1044.0, [M + 23], found 1065.9, $C_{55}H_{66}ClNO_{15}Si$: 1043.39.

2′-O-(tert-Butyldimethylsilyl)-2-debenzoyl-2-(3-trifluoromethylbenzoyl)-macrocyclic taxoid (**20e**). White solid; yield 26.7%; ^{1}H-NMR ($CDCl_3$, 400MHz) δ: 8.50 (s, 1H, Ar-H), 8.41 (d, J = 7.8 Hz, 1H, Ar-H), 7.92 (d, J = 7.9 Hz, 1H, Ar-H), 7.55–7.51 (m, 1H, Ar-H), 7.48–7.33 (m, 8H, Ar-H), 7.09 (d, J = 9.0 Hz, 1H, NH), 6.26–6.21 (m, 1H, H-13), 5.76 (dd, J =1.4, 9.1 Hz, 1H, H-3′), 5.64 (d, J = 7.8 Hz, 1H, H-2), 4.89–4.83 (m, 2H, H-5, H-3), 4.69–4.63 (m, 2H, $O\underline{CH_2}CH_2CH_2OCO$, H-2′), 4.60–4.55 (m, 1H, $OCH_2CH_2\underline{CH_2}OCO$), 4.49–4.43 (m, 2H, $OCH_2CH_2\underline{CH_2}OCO$, H-20a), 4.37 (d, J = 8.0 Hz,1H, H-20b), 4.13 (t, J = 7.7 Hz, 2H, H-7a, $OCH_2CH_2CH_2OCO$), 2.75–2.67 (m, 1H, H-6a), 4.02–3.96 (m, 1H, H-7b), 2.58 (s, 3H, CH_3), 2.53 (s, 3H, CH_3), 2.45–2.18 (m, 5H, H-6b, H-14a, H-14b, $OCH_2\underline{CH_2}CH_2O$), 1.84 (d, J =1.0 Hz, 1H, CH_3), 1.26 (s, 3H, CH_3), 1.25 (s, 3H, CH_3), 1.20 (s, 3H, CH_3), 0.83 (s, 9H, $SiC(CH_3)_3$), −0.006 (s, 3H, $Si(CH_3)$), −0.25 (s, 3H, $Si(CH_3)$); ^{13}C-NMR ($CDCl_3$, 100 MHz) δ: 191.7, 171.1, 167.0, 165.5, 153.9, 152.7, 135.4, 134.3, 133.6, 131.8, 131.4 (q, ^2J = 33.3 Hz), 130.9, 130.3 (q, ^3J = 3.9 Hz), 130.2, 129.7, 128.8, 128.0, 127.0, 126.9 (q, ^3J = 3.8 Hz), 126.5, 123.7 (q, ^1J = 273.8 Hz), 90.6, 84.7, 78.7, 76.2, 75.8, 75.3, 70.8, 69.2, 66.0, 64.5, 55.7, 42.9, 42.8, 36.5, 31.0, 29.0, 26.1, 22.6, 21.6, 18.2, 14.6, 14.4, −5.2, −5.8; LC-MS (ESI, *m/z*): [M + 1], found 1078.4, [M + 23], found 1100.4, $C_{56}H_{66}F_3NO_{15}Si$: 1077.42.

3.1.10. General Procedure for the Syntheses of Compounds **22a–e**

Macrocyclic taxoid (**22a**)

To a solution of of **20a** (29.6 mg, 0.0293 mmol) in THF (8 mL) was added, dropwise, 0.47 mL of HF-pyridine (*v/v* = 1:2) at 0 °C, and the reaction mixture was stirred at room temperature for 30 h. The reaction was quenched with saturated aqueous $NaHCO_3$, diluted with ethyl acetate, and washed with saturated NH_4Cl. The organic layer was dried over anhydrous Na_2SO_4 and then concentrated under reduced pressure. Purification of the crude product by silica gel chromatography (ethyl acetate: petroleum ether = 2:1) gave product **22a** as a white solid (13.4 mg, 51.0% yield). ^{1}H-NMR ($CDCl_3$, 400 MHz) δ: 7.16 (d, J = 7.1 Hz, 2H, Ar-H), 7.75 (d, J = 7.0 Hz, 2H, Ar-H), 7.64 (t, J = 7.5 Hz, 1H, Ar-H), 7.54–7.50 (m, 3H, Ar-H), 7.49–7.47 (m, 2H, Ar-H), 7.43–7.39 (m, 4H, Ar-H), 7.36–7.32 (m,1H, Ar-H), 7.04 (d, J = 9.1 Hz, 1H, NH), 6.18 (dd, J = 8.7 Hz, 1H, H-13), 5.81 (dd, J = 2.4, 9.1 Hz, 1H, H-3′), 5.59 (d, J = 7.7 Hz, 1H, H-2), 4.81–4.79 (overlap, 3H, H-5, H-3, H-2′), 4.61 (dt, J = 5.4, 11.0 Hz, 1H, $O\underline{CH_2}CH_2CH_2OCO$), 4.52 (dt, J = 6.9, 12.0 Hz, 1H, $OCH_2CH_2\underline{CH_2}OCO$), 4.44 (overlap, 2H, H-20a, $OCH_2CH_2\underline{CH_2}OCO$), 4.41–4.33 (m, 1H, H-20b), 4.34–4.28 (overlap, J = 6.7 Hz, H-7a), 4.08 (overlap, 2H, H-7a, $O\underline{CH_2}CH_2CH_2OCO$), 3.95 (m, 1H, H-7b), 3.58 (brs, 1H, OH-2′), 2.66–2.61 (m, 1H, H-6a), 2.55 (s, 3H, CH_3), 2.37–2.33 (brs, 3H, CH_3), 2.30–2.12 (overlap, 3H, H-6b, H-14a, H-14b), 1.67 (brs, 2H, $OCH_2\underline{CH_2}CH_2OCO$), 1.23 (s, 3H, CH_3), 1.16 (s, 3H, CH_3); ^{13}C-NMR ($CDCl_3$, 100 MHz) δ: 191.6, 172.4, 169.8, 167.0, 166.9, 153.8, 152.6, 144.6, 138.0 (2C), 136.1, 133.9, 133.7, 130.2 (2C), 129.1, 129.0 (2C), 128.9, 128.8 (2C), 128.7 (2C), 128.3, 127.0 (2C), 90.5, 84.7, 78.5, 76.3, 75.3, 73.2, 71.7, 69.2, 65.6, 64.4, 54.8, 42.9, 42.7, 36.5, 31.0, 29.0, 26.2, 22.4, 21.3, 14.7, 14.0; LC-MS (ESI, *m/z*): [M + 1], found 896.3, [M + 23], found 918.3, $C_{49}H_{53}NO_{15}$: 895.34.

2-Debenzoyl-2-(3-methoxybenzoyl)-macrocyclic taxoid (**22b**). White solid; yield 59.2%; ^{1}H-NMR ($CDCl_3$, 400 MHz) δ: 7.75 (d, J = 7.4 Hz, 3H, Ar-H), 7.65 (dd, J =1.42, 2.3 Hz, 1H, Ar-H), 7.52–7.38 (m, 9H, Ar-H), 7.17 (dd, J = 2.1, 8.2 Hz, 1H, Ar-H), 7.06 (d, J = 9.0 Hz, 1H, NH), 6.15 (t, J = 8.2 Hz, 1H, H-13), 5.78 (dd, J = 2.1, 8.9 Hz, 1H, H-3′), 5.59 (d, J = 7.6 Hz, 1H, H-2), 4.80–4.76 (overlap, 3H, H-5, H-3, H-2′), 4.60 (dt, J = 5.6, 11.2 Hz, 1H, $O\underline{CH_2}CH_2CH_2OCO$), 4.51 (dt, J = 5.7, 11.2 Hz, 1H, $OCH_2CH_2\underline{CH_2}OCO$), 4.44–4.37 (overlap, J = 5.6 Hz, 2H, $OCH_2CH_2\underline{CH_2}OCO$, H-20a), 4.36 (d, J = 8.3 Hz, 1H, H-20b), 4.07 (overlap, 2H, H-7a, $O\underline{CH_2}CH_2CH_2OCO$), 3.97–3.91 (m, 1H, H-7b), 3.87 (s, 3H, OCH_3), 3.66 (d, J = 4.1 Hz, 1H, OH-2′),

2.67–2.56 (m, 1H, H-6a), 2.55 (s, 3H, CH_3), 2.34 (s, 3H, CH_3), 2.40–2.30 (m, 2H, $OCH_2\underline{CH_2}CH_2OCO$), 2.28–2.12 (m, 3H, H-6b, H-14a, H-14b), 2.02 (brs, 1H, OH-1), 1.65 (s, 3H, CH_3), 1.22 (s, 3H, CH_3), 1.15 (s, 3H, CH_3); ^{13}C-NMR ($CDCl_3$, 100 MHz) δ: 191.6, 172.3, 169.8, 167.0, 166.8, 159.8, 153.7, 152.6, 144.6, 138.1, 137.9, 136.1, 133.7, 132.0, 130.3, 129.8, 129.0, 128.7, 128.3, 127.1, 127.0, 122.4, 112.0, 115.0, 90.4, 84.7, 78.4, 76.3, 75.3, 73.3, 71.7, 69.2, 66.0, 64.4, 55.5, 54.9, 42.8, 42.7, 36.5, 31.0, 29.0, 26.1, 22.4, 21.2, 14.7, 14.0; LC-MS (ESI, *m/z*): [M + 1], found 926.3, [M + 23], found 948.3, $C_{50}H_{55}NO_{16}$: 925.35.

2-Debenzoyl-2-(3-fluorobenzoyl)-macrocyclic taxoid (**22c**). White solid; yield 51.5%; ^{1}H-NMR ($CDCl_3$, 400 MHz) δ: 7.96 (d, J = 7.69 Hz, 1 H, Ar-H), 7.84 (d, J = 9.1 Hz, 1H, Ar-H), 7.74 (d, J = 7.7 Hz, 2H, Ar-H), 7.53–7.46 (m, 4 H, Ar-H), 7.40 (t, J = 7.5 Hz, 4H, Ar-H), 7.36–7.32 (m, 2H, Ar-H), 7.05 (d, J = 9.0 Hz, 1H, NH), 6.15 (t, J = 8.6 Hz, 1H, H-13), 5.78 (dd, J = 2.0, 9.0 Hz, 1H, H-3′), 5.57 (d, J = 7.7 Hz, 1H, H-2), 4.81–4.79 (overlap, 3H, H-5, H-3, H-2′), 4.60 (dt, J = 5.3, 10.7 Hz, 1H, $O\underline{CH_2}CH_2CH_2OCO$), 4.52 (dt, J = 5.4, 10.8 Hz, 1H, $OCH_2CH_2\underline{CH_2}OCO$), 4.44–4.40 (ovelap, 2H, H-7a, $OCH_2CH_2\underline{CH_2}OCO$), 4.40 (d, J = 8.0 Hz, 1H, H-20a), 4.32 (d, J = 8.1 Hz, 1H, H-20b), 4.07 (t, J = 7.5 Hz, 2H, $O\underline{CH_2}CH_2CH_2OCO$), 3.93 (dt, J = 5.9, 11.9 Hz, 1H, H-7b), 3.69 (brs, 1H, OH-2′), 2.68–2.58 (m, 1H, H-6a), 2.54 (s, 3H, CH_3), 2.34 (s, 3H, CH_3), 2.33–2.26 (m, 2H, $OCH_2CH_2CH_2OCO$), 2.24–2.16 (m, 3H, H-6b, H-14a, H-14b), 1.97 (brs, 1H, OH-1), 1.65 (br, 3H, CH_3), 1.22 (s, 3H, CH_3), 1.15 (s, 3H, CH_3); ^{13}C-NMR ($CDCl_3$, 100 MHz) δ: 191.5, 172.4, 169.7, 167.0, 165.7 (d, $J_{C\text{-}F}$ = 2.8 Hz, CO), 162.6 (d, $^1J_{C\text{-}F}$ =247.9 Hz), 153.8, 152.6, 144.5, 138.1 (2C), 135.9, 133.8, 131.9, 131.3 (d, $^3J_{C\text{-}F}$ = 7.5 Hz), 130.5 (d, $^3J_{C\text{-}F}$ = 7.6 Hz), 129.0, 128.7, 128.3, 127.0 (2C), 126.0 (d, $^4J_{C\text{-}F}$ = 2.9 Hz), 121.0 (d, $^2J_{C\text{-}F}$ = 21.3 Hz), 116.9 (d, $^2J_{C\text{-}F}$ = 23.3 Hz), 90.5, 84.6, 78.5, 76.2, 75.6, 73.3, 71.6, 69.2, 66.0, 64.4, 55.0, 42.8, 42.7, 36.4, 30.9, 29.3, 29.0, 26.1, 22.3, 21.3, 14.6, 14.0; LC-MS (ESI, *m/z*): [M + 1], found 914.3, [M + 23], found 936.3, $C_{49}H_{52}FNO_{15}$: 913.33.

2-Debenzoyl-2-(3-chlorobenzoyl)-macrocyclic taxoid (**22d**). White solid; yield 65.4%; ^{1}H-NMR ($CDCl_3$, 400 MHz) δ: 8.16 (t, J = 1.8 Hz, 1H, Ar), 8.06–8.04 (m, 1 H, Ar-H), 7.75–7.73 (m, 2H, Ar-H), 7.61 (ddd, J =1.0, 2.0, 8.0 Hz, 1H, Ar-H), 7.43–7.39 (m, 4H, Ar-H), 7.52–7.45 (m, 4 H, Ar-H), 7.37–7.32 (m, 1H, Ar-H), 7.01 (d, J = 9.0 Hz, 1H, NH), 6.15 (dd, J = 7.4, 8.7 Hz, 1H, H-13), 5.78 (dd, J = 2.3, 9.0 Hz, 1H, H-3′), 5.57 (d, J = 7.7 Hz, 1H, H-2), 4.81–4.79 (overlap, 3H, H-5, H-3, H-2′), 4.60 (dt, J = 5.3, 10.7 Hz, 1H, $O\underline{CH_2}CH_2CH_2OCO$), 4.53 (dt, J = 5.5, 11.3 Hz, 1H, $OCH_2CH_2\underline{CH_2}OCO$), 4.45–4.44 (m, 1H, $OCH_2CH_2\underline{CH_2}OCO$), 4.39 (d, J = 8.2 Hz, 1H, H-20a), 4.33 (d, J = 8.2 Hz, 1H, H-20b), 4.08 (overlap, J = 7.62 Hz, 2H, H-7a, $O\underline{CH_2}CH_2CH_2OCO$), 3.96–3.90 (m, 1H, H-7b), 3.60 (brs, 1H, OH-2′), 2.68–2.58 (m, 1H, H-6a), 2.54 (s, 3H, CH_3), 2.35 (s, 3H, CH_3), 2.44–2.30 (m, 2H, $OCH_2\underline{CH_2}CH_2OCO$), 2.28–2.16 (m, 3H, H-6b, H-14a, H-14b), 1.97 (brs, 1H, OH-1), 1.65 (d, J =1.7 Hz, 3H, CH_3), 1.23 (s, 3H, CH_3), 1.16 (s, 3H, CH_3); ^{13}C-NMR ($CDCl_3$, 100 MHz) δ: 191.5, 172.4, 169.7, 167.0, 165.5, 153.8, 152.6, 144.5, 138.0, 135.9, 134.8, 133.8, 133.7, 132.0, 130.9, 130.2 (2C), 129.0, 128.7, 128.4, 127.1, 127.0, 90.4, 84.6, 78.5, 76.1, 75.5, 73.2, 71.7, 69.2, 65.9, 64.4, 55.0, 42.8, 42.7, 36.4, 30.9, 29.0, 26.1, 22.3, 21.2, 14.6, 14.0; LC-MS (ESI, *m/z*): [M + 1], found 930.3, [M + 23], found 952.3, $C_{49}H_{52}ClNO_{15}$: 929.30.

2-Debenzoyl-2-(3-trifluoromethylbenzoyl)-macrocyclic taxoid (**22e**). White solid; yield 59.5%; ^{1}H-NMR ($CDCl_3$, 400 MHz) δ: 8.46 (s, 1 H, Ar), 8.36 (d, J = 7.8 Hz, 1H, Ar-H), 7.90 (d, J =7.7 Hz, 1H, Ar-H), 7.73–7.67 (m, 3 H, Ar-H), 7.51–7.47 (m, 3H, Ar-H), 7.42–7.32 (m, 5H, Ar-H), 6.98 (d, J = 9.0 Hz, 1H, NH), 6.15 (t, J = 8.1 Hz, 1H, H-13), 5.77 (dd, J = 2.0, 9.0 Hz, 1H, H-3′), 5.61 (d, J = 7.7 Hz, 1H, H-2), 4.84–4.78 (overlap, 3H, H-5, H-3, H-2′), 4.62–4.51 (m, 2H, $O\underline{CH_2}CH_2\underline{CH_2}OCO$), 4.45–4.41 (m, 2H, H-7a, $OCH_2CH_2\underline{CH_2}OCO$), 4.39 (d, J = 8.0 Hz, 1H, H-20a), 4.31 (d, J = 8.2 Hz, 1H, H-20b), 4.07 (t, J = 7.6 Hz, 1H, $OCH_2\underline{CH_2}CH_2OCO$), 3.93 (dt, J = 6.9, 11.6 Hz, 1H, H-7b), 3.62 (brs, 1H, OH-2′), 2.66–2.58 (m, 1H, H-6a), 2.54 (s, 3H, CH_3), 2.44–2.35 (m, 2H, $OCH_2\underline{CH_2}CH_2OCO$), 2.32 (s, 3H, CH_3), 2.28–2.16 (m, 3H, H-6b, H-14a, H-14b), 1.97 (brs, 1H, OH-1), 1.67 (br, 3H, CH_3), 1.23 (s, 3H, CH_3), 1.17 (s, 3H, CH_3); ^{13}C-NMR ($CDCl_3$, 75 MHz) δ: 191.6, 172.4, 169.7, 167.0, 165.4, 153.7, 152.6, 144.5, 138.1 (2C), 135.8, 133.7, 133.6, 131.9, 131.3 (d, $^2J_{C\text{-}F}$ = 33.2 Hz), 130.3 (d, $^3J_{C\text{-}F}$ = 3.7 Hz), 130.1, 129.6, 129.0, 128.7, 128.4, 127.1, 127.0, 126.9 (d, $^3J_{C\text{-}F}$ = 3.2 Hz), 125.5, 90.5, 84.6, 78.5, 76.1, 75.6, 73.1, 71.7, 69.2, 66.0, 64.4, 55.0, 42.8, 42.7, 36.3, 30.9, 29.3, 28.9, 26.1, 22.2, 21.2, 14.6, 14.0; LC-MS (ESI, *m/z*): [M + 1], found 964.4, [M + 23], found 986.3, $C_{50}H_{52}F_3NO_{15}$: 963.33.

3.2. *Cell Assays*

Cell viability after taxoids treatment was evaluated using CCK-8 assay. Briefly, 3000 cells per well were seeded in 96-well plates and incubated under normal conditions for 24 h. Cells were treated with different concentrations of the test agent for 72 h, then the medium was removed, 100 μL of CCK-8 working solution was added to each well for 1 h at 37 °C. The absorbance was measured at 450 nm with a microplate reader (Tecan Trading, AG, Switzerland). Vehicle-only treated cells served as the indicator of 100% cell viability. The 50% inhibitory concentration (IC_{50}) was defined as the concentration that reduced the absorbance of the vehicle-only treated wells by 50% in the 3-(4,5-dimethylthiazol-2-yl)-2,5-diphenyltetrazolium bromide (MTT) assay.

3.3. *Model Building and Molecular Dynamics Simulations*

The X-ray crystal structure of paclitaxel provided a template for the construction of **18b** and **22b** using the molecular editing tools implemented in PyMOL [17]. Geometry optimization of **18b** and **22b** was achieved by means of the updated AM1 hamiltonian implemented in the *sqm* program, which also produced atomic charge distributions for both ligands that can reproduce the molecular electrostatic potential. The ff14SB AMBER force field was used to assign bonded and non-bonded parameters to protein and ligand atoms [18,19]. **18b** was immersed in a cubic box containing TIP3P water molecules and simulated under periodic boundary conditions for 50 ns at 300 K. Subsequent gradual cooling, from 300 to 273 K over 1 ns, of snapshots taken regularly every 2.5 ns, followed by energy minimization until the root-mean-square of the Cartesian elements of the gradient was less than 0.1 kcal·mol^{-1}·Å^{-1}, provided representative structures of this molecule; those displaying the shortest distance between the free hydroxyl groups were chosen to build **22b** by means of a C=O linkage. The simulated macromolecular ensemble representing a short piece of a microtubule with bound **22b** was constructed as previously reported for D-seco taxol derivatives [20].

4. Conclusions

In summary, this study demonstrated that C-seco taxoids conformationally constrained via carbonate-containing linked macrocyclization display increased cytotoxicity on drug-resistant tumors overexpressing both βIII and P-gp, compared to the non-cyclized C-seco taxoid counterparts Among them, compound **22b**, bearing a 2-*m*-methoxybenzoyl group together with a five-atom linker, was identified as the most potent compound in the series.

Author Contributions: Y.Z. performed most of the experiments; T.-N.W. carried out the bioassays; A.M. and F.G. carried out the molecular modeling studies; writing—original draft preparation, Y.Z., T.-N.W. and A.M.; writing—review and editing, W.-S.F. and F.G.; W.-S.F. planned, designed, and organized the whole research of this study. All authors read and approved the final version of the manuscript.

References

1. Fojo, T.; Coley, H.M. The role of efflux pumps in drug-resistant metastatic breast cancer: New insights and treatment strategies. *Clin. Breast Cancer* **2007**, *7*, 749–756. [CrossRef] [PubMed]
2. Kavallaris, M. Microtubules and resistance to tubulin-binding agents. *Nat. Rev. Cancer* **2010**, *10*, 194–204. [CrossRef] [PubMed]
3. Kamath, K.; Wilson, L.; Cabral, F.; Jordan, M.A. βIII-tubulin induces paclitaxel resistance in association with reduced effects on microtubule dynamic instability. *J. Biol. Chem.* **2005**, *280*, 12902–12907. [CrossRef] [PubMed]

4. Orr, G.A.; Verdier-Pinard, P.; McDaid, H.; Horwitz, S.B. Mechanisms of Taxol resistance related to microtubules. *Oncogene* **2003**, *22*, 7280–7295. [CrossRef] [PubMed]
5. Ferlini, C.; Gallo, D.; Scambia, G. New taxanes in development. *Expert Opin. Investig. Drugs* **2008**, *17*, 335–347. [CrossRef] [PubMed]
6. Ojima, I.; Lichtenthal, B.; Lee, S.; Wang, C.; Wang, X. Taxane anticancer agents: A patent perspective. *Expert Opin. Ther. Pat.* **2016**, *26*, 1–20. [CrossRef] [PubMed]
7. Paradiso, A.; Mangia, A.; Chiratti, A.; Tommasi, S.; Zito, A.; Latorre, A.; Schittulli, F.; Lorusso, V. Biomarkers predictive for clinical efficacy of taxol-based chemotherapy in advanced breast cancer. *Ann. Oncol.* **2005**, *16*, 14–19. [CrossRef] [PubMed]
8. Seve, P.; Mackey, J.; Isaac, S.; Tredan, O.; Souquet, P.-J.; Perol, M.; Lai, R.; Voloch, A.; Dumontet, C. Class III β-tubulin expression in tumor cells predicts response and outcome in patients with non-small cell lung cancer receiving paclitaxel. *Mol. Cancer Ther.* **2005**, *4*, 2001–2007. [CrossRef] [PubMed]
9. Mozzett, S.; Ferlini, C.; Conocolino, P.; Filippetti, F.; Raspaglio, G.; Prislei, S.; Gallo, D.; Martinelli, E.; Ranelletti, F.O.; Ferrandina, G.; et al. Class III β-tubulin overexpression is a prominent mechanism of paclitaxel resistance in ovarian cancer patients. *Clin. Cancer Res.* **2005**, *11*, 298–305.
10. Ferrandina, G.; Zannoni, G.F.; Martinelli, E.; Paglia, A.; Gallotta, V.; Mozzetti, S.; Scambia, G.; Ferlini, C. Class III β-tubulin overexpression is a marker of poor clinical outcome in advanced ovarian cancer patients. *Clin. Cancer Res.* **2006**, *12*, 2774–2779. [CrossRef]
11. Ferlini, C.; Raspaglio, G.; Mozzetti, S.; Cicchillitti, L.; Filippetti, F.; Gallo, D.; Fattorusso, C.; Campiani, G.; Scambia, G. The Seco-Taxane IDN5390 Is able to target class III β-Tubulin and to overcome paclitaxel resistance. *Cancer Res.* **2005**, *65*, 2397–2405. [CrossRef]
12. Tang, Y.; Rodriguez-Salarichs, J.; Zhao, Y.; Cai, P.; Estevez-Gallego, J.; Balaguer-Perez, F.; Horcajo, M.R.; Lucena-Agell, D.; Barasoain, I.; Diaz, J.F.; et al. Modification of C-seco taxoids through ring tethering and substituent replacement leading to effective agents against tumor drug resistance mediated by βIII-Tubulin and P-glycoprotein (P-gp) overexpressions. *Eur. J. Med. Chem.* **2017**, *137*, 488–503. [CrossRef] [PubMed]
13. Pepe, A.; Sun, L.; Zanardi, I.; Wu, X.Y.; Ferlini, C.; Fontana, G.; Bombardelli, E.; Ojima, I. Novel C-seco-taxoids possessing high potency against paclitaxel-resistant cancer cell lines overexpressing class III β-tubulin. *Bioorg. Med. Chem. Lett.* **2009**, *19*, 3300–3304. [CrossRef] [PubMed]
14. Alushin, G.M.; Lander, G.C.; Kellogg, E.H.; Zhang, R.; Baker, D.; Nogales, E. High resolution microtubule structures reveal the structural transitions in alpha-beta tubulin upon GTP hydrolysis. *Cell* **2014**, *157*, 1117–1129. [CrossRef] [PubMed]
15. Chaudhary, A.G.; Gharpure, M.M.; Rimoldi, J.M.; Chordia, M.D.; Gunatilaka, A.A.L.; Kingston, D.G.I. Unexpectedly facile hydrolysis of the 2-benzoate group of taxol and syntheses of analogs with increased activities. *J. Am. Chem. Soc.* **1994**, *116*, 4097–4098. [CrossRef]
16. Kingston, D.G.I.; Chaudhary, A.G.; Chordia, M.D. Synthesis and biological evaluation of 2-acyl analogues of paclitaxel (taxol). *J. Med. Chem.* **1998**, *41*, 3715–3726. [CrossRef] [PubMed]
17. Vella-Zarb, L.; Baisch, U.; Dinnebier, R.E. Small molecule, big difference: The role of water in the crystallization of paclitaxel. *J. Pharm. Sci.* **2013**, *102*, 674–683. [CrossRef]
18. Walker, R.C.; Crowley, M.F.; Case, D.A. The implementation of a fast and accurate QM/MM potential method in Amber. *J. Comput. Chem.* **2008**, *29*, 1019–1031. [CrossRef]
19. Kaus, J.W.; Pierce, L.T.; Walker, R.C.; McCammon, J.A. Improving the efficiency of free energy calculations in the Amber molecular dynamics package. *J. Chem. Theory Comput.* **2013**, *9*, 4131–4139. [CrossRef]
20. Wang, S.R.; Yang, C.G.; Sánchez-Murcia, P.A.; Snyder, J.P.; Yan, N.; Sáez-Calvo, G.; Díaz, J.F.; Gago, F.; Fang, W.S. Restoration of Microtubule Interaction and Cytotoxicity in D-seco Taxanes upon Incorporation of 20-Hydroxymethyl-4-allyloxy Groups. *Org. Lett.* **2015**, *17*, 6098–6101. [CrossRef]
21. Cai, P.; Lu, P.; Sharom, F.J.; Fang, W.S. A semisynthetic taxane Yg-3-46a effectively evades P-glycoprotein and beta-III tubulin mediated tumor drug resistance in vitro. *Cancer Lett.* **2013**, *341*, 214–223. [CrossRef] [PubMed]

Permissions

All chapters in this book were first published by MDPI; hereby published with permission under the Creative Commons Attribution License or equivalent. Every chapter published in this book has been scrutinized by our experts. Their significance has been extensively debated. The topics covered herein carry significant findings which will fuel the growth of the discipline. They may even be implemented as practical applications or may be referred to as a beginning point for another development.

The contributors of this book come from diverse backgrounds, making this book a truly international effort. This book will bring forth new frontiers with its revolutionizing research information and detailed analysis of the nascent developments around the world.

We would like to thank all the contributing authors for lending their expertise to make the book truly unique. They have played a crucial role in the development of this book. Without their invaluable contributions this book wouldn't have been possible. They have made vital efforts to compile up to date information on the varied aspects of this subject to make this book a valuable addition to the collection of many professionals and students.

This book was conceptualized with the vision of imparting up-to-date information and advanced data in this field. To ensure the same, a matchless editorial board was set up. Every individual on the board went through rigorous rounds of assessment to prove their worth. After which they invested a large part of their time researching and compiling the most relevant data for our readers.

The editorial board has been involved in producing this book since its inception. They have spent rigorous hours researching and exploring the diverse topics which have resulted in the successful publishing of this book. They have passed on their knowledge of decades through this book. To expedite this challenging task, the publisher supported the team at every step. A small team of assistant editors was also appointed to further simplify the editing procedure and attain best results for the readers.

Apart from the editorial board, the designing team has also invested a significant amount of their time in understanding the subject and creating the most relevant covers. They scrutinized every image to scout for the most suitable representation of the subject and create an appropriate cover for the book.

The publishing team has been an ardent support to the editorial, designing and production team. Their endless efforts to recruit the best for this project, has resulted in the accomplishment of this book. They are a veteran in the field of academics and their pool of knowledge is as vast as their experience in printing. Their expertise and guidance has proved useful at every step. Their uncompromising quality standards have made this book an exceptional effort. Their encouragement from time to time has been an inspiration for everyone.

The publisher and the editorial board hope that this book will prove to be a valuable piece of knowledge for researchers, students, practitioners and scholars across the globe.

List of Contributors

Mohamed El-Naggar
Chemistry Department, Faculty of Sciences, University of Sharjah, Sharjah 27272, UAE

Abd El-Galil E. Amr
Drug Exploration & Development Chair (DEDC), Pharmaceutical Chemistry Department, College of Pharmacy, King Saud University, Riyadh 11451, Saudi Arabia
Applied Organic Chemistry Department, National Research Center, Cairo 12622, Egypt

Ahmed A. Fayed
Applied Organic Chemistry Department, National Research Center, Cairo 12622, Egypt
Respiratory Therapy Department, College of Medical Rehabilitation Sciences, Taibah University, Madinah Munawara 22624, Saudi Arabia

Elsayed A. Elsayed
Zoology Department, Bioproducts Research Chair, College of Science, King Saud University, Riyadh 11451, Saudi Arabia
Chemistry of Natural and Microbial Products Department, National Research Centre, Cairo 12622, Egypt

Mohamed A. Al-Omar
Drug Exploration & Development Chair (DEDC), Pharmaceutical Chemistry Department, College of Pharmacy, King Saud University, Riyadh 11451, Saudi Arabia

Mohamed M. Abdalla
Atos Pharma, Elkatyba Land, Belbis 44621, El Sharkya, Egypt

Murat Bingul
School of Chemistry, UNSW Sydney, Sydney, NSW 2052, Australia
Children's Cancer Institute, Lowy Cancer Research Centre, UNSW Sydney, Sydney, NSW 2052, Australia
School of Pharmacy, Dicle University, 21280 Diyarbakır, Turkey

Greg M. Arndt
Children's Cancer Institute, Lowy Cancer Research Centre, UNSW Sydney, Sydney, NSW 2052, Australia
ACRF Drug Discovery Centre for Childhood Cancer, Children's Cancer Institute, Lowy Cancer Research Centre, UNSW Sydney, Sydney, NSW 2052, Australia

Glenn M. Marshall
Children's Cancer Institute, Lowy Cancer Research Centre, UNSW Sydney, Sydney, NSW 2052, Australia
Kids Cancer Centre, Sydney Children's Hospital, Randwick, NSW 2031, Australia

Belamy B. Cheung
Children's Cancer Institute, Lowy Cancer Research Centre, UNSW Sydney, Sydney, NSW 2052, Australia
School of Women's and Children's Health, UNSW Sydney, Sydney, NSW 2052, Australia

Naresh Kumar and David StC. Black
School of Chemistry, UNSW Sydney, Sydney, NSW 2052, Australia

Thi Thao Do
Institute of Biotechnology, Vietnam Academy of Science and Technology, 18 Hoang Quoc Viet Road, Hanoi 10000, Vietnam
Graduate University of Science and Technology, Vietnam Academy of Science and Technology, 18 Hoang Quoc Viet Road, Hanoi 10000, Vietnam

Thi Nga Nguyen, Thi Phuong Do, Thi Cuc Nguyen, Ha Phuong Trieu and Phuong Thi Thu Vu
Institute of Biotechnology, Vietnam Academy of Science and Technology, 18 Hoang Quoc Viet Road, Hanoi 10000, Vietnam

Tuan Anh Hoang Le
Center for Research and Technology Transfer, Vietnam Academy of Science and Technology, 18 Hoang Quoc Viet Road, Hanoi 10000, Vietnam

Jiawen Wang
Graduate Institute, Tianjin University of Traditional Chinese Medicine, Tianjin 301617, China

Ge Hong
Tianjin Key Laboratory of Biomedical Materials, Institute of Biomedical Engineering, Chinese Academy of Medical Sciences & Peking Union Medical College, Tianjin 300192, China
State Key Laboratory of Bioactive Substances and Functions of Natural Medicines, Institute of Materia Medica, Chinese Academy of Medical Sciences and Peking Union Medical College, Beijing 100050, China

Guoliang Li and Wenzhi Wang
Tianjin Key Laboratory of Biomedical Materials, Institute of Biomedical Engineering, Chinese Academy of Medical Sciences & Peking Union Medical College, Tianjin 300192, China

Tianjun Liu
Graduate Institute, Tianjin University of Traditional Chinese Medicine, Tianjin 301617, China
Tianjin Key Laboratory of Biomedical Materials, Institute of Biomedical Engineering, Chinese Academy of Medical Sciences & Peking Union Medical College, Tianjin 300192, China
State Key Laboratory of Bioactive Substances and Functions of Natural Medicines, Institute of Materia Medica, Chinese Academy of Medical Sciences and Peking Union Medical College, Beijing 100050, China

Luiz Antonio Lupi, Maira Smaniotto Cucielo, Raquel Fantin Domeniconi, Francisco Eduardo Martinez and Luiz Gustavo de Almeida Chuffa
Department of Anatomy, UNESP-São Paulo State University, Institute of Biosciences, Botucatu, 18618-689 São Paulo, Brazil

Flávia Karina Delella
Department of Morphology, UNESP-São Paulo State University, Institute of Biosciences, Botucatu, 18618-689 São Paulo, Brazil

Graziela Gorete Romagnoli and Ramon Kaneno
Department of Microbiology and Immunology, UNESP-São Paulo State University, Institute of Biosciences, Botucatu, 18618-689 São Paulo, Brazil

Iseu da Silva Nunes
Farmabrasilis R&D Division, Campinas, 13279-020 SP, Brazil

Marcelo Martinez
Department of Morphology and Pathology, Federal University of São Carlos, 13565-905 São Paulo, Brazil

Wagner José Fávaro
Department of Structural and Functional Biology, UNICAMP-University of Campinas, Campinas, 13083-970 São Paulo, Brazil

Valéria Verebová
Department of Chemistry, Biochemistry and Biophysics, University of Veterinary Medicine & Pharmacy, Komenského 73, 041 81 Košice, Slovakia

Jiří Beneš
Institute of Biophysics and Informatics, First Faculty of Medicine, Charles University, Kateřinská 1, 121 08 Prague, Czech Republic

Jana Staničová
Department of Chemistry, Biochemistry and Biophysics, University of Veterinary Medicine & Pharmacy, Komenského 73, 041 81 Košice, Slovakia
Institute of Biophysics and Informatics, First Faculty of Medicine, Charles University, Kateřinská 1, 121 08 Prague, Czech Republic

Guanglin Chen, Ziran Jiang and Qiao-Hong Chen
Department of Chemistry, California State University, Fresno, CA 93740, USA

Qiang Zhang and Guangdi Wang
Department of Chemistry and RCMI Cancer Research Center, Xavier University of Louisiana, New Orleans, LA 70125, USA

Amira A. El-Sayed and Mahmoud F. Ismail
Department of Chemistry, Faculty of Science, Ain Shams University, 11566 Abbassia, Cairo 11566, Egypt

Ahmed M. Naglah
Pharmaceutical Chemistry Department, Drug Exploration & Development Chair (DEDC), College of Pharmacy, King Saud University, Riyadh 11451, Saudi Arabia
Peptide Chemistry Department, Chemical Industries Research Division, National Research Centre, Dokki, Cairo 12622, Egypt

Thitiya Luetragoon
Cellular and Molecular Immunology Research Unit, Faculty of Allied Health Sciences, Naresuan University, Phitsanulok 65000, Thailand
Faculty of Medicine, School of Human Development and Health, University of Southampton, Southampton SO16 6YD, UK

Rungnapa Pankla Sranujit and Chanai Noysang
Thai Traditional Medicine College, Rajamangala University of Technology Thanyaburi, Pathum Thani 12130, Thailand

Yordhathai Thongsri, Pachuen Potup and Kanchana Usuwanthim
Cellular and Molecular Immunology Research Unit, Faculty of Allied Health Sciences, Naresuan University, Phitsanulok 65000, Thailand

Nungruthai Suphrom
Department of Chemistry, Faculty of Science and Center of Excellence for Innovation in Chemistry, Naresuan University, Phitsanulok 65000, Thailand

Nitra Nuengchamnong
Science Laboratory Centre, Faculty of Science, Naresuan University, Phitsanulok 65000, Thailand

Gloria C. Bonel-Pérez, Isabel Gris-Cárdenas, Alberto M. Parra-Pérez, José Antonio Lupiáñez, Fernando J. Reyes-Zurita and Eva E. Rufino-Palomares
Department of Biochemistry and Molecular Biology I, Faculty of Sciences, University of Granada, Avenida Fuentenueva, 1, 18071 Granada, Spain

Amalia Pérez-Jiménez
Department of Zoology, Faculty of Sciences, University of Granada, Avenida Fuentenueva, 1, 18071 Granada, Spain

Eva Siles and Juan Peragón
Department of Experimental Biology, University of Jaen, Campus Las Lagunillas s/n. 23071 Jaén, Spain

René Csuk
Berreich Organische Chemie, Martin Luther University Halle-Wittenberg, 06120 Halle (Saale), Germany

Sheng-You Li
College of Pharmacy, Guizhou University, Huaxi Avenue South, Guiyang 550025, China
State Key Laboratory of Functions and Applications of Medicinal Plants, Guizhou Medical University, 3491 Baijin Road, Guiyang 550014, China

Ze-Kun Sun
State Key Laboratory of Functions and Applications of Medicinal Plants, Guizhou Medical University, 3491 Baijin Road, Guiyang 550014, China
School of Medicine, Guizhou University, Huaxi Avenue South, Guiyang 550025, China

Xue-Yi Zeng, Meng-Ling Wang, Jun-Rong Song, Chao Chen and Heng Luo
State Key Laboratory of Functions and Applications of Medicinal Plants, Guizhou Medical University, 3491 Baijin Road, Guiyang 550014, China
The Key Laboratory of Chemistry for Natural Products of Guizhou Province and Chinese Academy of Sciences, 3491 Baijin Road, Guiyang 550014, China

Yue Zhang
State Key Laboratory of Functions and Applications of Medicinal Plants, Guizhou Medical University, 3491 Baijin Road, Guiyang 550014, China
College of Agriculture, Guizhou University, Huaxi Avenue South, Guiyang 550025, China

Sheng-Cao Hu and Jun Luo
The Key Laboratory of Chemistry for Natural Products of Guizhou Province and Chinese Academy of Sciences, 3491 Baijin Road, Guiyang 550014, China

Wei-Dong Pan
College of Pharmacy, Guizhou University, Huaxi Avenue South, Guiyang 550025, China
State Key Laboratory of Functions and Applications of Medicinal Plants, Guizhou Medical University, 3491 Baijin Road, Guiyang 550014, China
The Key Laboratory of Chemistry for Natural Products of Guizhou Province and Chinese Academy of Sciences, 3491 Baijin Road, Guiyang 550014, China

Yu Zhao, Tian-En Wang and Wei-Shuo Fang
State Key Laboratory of Bioactive Substances and Functions of Natural Medicines, Institute of Materia Medica, Chinese Academy of Medical Sciences and Peking Union Medical College, 2A Nan Wei Road, Beijing 100050, China

Alberto Mills and Federico Gago
Department of Biomedical Sciences and "Unidad Asociada IQM-CSIC", School of Medicine and Health Sciences, University of Alcalá, E-28805 Alcalá de Henares, Madrid, Spain

Index

www.ingramcontent.com/pod-product-compliance
Lightning Source LLC
LaVergne TN
LVHW060537210926
848485LV00005B/1218